AAOS
Comprehensive
Orthopaedic
Review

AAOS

AMERICAN ACADEMY OF
ORTHOPAEDIC SURGEONS

AAOS

Comprehensive Orthopaedic Review

Volume 1

Editor

Jay R. Lieberman, MD

Director, New England Musculoskeletal Institute
Professor and Chairman, Department of Orthopaedic Surgery
University of Connecticut Health Center
Farmington, Connecticut

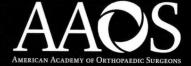

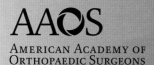

AMERICAN ACADEMY OF ORTHOPAEDIC SURGEONS

The material presented in the **AAOS Comprehensive Orthopaedic Review** has been made available by the American Academy of Orthopaedic Surgeons for educational purposes only. This material is not intended to present the only, or necessarily best, methods or procedures for the medical situations discussed, but rather is intended to represent an approach, view, statement, or opinion of the author(s) or producer(s), which may be helpful to others who face similar situations.

Some drugs or medical devices demonstrated in Academy courses or described in Academy print or electronic publications have not been cleared by the Food and Drug Administration (FDA) or have been cleared for specific uses only. The FDA has stated that it is the responsibility of the physician to determine the FDA clearance status of each drug or device he or she wishes to use in clinical practice.

Furthermore, any statements about commercial products are solely the opinion(s) of the author(s) and do not represent an Academy endorsement or evaluation of these products. These statements may not be used in advertising or for any commercial purpose.

Published 2009 by the
American Academy of Orthopaedic Surgeons
6300 North River Road
Rosemont, IL 60018

Second printing, 2009

Copyright 2009
by the American Academy of Orthopaedic Surgeons

ISBN: 978-0-89203-362-1

Printed in the USA

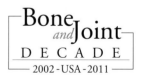

Acknowledgments

Contributors

Yousef Abu-Amer, PhD
Associate Professor
Washington University Departments of
*   Orthopaedics and Cell Biology and Physiology*
Washington University School of Medicine
St. Louis, Missouri

Christopher S. Ahmad, MD
Assistant Professor
Center for Shoulder, Elbow, and Sports Medicine
Department of Orthopaedic Surgery
Columbia University
New York, New York

Jay C. Albright, MD
Director, Pediatric Sports Medicine
Pediatric Specialty Practice
Arnold Palmer Hospital for Children
Orlando, Florida

Annunziato Amendola, MD
Professor, and Director, University of Iowa
*   Sports Medicine*
Department of Orthopaedic Surgery
University of Iowa
Iowa City, Iowa

John G. Anderson, MD
Associate Professor
Michigan State University
College of Human Medicine
Orthopaedic Associates of Grand Rapids
Co-Director, Grand Rapids Foot and Ankle
*   Fellowship*
Grand Rapids, Michigan

Jack Andrish, MD
Orthopaedic Surgeon
Department of Orthopaedics
Cleveland Clinic
Cleveland, Ohio

Robert A. Arciero, MD
Professor and Director
Orthopaedic Sports Medicine Fellowship
Department of Orthopaedics
University of Connecticut
Farmington, Connecticut

Elizabeth A. Arendt, MD
Professor and Vice Chair
Department of Orthopaedic Surgery
University of Minnesota
Minneapolis, Minnesota

April D. Armstrong, BSc(PT), MD, MSc, FRCSC
Assistant Professor
Department of Orthopaedics and Rehabilitation
Penn State Milton S. Hershey Medical Center
Hershey, Pennsylvania

Edward A. Athanasian, MD
Associate Professor
Cornell Weill Medical College
Hospital for Special Surgery
Memorial Sloan-Kettering Cancer Center
New York, New York

Andrew Auerbach, MD, MPH
Associate Professor of Medicine
Department of Medicine
University of California, San Francisco
San Francisco, California

Donald S. Bae, MD
Instructor in Orthopaedic Surgery
Harvard Medical School
Department of Orthopaedic Surgery
Children's Hospital Boston
Boston, Massachusetts

Hyun Bae, MD
Research Director
The Spine Institute
Santa Monica, California

Kelley Banagan, MD
Resident, Orthopaedic Surgery
University of Maryland
Department of Orthopaedics
Baltimore, Maryland

Paul E. Beaulé, MD, FRCSC
Associate Professor
Head, Adult Reconstruction
Department of Orthopaedic Surgery
University of Ottawa
Ottawa, Ontario, Canada

Kathleen Beebe, MD
Assistant Professor
Department of Orthopaedics
University of Medicine and Dentistry of
*   New Jersey–New Jersey Medical School*
Newark, New Jersey

Keith R. Berend, MD
Vice Chairman, Board of Directors
New Albany Surgical Hospital
New Albany, Ohio

Gregory C. Berlet, MD, FRCSC
Chief, Foot and Ankle
Department of Orthopaedics
The Ohio State University
Orthopedic Foot and Ankle Center
Columbus, Ohio

Bruce D. Beynnon, PhD
Director of Research
Department of Orthopaedics and Rehabilitation
University of Vermont
Burlington, Vermont

Mohit Bhandari, MD, MSc, FRCSC
Toronto, Ontario, Canada

Nitin N. Bhatia, MD
Chief, Spine Service
Assistant Professor
Department of Orthopaedic Surgery
University of California, Irvine
Orange, California

Jesse E. Bible, BS
Orthopaedic Research Fellow
Department of Orthopaedics
Yale University School of Medicine
New Haven, Connecticut

Debdut Biswas, BA
Orthopaedic Research Fellow
Department of Orthopaedics
Yale University School of Medicine
New Haven, Connecticut

Donald R. Bohay, MD, FACS
Associate Professor
Department of Orthopaedic Surgery
Michigan State University
Orthopaedic Associates of Michigan
Grand Rapids, Michigan

Michael Paul Bolognesi, MD
Assistant Professor and Director,
  Adult Reconstructive Surgery
Division of Orthopaedic Surgery
Duke University Medical Center
Durham, North Carolina

Deanna M. Boyette, MD
Department of Orthopaedic Surgery
East Carolina University
Greenville, North Carolina

William Bugbee, MD
Division of Orthopaedic Surgery
Scripps Clinic
Associate Adjunct Professor
Department of Orthopaedics
University of California, San Diego
La Jolla, California

R. Stephen J. Burnett, MD, FRCSC
Adult Reconstructive Surgery—Hip and Knee
Division of Orthopaedic Surgery
Vancouver Island Health
Royal Jubilee Hospital
Victoria, British Columbia, Canada

Lisa K. Cannada, MD
Assistant Professor
Department of Orthopaedic Surgery
University of Texas Southwestern Medical Center
Dallas, Texas

Robert V. Cantu, MD
Division Leader of Orthopaedic Trauma
Department of Orthopaedics
Dartmouth-Hitchcock Medical Center
Lebanon, New Hampshire

Kevin M. Casey, MD
Fellow, Lower Extremity Reconstruction
Department of Orthopaedic Surgery
Scripps Clinic
Torrey Pines, California

Paul D. Choi, MD
Assistant Professor of Clinical Orthopaedics
Children's Hospital Los Angeles
Keck School of Medicine
University of Southern California
Los Angeles, California

Charles Day, MD, MBA
Chief, Hand and Upper Extremity Surgery
Department of Orthopedic Surgery
Beth Israel Deaconess Medical Center
Harvard Medical School
Boston, Massachusetts

Craig J. Della Valle, MD
Assistant Professor
Department of Orthopaedic Surgery
Rush University Medical Center
Chicago, Illinois

Mohammad Diab, MD
Associate Professor
Department of Orthopaedic Surgery
University of California, San Francisco
San Francisco, California

Benedict F. DiGiovanni, MD
Associate Professor
Division of Foot and Ankle Surgery
Department of Orthopaedics
University of Rochester School of Medicine
Rochester, New York

Jon Divine, MD

Seth D. Dodds, MD
Assistant Professor
Hand and Upper Extremity Surgery
Department of Orthopaedics and Rehabilitation
Yale University School of Medicine
New Haven, Connecticut

Warren R. Dunn, MD, MPH
Assistant Professor, Orthopaedics and
*   Rehabilitation*
Assistant Professor, General Internal Medicine and
*   Public Health*
Department of Orthopaedics and Rehabilitation,
*   Sports Medicine*
Vanderbilt University Medical Center
Nashville, Tennessee

Mark E. Easley, MD
Assistant Professor
Division of Orthopaedic Surgery
Duke University Medical Center
Durham, North Carolina

Kenneth Egol, MD
Associate Professor and Vice Chairman
Department of Orthopaedic Surgery
NYU Hospital for Joint Diseases
New York, New York

Howard R. Epps, MD
Fondren Orthopedic Group, LLP
Houston, Texas

Greg Erens, MD
Assistant Professor
Department of Orthopaedic Surgery
Emory University School of Medicine
Atlanta, Georgia

Justin S. Field, MD
Orthopaedic Spine Surgeon
Desert Institute for Spine Care
Phoenix, Arizona

Robert Warne Fitch, MD
Assistant Professor of Emergency Medicine
Assistant Professor of Orthopedics
Department of Sports Medicine
Vanderbilt University
Nashville, Tennessee

Vijay K. Goel, PhD
Professor
Department of Bioengineering
The University of Toledo
Toledo, Ohio

Charles A. Goldfarb
Assistant Professor of Orthopedic Surgery
Department of Orthopedic Surgery
Washington University School of Medicine
Saint Louis, Missouri

Gregory D. Gramstad, MD
Shoulder and Elbow Surgeon
Rebound Orthopedics
Vancouver, Washington

Andrew Green, MD
Associate Professor
Department of Orthopaedic Surgery
Warren Alpert Medical School
Brown University
Providence, Rhode Island

Amit Gupta, MD, FRCS
Assistant Clinical Professor
Department of Orthopaedic Surgery
University of Louisville
Louisville, Kentucky

Ranjan Gupta, MD
Professor and Chair
Department of Orthopaedic Surgery
University of California, Irvine
Irvine, California

David A. Halsey, MD
Chief Quality Medical Officer
Springfield Hospital
Springfield Medical Care Systems
Springfield, Vermont

Mark E. Halstead, MD
Clinical Instructor
Team Physician, St. Louis Rams
Departments of Orthopedics and Pediatrics
Washington University School of Medicine
St. Louis, Missouri

Lance Hamlin, PA-C
Physician Assistant
Spine Colorado/Durango Orthopedic Associates, PC
Mercy Regional Medical Center
Durango, Colorado

Timothy J. Hannon, MD, MBA
Medical Director, Blood Management Program
Department of Anesthesiology
St. Vincent Hospital
Indianapolis, Indiana

Timothy E. Hewett, PhD
Director, Associate Professor
Sports Medicine Biodynamics Center
Cincinnati Children's Hospital Medical Center
Cincinnati, Ohio

Alan S. Hilibrand, MD
Associate Professor of Orthopaedic Surgery and
  Neurosurgery
Rothman Institute at Thomas Jefferson University
  Hospital
Philadelphia, Pennsylvania

Jason L. Hurd, MD
Shoulder and Elbow Fellow
Department of Orthopaedics
NYU Hospital for Joint Diseases
New York, New York

Morgan Jones, MD
Associate Staff
Department of Orthopaedic Surgery
Cleveland Clinic
Cleveland, Ohio

Christopher Kaeding, MD
Professor of Orthopaedics
Department of Orthopaedics
Medical Director, OSU Sports Medicine Center
The Ohio State University
Columbus, Ohio

Mary Ann Keenan, MD
Chief, Neuro-Orthopaedics Service
Professor and Vice Chair for Graduate Medical
  Education
Department of Orthopaedic Surgery
University of Pennsylvania
Philadelphia, Pennsylvania

Ali Kiapour, MSc
Department of Bioengineering
The University of Toledo
Toledo, Ohio

Thorsten Kirsch, PhD
Professor
Department of Orthopaedics
University of Maryland School of Medicine
Baltimore, Maryland

John E. Kuhn, MD
Associate Professor
Chief of Shoulder Surgery
Vanderbilt Sports Medicine
Vanderbilt University Medical Center
Nashville, Tennessee

Young W. Kwon, MD, PhD
Assistant Professor
Department of Orthopaedic Surgery
NYU Hospital for Joint Diseases
New York, New York

Mario Lamontagne, PhD
Professor
School of Human Kinetics
University of Ottawa
Ottawa, Ontario, Canada

Francis Y. Lee, MD

Simon Lee, MD
Assistant Professor of Orthopaedics
Department of Orthopaedic Surgery
Rush University Medical Center
Chicago, Illinois

Yu-Po Lee, MD
Assistant Clinical Professor
Department of Orthopaedic Surgery
University of California, San Diego
San Diego, California

Joseph R. Leith, MD
Fellow
Joint Implant Surgeons, Inc.
New Albany, Ohio

Fraser J. Leversedge, MD
Assistant Clinical Professor
Department of Orthopaedic Surgery
University of Colorado Health Sciences Center
Hand Surgery Associates
Denver, Colorado

Johnny Lin, MD
Assistant Professor
Department of Orthopaedic Surgery
Rush University Medical Center
Chicago, Illinois

Sheldon Lin, MD
Associate Professor
Chief, Division of Foot and Ankle
Department of Orthopaedics
University of Medicine and Dentistry of
    New Jersey—New Jersey Medical School
Newark, New Jersey

Dieter Lindskog, MD
Assistant Professor
Department of Orthopaedics and Rehabilitation
Yale University School of Medicine
New Haven, Connecticut

Frank A. Liporace, MD
Assistant Professor
Department of Orthopaedic Surgery
University of Medicine and Dentistry of New
    Jersey—New Jersey Medical School
Newark, New Jersey

Adolph V. Lombardi, Jr, MD, FACS
Clinical Assistant Professor
Department of Orthopaedics
Department of Biomedical Engineering
The Ohio State University
Columbus, Ohio

David W. Lowenberg, MD
Chairman
Department of Orthopaedic Surgery
California Pacific Medical Center
San Francisco, California

Scott J. Luhmann, MD
Associate Professor
Department of Orthopaedic Surgery
St. Louis Children's Hospital
Shriners Hospital for Children
Washington University School of Medicine
St. Louis, Missouri

C. Benjamin Ma, MD
Assistant Professor in Residence
Chief, Shoulder and Sports Medicine
Department of Orthopaedic Surgery
University of California, San Francisco
San Francisco, California

David Maish, MD
Assistant Professor
Department of Orthopaedic Surgery
Penn State Hershey Medical Center
Hershey, Pennsylvania

Peter J. Mandell, MD
Assistant Clinical Professor
Department of Orthopaedic Surgery
University of California, San Francisco
San Francisco, California

Robert G. Marx, MD, MSc, FRCSC
Associate Professor of Orthopaedic Surgery
Weill Medical College of Cornell University
Hospital for Special Surgery
New York, New York

Matthew J. Matava, MD
Associate Professor
Department of Orthopaedic Surgery
Washington University School of Medicine
St. Louis, Missouri

Augustus D. Mazzocca, MS, MD
Assistant Professor of Orthopaedic Surgery
University of Connecticut
Farmington, Connecticut

David R. McAllister, MD
Associate Professor
Chief, Sports Medicine Service
Department of Orthopaedic Surgery
David Geffen School of Medicine
University of California, Los Angeles
Los Angeles, California

Eric C. McCarty, MD
Associate Professor
Chief, Sports Medicine and Shoulder Surgery
Department of Orthopaedics
University of Colorado School of Medicine
Denver, Colorado

Michael David McKee, MD, FRCSC
Associate Professor
Division of Orthopaedic Surgery
Department of Surgery
St. Michael's Hospital
University of Toronto
Toronto, Ontario, Canada

Michael J. Medvecky, MD
Assistant Professor
Department of Orthopaedics and Rehabilitation
Yale University School of Medicine
New Haven, Connecticut

Ankit Mehta, BS
Department of Bioengineering
The University of Toledo
Toledo, Ohio

Steven L. Moran, MD
Associate Professor of Plastic Surgery and
Orthopedic Surgery
Division of Hand Surgery
Mayo Clinic
Rochester, Minnesota

Steven J. Morgan, MD
Associate Professor
Department of Orthopaedics
University of Colorado School of Medicine
Denver Health Medical Center
Denver, Colorado

Thomas E. Mroz, MD
Staff, Spine Surgery
Neurological Institute
Center for Spine Health
Cleveland Clinic
Cleveland, Ohio

Anand M. Murthi, MD
Assistant Professor
Chief, Shoulder and Elbow Service
Department of Orthopaedics
University of Maryland School of Medicine
Baltimore, Maryland

Wendy M. Novicoff, PhD
Manager, Department of Orthopaedic Surgery
Assistant Professor, Department of
Public Health Sciences
University of Virginia Health System
Charlottesville, Virginia

Robert F. Ostrum, MD
Professor, Department of Orthopaedic Surgery
University of Medicine and Dentistry of New
Jersey—Robert Wood Johnson Medical School
Director of Orthopaedic Trauma,
Cooper University Hospital
Camden, New Jersey

Thomas Padanilam, MD
Department of Orthopaedic Surgery
The University of Toledo
Toledo, Ohio

Richard D. Parker, MD
Education Director
Cleveland Clinic Sports Health
Department of Orthopaedics
Cleveland Clinic
Cleveland, Ohio

Michael L. Parks, MD
Assistant Professor
Hospital for Special Surgery
Cornell Weill Medical Center
New York, New York

Javad Parvizi, MD
Director of Clinical Research
Associate Professor
Department of Orthopaedic Surgery
Rothman Institute at Thomas Jefferson
University Hospital
Philadelphia, Pennsylvania

Nikos K. Pavlides, MD
Pottstown, Pennsylvania

Terrence M. Philbin, DO
Chief, Division of Orthopedic Foot and
Ankle Surgery
Grant Medical Center
Columbus, Ohio

Jeffery L. Pierson, MD
Medical Director
St. Vincent Orthopedic Center
Joint Replacement Surgeons of Indiana
Indianapolis, Indiana

Kornelis A. Poelstra, MD, PhD
Assistant Professor
Department of Orthopaedics
University of Maryland
Baltimore, Maryland

Ben B. Pradhan, MD, MSE
Pasadena, California

Steven M. Raikin, MD
Associate Professor of Orthopaedic Surgery
Director, Foot and Ankle Service
Rothman Institute at Thomas Jefferson
University Hospital
Philadelphia, Pennsylvania

Gannon B. Randolph, MD
Attending Surgeon
Boise Orthopedic Clinic
Boise, Idaho

Joshua Ratner, MD
The Philadelphia Hand Center, PC
Atlanta, Georgia

David R. Richardson, MD
Intructor
Department of Orthopaedic Surgery
Director, Orthopaedic Residency Program
University of Tennessee—Campbell Clinic
Memphis, Tennessee

E. Greer Richardson, MD
Professor
Department of Orthopaedic Surgery
University of Tennessee College of Medicine
Director of Fellowship and Foot and Ankle Service,
* Campbell Clinic*
Memphis, Tennessee

Michael D. Ries, MD
Professor of Orthopaedic Surgery
Chief of Arthroplasty
University of California, San Francisco
San Francisco, California

K. Daniel Riew, MD
St. Louis, Missouri

Marco Rizzo, MD
Associate Professor
Department of Orthopedic Surgery
Mayo Clinic
Rochester, Minnesota

Tamara D. Rozental, MD
Instructor
Department of Orthopaedic Surgery
Harvard Medical School
Boston, Massachusetts

Khaled J. Saleh, MD, MSc(Epid), FRCSC
Professor and Adult Reconstruction Division Chief
* and Fellowship Director*
Department of Orthopaedic Surgery
University of Virginia
Charlottesville, Virginia

Vincent James Sammarco, MD
Director, Foot and Ankle Fellowship
Cincinnati Sports Medicine and Orthopaedic Center
Cincinnati, Ohio

David Sanders, MD, MSc, FRCSC
Associate Professor
Department of Orthopaedic Surgery
University of Western Ontario
Victoria Hospital
London, Ontario, Canada

Anthony A. Scaduto, MD
Los Angeles, California

Perry L. Schoenecker, MD
Professor
Department of Orthopaedic Surgery
Washington University School of Medicine
St. Louis, Missouri

Thomas Scioscia, MD
West End Orthopaedic Clinic
Richmond, Virginia

Jon K. Sekiya, MD
Associate Professor
MedSport—Department of Orthopaedic Surgery
University of Michigan
Ann Arbor, Michigan

Sung Wook Seo, MD
New York, New York

Arya Nick Shamie, MD
Associate Clinical Professor
Chief, Wadsworth Spine Service
Department of Orthopaedic Surgery and
* Neurosurgery*
David Geffen School of Medicine at UCLA
Los Angeles, California

Alexander Y. Shin, MD
Consultant and Professor of Orthopedic Surgery
Department of Orthopedic Surgery
Mayo Clinic
Rochester, Minnesota

Beth E. Shubin Stein, MD
Assistant Professor, Orthopaedic Surgery
Sports Medicine and Shoulder Department
Weill Medical College, Cornell University
Hospital for Special Surgery
New York, New York

Kern Singh, MD
Assistant Professor
Department of Orthopaedic Surgery
Rush University Medical Center
Chicago, Illinois

Douglas G. Smith, MD
Seattle, Washington

Nelson Fong SooHoo, MD
Assistant Professor
Department of Orthopaedic Surgery
University of California, Los Angeles
Los Angeles, California

Jeffrey T. Spang, MD
Department of Orthopaedics
University of Connecticut
Farmington, Connecticut

Samantha A. Spencer, MD
Instructor in Orthopaedic Surgery
Harvard Medical School
Staff Physician
Children's Hospital Boston
Department of Orthopaedic Surgery
Boston, Massachusetts

Lynne Steinbach, MD
Professor
Chief, Musculoskeletal Imaging
Department of Radiology
University of California, San Francisco
San Francisco, California

Michael Steinmetz, MD
Assistant Professor
Center for Spine Health
Cleveland Clinic
Cleveland, Ohio

John S. Taras, MD
Associate Professor
Division of Hand Surgery
Department of Orthopaedic Surgery
The Philadelphia Hand Center, P.C.
Philadelphia, Pennsylvania

Ross Taylor, MD
Attending Orthopaedic Surgeon
Department of Orthopaedic Surgery
Coastal Orthopaedic Associates
Conway, South Carolina

Stavros Thomopoulos, PhD
Assistant Professor
Department of Orthopaedic Surgery and
*   Biomedical Engineering*
Washington University
St. Louis, Missouri

Jeffry T. Watson, MD
Assistant Professor
Department of Orthopaedics
Vanderbilt University
Nashville, Tennessee

Peter G. Whang, MD
Assistant Professor
Department of Orthopaedics and Rehabilitation
Yale University School of Medicine
New Haven, Connecticut

Glenn N. Williams, PhD, PT, ATC
Director of Research, University of Iowa Sports
*   Medicine Center*
Assistant Professor, Physical Therapy and
*   Rehabilitation Sciences, and Orthopaedics*
*   and Rehabilitation*
University of Iowa
Iowa City, Iowa

Brian R. Wolf, MD, MS
Assistant Professor
Team Physician, University of Iowa
Department of Orthopaedics and Rehabilitation
University of Iowa
Iowa City, Iowa

Philip Wolinsky, MD
Professor of Orthopaedic Surgery
Department of Orthopaedic Surgery
University of California at Davis
Sacramento, California

Rick Wright, MD
Associate Professor
Department of Orthopaedics
Washington University School of Medicine
St. Louis, Missouri

Dane K. Wukich, MD
Medical Director
UPMC Comprehensive Foot and Ankle Center
University of Pittsburgh Medical Center
Pittsburgh, Pennsylvania

S. Tim Yoon, MD, PhD
Assistant Professor
Department of Orthopaedic Surgery
Emory University
Atlanta, Georgia

Jim A. Youssef, MD
Senior Partner
Spine Colorado/Durango Orthopedic Associates, PC
Mercy Regional Medical Center
Durango, Colorado

Warren D. Yu, MD
Assistant Professor
Department of Orthopaedic Surgery
George Washington University
Medical Faculty Associates
Washington, D.C.

M. Siobhan Murphy Zane, MD
Assistant Professor
Division of Pediatric Orthopaedic Surgery
Department of Orthopaedic Surgery
Tufts University School of Medicine
Tufts-New England Medical Center
The Floating Hospital for Children
Boston, Massachusetts

Preface

The *AAOS Comprehensive Orthopaedic Review* is designed to facilitate studying for board examinations and the Orthopaedic In-Training Examination (OITE). This review text involves the work of more than 150 experts in various fields of orthopaedic surgery and musculoskeletal health. The goal is to provide busy orthopaedic surgeons with a text that is both comprehensive and easy to read and that will facilitate preparation for the aforementioned examinations.

This comprehensive review text has several unique features that set it apart from other texts on the market. First, the information is presented in a consise, short-statement format that is easy to read. Second, top testing facts appear at the end of each chapter; these items provide the reader with the essential information that should have been mastered after reading the chapter. Third, the *AAOS Comprehensive Orthopaedic Review* includes many color illustrations and photographs to enhance learning. Finally, the book is accompanied by a booklet containing hundreds of study questions that have been validated and created for this text and other AAOS publications. These questions and the accompanying answers provide the reader with a means of assessing his or her knowledge and identifying subjects that may require further review. Purchasers of the text may also access it online in a fully searchable format. All of these features make this book the most comprehensive board review text for orthopaedic surgery that has been published to date.

The text is divided into 12 sections: *Basic Science, General Knowledge, Pediatrics, Orthopaedic Oncology and Systemic Disease, Sports Medicine, Trauma, Spine, Shoulder and Elbow, Hand and Wrist, Total Joint Arthroplasty/Joint Salvage, Knee,* and *Foot and Ankle.*

I owe a significant debt of gratitude to the section editors. The book would have fallen far short of its objectives without the contributions of the following section editors (listed in alphabetical order): Martin Boyer, MD (Hand and Wrist);

Kevin Bozic, MD (General Knowledge); John Clohisy, MD, and Jonathan Grauer, MD (Basic Science); Brian Donley, MD (Foot and Ankle); Leesa Galatz, MD (Shoulder and Elbow); Ken Koval, MD (Trauma); David Skaggs, MD, and Robert Kay, MD (Pediatrics); Kurt Spindler, MD (Sports Medicine; Knee); Thomas Vail, MD (Total Joint Arthroplasty/Joint Salvage); Jeffrey Wang, MD (Spine); and Kristy Weber, MD, and Frank Frassica, MD (Orthopaedic Oncology and Systemic Disease). These section editors chose the chapter authors and participated in the intensive editorial process. Each chapter has been reviewed multiple times by the section editors and me in order to provide the reader with accurate data and in a format that facilitates learning.

This text has been 2 years in the making. I especially want to thank Laurie Braun, Managing Editor, for her hard work, patience, and commitment to quality in editing this book. I also want to thank Mary Steermann Bishop, Senior Manager, Production and Archives, and her staff for their fine work with respect to layout and the production of the numerous illustrations used in this text. Finally, I would be remiss if I did not thank Marilyn Fox, PhD, Director, Department of Publications, for her vision to create this text and her support, which allowed us to include the full-color illustrations and the study questions.

The section editors and I hope you will agree that we have accomplished our goal of creating a comprehensive review text that will enhance your understanding of musculoskeletal medicine and facilitate your preparation for the critical examinations you face as you pursue your career in orthopaedic surgery.

Jay R. Lieberman, MD
Director, New England Musculoskeletal Institute
Professor and Chairman,
Department of Orthopaedic Surgery
University of Connecticut Health Center
Farmington, Connecticut

Table of Contents

VOLUME 1

Section 1

Basic Science

Section Editors

John C. Clohisy, MD

Jonathan N. Grauer, MD

Chapter 1
Cellular and Molecular Biology, Immunology, and Genetics

Sung Wook Seo, MD   Francis Y. Lee, MD

1: Basic Science

I. Terminology and Definitions

A. Nuclear structure of cells

1. DNA-related terms

    a. DNA—A double-stranded deoxyribose that contains pairs of nucleotides connected by hydrogen bonds. Four nitrogenous bases (adenine, guanine, cytosine, thymine) are found in DNA. DNA contains biologic information for replication and regulation of gene expression. The nucleotide sequence in DNA determines the specific information.

    b. Genome—Complete complement of genetic information of an organism.

    c. Chromosome—Nuclear structure containing a linear strand of DNA; humans have 46 chromosomes (23 pairs).

    d. Solenoid—Three-dimensional shape found in cells that resembles an electromagnetic coil wrapped around a core.

    e. Nucleosome—DNA/histone complex consisting of DNA wrapped around four pairs of proteins called histones (**Figure 1**).

    f. Gene—Specific segment of DNA that contains all the information required for synthesis of a protein, including both coding and noncoding sequences.

    g. Recombinant DNA—DNA artificially made by recombinant technique (manipulation of a DNA segment).

    h. Exon—Portion of a gene that codes for messenger RNA (mRNA).

    i. Intron—Portion of a gene that does not code for mRNA.

    j. Gene promoter—Regulatory portion of DNA that controls initiation of transcription adjacent to the transcription start site of a gene.

    k. Promoter DNA sequences—DNA sequences that are upstream of the coding sequences that are necessary for binding of transcription factors. Each transcription factor has a strong affinity for specific sequences (**Figure 2**).

    l. Gene enhancer—Regions of a gene that positively regulate rates of transcription.

    m. Transgene—A gene that is artificially placed into a single-celled embryo and is present in all cells of that organism.

2. RNA-related terms

    a. RNA—Nucleic acid composed of ribonucleotide monomers, each of which contains ribose, a phosphate group, and a purine or pyrimidine.

    b. Messenger RNA (mRNA)—Translates and transmits DNA information into protein synthesis machinery.

    c. Small interfering RNA (siRNA)—Short double-stranded RNA that interferes with the expression of a specific gene.

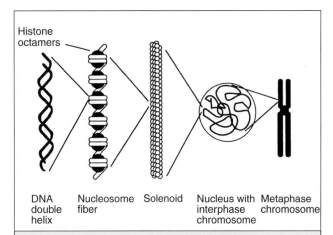

Histone octamers

| DNA double helix | Nucleosome fiber | Solenoid | Nucleus with interphase chromosome | Metaphase chromosome |

Figure 1 DNA wraps around histone octamers to create a histone/DNA complex called a nucleosome, which is wound further into a solenoid form. The solenoid form is packed into the chromosome. (*Adapted with permission from Shore EM, Kaplan FS: Tutorial: Molecular biology for the clinician: Part I. General principles. Clin Orthop 1994:306:264-283.*)

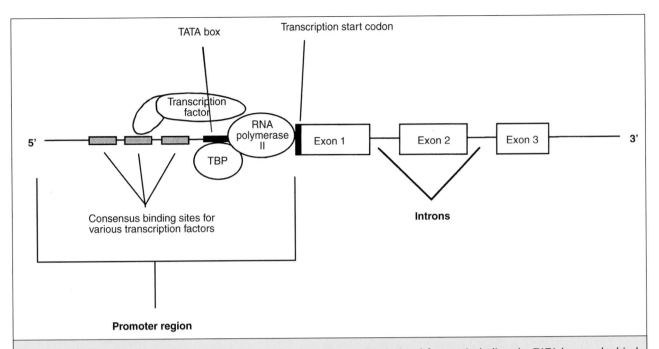

Figure 2   The promoter region includes the binding site for various transcriptional factors, including the TATA box, and a binding site for RNA polymerase II. TBP = TATA-binding protein. (*Reprinted from Buckwalter JA (ed): Orthopaedic Basic Science: Biology and Biomechanics of the Musculoskeletal System, ed 2. Rosemont, IL, American Academy of Orthopaedic Surgeons, 2000, p 30.*)

d. Ribosomal RNA (rRNA)—Major constituent of the ribosome, which is the cell machinery for synthesizing proteins.

e. Transfer RNA (tRNA)—Transfers a specific amino acid to mRNA.

f. RNA polymerase RNAP I (Pol I)—Transcribes the rRNA genes.

g. RNAP II (Pol II)—Transcribes protein-encoding genes into mRNA.

h. RNAP III (Pol III)—Transcribes all the tRNA genes.

B. Gene expression (transcription; DNA → mRNA) (**Figure 3**)

1. Transcription—Process of reading DNA information by RNA polymerase to make specific mRNA.

2. Translation—Building a protein from amino acids by specific mRNA. tRNA interprets the code on the mRNA and delivers the amino acids.

3. Transformation—Inserting a plasmid into a bacterium with added recombinant DNA.

4. Splicing—Removal of intronic sequences from newly transcribed RNA, resulting in the production of mRNA.

5. Transcription factor—Protein that can initiate transcription.

C. Protein expression (translation; mRNA → peptides)—

tRNA interprets the code on the mRNA and delivers amino acids to the peptide chain, which is mediated by the ribosome machinery.

D. Cell division and cell cycle

1. Haploid—Amount of DNA in a human egg or sperm cell, or half the DNA in a normal cell.

2. Diploid—Twice haploid; the amount of DNA in a normal resting human cell (the G0/G1 phase of the cell cycle).

3. Tetraploid—Four times haploid, or twice the amount of DNA in a resting cell; the amount of DNA in a cell in the G2 phase of the cell cycle.

4. Point mutation—An alteration in the genomic DNA at a single nucleotide.

E. Extracellular matrix

1. Extracellular matrix (ECM)—The noncellular portion of a tissue that provides structural support and affects the development and biochemical functions of cells (**Table 1**).

2. Collagen—Triple-helix proteins that form most of the fibrils in the ECM (**Table 1**). Consists of various combinations of α1, α2, and α3 chains.

3. Glycosaminoglycans (GAGs)—Structural polysaccharides in the ECM. A GAG is composed of a repeating disaccharide. These include hyaluronic acid, dermatan sulfate, chondroitin sulfate, heparin, heparan sulfate, and keratan sulfate. Most

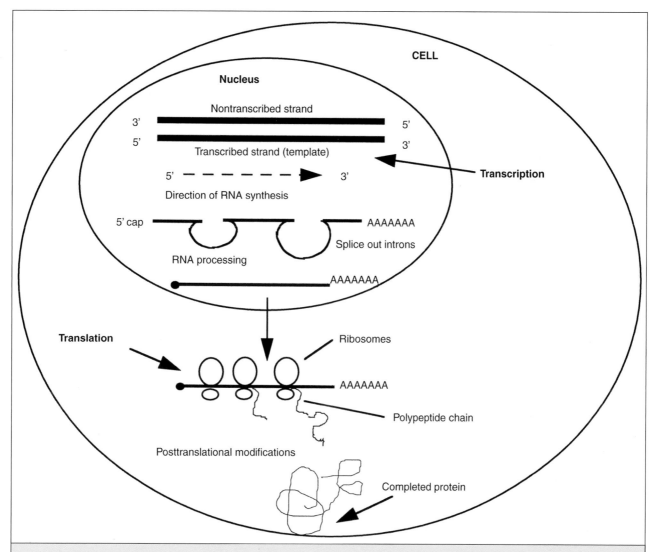

Figure 3 The general flow of gene expression (from DNA to RNA to protein). (*Reprinted from Buckwalter JA (ed): Orthopaedic Basic Science: Biology and Biomechanics of the Musculoskeletal System, ed 2. Rosemont, IL, American Academy of Orthopaedic Surgeons, 2000, p 28.*)

GAGs attach covalently to a protein core to become a proteoglycan. Hyaluronic acid, a nonsulfated GAG, does not attach to proteins, but proteoglycans are linked to hyaluronic acid to form giant molecules that act as excellent lubricators or shock absorbers.

4. Fibronectin—The role of fibronectin is to attach cells to various fibrous collagens (type I, II, III, V) in the ECM. Fibronectin is composed of several functional units that contain binding sites for ECM molecules such as heparin, collagen, and fibrin. Fibronectin also contains cell-binding domains, which have RGD (Arg-Gly-Asp) integrin-binding sequences. Fibronectin has been known to regulate cell migration and differentiation.

5. Laminin—An important component of the basal lamina. Laminin and type IV collagen form a network for the basement membrane scaffold.

Table 1

Collagen Types and Representative Tissues

Type	Tissues
I	Skin, tendon, bone, annulus of intervertebral disk
II	Articular cartilage, vitreous humor, nucleus pulposus of intervertebral disk
III	Skin, muscle, blood vessels
IX	Articular cartilage
X	Articular cartilage, mineralization of cartilage in growth plate
XI	Articular cartilage

1: Basic Science

Table 2

Genetic Defects Associated With Skeletal Dysplasias

Genetic Disorder	Genetic Mutation	Functional Defect	Characteristic Phenotypes
Achondroplasia	FGFR-3	Inhibition of chondrocyte proliferation	Short stature (skeletal dysplasia), normal- to large-sized head, rhizomelic shortening of the limbs, shortened arms and legs (especially the upper arm and thigh), a normal-sized trunk
Thanatophoric dysplasia	FGFR-3	Inhibition of chondrocyte proliferation	Severe dwarfism (marked limb shortening, a small chest, and a relatively large head). Lethal after birth because of respiratory compromise
Hypochondroplasia	FGFR-3	Inhibition of chondrocyte proliferation	Milder dwarfism than achondroplasia
Pseudoachondroplasia	COMP	Abnormality of cartilage formation	Short stature (skeletal dysplasia) Rhizomelic limb shortening, similar body proportion as achondroplasia; lack the distinct facial features characteristic of achondroplasia Early-onset osteoarthritis
Multiple epiphyseal dysplasia	COMP or type IX collagen	Abnormality of cartilage formation	Short stature (skeletal dysplasia) Early-onset osteoarthritis
Spondyloepiphyseal dysplasia	Type II collagen	Defect in cartilage matrix formation	Short stature (skeletal dysplasia), short trunk Spine malformation, coxa vara, myopia, and retinal degeneration
Diatrophic dysplasia	Sulfate transporter	Defect in sulfation of proteoglycan	Fraccato-type achondroplasia, dwarfism, fetal hydrops
Schmid metaphyseal chondrodysplasia	Type X collagen	Defect in cartilage matrix formation	Short stature, coxa vara, genu varum, involvement in metaphyses of the long bones but not in the spine Less severe than in the Jansen type—None of the disorganized metaphyseal calcification that occurs in the Jansen type
Jansen metaphyseal chondrodysplasia	PTH/PTHrP receptor	Functional defect of parathyroid hormone	Short limbs, characteristic facial abnormalities, and additional skeletal malformations Sclerotic bones in the back cranial bones, which may lead to blindness or deafness Hypercalcemia
Cleidocranial dysplasia	Runx2 (cbfa-1)	Impaired intramembranous ossification	Hypoplasia or aplasia of the clavicles, open skull suture, mild facial hypoplasia, wide symphysis pubis, mild short stature, dental abnormality, vertebral abnormality

FGFR-3 = fibroblast growth factor receptor 3; COMP = cartilage oligomeric matrix protein; PTH = parathyroid hormone; PTHrP = parathyroid hormone–related proton.

II. Basic Genetics

A. Genomic DNA

1. Human chromosomes contain 6 billion base pairs, which encode approximately 50,000 to 100,000 individual genes. All the genetic information present in a single haploid set of chromosomes constitutes the genome for a human being. A variety of orthopaedic disorders are secondary to genetic mutation (**Tables 2 through 5**).

2. Only 5% to 10% of genomic DNA in humans is transcribed. Genes in DNA are organized into introns, or noncoding sequences, and exons, which contain the code for the mRNA to produce the proteins as a gene product.

3. The noncoding sequences contain promoter regions, regulatory elements, and enhancers. About half of the coding genes in human genomic DNA are solitary genes, and their sequences occur only once in the haploid genome.

4. Directionality—Single-strand nucleic acid is syn-

Table 3

Genetic Defects Associated with Metabolic Bone Diseases and Connective Tissue Disorders

Genetic Disorder	Genetic Mutation	Functional Defect	Characteristic Phenotypes
Metabolic Bone Diseases			
X-linked hypophosphatemic rickets	A cellular endopeptidase	Vitamin D–resistant rickets	Rickets, short stature, and impaired renal phosphate reabsorption and vitamin D metabolism
Hypophosphatasia	Alkaline phosphatase gene	Generalized impairment of skeletal mineralization	Rickets, bow leg, loss of teeth, short stature
Familial osteolysis	OPGL; RANKL	Idiopathic multicentric osteolysis	Typical facies with a slender nose, maxillary hypoplasia, and micrognathia; rheumatoid arthritis–like hand deformities
Mucopolysaccharidosis type I (MPS I)	α-L-iduronidase	Deficiency of α-L-iduronidase (lysosomal enzymes for breaking glycosaminoglycans)	Hurler syndrome; progressive cellular damage that affects the development of neurologic and musculoskeletal system (short stature and bone dysplasia)
Mucopolysaccharidosis type II (MPS II)	Iduronate sulfatase; X-linked recessive	Deficiency of iduronate sulfatase	Hunter syndrome; mild to moderate features of MPS
Mucopolysaccharidosis type III (MPS III)	Heparan N-sulfatase or N-acetylglucosamine 6-sulfatase	Deficiency of heparan N-sulfatase (IIIA); α-N-acetylglucosaminidase (IIIB); acetyl-coenzyme A:α-glucosaminide-N-acetyltransferase (IIIC); N-acetylglucosamine 6-sulfatase (IIID)	Sanfilippo syndrome; severe neurologic syndrome with mild progressive musculoskeletal syndrome
Mucopolysaccharidosis type IV (MPS IV)	Deficient enzymes N-acetylgalactosamine 6-sulfatase (type A) or β-galactosidase (type B)	Deficiency of lysosomal enzymes for breaking keratin sulfate	Morquio syndrome; bell-shaped chest, anomaly of spine, shortened long bones, and dysplasia of the hips, knees, ankles, and wrists Odontoid hypoplasia
Connective Tissue Disorders			
Osteogenesis imperfecta	Type I collagen	Decreased amount and poorer quality of collagen than normal	Common characteristics: fragile bone, low muscle tone, possible hearing loss, dentinogenesis imperfecta Type I: most common, mildest; blue sclera Type II: most severe, lethal after birth because of respiratory problem Type III: significantly shorter than normal, blue sclera Type IV: normal sclera
Ehlers-Danlos syndrome	Fibrillar collagen gene	Laxity and weakness of connective tissue	Lax joint, hyperextensible skin
Marfan syndrome	Fibrillin	Abnormality of connective tissue	Tall, scoliosis, myopia, lens dislocation, aortic aneurysm, mitral valve prolapse

OPGL = osteoprotegerin ligand; RANKL = receptor activator for nuclear factor κB ligand.

1: Basic Science

Table 4

Genetic Defects Associated With Musculoskeletal Tumors

Genetic Disorder	Genetic Mutation	Functional Defect	Characteristic Phenotypes
Bloom syndrome	Mutation in BLM gene located on chromosome 15, in band q26.1	Helicase dysfunction (unwinding DNA and RNA)	Short stature and a predisposition to various types of cancer and sarcoma
Rothmund-Thompson syndrome	RecQ helicase	Defect in DNA replication and cell proliferation	Short stature; cataracts; pigmentation of skin; baldness; abnormalities of bones, nails, and teeth; high incidence of sarcoma
Li-Fraumeni syndrome	P53 tumor suppressor gene	Increased susceptibility to cancer	Various cancers; osteosarcoma and liposarcoma at early age
Fibrous dysplasia	Gsα (receptor-coupled signaling protein)	Inappropriate stimulation of adenyl cyclase	McCune-Albright syndrome: fibrous dysplasia, skin pigmentation, and endocrine abnormalities
Multiple hereditary exostoses	EXT1, EXT2 genes	Dysfunction of tumor suppressor gene	Noticeable exostoses
Ewing sarcoma	t(11;22): EWS gene of chromosome 22 fuses FLI gene on chromosome	Primitive neuroectodermal tumor in the bone and soft tissue	Commonly occurs in long bone diaphysis
Synovial sarcoma	T(X;18): SYT-SSX fusion gene	Dysregulation of gene expression (SYT-SSX fusion protein)	Sarcoma adjacent to joints
Myxoid liposarcoma	T(12;16)(q13:p11): FUS-DDIT3 chimeric gene	Cytogenic abnormality	Lipogenic tumor in the soft tissue

Table 5

Genetic Defects Associated With Other Musculoskeletal Disorders

Genetic Disorder	Genetic Mutation	Functional Defect	Characteristic Phenotypes
Duchenne muscular dystrophy	Dystrophin	Absence of dystrophin in muscle	Progressive weakness and degeneration of muscle, short life expectancy
Osteopetrosis	Carbonic anhydrase type II; proton pump (human) c-src, MCSF, β3 integrin (mouse)	Osteoclast dysfuction	Fragile bone, anemia, immune problem because of bone marrow deficiency
Fibrodysplasia ossificans progressiva	Mutation of the noggin, BMP-1 receptor	Heterotopic ossification	Heterotopic ossification and rigidity of joints

MCSF = macrophage colony–stimulating factor; BMP-1 = bone morphogenetic protein 1.

thesized in vivo in a 5' to 3' direction, meaning from the fifth to the third carbon in the nucleotide sugar ring (**Figure 3**).

5. Simple-sequence repeated DNA in long tandem array is located in centromeres, telomeres, and specific locations within the arms of particular chromosomes. Because a particular simple-sequence tandem array is variable between individuals, these differences form the basis for DNA fingerprinting for identifying individuals.

6. Mitochondrial DNA (mtDNA) encodes rRNA, tRNA, and proteins for electron transport and adenosine triphosphate (ATP) synthesis. mtDNA originates from egg cells. Mutations in mtDNA can cause neuromuscular disorders.

B. Control of gene expression

1. Transcription—Transcriptional control is the

primary step for gene regulation (**Figure 2**). A transcription process means the synthesis of complementary RNA by RNA polymerase from a strand of DNA molecule. Transcription is controlled by a regulatory sequence in DNA called the cis-acting sequence, which includes enhancer and promoter sites. Trans-acting factors bind to the cis-acting sequence and regulate gene expression. The trans-acting factor is usually a protein such as a transcriptional factor. Promoter regions include the binding site for various transcriptional factors, including the TATA box, and a binding site for RNA polymerase II. The TATA-binding protein, together with other transcriptional proteins, initiates transcription, followed by binding of RNA polymerase. RNA polymerase II generates mRNA template.

2. Translation (**Figure 3**)—The ribosome binds to the translation start sites of the mRNA and initiates protein synthesis. tRNA interprets the code on the mRNA and delivers amino acids to the peptide chain. Each amino acid is encoded by a 3-nucleotide sequence (codon). For example, UUC is a codon for lysine, and GGG or GGU are codons for glycine. UGA, UUA, and UAG are codons that stop translation.

C. Inheritance patterns of genetic disease

1. Autosomal mutation—A gene mutation that is located on a chromosome other than the X or Y chromosome.

2. Sex-linked mutation—A gene mutation that is located on the X or Y chromosome.

3. Dominant mutation—A mutation of one allele is sufficient to cause an abnormal phenotype.

4. Recessive mutation—A mutation of both alleles is necessary to cause an abnormal phenotype.

D. Musculoskeletal genetic disorders are listed in **Tables 2 through 5**.

III. Extracellular Signaling (cell-to-cell interaction)

A. Signaling by secretary molecules

1. Endocrine signaling—Hormones secreted from distant endocrine cells are carried by the blood to its target cells. Some lipophilic hormones (steroid hormone, thyroxine, and retinoids) can diffuse across the cell membrane and bind to specific receptors in the cytosole or nucleus. The hormone-receptor complex affects DNA by altering the transcription of specific genes.

2. Paracrine signaling—Water-soluble hormones (peptide hormones such as insulin and glucagons, catecholamines) and some lipophilic hormones (prostaglandins) bind to cell-surface receptors of

neighboring cells to affect their growth and proliferation.

3. Autocrine signaling—Some kinds of growth factors are secreted from cells to stimulate their own growth and proliferation.

B. Signaling by membrane-bound protein—Certain membrane-bound proteins on cells can bind directly to specific receptors on adjacent cells to transfer signals.

IV. Intracellular Signaling

A. Cell response—Cells express specific genes in response to extracellular influences such as mechanical forces; extracellular matrices; and contact with other cells, hormones, and cytokines. External influences are used by cells to coordinate intracellular signaling events and regulate the synthesis of specific genes that impact cell proliferation, differentiation, and paracrine function (**Figures 4 and 5**).

B. Signal transduction—The process of converting extracellular signals to cell response.

1. Initiation of signal transduction—Binding of the ligand to a specific receptor initiates signal transduction in various ways, depending on the type of receptor.

    a. G protein-coupled receptors—Binding the ligand to the receptor activates a G protein. The G protein modulates a specific second messenger or an ion channel.

    b. Ion-channel receptors—Ligand binding alters the conformation of a specific ion channel. The resultant ion movement across the cell membrane activates a specific intracellular molecule.

    c. Tyrosine kinase–linked receptors—Binding the ligand activates cytosolic protein-tyrosine kinase.

    d. Receptors with intrinsic enzyme activity—Some receptors have intrinsic catalytic activity. Some have guanine cyclase activity to convert guanosine triphosphate (GTP) to cyclic guanosine monophosphate (cGMP). The others have tyrosine kinase activity to phosphorylate various protein substrates (referred to as receptor tyrosine kinase).

2. Secondary messengers—Intracellular signaling molecules, the concentration of which is controlled by binding the ligand to a membrane receptor. The elevated concentration of secondary messengers activates other signaling molecules. These include cyclic adenosine monophosphate (cAMP), cGMP, diacylglycerol (DAG), IP3, phosphoinositides, and Ca^{2+}.

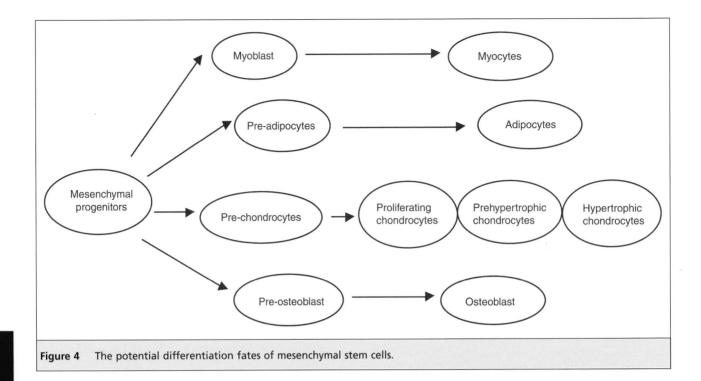

Figure 4   The potential differentiation fates of mesenchymal stem cells.

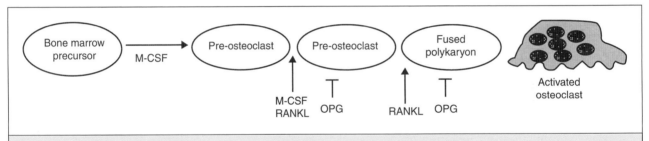

Figure 5   The differentiation schema of bone marrow precursor cells into osteoclasts. Cortical cytokine regulators are indicated. M-CSF = macrophage colony–stimulating ligand; RANKL = receptor activator for nuclear factor κB ligand; OPG = osteoprotegerin.

3. Other intracellular signaling proteins—In addition to secondary messengers, GTP-binding proteins such as Ras and protein kinases can accomplish the signal transduction without secondary messengers, through kinase cascades.

4. Activation and translocation of a protein kinase to the nucleus activates transcription factors, which regulate gene expression.

V. Immunology

A. Innate and adaptive immunity—Defense against foreign pathogens is mediated early by innate immunity and later by adaptive immunity.

1. Innate immunity, which provides the early defense line, is stimulated by a certain structure shared by a group of microbes. It responds rap-

idly to infection, and will respond in the same way to repeated infections. Physical barriers: epidermis, dermis, mucosa; cellular barriers: phagocytotic cells and natural killer (NK) cells; chemical barriers: antimicrobial substances, blood proteins (complement system), and cytokines.

2. Adaptive immunity memorizes the specific antigens of foreign pathogens. It is able to recognize diverse and specific antigens. Successive exposure to antigens increases the magnitude of the immune reaction. The two types of adaptive immune responses are humoral immunity and cell-mediated immunity.

a. Humoral immunity—Mediated by antibodies produced by B lymphocytes.

b. Cell-mediated immunity—Mediated by T lymphocytes (T cells). T cells can activate macrophages to kill phagocytosed antigens or can destroy infected cells directly. Example: An

Cloning a DNA Fragment

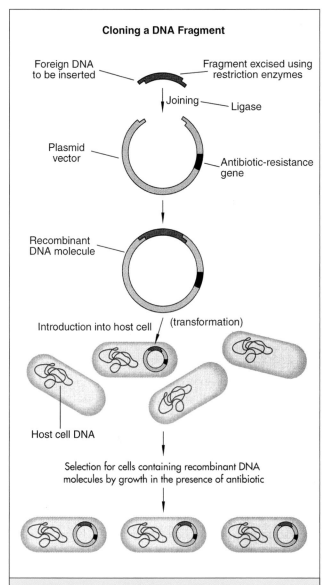

Figure 6 The general sequence of events for cloning a DNA fragment: Transformation means the introduction of recombinant DNA into host cells. *(Adapted with permission from Watson JD, Gilman M, Witkowski J, Zoller M (eds): Recombinant DNA, ed 2. New York, NY, WH Freeman, 1992, p 74.)*

individual who has had chicken pox has immunity against chicken pox.

B. Immune mediators and regulation of bone mass

1. Inflammatory bone destruction or osteolysis is seen clinically in rheumatoid arthritis, chronic inflammatory disease, periodontitis, and wear particle-induced osteolysis. Osteoblasts and osteoclasts communicate in the regulation of bone mass.

2. Inflammatory stimuli may stimulate osteoblasts to express receptor activator of nuclear factor κB ligand (RANKL), a member of the tumor necrosis

factor (TNF) superfamily of proteins. RANKL is the key molecule that induces osteoclastogenesis.

3. Anabolic factors such as transforming growth factor-β (TGF-β) and bone morphogenetic proteins (BMPs) may stimulate osteoblatic precursors to differentiate into osteoblasts.

VI. Experimental Methods

A. Recombinant technology (**Figure 6**)

1. Definition—Manipulation of DNA or RNA segments, including production of specific desired DNA, RNA, or amino acids

2. Recombinant protein—A desired protein can be made by introducing the genetic sequence coding the specific protein into the genome of an organism.

3. Recombinant DNA—A DNA fragment that is removed from its original genome and ligated into the other genome.

4. Manipulation of DNA (cutting, pasting, copying)

   a. Restriction digestion (cutting DNA)—Restriction enzyme is used to cut double-stranded DNA at a specific sequence of DNA.

   b. Ligation (pasting a DNA fragment)—Can be accomplished using enzymes called ligases, which make complete covalent phosphate bonds between nucleotides.

   c. Hybridization techniques—Each base of DNA or RNA pairs with a complementary base by hydrogen bonding. A probe (labeled segment of DNA or RNA) enables detection of complementary sequences of either DNA or RNA.

5. Southern blotting—DNA is subjected to agarose gel electrophoresis to identify specific DNA fragments by the size of base pairs.

6. Northern blotting—Used to identify and quantify specific RNA. As with Southern blotting, RNA is subjected to agarose gel electrophoresis and separated by size.

7. DNA sequencing—Several methods have been developed for detection of the nucleotide sequences of DNA. The Sanger method uses dideoxynucleotides (a, c, g, t instead of A,C,G,T) during DNA polymerization. Because dideoxynucleotides do not have a 3' OH group to link the next nucleotide, they stop DNA synthesis. One dideoxynucleotide (eg, a instead of A) is mixed with the other three deoxynucleotides (C, G, T) in the DNA synthesis; this reaction will stop at the a-site, indicating that there is A at this location.

8. Polymerase chain reaction (PCR)—Method of

1: Basic Science

amplifying a sequence of DNA to a significantly detectable level by repeating a thermal cycle. A DNA template with two primers (forward and reverse) complementary to the target sequence is incubated with nucleotides and polymerase.

B. Methods of protein detection

1. Western blotting—Proteins are separated by sodium dodecyl sulfate polyacrylamide gel electrophoresis (SDS/PAGE) according to molecular weight, confirmation, and charge. A specific antibody is used to recognize the protein of interest.

2. Immunohistochemistry—Method to detect and localize a target protein in the cells or tissue using a specific antibody for the protein of interest.

3. ELISA (enzyme-linked immunosorbent assay)—Method to detect and quantify a specific soluble protein.

C. Modulation of gene expression

1. Transfection—Method to introduce a foreign DNA into a cell or organism using vectors such as plasmid DNA, retroviruses, and adenovirouses, where a specific gene is incorporated.

2. Antisense strategies—Method to introduce an RNA or DNA complementary to an mRNA of interest. The antisense sequence will bind to a specific mRNA and inhibit its translation. Referred to as "gene knockdown" because it reduces the expression level of the target gene.

3. Transgenics—Technique to generate a transgenic animal by introducing a cloned gene into a fertilized ovum. Accomplished by microinjection or by transfection of embryonic stem cells in an embryo.

VII. Pharmaceutical Interventions

A. Anti-TNF—TNF inhibitors reportedly reduce erosive damage and disability in patients with rheumatoid arthritis (RA). Three anti-TNFs have been approved for the treatment of RA:

1. Infliximab and adalimumab—Monoclonal anti–TNF-α antibodies with high a affinity for TNF-α; they prevent TNF-α from binding to its receptors.

2. Etanercept—A fusion protein that binds to TNF-α and prevents it from interacting with its receptors.

B. Osteoclast inhibitors—Control excessive osteoclastogenesis

1. DNA vaccination against RANKL has been tried on an experimental basis in animals.

2. Anti-RANKL antibody has been tried clinically for treatment of osteoporosis.

3. Osteoprotegerin (OPG)—OPG binds to RANKL, preventing its binding to receptor activator of nuclear factor κB (RANK), a receptor for osteoclast differentiation. Direct OPG injection and modulation of OPG expression in cells are being considered as therapeutic strategies.

4. Other inhibitors of osteoclast—Cathepsin K inhibitors, αvβ3 integrin receptor blockers, and an osteoclast-selective H1-ATPase inhibitor could potentially be used to block bone resorption.

Top Testing Facts

1. DNA is a double-stranded deoxyribose. An exon is a portion of a gene that codes for mRNA.

2. mRNA translates and transfers DNA information into protein synthesis machinery. tRNA transfers amino acid to mRNA.

3. Transcription: DNA → mRNA; translation: mRNA → protein.

4. Achondroplasia is related to a defect in FGF receptor 3.

5. Signal transduction is the process of converting extracellular signals to cell response.

6. Inflammatory stimuli may stimulate osteoblasts to express RANKL, a key molecule of osteoclastogenesis.

7. Recombinant technology is manipulation of DNA or RNA segments to produce specific desired DNA, RNA, or amino acids.

8. Infliximab is a monoclonal antibody for TNF-α; it prevents TNF-α from binding to its receptors.

9. Etanercept is a competitive inhibitor of TNF-α signaling; it is a fusion protein that combines the ligand-binding domain of the TNF-α receptor.

10. OPG, anti-TNFs, and anti-RANKLs can control excessive osteoclastogenesis.

Bibliography

Alberts B, Bray D, Lewis J, Raff M, Roberts K, Watson JD: *Molecular Biology of the Cell*, ed 4. New York, NY, Garland Publishing, 2002.

Shore EM, Kaplan FS: Tutorial. Molecular biology for the clinician: Part II. Tools of molecular biology. *Clin Orthop Relat Res* 1995;320:247-278.

Zuscik MJ, Drissi MH, Chen D, Rosier RN: Molecular and Cell Biology in Orthopaedics, in Einhorn TA, O'Keefe RJ, Buckwalter JA, (eds): *Orthopaedic Basic Science*, ed 3. Rosemont, IL, American Academy of Orthopaedic Surgeons, 2000, pp 3-23.

1: Basic Science

Chapter 2
Biomechanics

Vijay K. Goel, PhD   Ankit Mehta, BS   Ali Kiapour, MSc   Jonathan N. Grauer, MD

I. Introduction

A. Biomechanics combines the fundamentals of multiple fields to predict the effects of energy and forces on biologic systems.

   1. The static and/or dynamic behavior of a body is characterized in response to internal and external factors.

   2. Principles of biomechanics can be used to help understand normal forces and motions, altered situations such as responses to injury or surgery, and design considerations of orthopaedic implants and equipment.

B. Definitions and basic concepts

   1. Rigid body—Maintains the relative position of any two particles inside it when subjected to external loads. All objects deform to some degree in response to their environment, but for rigid bodies, these deformations are so small compared to the size of the body that they can be ignored. For example, the small deformations that occur in bone under standard conditions are ignored, and bone is considered to be a rigid body.

   2. Deformable body—Unlike a rigid body, a deformable body undergoes significant changes when subjected to external loads. For example, intervertebral disks are considered to be deformable bodies. Deformable body mechanics describes internal force density (stress) and the related deformation (strain). These terms are described in detail in the chapter on biomaterials.

   3. Force—The physical quantity that changes the state of rest or state of uniform motion of a body and/or deforms its shape.

     a. Forces exist as a result of interaction and are not necessarily associated with motion; for example, a person sitting on a chair exerts a force on the chair but the chair does not move.

     b. Force is a vector quantity, which has both magnitude and direction. The International System of Units (SI) unit for force is the newton (N), with 1 N being the force required to give a 1-kg mass an acceleration of 1 m/s².

   4. Resultant force—If more than one force is applied to a body, the resultant force will be the vector sum of all the forces.

     a. A force vector can be represented graphically by an arrow, where the orientation of the arrow indicates the line of action of the force vector, the base of the arrow represents the point of application of the force, the head of the arrow identifies the direction along which the force is acting, and the length of the arrow is proportional to the magnitude of the force it represents.

     b. Graphic and trigonometric methods can be used to add forces (**Figure 1**).

   5. Mass—Represents the amount of matter physical objects contain. The SI unit of mass is the kilogram (kg).

   6. Velocity—The rate of positional or angular change of an object's position with time. The SI unit for velocity is meters per second (m/s) for linear velocity and radians per second (rad/s) for angular velocity.

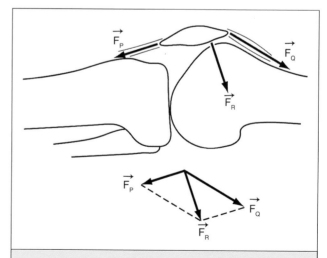

Figure 1   The forces applied on the patella by the quadriceps ($\vec{F}_Q$) and patellar tendon ($\vec{F}_P$) and the resultant force ($\vec{F}_R$). *(Adapted from Mow VC, Flatow EL, Ateshian GA: Biomechanics, in Buckwalter JA, Einhorn TA, Simon SR (eds): Orthopaedic Basic Science: Biology and Biomechanics of the Musculoskeletal System, ed 2. Rosemont, IL, American Academy of Orthopaedic Surgeons, 2000, p134.)*

Table 1

Joint Reaction and Muscle Forces for Various Activities

Joint	Activity	Joint Reaction Force/ Contact Force	Muscle Force
Elbow	Elbow flexed at right angle holding an object weighing approximately 0.06 times body weight	Force at elbow joint: 0.5 times body weight	Biceps muscle force: approximately 0.6 times body weight
Shoulder	Arm abducted to horizontal position and holding a dumbbell of 0.08 times body weight to exercise shoulder muscles	Force at shoulder joint: approximately 1.5 times body weight	Deltoid muscle force: approximately 1.5 times body weight
Spinal Column	Weightlifter bent forward by 45° and lifting a weight equal to his or her body weight	Compressive force generated at the union of L5-S1, approximately 10 times body weight	Erector spinae muscle (supporting the trunk) force: approximately 12 times body weight
Hip	Single-leg stance during walking	Force at hip joint: approximately 3 times body weight	Hip abductor muscles force: approximately 3 times body weight
Knee	Person wearing a weight boot and doing leg raise from a sitting position	Force at tibiofemoral joint: approximately 1 times body weight	Quadriceps muscles force: approximately 1 times body weight

7. Acceleration—The rate at which the velocity of an object changes with time. Like velocity, acceleration can be either linear or angular. The SI units for linear acceleration and angular acceleration are m/s^2 and rad/s^2, respectively.

8. Moment—A measure of the ability of a force to generate rotational motion.

   a. The axis the object rotates about is called the instantaneous axis of rotation (IAR).

   b. The shortest distance between the IAR and the point of load application is called the moment arm.

   c. The magnitude of the moment generated by a force is the magnitude of the force times its moment arm. The SI unit for moment is the newton-meter (N·m).

9. Torque—A rotational moment.

10. Mechanical equilibrium—A system is in mechanical equilibrium when the sums of the forces and moments are zero.

   a. A body in mechanical equilibrium is undergoing neither linear nor rotational acceleration; however, it could be translating or rotating at a constant velocity.

   b. Static equilibrium describes the special case of mechanical equilibrium of an object that is at rest.

11. Free body diagrams—Drawings used to show the location and direction of all known forces and moments acting upon an object in a given situation. They are useful to identify and evaluate the unknown forces and moments acting on individual parts of a system in equilibrium.

12. Degrees of freedom (DOF)—The number of parameters that it takes to uniquely specify the position and movement of a body.

   a. For a body moving in three-dimensional space, there are six DOF, three translational and three rotational.

   b. For a body moving in two dimensions, there are three DOF (eg, two translational and one rotational).

   c. Clinical examples

      i. A hinge joint such as the elbow has one DOF; the geometric constraints of the joint permit only one rotational motion about its axis of rotation.

      ii. A ball-and-socket joint such as the hip has three rotational DOF.

13. In biomechanics, the three-dimensional motion of a body segment is generally expressed using a Cartesian coordinate system (*x*, *y*, and *z* axes).

   a. Sagittal (divides the body into right and left sides)

   b. Coronal (divides the body into anterior and posterior parts)

   c. Transverse (divides the body into upper and lower parts)

II. Kinematics and Kinetics

A. Kinematics describes the motion of objects without regard to how that motion is brought about.

   1. In general, kinematics is concerned with the geometric and time-dependent aspects of motion without considering the forces or moments responsible for the motion.

   2. Kinematics principally involves the relationships among position, velocity, and acceleration.

   3. Knowledge of joint kinematics helps in understanding an articulation. As an example, this is important for the design of prosthetic implants to restore function and to understand joint wear, stability, and degeneration.

B. Kinetics involves analysis of the effects of the forces or moments that are responsible for the motion.

C. Kinematics and kinetics involve categorizing motion into translational components, rotational components, or both.

III. Joint Mechanics

A. Each joint provides various degrees of mobility and stability based on specific structural considerations (Table 1). These are acted on by internal and external loads.

B. Mechanics of the elbow joint—Figure 2 shows a free body diagram in the x-y plane (two-dimensional problem) for the forearm at 90° of flexion and holding a weight in the hand.

   1. The forces acting on the forearm are the total weight of the forearm (W_f), the weight of the object in the hand (W_o), the magnitude of the force exerted by the biceps on the forearm (F_{muscle}), and the magnitude of the joint reaction force at the elbow (F_{joint}).

   2. Point O is the IAR of the elbow joint, P is the point of attachment of the biceps on the radius, Q represents the center of gravity of the forearm, and R lies on the vertical line passing through the center of gravity of the weight held in the hand.

   3. The distances from these points to the center of rotation (moment arms) are shown in the figure and are assumed to be known from the anatomy. The direction of the muscle force is also known; in this problem, it is assumed to be vertical.

   4. Considering the rotational equilibrium of the forearm about O,
   $$\sum \vec{M} = 0 \rightarrow p F_{muscle} = q W_f + r W_o.$$

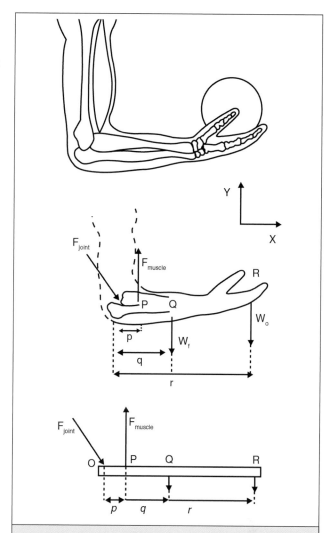

Figure 2 Free body diagram for an arm holding a weight in the hand.

   5. Because the forearm is in translational equilibrium, the sum of the forces is zero:
   $$\sum \vec{F} = 0$$

   6. Breaking down the vector into the components along the Cartesian axes,
   $$\sum F_x = 0 \rightarrow F_{Xjoint} = 0$$
   (There is no joint reaction force along the x axis.)
   $$\sum F_y = 0 \rightarrow F_{Yjoint} = F_{joint} = F_{muscle} - (W_f + W_o).$$

   7. The above equations can be solved for the muscle force and the joint reaction force for given geometric parameters and weights. By assuming that $W_f = 25$ N, $W_o = 100$ N, $P = 5$ cm, $q = 12$ cm, and $r = 40$ cm, the muscle force and joint reaction force can be calculated as follows:
   $$F_{muscle} = (1/0.05)[(0.12 \times 25) + (0.4 \times 100)]$$
   $$= 860 \text{ N}\uparrow$$
   $$F_{joint} = (860 - 25) - 100 = 735 \text{ N}\downarrow.$$

1: Basic Science

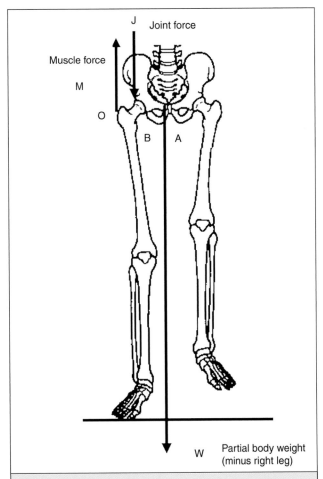

Figure 3   Forces acting across the hip joint during single-limb stance.

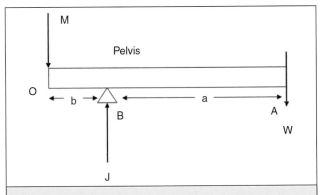

Figure 4   The free body diagram for the problem defined in Figure 3.

C. Mechanics of the hip joint—**Figures 3 and 4** show the forces acting across the hip joint during single-limb stance (2-dimensional problem). During walking and running, all the body weight is momentarily on one leg.

1. The forces acting on the leg carrying the total body weight during such a single-leg stance are shown in **Figure 3**, where M is the magnitude of the resultant force exerted by the hip abductor muscles, assumed vertical; J is the magnitude of the joint reaction force applied by the pelvis on the femur, again assumed vertical; and W is the partial body weight (body weight minus weight of the right leg).

2. The free body diagram of the body without the supported leg is shown in **Figure 4**, where O is the point where the hip abductor muscles attach to the femur; B is a point along the IAR of the hip joint; and A is the center of gravity of the body without the supported leg.

3. The distances between O and B and between A and B are specified as b and a, respectively.

4. To find the magnitude of the force M exerted by the hip abductor muscles, the condition of the rotational equilibrium of the leg about B can be applied. (Assumption: Clockwise moments are positive.)

$$(W \cdot a) - (M \cdot b) = 0$$
$$M = (W \cdot a)/b$$

For $W = 600$ N, $b = 50$ mm, and $a = 100$ mm,

$$M = (600 \cdot 100)/(50)$$
$$M = 1200 \text{ N} \downarrow$$

5. To calculate the joint reaction force J, consider force equilibrium along the y axis. (Assumption: Forces acting downward are negative.)

$$\Sigma F_y = 0$$
$$J - M - W = 0$$
$$J = M + W = 1200 + 600$$
$$J = 1800 \text{ N} \uparrow$$

Top Testing Facts

1. Mechanical equilibrium is when the sums of all forces and moments are zero.

2. Free body diagrams show the locations and directions of all forces and moments acting on a body.

3. Kinematics describes the motion of objects without regard to how that motion is brought about.

4. Kinetics involves analysis of the effects of forces and/or moments that are responsible for motion.

5. Each joint has specific load interactions because of the particular characteristics of the joint and the muscle actions that cross the joint.

Bibliography

Ashton-Miller JA, Schultz AB: Basic orthopaedic biomechanics, in Mow VC, Hayes WC (eds): *Biomechanics of the Human Spine*, ed 2. Philadelphia, PA, Lippincott-Raven, 1997, pp 353-385.

Lu LL, Kaufman KR, Yaszemski MJ: Biomechanics, in Einhorn TA, O'Keefe RJ, Buckwalter JA (eds): *Orthopaedic Basic Science: Foundations of Clinical Practice,* ed 3. Rosemont, IL, American Academy of Orthopaedic Surgeons, 2007, pp 49-64.

Panjabi MM, White AA (eds): *Biomechanics in the Musculoskeletal System.* New York, NY, Churchill Livingstone, 2001.

1: Basic Science

Chapter 3
Biomaterials

Kern Singh, MD

I. General Information

A. Biomaterials are synthetic or naturally derived materials that are used in vivo to replace or augment function.

B. Uses—Biomaterials are used for internal fixation of fractures, osteotomies and arthrodeses, wound closure, tissue substitution, and total joint arthroplasty.

C. Orthopaedic requirements—Orthopaedic biomaterials must be biocompatible (able to function in vivo without eliciting detrimental local or systemic responses), resistant to corrosion and degradation (able to withstand the in vivo environment), and have adequate mechanical and wear properties.

II. Biocompatibility

A. Inert—Little or no host response.

B. Interactive—Designed to elicit specific beneficial responses such as tissue ingrowth (porous tantalum).

C. Viable—Incorporates and attracts cells that are then resorbed and remodeled (biodegradable polymeric scaffolds for functional tissue engineering).

D. Replant—Native tissue that has been cultured in vitro from cells obtained from a specific patient (chondroplasty).

E. Not biocompatible—Elicits unacceptable biologic reactions.

III. Corrosion and Degradation Resistance

A. The in vivo environment of the human body can be highly corrosive.

B. Corrosion can weaken implants and release products that can adversely affect biocompatibility and cause pain, swelling, and destruction of nearby tissue.

C. Orthopaedic devices can be susceptible to several modes of corrosion.

1. Galvanic corrosion is the result of the electrochemical potential created between two metals in a conductive medium such as serum or interstitial fluid.

   a. Galvanic corrosion is seen in fracture fixation plates at the interface between the plate and the screws or constructs when different metals are used.

   b. It is best avoided by minimizing impurities that can enter the material during manufacturing and by ensuring consistent preparation of implant materials.

2. Fretting corrosion results at contact sites between materials that are subject to relative micromotion when under load.

   a. Fretting corrosion is seen in modular arthroplasty devices that make use of tapered junctions.

   b. It is best prevented by avoiding implant junctions and/or micromotion.

3. Crevice corrosion results from differences in oxygen tension within and outside of a crevice with an associated differential in electrolytes and pH

   a. Crevice corrosion is seen at holes in devices such as plates and uncemented acetabular components.

   b. It is best avoided by minimizing surface defects that might be created during manufacturing and intraoperative handling.

4. Pitting corrosion is a form of localized, symmetric corrosion in which pits form on the metal surface.

5. Degradation of orthopedic biomaterials such as polymers

   a. This is a form of corrosion resulting from exposure to harsh environments.

   b. Most common: oxidating degradation of ultra-high-molecular-weight polyethylene (UHMWPE) components for total joint arthroplasty.

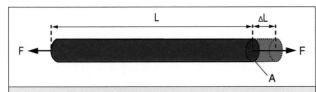

Figure 1 Stress and deformation in a material subjected to axial tensile force. F = force; A = area; L = length; ΔL = change in length.

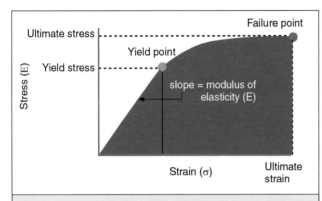

Figure 2 The stress-strain curve can be divided into two distinct deformation regions, elastic and plastic. The yield stress defines the transition point from elastic to plastic deformation, where a material is no longer able to recover to its preloading condition. The slope of the stress-strain curve in the elastic deformation region is the modulus of elasticity.

IV. Mechanical Properties

A. Performance factors—The mechanical performance of an orthopaedic device depends on several factors:

1. The forces to which it is subjected

2. The mechanical burdens of those forces

3. The ability of the materials to withstand those burdens over the device lifetime

B. Definitions

1. Load—The force that acts on a body.

    a. Compression/tension—Forces perpendicular to the surface of application.

    b. Shear—Forces parallel to the surface of application.

    c. Torsion—Force that causes rotation.

2. Stress—intensity of a force over a cross section

    a. Stress (E) = force (F)/cross-sectional area (A) (**Figure 1**).

    b. The SI unit for stress is newtons/meter^2 (N/m^2) or Pascals (Pa).

Table 1

Orthopaedic Materials in Order of Modulus of Elasticity (E)

Cancellous bone	(Low E)
PMMA	
Cortical bone	
Titanium	
Stainless steel	
Co-Cr-Mo (alloy)	
Al$_2$O$_3$ (ceramic)	
Tantalum	(High E)

PMMA = polymethylmethacrylate

c. A force that acts perpendicularly to a surface results in a normal stress.

d. A force that acts tangentially to a surface results in a shear stress.

e. A stress is tensile if the material is stretched by the force and compressive if the material is compressed by the force.

3. Strain—Deformation of the material due to a force application.

    a. Strain (σ) = change in length (ΔL)/original length (L).

    b. The types of strain associated with normal and shear stress are called normal strain and shear strain, respectively.

    c. Like stress, strain can be either tensile or compressive.

4. Stress-strain curve

    a. A typical stress-strain diagram for a material is shown in **Figure 2**.

    b. The stress-strain ratio, or modulus of elasticity (E), is the slope of a stress-strain curve. This is unique to each material. The modulus of elasticity is a measure of an object's ability to resist deformation under the application of an external load (**Table 1**).

    c. A higher modulus of elasticity indicates a material that is stiffer and more resistant to deformation.

    d. As the stress increases, the slope of the stress-strain curve changes when it reaches the point called yield stress. Up to this point, the material has been in its elastic area, which means that if the specimen unloads gradually, the strain decreases until the material reaches its original shape.

    e. The yield stress is the transition point between elastic and plastic deformation. When the stress reaches the yield point, yielding occurs

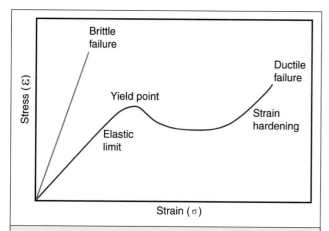

Figure 3 Typical stress-strain curves for brittle materials (red) and ductile materials (blue). Brittle materials demonstrate little plastic deformation, and they fail at a relatively low strain. Ductile materials undergo large strains during plastic deformation before failure.

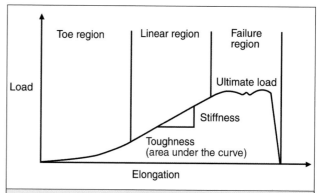

Figure 4 Biologic materials demonstrate viscoelastic properties. Because of the uncrimping of collagen fibers and the elasticity of elastin, the initial portion of a stress-strain curve for a biologic sample has a high deformation/low force characteristic known as the toe region. In the linear region, slippage initially occurs within collagen fibrils, then between collagen fibrils; finally, tearing of the fibrils and tissue failure occurs. From this curve, the stiffness (slope of the curve), the ultimate load (load at failure), and the energy absorbed to failure (toughness, area under the curve) can be calculated.

and the material starts demonstrating plastic behavior. Beyond the yield point, the stress either does not increase or it increases only slightly, but considerable elongation occurs.

f. The maximum stress a material can support is called the ultimate stress. Beyond the ultimate stress, the stress decreases while the material elongates, until fracture or failure occurs.

g. A material can be classified as either brittle or ductile, based on the characteristics of the stress-strain curve.

   i. A brittle material exhibits very little plastic deformation before fracture, and it fails in tension at relatively low strain (**Figure 3**). Examples of brittle materials are concrete, stone, cast iron, glass, ceramic materials, and many common metallic alloys.

   ii. In contrast, ductile materials undergo large strains during plastic deformation before failure. Mild steel, aluminum, copper, magnesium, lead, nickel, brass, bronze, nylon, and Teflon are examples of ductile materials.

h. Toughness is represented by the area under the stress-strain curve; it is an indication of the amount of energy the material can withstand before rupture.

i. Fatigue failure is failure related to cyclic loading.

   i. This is the most common mode of failure in orthopaedic applications.

   ii. When a material is subjected to a dynamic load with a large number of loading cycles, failure will occur at a lower stress than the

ultimate stress of static loading. The stress at failure decreases as the number of cycles increases.

   iii. Fatigue failure consists of three steps: the initiation of a crack, the propagation of the crack, and catastrophic failure.

   iv. The endurance limit (fatigue strength) is the stress at which the material can withstand 10 million stress cycles.

j. Isotropic materials have the same mechanical properties in all directions (eg, stainless steel, titanium alloys).

k. Anisotropic materials exhibit varying mechanical properties with different directions of loading (eg, bone, cartilage, muscle, ligament). This anisotropic behavior is a result of specifically oriented constituent parts such as collagen fibrils and/or hydroxyapatite (HA) crystals.

l. Viscoelastic materials exhibit stress-strain curve patterns that are time/rate dependent as a result of the internal friction of a material (eg, ligaments, tendons) (**Figure 4**).

   i. The modulus of elasticity of a viscoelastic material increases as the strain rate increases.

   ii. Hysteresis is the area between the load and unload portions of a stress-strain curve.

   iii. Creep is increased displacement of a material over time due to a constant force.

1: Basic Science

iv. Stress relaxation is a decrease in stress over time due to a constant displacement.

v. Polar moment of inertia is the quantity that is determined by the cross-sectional area and distribution of tissue around a neutral axis in torsional loading. The larger the polar moment of inertia, the stiffer and stronger the material.

V. Biomechanical Properties of Specific Compounds

A. Host tissue

1. Bone

   a. Bone is a composite of inorganic mineral salts (mainly calcium and phosphate) and organic matrix (mainly type I collagen and ground substance). The inorganic component makes bone hard and rigid, whereas the organic component gives bone its flexibility.

   b. Bone is anisotropic as a result of the orientation of its components.

   c. Bone is stiffer and stronger and stores more energy when loaded at higher rates (viscoelastic).

   d. Macroscopically, skeletal tissue is composed of cortical and cancellous (trabecular) bone. Bone of both types can be considered as one material with widely varying porosity and density.

   e. The apparent density of bone is determined by the mass of bone tissue divided by the volume of the specimen.

      i. The apparent density of cortical bone is approximately 1.8 g/cm^3.

      ii. The apparent density of trabecular bone ranges from 0.1 g/cm^3 to 1.0 g/cm^3.

   f. With aging, a progressive net loss of bone mass occurs beginning in the fifth decade and proceeding at a faster rate in women. This results in reduced bone strength, a reduced modulus of elasticity, and increased likelihood of fractures.

   g. Several radiographic studies have suggested that aging is associated with bone remodeling that affects force distribution.

      i. Subperiosteal apposition of bone occurs along with endosteal absorption in tubular bones, creating a cylinder of larger diameter.

      ii. This remodeling of the diaphysis is hypothesized to serve as a mechanical "compensatory" function by increasing the moment of inertia as the cortex thins with aging. Essentially, the effective bone is shifted to a more peripheral location.

      iii. The increase in outer diameter from bone apposition is much smaller in women than in men, potentially predisposing women to an increased rate of fracture.

2. Tendons

   a. Tendons consist predominantly of type I collagen.

   b. Tendons transmit muscle forces to bone.

      i. Tendons center the action of several muscles into a single line of pull (eg, Achilles tendon)

      ii. They distribute the contractile force of one muscle to several bones (eg, posterior tibialis).

      iii. Tendons allow the direction of pull to be changed in conjunction with a pulley (eg, posterior tibialis tendon around the medial malleolus).

   c. Tendons are anisotropic as a result of the orientation of their components.

   d. Tendons are viscoelastic.

      i. Under low loading conditions, tendons are relatively compliant.

      ii. With increasing loads, tendons become increasingly stiff until they reach a range where they exhibit nearly linear stiffness.

   e. Many tendons are composed of portions of varying orientation that may experience variable loads with any action. Loads applied obliquely during eccentric contractions pose the highest risk of tendon ruptures.

   f. The ultimate load of the tendon usually is greater than that of the muscle or its insertion; thus, muscle ruptures or tendon avulsions are more common than ruptures of the tendon itself. Midsubstance disruptions of a tendon usually occur only in a tendon with pre-existing disease before tensile overload (eg, Achilles tendon with tendinosis).

3. Ligaments

   a. Ligaments are composed predominantly of type I collagen.

   b. Ligaments connect bones to bones.

      i. The bony attachment of ligaments is very important to their structural strength.

      ii. Forces directed perpendicular to the insertions have been shown to cause shear failure of the ligament at the bony interface at relatively low loads.

   c. Similar to tendons, ligaments are viscoelastic, with properties dependent on the rate of load application.

Table 2

Metals Used in Orthopaedic Applications

Metal	Properties	Applications
Stainless steel	Predominantly an iron-carbon alloy with smaller amounts of molybdenum, chromium, manganese, and silicon. Carbon is added to form metallic carbides that impart strength to the material. Chromium provides the stainless quality to stainless steel by forming a strongly adherent oxide on the surface. Susceptible to galvanic and crevice corrosion.	Implants such as fracture plates and screws.
Cobalt alloys	Composed of three basic elements: cobalt, chromium, and molybdenum. Chromium is added for increased hardness and corrosion resistance, particularly resistance to crevice corrosion. Molybdenum is added for increased strength. Cobalt alloys are among the strongest materials used for orthopaedic implants.	High-load applications that require longevity, such as joint arthroplasty devices.
Titanium and titanium alloys	Titanium and titanium alloys have unique tissue biocompatibility due to an adherent passive layer of titanium oxide (TiO_2) that forms on the surface (passivation). Uniform corrosion is extremely limited, even in saline solutions, and resistance to pitting and crevice corrosion is excellent. Titanium alloy has an elastic modulus roughly half that of stainless steel and cobalt alloy. Ti-6Al-4V alloy is notch sensitive (ie, sharp corners, holes, notches, and other stress concentrations lower the strength of the metal).	Pure titanium is used for low-load fracture fixation (eg, phalangeal fractures). For higher strength applications (eg, hip and knee implants), titanium alloys (eg, titanium-aluminum-vanadium, Ti-6Al-4V) must be used.
Tantalum	Highly biocompatible, corrosion resistant, and osteoconductive	Porous forms of tantalum deposited on pyrolytic carbon backbones have been promoted as superior structures for bone ingrowth. Possible orthopaedic applications include coatings for joint arthroplasty components (acetabular cups).

1: Basic Science

B. Metals

1. Metals are crystalline arrays. Within each crystal, the atoms are regularly spaced and packed in specific configurations, allowing for the sharing of outer electrons that give rise to excellent heat and electrical conductivity.

2. Alloys are mixtures of metals or of metals and nonmetallic elements.

3. Metals are typically fabricated by casting, forging, or extrusion.

   a. Casting—Molten metal is poured into a mold.

   b. Forging—One half of a die is attached to a hammer and held and heated metal is worked with an anvil.

   c. Extrusion—Metal is heated and forced through a hole to obtain a long piece with a uniform cross section.

4. Several alloys are commonly used in orthopaedics (**Table 2**).

a. Stainless steel (most common alloy is 316L)

   i. The ductility of stainless steel is important in applications such as bone screws where a definite yield point allows the surgeon to feel the onset of plastic deformation.

   ii. Carbon is added to form metallic carbides that impart strength to the material. If carbide concentrations are too high, however, carbides segregate at the grain boundaries, significantly weakening the steel by making it prone to corrosion-related fracture.

   iii. Stainless steel is susceptible to galvanic and crevice corrosion, although corrosion resistance can be improved by increasing chromium, molybdenum, and nitrogen concentrations.

b. Cobalt alloys

   i. The predominant fabrication technique is casting.

---

ii. Cobalt alloys are among the strongest orthopaedic implant materials and are suitable for high-load applications that require longevity.

c. Titanium and its alloys

   i. Pure titanium is typically used for fracture fixation where large loads are not expected (eg, maxillofacial, wrist, phalanges). Pure titanium is less ductile than stainless steel, however, and increased incidence of screw breakage is often noted.

   ii. For higher-strength applications, titanium alloys must be used (eg, titanium-aluminum-vanadium, Ti-6Al-4V, which has a high strength-to-weight ratio).

d. Tantalum

   i. A transitional metal that is highly corrosion resistant

   ii. Facilitates bony ingrowth

C. Polymers

1. Polymers are large molecules made from combinations of smaller molecules. The properties of a polymer are dictated by

   a. Its chemical structure (the monomer)

   b. The molecular weight (the number of monomers)

   c. The physical structure (the way monomers are attached to each other)

   d. Isomerism (the different orientation of atoms in some polymers)

   e. Crystallinity (the packing of polymer chains into ordered atomic arrays)

2. Polymethylmethacrylate (PMMA) is the most commonly used polymer in orthopaedics.

   a. PMMA is produced from two components, a liquid and a powder.

      i. The liquid component is predominantly a methylmethacrylate monomer and does not polymerize until it comes into contact with the initiator.

      ii. The powder is composed mainly of a polymerized PMMA or a blend of PMMA with a copolymer of both PMMA and polystyrene or PMMA and methacrylic acid. The powder also contains the initiator, dibenzoyl peroxide.

      iii. Mixing the two components results in an exothermic reaction.

   b. Antibiotics can be added to PMMA bone cement to provide prophylaxis or aid in the treatment of infection. Adding antibiotics during the mixing process, however, can negatively affect the properties of PMMA bone cement by interfering with the crystallinity of the polymer.

   c. The performance of PMMA cement has been enhanced by improved protocols in handling, bone preparation, and cement delivery.

   d. Vacuum mixing or centrifugation of the cement may decrease the porosity of PMMA cement, increasing ultimate tensile strength by ~ 40%.

3. UHMWPE is another polymer commonly used in orthopaedics.

   a. This long polyethylene polymer has a very high molecular weight, imparting significantly higher impact strength, toughness, and better abrasive wear characteristics than polyethylenes of lesser weights.

   b. Three methods are used to fabricate orthopaedic components from UHMWPE.

      i. Ram extrusion—The resin is extruded through a die under heat and pressure to form a cylindrical bar that in turn is machined into the final shape.

      ii. Compression molding—The resin is modeled into a large sheet that is cut into smaller pieces to use in machining the final components.

      iii. Direct molding—The resin is directly molded into the finished part.

   c. The most common method for sterilizing UHMWPE components is by exposure to gamma radiation.

   d. Postirradiation oxidation adversely affects the material properties of UHMWPE by increasing the modulus of elasticity, decreasing the elongation to break, and decreasing the toughness. Free radicals generated from radiation may follow one of several paths:

      i. Recombination—The bonds that were broken are simply re-formed; no net change in chemistry.

      ii. Chain scission—Free radicals may react with oxygen, fragmenting the polymer chain. The resulting polyethylene will have a lower molecular weight and increased density.

      iii. Cross-linking—Free radicals from different polymer sections combine to form chemical bonds between two polymer chains. A cross-linked polymer may be harder and more abrasion resistant. Extremely high levels of cross-links may result in the material becoming increasingly brittle. Increased cross-linking with either gamma or electron beam irradiation improves wear resistance in polyethylene components used in total joint arthroplasty. However, the process has a negative effect on fracture and fatigue properties.

    iv. Degradation is a breakdown of the polymer chain. This may be avoided or minimized in two ways.

        (a) Sterilization methods that do not involve irradiation, such as ethylene oxide or gas plasma, do not generate free radicals and therefore do not create any crosslinking. However, recent clinical studies of total hip arthroplasty patients have demonstrated significantly less wear with radiation sterilization than with sterilization using ethylene oxide or gas plasma.

        (b) Irradiation in the absence of oxygen with nitrogen or argon minimizes free radical formation.

4. Biodegradable polymers that degrade chemically and/or physically in a controlled manner over time can be synthesized.

    a. Examples include variations of polylactic acid (PLA), polyglycolic acid (PGA), polydioxanone, and polycaprolactone. PLA has been a desirable choice because its degradation product is lactic acid, a natural constituent of the Krebs cycle.

    b. These polymers are resorbed at different rates.

      i. PLA resorbs faster than PGA.

      ii. Composite products may have intermediate properties.

    c. Resorption allows the host tissue to assume its normal role as the load-sharing capabilities of the polymer decrease. This must be balanced with the need for maintaining mechanical properties.

    d. Resorbable polymers can also be used in drug delivery, releasing the drug as the polymer degrades.

5. Hydrogels—Networks of polymer chains that have been considered for use in a wide range of applications, including tissue engineering.

    a. These materials are soft, porous, permeable polymers that absorb water readily.

    b. Hydrogels have low coefficients of friction and time-dependent mechanical properties that can be varied through altering the material's composition and structure.

D. Ceramics

1. Ceramics are solid, inorganic compounds consisting of metallic and nonmetallic elements held together by ionic or covalent bonds.

2. Ceramics include compounds such as silica (SiO_2) and alumina (Al_2O_3).

3. Ceramics are typically three-dimensional arrays of positively charged metal ions and negatively charged nonmetal ions such as oxygen.

4. When processed to high purity, ceramics possess excellent biocompatibility because of their insolubility and chemical inertness.

5. Ceramic materials are very stiff and brittle but are very strong under compressive loads.

6. Ceramics have gained favor for two different orthopaedic applications: total joint arthroplasty (TJA) components and bone graft substitutes.

    a. Bearings—ceramic-on-polyethylene and ceramic-on-ceramic bearings are becoming more widely used in TJA.

      i. Ceramics have high hardness and a high modulus of elasticity, allowing them to be polished to a very smooth finish and to resist roughening while in use as a bearing surface.

      ii. Ceramics also have good wettability, suggesting the possibility of forming lubricating layers between ceramic couplings to reduce adhesive forms of wear.

      iii. Alumina, in the form of aluminum oxide, has shown lower wear rates than conventional metal-on-polyethylene bearings. Although early clinical experience showed fracture of alumina femoral heads to be a significant complication, this problem appears to be design related, and newer-generation designs have shown significantly lower fracture rates.

      iv. Zirconia, in the form of zirconia oxide, has shown less clinical success than alumina when used as a bearing surface against polyethylene. Zirconia oxide has lower toughness, which makes the material more susceptible to roughening and increased wear.

    b. Bone substitutes

      i. Certain ceramics have been found to be osteoconductive in nature and have accordingly been developed as bone graft materials.

      ii. Hydroxyapatite (HA)

        (a) HA is a hydrated calcium phosphate that is similar in crystalline structure to the mineral of bone.

(b) Its structural and inorganic components differ from those of bone.

(c) HA is very slow to resorb.

iii. β-tricalcium phosphate (β-TCP) and calcium sulfate are other alternatives. These materials have less strength and faster resorption than HA products.

iv. Other molecules, such as silicone (Si), have been shown to induce bone formation when combined with other ceramics.

Top Testing Facts

1. Stress—Force per unit area.

2. Strain energy is the amount of energy stored in a loaded material. In a stress-strain curve, it represents the area under the curve.

3. Modulus of elasticity is the ratio of stress to strain; it measures the ability of a material to maintain its shape under the application of external load. The higher the modulus of elasticity, the stiffer the material.

4. Polar moment of inertia is the quantity that is determined by the cross-sectional area and distribution of tissue around a neutral axis in torsional loading. The larger the polar moment of inertia, the stiffer and stronger the material.

5. A viscoelastic material has properties that are rate dependent or have time-dependent responses to applied forces.

6. An isotropic material has the same mechanical properties in all directions. In general, ceramics and metals are isotropic.

7. An anisotropic material has properties that differ depending on the direction of load. Bone, muscle, ligament, and tendon all are anisotropic.

8. Alloys are metals composed of mixtures or solutions of metallic and nonmetallic elements that are varied to influence their biomechanical properties, including strength, stiffness, corrosion resistance, and ductility.

9. The properties of a polymer are dictated by its chemical structure (the monomer), the molecular weight (the number of monomers), the physical structure (the way monomers are attached to each other), isomerism (the different orientation of atoms in some polymers), and crystallinity (the packing of polymer chains into ordered atomic arrays).

10. Ceramics are solid, inorganic compounds consisting of metallic and nonmetallic elements held together by ionic or covalent bonds.

Bibliography

Behravesh E, Yasko AW, Engel PS, Mikos AG: Synthetic biodegradable polymers for orthopedic applications. *Clin Orthop Relat Res* 1999;367:S118-S129.

Einhorn TA, O'Keefe RJ, Buckwalter JA (eds): *Orthopaedic Basic Science: Foundations of Clinical Practice*, ed 3. Rosemont, IL, American Academy of Orthopaedic Surgeons, 2007.

Hamadouche M, Sedel L: Ceramics in orthopaedics. *J Bone Joint Surg Br* 2000;82:1095-1099.

Jacobs JJ, Gilbert JL, Urban RM: Corrosion of metal orthopedic implants. *J Bone Joint Surg Am* 1998;80:268-282.

Lewis G: Properties of acrylic bone cement: State of the art review. *J Biomed Mater Res* 1997;38:155-182.

Li P: Bioactive ceramics: State of the art and future trends. *Semin Arthroplasty* 1998;9:165-175.

Morita M, Sasada T, Hayashi H, Tsukamoto Y: The corrosion fatigue properties of surgical implants in a living body. *J Biomed Mater Res* 1988;22:529-540.

1: Basic Science

Chapter 4

Skeletal Development

Kelley Banagan, MD   Thorsten Kirsch, PhD   Kornelis A. Poelstra, MD, PhD

I. Cartilage and Bone Development

A. Formation of the bony skeleton

1. Intramembranous bone formation is achieved through osteoblast activity and is characterized by the formation of a calcified osteoid matrix in a cartilage framework. This type of bone formation can be found at the periosteal surfaces of bone as well as parts of the pelvis, scapula, clavicles, and the skull.

2. Endochondral ossification occurs at the growth plates and within fracture callus and is characterized by osteoblast production of osteoid on, not within, a cartilaginous framework.

B. Vertebral and limb bud development (**Table 1**)

1. 4 weeks of gestation

a. The vertebrate limb begins as an outpouching of the lateral body wall.

b. Formation of the limb is controlled along three cardinal axes of the limb bud: proximal-distal, anterior-posterior, and dorsal-ventral.

c. Interactions between the ectoderm and mesoderm characterize development along each axis and are governed by the interaction of fibroblast growth factors, bone morphogenetic proteins, and several homeobox genes.

2. 6 weeks of gestation

a. The mesenchymal condensations that represent the limbs and digits chondrify.

b. The mesenchymal cells differentiate into chondrocytes.

3. 7 weeks of gestation

a. The chondrocytes hypertrophy and the local matrix begins to calcify.

b. A periosteal sleeve of bone forms in a circumferential fashion around the midshaft of each anlage, and intramembranous bone formation begins to occur via direct ossification.

4. 8 weeks of gestation

a. Vascular invasion into the cartilaginous anlage occurs as capillary buds expand through the periosteal sleeve.

b. The capillaries deliver the blood-borne precursors of osteoblasts and osteoclasts and thus create a primary center of ossification. This process occurs first at the humerus, and signals the transition from the embryonic to the fetal period.

C. Formation of endochondral bone and ossification centers

1. As development continues, the osteoblasts produce an osteoid matrix on the surface of the calcified cartilaginous bars and form the primary trabeculae of endochondral bone.

2. The osteoblasts create the medullary canal by the removal of the primary trabecular bone. This process of formation and absorption enlarges the primary center of ossification so that it may become the growth region.

Table 1	
Limb Bud Development	
Weeks of Gestation	**Major Biologic Events**
4	Limb begins as outpouching from lateral body wall
6	Mesenchymal condensations that represent limbs and digits develop Mesenchymal cells differentiate into chondrocytes
7	Chondrocytes hypertrophy; local matrix begins to calcify Periosteal sleeve of bone forms around midshaft of each anlage Intramembranous bone formation begins via direct ossification
8	Vascular invasion into the cartilaginous anlage Capillaries deliver precursor cells; primary center of ossification develops

1: Basic Science

3. These growth regions differentiate further and become well-defined growth plates.

4. Division within the growth plate is coupled with the deposition of bone at the metaphyseal side of the bud, and long-bone growth begins.

5. At a specific time in the development of each long bone, a secondary center of ossification develops within the chondroepiphysis.

6. The secondary center of ossification typically grows in a spherical fashion and accounts for the centripetal growth of the long bone.

7. The rates of division within the centers of ossification ultimately determine the overall contour of each joint.

II. Normal Growth Plate

A. Structure, organization, and function

1. The function of the growth plate is related to its structure. In its simplest form, the growth plate comprises three histologically distinct zones surrounded by a fibrous component and bounded by a bony metaphyseal component.

2. The three cellular zones of the growth plate are the reserve, proliferative, and hypertrophic zones (**Figure 1**).

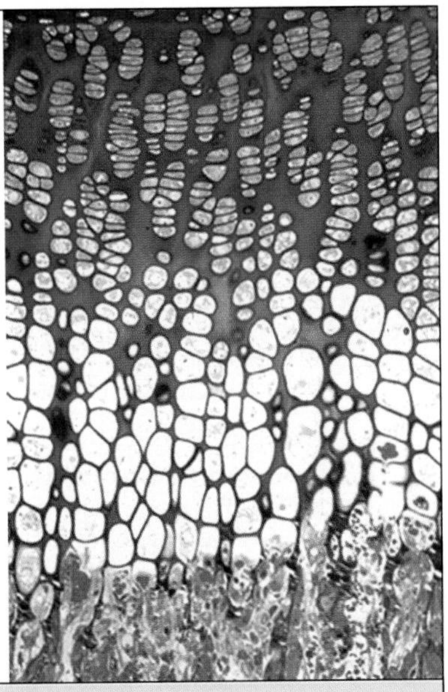

Figure 1 Photomicrograph showing the structure and zones of the growth plate, x220. (*Adapted with permission from Farnum CE, Nixon A, Lee AO, Kwan DT, Belanger L, Wilsman NJ: Quantitative three-dimensional analysis of chondrocytic kinetic responses to short-term stapling of the rat proximal tibial growth plate. Cells Tissues Organs 2000;167:247-258.*)

a. The reserve zone is adjacent to the secondary center of ossification and is characterized by a sparse distribution of cells in a vast matrix.

   i. Cellular proliferation in this zone is sporadic, and the chondrocytes in this region do not contribute to longitudinal growth.

   ii. Type II collagen content is highest here.

   iii. Blood supply to this zone is via the terminal branches of the epiphyseal artery, which enter the secondary center of ossification.

b. The proliferative zone is characterized by longitudinal columns of flattened cells. The uppermost cell in each column is the progenitor cell, which is responsible for longitudinal growth.

   i. The total longitudinal growth of the growth plate depends on the number of cell divisions of the progenitor cell.

   ii. The rate at which the cells divide is influenced by mechanical and hormonal factors.

   iii. The matrix of the proliferative zone comprises a nonuniform array of collagen fibrils and matrix vesicles.

   iv. Proliferative zone chondrocytes are also supplied by the terminal branches of the epiphyseal artery; however, these vessels do not penetrate the proliferative zone but rather terminate at the uppermost cell. These vessels deliver the oxygen and nutrients that facilitate the cellular division and matrix production that occur within this zone.

c. The cells in the hypertrophic zone are 5 to 10 times the size of those in the proliferative zone.

   i. The role of the hypertrophic zone chondrocytes is the synthesis of novel matrix proteins.

   ii. The hypertrophic zone has the highest content of glycolytic enzymes, and the chondrocytes participate in matrix mineralization through the synthesis of alkaline phosphatase, neutral proteases, and type X collagen.

   iii. The hypertrophic zone is avascular.

3. Metaphysis

a. The metaphysis begins distal to the hypertrophic zone and removes the mineralized cartilaginous matrix of the hypertrophic zone.

b. The metaphysis is also involved in bone formation and the histologic remodeling of cancellous trabeculae.

c. The main nutrient artery of the long bone enters at the mid-diaphysis, then bifurcates and sends a branch within the medullary canal to each metaphysis.

d. The capillary loops of these arteries terminate at the bone-cartilage interface of the growth plate (**Figure 2**).

4. Surrounding the periphery of the growth plate is the groove of Ranvier and the perichondral ring of LaCroix.

   a. There are three cell types in the groove of Ranvier: an osteoblast-type cell, a chondrocyte-type cell, and a fibroblast-type cell.

   b. These cells are active in cell division and contribute to bone formation, latitudinal growth, and anchorage to the perichondrium.

   c. The ring of LaCroix is a fibrous collagenous network that is continuous with both the groove of Ranvier and the metaphysis and functions as mechanical support at the bone-cartilage junction.

B. Biochemistry

1. Reserve zone

   a. Has the lowest intracellular and ionized calcium content.

   b. Oxygen tension is low.

2. Proliferative zone

   a. Oxygen tension is highest in this zone secondary to its rich vascular supply.

   b. The presence of abundant glycogen stores and a high oxygen tension supports aerobic metabolism in the proliferative chondrocyte.

3. Hypertrophic zone

   a. Oxygen tension in the hypertrophic zone is low, secondary to the avascular nature of the region. Because of this low oxygen tension, energy production in the hypertrophic zone occurs via anaerobic glycolysis of the glycogen stored in the proliferative zone.

   b. In the upper hypertrophic zone, a switch from adenosine triphosphate (ATP) production to calcium production occurs. Once the glycogen stores have been depleted, calcium is released. This is the mechanism by which the matrix is calcified.

   c. The region of the hypertrophic zone where mineralization occurs is known as the zone of provisional calcification.

   d. Slipped capital femoral epiphysis (SCFE) involves the hypertrophic zone.

4. Cartilage matrix turnover

   a. Several enzymes are involved in this process, including metalloproteinases, which depend on the presence of calcium and zinc for activity. Collagenese, gelatinase, and stromelysin are

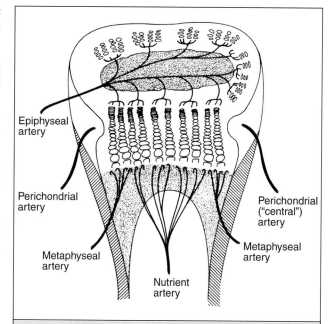

Figure 2   Structure and blood supply of a typical growth plate. *(Reproduced with permission from Brighton CT: Structure and function of the growth plate. Clin Orthop 1978;136:24.)*

produced by the growth plate chondrocytes in an inactive form and are then activated by interleukin-1, plasmin, or tissue inhibitor of metalloproteinases.

   b. The metaphysis removes the mineralized cartilage matrix as well as the unmineralized last transverse septum of the hypertrophic zone.

   c. The unmineralized portion is removed via lysosomal enzymes, and the cartilaginous lacunae are invaded by endothelial and perivascular cells.

3. Metaphysis

   a. Characterized by anaerobic metabolism, vascular stasis, and low oxygen tension. This is secondary to the blood supply to the region.

   b. After the removal process is complete, osteoblasts begin the remodeling process, in which the osteoblasts progressively lay down bone on the cartilage template, creating an area of woven bone on a central core that is known as primary trabecular bone. The primary trabecular bone is resorbed via osteoclastic activity and replaced by lamellar bone, which represents the secondary bony trabeculae.

   c. This remodeling process occurs around the periphery and subperiosteal regions of the metaphysis and results in funnelization, a narrowing of the diameter of the metaphysis to meet the diaphysis.

Table 2

Skeletal Dysplasias Associated With Genetic Defects

Genetic Disorder	Genetic Mutation	Functional Defect	Characteristic Phenotypes
Achondroplasia	FGFR-3	Inhibition of chondrocyte proliferation	Short stature (skeletal dysplasia), normal- to large-sized head, rhizomelic shortening of the limbs (especially the upper arm and thigh), a normal-sized trunk
Thanatophoric dysplasia	FGFR-3	Inhibition of chondrocyte proliferation	Severe dwarfism (marked limb shortening, a small chest, and a relatively large head) Lethal after birth because of respiratory compromise
Hypochondroplasia	FGFR-3	Inhibition of chondrocyte proliferation	Milder dwarfism than achondroplasia
Pseudoachondroplasia	COMP	Abnormality of cartilage formation	Short stature (skeletal dysplasia) Rhizomelic limb shortening, similar body proportion as achondroplasia; lacks the distinct facial features characteristic of achondroplasia Early-onset osteoarthritis
Multiple epiphyseal dysplasia	COMP or type IX collagen	Abnormality of cartilage formation	Short stature (skeletal dysplasia) Early-onset osteoarthritis
Spondyloepiphyseal dysplasia	Type II collagen	Defect in cartilage matrix formation	Short stature (skeletal dysplasia), short trunk Spine malformation, coxa vara, myopia, and retinal degeneration
Diatrophic dysplasia	Sulfate transporter	Defect in sulfation of proteoglycan	Fraccato-type achondroplasia, dwarfism, fetal hydrops
Schmid metaphyseal chondrodysplasia	Type X collagen	Defect in cartilage matrix formation	Short stature, coxa vara, genu varum, involvement in metaphyses of the long bones but not in the spine Less severe than in the Jansen type—none of the disorganized metaphyseal calcification that occurs in the Jansen type
Jansen metaphyseal chondrodysplasia	PTH/PTHrP receptor	Functional defect of parathyroid hormone	Short limbs, characteristic facial abnormalities, and additional skeletal malformations Sclerotic bones in the back cranial bones, which may lead to blindness or deafness Hypercalcemia
Cleidocranial dysplasia	Runx2 (cbfa-1)	Impaired intramembranous ossification	Hypoplasia or aplasia of the clavicles, open skull suture, mild facial hypoplasia, wide symphysis pubis, mild short stature, dental abnormality, vertebral abnormality

FGFR-3 = fibroblast growth factor receptor 3; COMP = cartilage oligomeric matrix protein; PTH = parathyroid hormone; PTHrP = parathyroid hormone–related proton.

C. Pathophysiology

1. Overview

a. Most growth plate abnormalities can be attributed to a defect within a specific zone or to a particular malfunction in the system.

b. Most growth plate abnormalities affect the reserve zone; however, there is currently no evidence to suggest that any disease state originates from cytopathology unique to the reserve zone.

c. However, any disease state that affects the matrix will have an impact on the proliferative zone.

2. Achondroplasia (Table 2 and Figure 3)

a. Originates in the chondrocytes of the proliferative zone.

b. The disorder usually results from a single amino acid substitution, which causes a defect in fibroblast growth factor receptor 3 (FGFR-3).

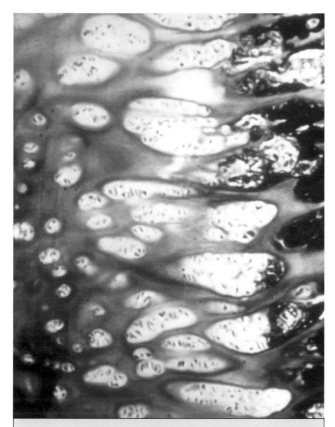

Figure 3 Histologic image showing the disorganized arrangement seen with achondroplasia. *(Reproduced from Iannotti JP et al: The formation and growth of skeletal tissues, in Buckwalter JA, Einhorn TA, Simon SR (eds): Orthopaedic Basic Science: Biology and Biomechanics of the Musculoskeletal System, ed 2. American Academy of Orthopaedic Surgeons, Rosemont, IL, 2000, p 103.)*

3. Jansen dysplasia

   a. A mutation in the parathyroid hormone-related protein (PTHrP) receptor affects the negative feedback loop in which PTHrP slows down the conversion of proliferating chondrocytes to hypertrophic chondrocytes.

   b. The mutation in the receptor results in a constitutively active state that is the molecular basis for Jansen chondrometaphyseal dysplasia.

   c. Because this receptor is the shared receptor for PTH, hypercalcemia and hypophosphatemia can occur in Jansen dysplasia.

D. Growth plate mineralization

   1. Growth plate mineralization is a unique process because of the specialized blood supply to the growth plate, its unique energy metabolism, and its handling of intracellular calcium stores.

   2. The major factors that affect growth plate mineralization are intracellular calcium homeostasis

and the extracellular matrix vesicles and extracellular macromolecules. Various microenvironmental factors and systemic hormones also modulate this process.

   a. Intracellular calcium

      i. The role of intracellular calcium in matrix mineralization is so significant that the mitochondria in the chondrocytes are specialized for calcium transport.

      ii. Compared to nonmineralizing cells, the chondrocyte mitochondria have a greater capacity for calcium accumulation as well as the ability to store calcium in a labile form so that it can be used for release.

      iii. Histologic studies have demonstrated that mitochondrial calcium accumulates in the upper two thirds of the hypertrophic zone and is depleted in the lower chondrocytes.

      iv. When the mitochondrial calcium is released in the lower cells, matrix mineralization occurs (**Figure 4**).

   b. Extracellular matrix vesicles

      i. The initial site for matrix calcification is unclear, though data exist to support the role of the matrix vesicle in this process.

      ii. The matrix vesicles are rich in alkaline phosphatase and neutral proteases, which are critical to promote mineralization.

   c. Extracellular macromolecules

      i. The major collagen in the hypertrophic zone is type II; however, the terminal hypertrophic chondrocytes also produce and secrete type X collagen.

      ii. The appearance of this collagen in the matrix initiates the onset of endochondral ossification.

III. Effects of Hormones and Growth Factors on the Growth Plate

A. Influence on growth plate mechanics

   1. Hormones, growth factors, and vitamins have been shown to influence the growth plate through mechanisms such as chondrocyte proliferation and maturation, macromolecule synthesis, intracellular calcium homeostasis, or matrix mineralization.

   2. Each growth plate zone may be targeted by one or more factors that help to mediate the cytologic characteristics unique to that zone. These factors may be exogenous or endogenous to the growth plate.

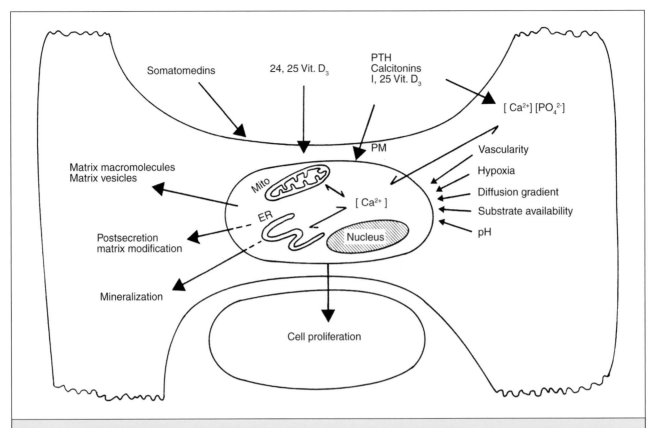

Figure 4   The factors influencing growth plate chondrocyte function and matrix mineralization. ER = endoplasmic reticulum, N = nucleus, PM = plasma membrane, Mito = mitochondria. *(Adapted with permission from Iannotti JP: Growth plate physiology and pathology.* Orthop Clin North Am *1990;21:1-17.)*

a. Paracrine factors are produced by the cell within the growth plate and act within the growth plate, but on another cell type.

b. Autocrine factors act on the cells that produced them.

B. Thyroid hormones and PTH

1. The thyroid hormones, thyroxine (T4) and tri-iodothyronine (T3), act on the proliferative and upper hypertrophic zone chondrocytes through a systemic endocrine effect.

a. Thyroxine is essential for cartilage growth. It increases DNA synthesis in the cells of the proliferative zone and affects cell maturation by increasing glycosaminoglycan synthesis, collagen synthesis, and alkaline phosphatase activity.

b. Excess T4 results in protein catabolism; a deficiency of T4 results in growth retardation, cretinism, and abnormal degradation of mucopolysaccharides.

2. PTH also acts on the proliferative and upper hypertrophic zone chondrocytes.

a. PTH has a direct mitogenic effect on epiphyseal chondrocytes. Furthermore, PTH stimulates proteoglycan synthesis through an increase in intracellular ionized calcium and the stimulation of protein kinase C.

b. PTHrP is a cytokine with autocrine or paracrine action.

c. The common PTHrP-PTH receptor has a role in the conversion of the small cell chondrocyte to the hypertrophic phenotype.

3. Calcitonin is a peptide hormone that is produced by the parafollicular cells of the thyroid and which acts primarily in the lower hypertrophic zone to accelerate growth plate calcification and cell maturation.

C. Adrenal corticoids

1. Adrenal corticoids, or glucocorticoids, are steroid hormones primarily produced by the adrenal cortex. These hormones primarily affect the zones of cellular differentiation and proliferation.

a. The primary influence of the glucocorticoids is a decrease in proliferation of the chondroprogenitor cells in the zone of differentiation.

b. Supraphysiologic amounts of these hormones result in growth retardation through a depression of glycolysis and a reduction of energy stores.

2. Sex steroids, or androgens, function as anabolic factors.

   a. The primary active androgen metabolite is postulated to be dihydrotestosterone, based on the presence of this receptor in both male and female growth plate tissue.

   b. The role of the androgens is to regulate mineralization in the lower part of the growth plate, increase the deposition of glycogen and lipids in cells, and increase the number of proteoglycans in the cartilage matrix.

D. Growth hormone (GH) and vitamins

1. Growth hormone

   a. GH is produced by the pituitary and is essential for growth plate function. The effects of GH are mediated by the somatomedins, a group of peptide factors.

   b. When GH binds to epiphyseal chondrocytes, insulin-like growth factor 1 (IGF-1) is released locally. Therefore, GH regulates not only the number of cells containing the IGF receptor, but also the synthesis of IGF-1 in all zones of the growth plate.

2. Vitamin D

   a. The active metabolites of vitamin D are the 1,25- and 24,25-dihydroxylated forms, both of which are produced by the liver and kidneys.

   b. A direct mitogenic effect has been reported with 24,25-dihydroxy vitamin D.

   c. The metabolite significantly increases DNA synthesis and inhibits proteoglycan synthesis.

   d. The highest level of vitamin D metabolites are found in the proliferative zone; no metabolites are found in the hypertrophic zone.

3. Vitamin A

   a. Vitamin A (the carotenes) are essential to the metabolism of epiphyseal cartilage.

   b. A deficiency of vitamin A results in impairment of cell maturation, which ultimately causes abnormal bone shape.

   c. Excessive vitamin A leads to bone weakness secondary to increases in lysosomal body membrane fragility.

4. Vitamin C

   a. Vitamin C is a cofactor in the enzymatic synthesis of collagen.

   b. It is therefore necessary for the development of the growth plate.

IV. Biomechanics of the Growth Plate

A. Growth plate injury

1. The weakest structure in the ends of the long bones is the growth plate, and the weakest region within the growth plate itself is the hypertrophic zone.

2. Growth plate injuries occur when the mechanical demands exceed the mechanical strength of the epiphysis–growth plate metaphysis complex.

3. The factors that determine the incidence of injury are the ability of the growth plate to resist failure and the nature of the stresses introduced to the bone.

4. The mechanical properties of the growth plate are described by the Hueter-Volkmann law, which states that increasing compression across a growth plate leads to decreasing growth (**Figure 5**).

B. Growth plate properties

1. The morphology of the growth plate allows it to adapt its form to follow the contours of principal tensile stresses. The contours allow the growth plate to be subjected to compressive stress.

2. The tensile properties of the growth plate have been determined by controlled uniaxial tension tests in the bovine femur. The ultimate strain at

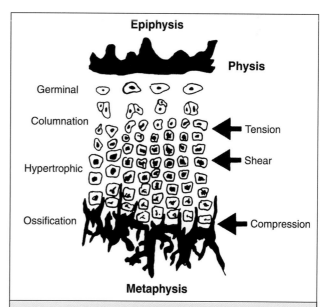

Figure 5   The histologic zone of failure varies with the type of load applied to the specimens. (*Reproduced with permission from Moen CT, Pelker RR: Biomechanical and histological correlations in growth plate failure. J Pediatr Orthop 1984;4:180-184.*)

1: Basic Science

failure has been shown to be uniform throughout the growth plate.

3. The growth plate has been shown to be stronger and stiffer in the anterior and inferior regions.

4. Mechanical forces can influence the shape and length of the growing bone, and studies have demonstrated that mechanical forces are present and can influence bone development during the earliest stages of endochondral ossification.

5. The biologic interface between the metaphyseal ossification front and the adjacent proliferative cartilage is partially determined by mechanical forces, initially in the form of muscle contractions.

6. Both the function of the growth plate and its mechanical properties appear to be influenced by both internal structure and external mechanical factors.

V. Pathologic States Affecting the Growth Plate

A. Genetic disorders (**Tables 3 and 4**)

1. Cartilage matrix defects—All produce some form of skeletal dysplasia, with varying degrees of impact on articular and growth plate cartilage.

   a. Abnormalities of type II collagen are the cause of Kniest dysplasia and of some types of Stickler syndrome and spondyloepiphyseal dysplasia.

   b. Abnormalities of type IX collagen are the cause of some forms of multiple epiphyseal dysplasia.

   c. Defects in type X collagen cause the Schmid-type metaphyseal chondrodysplasia.

2. Diastrophic dysplasia—Classic example of a defect in proteoglycan metabolism.

   a. The disorder is caused by a mutation in the sulfate transporter molecule, which results in undersulfation of the proteoglycan matrix.

   b. The phenotype is short stature and characteristic severe equinovarus feet.

3. Mucopolysaccharidoses—A group of disorders that result from defects in the proteoglycan metabolism (**Table 3**).

   a. These disorders are caused by a defect in the enzymes involved in proteoglycan metabolism with a resultant accumulation of undegraded glycosaminoglycans (**Table 4**).

   b. The clinical presentation of each mucopolysaccharidosis depends on the specific enzyme defect and the resultant glycoprotein accumulation.

   c. Common to all six disease states is a toxic effect on the central nervous system, skeleton, or ocular or visceral system.

4. Metabolic mineralization disorders

   a. Hypophosphatasia is an autosomal recessive defect in alkaline phosphatase with resultant normal serum levels of calcium and phosphate but inability of the matrix to calcify. The hypertrophic zone widens, but there is no mineralization of the osteoid that is laid down. The zone of provisional calcification never forms. The histologic appearance and effect are similar to nutritional rickets, with a resulting inhibition of growth.

   b. Hypophosphatemic familial rickets is a sex-linked dominant disorder characterized by low serum calcium and phosphorus. Alkaline phosphatase activity is high, with resultant abnormal conversion of vitamin D to its metabolites. The skeletal changes seen are those typical of nutritional rickets, which is discussed below.

B. Environmental factors

1. Infection

   a. The metaphyseal portion of the growth plate is typically affected by bacterial infection. This is due to the slow circulation, low oxygen tension, and deficiency of the reticuloendothelial system in this area.

   b. Bacteria become lodged in the vascular sinusoids, with the resultant production of small abscesses in the area.

   c. If the infection extends into the Haversian canals, osteomyelitis of the cortical bone ensues, with associated subperiosteal abscess.

   d. In the first year of life, cartilage canals may persist across growth plates and serve as an additional conduit for the spread of infection. Severe infection may cause local or total cessation of growth, and in most instances inhibited or angular growth results.

2. Irradiation—Depending on the dose, irradiation can result in shortened bones with increased width as a result of the preferential effect of irradiation on longitudinal chondroblastic proliferation, with sparing of latitudinal bone growth.

C. Nutritional disorders

1. Nutritional rickets

   a. Results from abnormal processing of calcium, phosphorus, and vitamin D

   b. The common disorder is failure to mineralize the matrix in the zone of provisional calcification.

Table 3

Genetic Abnormalities With Musculoskeletal Manifestations

Disease	Subtype	Inheritance Pattern	Affected Gene/Gene Product
Achondroplasia		AD	FGRC-3
Apert syndrome		AD	FGRC-2
Chondrodysplasia punctata		XLD	Unknown
Cleidocranial		AD	Unknown
Diastrophic dysplasia		AR	Diastrophic dysplasia sulfate transporter
Hypochondroplasia		AD	FGRC-3
Kniest syndrome		AD	Type II collagen
Metaphyseal chondrodysplasia			
	Jansen type	AD	Parathyroid hormone–related peptide receptor
	McKusick type	AR	Unknown
	Schmid type	AD	Type X collagen
McCune-Albright syndrome		Unknown	Guanine nucleotide-binding protein alpha
Mucopolysaccharidosis			
	Type I (Hurler)	AR	Alpha-L-iduronidase
	Type II (Hunter)	XLR	Sulfoiduronate sulfatase
	Type IA (Morquio)	AR	Galactosamine-6-sulfate-sulfatase, beta-galactosidase
Multiple epiphyseal dysplasia			
	Type I	AD	Cartilage oligomeric matrix protein
	Type II	AD	Type IX collagen
Nail-patella syndrome		AD	Unknown
Osteopetrosis		AR	Macrophage colony–stimulating factor
Pseudoachondroplasia		AD	Cartilage oligomeric matrix protein
Stickler syndrome		AD	Type II collagen
Spondyloepiphyseal dysplasia			
	Congenital	AD	Type II collagen
	Tarda	AR	Type II collagen
	X-linked	XLD	Unknown
Angelman syndrome		AR	Unknown
Dystrophinopathies			
	Duchenne muscular dystrophy	XLR	Dystrophin
	Becker muscular dystrophy	XLR	Dystrophin

AD = Autosomal dominant, XLD = X-linked dominant, AR = autosomal recessive, XLR = X-linked recessive.

(continued on next page)

1: Basic Science

1: Basic Science

Table 3

Genetic Abnormalities With Musculoskeletal Manifestations (continued)

Disease	Subtype	Inheritance Pattern	Affected Gene/Gene Product
Charcot-Marie-Tooth disease			
	Type IA	AD	Peripheral myelin protein-22
	Type IB	AD	Myelin protein zero
	Type IIA	AD	Unknown
	Type IVA	AR	Unknown
	X-linked	XL	Connexin-32
Friedreich ataxia		AR	Frataxin
Myotonic dystrophy		AD	Myotonin-protein kinase
Myotonia congenita		AD	Muscle chloride channel-1
Prader-Willi syndrome		AR	Unknown
Spinocerebellar ataxia			
	Type I	AD	Ataxin-1
	Type II	AD	MJD/SCA1
Spinal muscular atrophy		AR	Survival motor neuron
Ehlers-Danlos syndrome			
	Type IVA	AD	Type III collagen
	Type VI	AR	Lysine hydroxylase
	Type X	AR	Fibronectin-1
Marfan syndrome		AD	Fibrillin-1
Osteogenesis imperfecta			
	Type I	AD	Type I collagen (COL1A1, COL1A2)
	Type II	AR	Type I collagen (COL1A1, COL1A2)
	Type III	AR	Type I collagen (COL1A1, COL1A2)
	Type IVA	AD	Type I collagen (COL1A1, COL1A2)

AD = Autosomal dominant, XLD = X-linked dominant, AR = autosomal recessive, XLR = X-linked recessive.
A portion of this table was adapted with permission from Dietz FR, Matthews KD: Update on the genetic bases of disorders with orthopaedic manifestations. *J Bone Joint Surg Am* 1996;78:1583-1598.

c. The hypertrophic zone is greatly expanded, with widening of the growth plate and flaring of the metaphysis noted on plain radiographs (**Figure 6**).

2. Scurvy

a. Caused by vitamin C deficiency, with a resultant decrease in chondroitin sulfate and collagen synthesis.

b. The greatest deficiency in collagen synthesis is

seen in the metaphysis, where the demand for type I collagen is the highest during new bone formation.

c. Characteristic radiographic findings of scurvy are the line of Frankel (a dense white line that represents the zone of provisional calcification) and osteopenia of the metaphysis.

d. Clinical findings include microfractures, hemorrhages, and collapse of the metaphysis.

Table 4

Genetic Defects Associated With Metabolic Bone Diseases

Genetic Disorder	Genetic Mutation	Functional Defect	Characteristic Phenotypes
X-linked hypophosphatemic rickets	Acellular endopeptidase	Vitamin D–resistant rickets	Rickets, short stature, and impaired renal phosphate reabsorption and vitamin D metabolism
Hypophosphatasia	Alkaline phosphatase gene	Generalized impairment of skeletal mineralization	Rickets, bow leg, loss of teeth, short stature
Mucopolysaccharidosis type I (MPS I)	α-L-iduronidase	Deficiency of α-L-iduronidase (lysosomal enzymes for breaking glycosaminoglycans)	Hurler syndrome; progressive cellular damage that affects the development of neurologic and musculoskeletal system (short stature and bone dysplasia)
Mucopolysaccharidosis type II (MPS II)	Iduronate sulfatase; X-linked recessive	Deficiency of iduronate sulfatase	Hunter syndrome; mild to moderate features of MPS
Mucopolysaccharidosis type III (MPS III)	Heparan N-sulfatase or N-acetylglucosamine 6-sulfatase	Deficiency of heparan N-sulfatase (IIIA); α-N-acetylglucosaminidase (IIIB); acetyl coenzyme A: α-glucosaminide N-acetyltransferase (IIIC); N-acetylglucosamine 6-sulfatase (IIID)	Sanfilippo syndrome; severe neurologic syndrome with mild progressive musculoskeletal syndrome
Mucopolysaccharidosis type IV (MPS IV)	Deficient enzymes N-acetylgalactosamine 6-sulfatase (type A) or β-galactosidase (type B)	Deficiency of lysosomal enzymes for breaking keratin sulfate	Morquio syndrome; bell-shaped chest, anomaly of spine, shortened long bones, and dysplasia of the hips, knees, ankles, and wrists. Odontoid hypoplasia

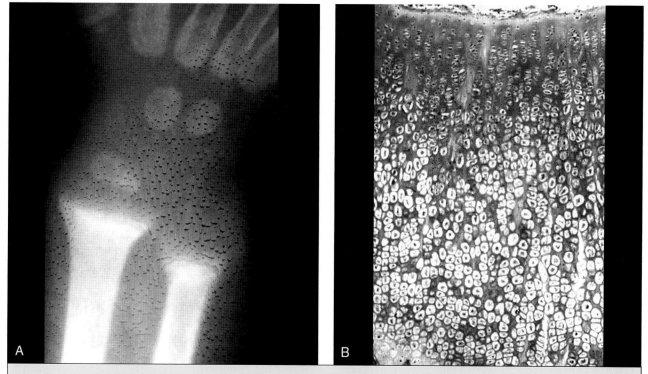

Figure 6 **A,** Radiographic features of rickets in the distal radius and ulna. Note the widened growth plates and flaring of the metaphyses. **B,** Histologic features of rickets. The zone of proliferation is largely unaffected, but the hypertrophic zone is markedly widened. *(Photographs courtesy of Dr. Henry J. Mankin.)*

1: Basic Science

Top Testing Facts

1. Formation of the bony skeleton occurs via either intramembranous bone formation or endochondral bone formation. Intramembranous bone formation occurs through osteoblast activity; endochondral ossification occurs at the growth plates and within fracture callus.

2. In the primary center of ossification, blood-borne precursors of osteoblasts and osteoclasts are delivered by the capillaries. This process signals the transition from the embryonic to the fetal period and occurs first at the humerus.

3. The total length of the growth plate depends on the number of cell divisions of the progenitor cell.

4. The region of the hypertrophic zone where mineralization occurs is known as the zone of provisional calcification.

5. SCFE involves the hypertrophic zone.

6. The genetic mutation in achondroplasia is a defect in FGFR-3.

7. Growth plate injuries occur when the mechanical demands of bone exceed the strength of the epiphysis–growth plate metaphysis complex. The Hueter-Volkmann law states that increasing compression across the growth plate leads to decreased growth.

8. Diastrophic dysplasia is a defect in proteoglycan sulfation.

9. Bacterial infection affects the metaphyseal portion of the growth plate.

10. Scurvy is caused by a vitamin C deficiency with resultant decrease in chondroitin sulfate and collagen synthesis.

Bibliography

Ballock RT, O'Keefe RJ: Growth and development of the skeleton, in Einhorn TA, O'Keefe RJ, Buckwalter JA (eds): *Orthopaedic Basic Science: Foundations of Clinical Practice*, ed 3. Rosemont, IL, American Academy of Orthopaedic Surgeons, 2007, pp 115-128.

Colnot C: Cellular and molecular interactions regulating skeletogenesis. *J Cell Biochem* 2005;95:688-697.

Ferguson C, Alpern E, Miclau T, Helms JA: Does adult fracture repair recapitulate embryonic skeletal formation? *Mech Dev* 1999;87:57-66.

Provot S, Schipani E: Molecular mechanisms of endochondral bone development. *Biochem Biophys Res Commun* 2005; 328:658-665.

Shimizu H, Yokoyama S, Asahara H: Growth and differentiation of the developing limb bud from the perspective of chondrogenesis. *Dev Growth Differ* 2007;49:449-454.

Chapter 5

Bone and Joint Biology

*John C. Clohisy, MD   *Dieter Lindskog, MD   Yousef Abu-Amer, PhD

I. Bone

A. Overview

1. Functions of bone—The unique composition and structure of bone enables this tissue to accomplish the following:

   a. Provide mechanical support

   b. Regulate mineral homeostasis

   c. House the marrow elements

2. Types of bones—long, short, and flat

3. Formation of bones

   a. Long bones are formed via endochondral ossification, which is formation of bone from a cartilage model.

   b. Flat bones are formed by intramembranous bone formation, which is the formation of bone through loose condensations of mesenchymal tissue.

B. Anatomy

1. Long bones are composed of three anatomic regions: the diaphysis, the metaphysis, and the epiphysis (**Figure 1**).

   a. Diaphysis—The shaft of a long bone, consisting of a tube of thick cortical bone surrounding a thin central canal of trabecular bone (the intramedullary canal).

      i. The inner aspect of the cortical bone is called the endosteal surface.

      ii. The outer region is called the periosteal surface. This surface is covered by the periosteal membrane, which is composed of an outer layer of fibrous connective tissue and an inner layer of undifferentiated, osteogenic progenitor cells.

   b. Metaphysis—Transition zone from epiphysis to diaphysis; composed of loose trabecular bone surrounded by a thin layer of cortical bone.

   c. Epiphysis—Specialized end of bone that forms the joint articulation.

      i. The growth plate (physis or physeal scar) divides the epiphysis from the metaphysis.

      ii. The epiphysis is composed of loose trabecular bone surrounded by a thin layer of cortical bone.

      iii. The articular portion of the bone has a specialized subchondral region underlying the articular cartilage.

2. Flat bones

   a. Flat bones include the pelvis, scapula, skull, and mandible.

   b. The composition of these bones varies from purely cortical in some regions to cortical bone with a thin inner region of trabecular bone.

3. Neurovascular anatomy of bone

   a. Innervation—The nerves that innervate bone derive from the periosteum and enter bone in tandem with blood vessels. Nerves are found in the haversian canals and Volkmann canals (**Figure 2**).

   b. Blood supply

      i. Nutrient arteries pass through the diaphyseal cortex and enter the intramedullary canal. These vessels provide blood supply to the inner two thirds of the cortical bone and are at risk during intramedullary reaming.

      ii. The outer one third of the cortical bone derives its blood supply from the periosteal membrane vessels. These vessels are at risk with periosteal stripping during surgical procedures.

B. Structure

1. Macroscopic level

   a. Cortical bone—A dense, compact bone with low porosity and no macroscopic spaces.

John C. Clohisy, MD, or the department with which he is affiliated has received research or institutional support from Wright Medical Technology and Zimmer and is a consultant or employee for Zimmer. Dieter Lindskog, MD, is a consultant or employee for Arthrocare.

1: Basic Science

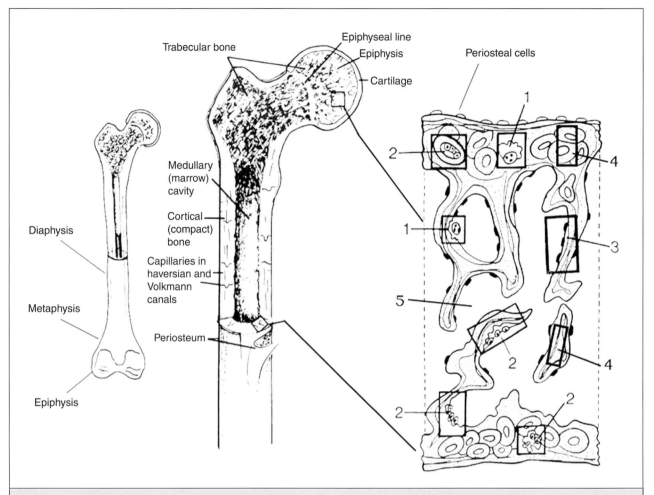

Figure 1   Schematic diagram of cortical and trabecular bone showing the different structures and cell types. 1 = osteoclasts, 2 = osteoblasts, 3 = bone lining cells, 4 = osteocytes, 5 = marrow space. *(Reproduced with permission from Hayes WC: Biomechanics of cortical and trabecular bone: Implications for assessment of fracture risk, in Basic Orthopaedic Biomechanics. New York, NY, Raven Press, 1991, pp 93-142 and Bostrom MPG, Boskey A, Kaufma JK, Einhorn TA: Form and function of bone, in Buckwalter JA, Einhorn TA, Simon SR (eds): Orthopaedic Basic Science: Biology and Biomechanics of the Musculoskeletal System, ed 2. Rosemont, IL, American Academy of Orthopaedic Surgeons, 2000, pp 320-369.)*

    i. In the diaphyseal region, cortical bone is load bearing.

    ii. In the metaphysis and epiphysis, cortical bone serves as a border to trabecular bone. It supports only a portion of the load, which is primarily carried by the trabecular bone in these regions.

  b. Trabecular bone—Bone composed of a loose network of bony struts (rods and plates). These struts have a maximum thickness of approximately 200 μm.

    i. Trabecular bone is porous, with a macroscopic porosity ranging from 30% to 90%, and houses the bone marrow contents.

    ii. In osteoporosis, the macroscopic porosity is increased because of thinning of the trabecular struts.

2. Microscopic level

  a. Woven bone is primary bone that is characterized by random orientation of collagen and mineral.

  b. Lamellar bone is secondary bone that results from the remodeling of woven bone into an organized bone tissue.

  c. Lacunae are ellipsoidal spaces in bone that are occupied by osteocytes. Small channels through the bone called canaliculi connect the lacunae and contain osteocyte cell processes that interact with other cells.

C. Composition of the extracellular matrix (ECM)—The ECM is composed of 60% to 70% mineral matrix and 20% to 25% organic matrix.

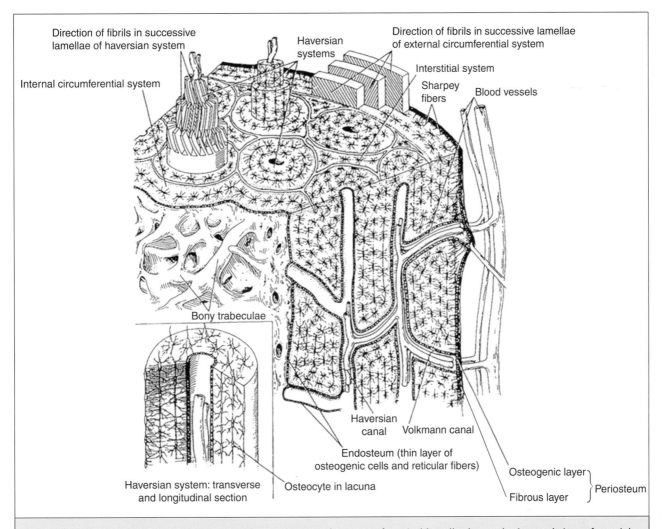

Figure 2 Diagram of the structure of cortical bone, showing the types of cortical lamellar bone: the internal circumferential system, interstitial system, osteonal lamellae, and outer circumferential system. The diagram also shows the intraosseous vascular system that serves the osteocytes and connects the periosteal and medullary blood vessels. The haversian canals run primarily longitudinally through the cortex, whereas the Volkmann canals create oblique connections between the haversian canals. Cement lines separate each osteon from the surrounding bone. Periosteum covers the external surface of the bone and consists of two layers: an osteogenic (inner) cellular layer and a fibrous (outer) layer. *(Reproduced with permission from Kessel RG, Kardon RH: Tissues and Organs: A Text-Atlas of Scanning and Microscopy. New York, NY, WH Freeman, 1979, p 25.)*

1. Mineral matrix

   a. Responsible for the compressive strength of bone

   b. Composed primarily of calcium and phosphate (but also some sodium, magnesium, and carbonate) in the form of hydroxyapatite and tricalcium phosphate

   c. The mineral component of bone is closely associated with collagen fibrils.

   d. Tropocollagen helices in the fibrils are organized in a quarter-staggered arrangement, with empty regions (hole zones) between the ends and pores running lengthwise between collagen fibrils (**Figure 3**).

   e. Mineral crystals form in the hole zones and pores.

2. Organic matrix—90% type I collagen; 5% other collagen types (III and IV), noncollagenous proteins, and growth factors; the remaining tissue volume is occupied by water.

   a. Collagen

      i. Type I collagen is the primary ECM protein of bone.

      ii. Type I collagen is fibril-forming, with a triple helical structure (three α chains) that contributes tensile strength to the ECM.

      iii. Fibrils are intrinsically stable because of noncovalent interconnections and covalent cross-links between lysine residues.

Mineral accretion: Biologic considerations

Heterogeneity within a collagen fibril

Progressively increasing mineral mass due to:

1. Increased number of new mineral phase particles (nucleation)
   a. Heterogeneous nucleation by matrix in collagen holes
   b. Secondary crystal-induced nucleation in holes and pores
2. Initial growth of particles to ~ 400 Å x 15-30 Å x 50-75 Å

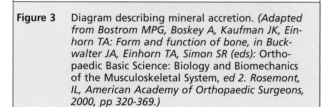

Figure 3 Diagram describing mineral accretion. *(Adapted from Bostrom MPG, Boskey A, Kaufman JK, Einhorn TA: Form and function of bone, in Buckwalter JA, Einhorn TA, Simon SR (eds): Orthopaedic Basic Science: Biology and Biomechanics of the Musculoskeletal System, ed 2. Rosemont, IL, American Academy of Orthopaedic Surgeons, 2000, pp 320-369.)*

iv. Small amounts of types III and IV collagen also are present in bone.

b. Noncollagenous ECM proteins

   i. Vitamin K–dependent proteins—Osteocalcin is the most common vitamin K–dependent, noncollagenous protein in bone and is a marker of osteoblast differentiation. Osteocalcin undergoes carboxylation in a vitamin K–dependent manner.

   ii. Adhesive proteins—Facilitate the interaction of cells (attachment and detachment) with the ECM via cell surface receptors called integrins. Fibronectin and vitronectin are common adhesive proteins of bone.

   iii. Matricellular proteins—Proteins that mediate cell-matrix interactions by modulating signaling from the matrix to the cell.

   iv. Phosphoproteins—Phosphorylated (negatively charged) extracellular proteins that interact with calcium and are thought to play a role in mineralization.

   v. Growth factors and cytokines—Biologically active proteins that are potent regulators of differentiation and activation. These include bone morphogenetic proteins (BMPs), transforming growth factor-β (TGF-β), basic fibroblast growth factor (bFGF), insulin growth factors (IGFs), and interleukins (ILs).

   vi. Proteoglycans—Molecules composed of protein core and glycosaminoglycan side chains. Proteoglycans provide tissue structure, bind to

growth factors, regulate proliferation, and act as cell surface receptors.

D. Composition of bone cells—The cells associated with the bone ECM include osteoblasts, osteocytes, and osteoclasts. Cells of the marrow and periosteum also contribute significantly to the process of bone remodeling.

1. Osteoblasts—Bone surface cells that form bone matrix and regulate osteoclast activity.

   a. Marker proteins include alkaline phosphatase, osteocalcin, osteonectin, and osteopontin.

   b. Osteoblasts have parathyroid hormone (PTH) receptors and secrete type I collagen.

   c. Differentiation

      i. Osteoblasts arise from marrow stromal cells and periosteal membrane cells. A series of cellular regulators serve as differentiation cues for osteoblast development from stem cell to mature osteoblast/osteocyte (**Figure 4**).

      ii. Cells committed to osteoblastic differentiation are called osteoprogenitor cells.

      iii. Each stage of differentiation has characteristic molecular markers, transcription factors, and secreted proteins.

      iv. Runx2 and osterix are essential transcription factors required for osteoblast cell function.

      v. The mature osteoblast has a lifespan of 100 days. It can then become a bone lining cell or an osteocyte, or it can undergo apoptosis. Bone lining cells are relatively inactive cells that cover the surfaces of bone. These cells likely have the ability to become reactivated as functional osteoblasts.

2. Osteocytes

   a. Active osteoblasts become embedded in the mineralized matrix and become osteocytes.

   b. Osteocytes reside in the lacunar spaces of trabecular and cortical bone. They are nonmitotic and are not highly synthetic.

   c. Distinct from the osteoblast, they do not express alkaline phosphatase.

   d. Osteocytes have numerous cell processes that communicate with other cells via the canaliculi.

   e. Signaling between osteocytes is mediated by protein complexes called gap junctions.

   f. Osteocytes contribute to regulation of bone homeostasis.

3. Osteoclasts—Multinucleated bone-resorbing cells.

   a. Marker proteins include tartrate-resistant acid

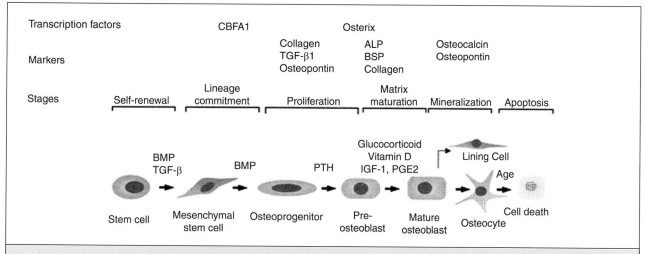

Figure 4 Osteoblast differentiation. This idealized depiction of the osteoblast developmental lineage illustrates the key concepts of early proliferation versus terminal phenotypic differentiation, the temporal onset of molecular markers, and important regulators of this process as well as the different fates possible for cells of the osteoblastic lineage. CBFA1 = core binding factor alpha 1, ALP = alkaline phosphatase, BSP = bone sialoprotein, PGE2 = prostaglandin E2. *(Adapted with permission from Lian JB, Stein GS, Aubin JE: Bone formation: Maturation and functional activities of osteoblast lineage cells, in Favus MJ (ed): Primer on the Metabolic Bone Diseases and Disorders of Mineral Metabolism, ed 5. Washington, DC, American Society for Bone and Mineral Research, 2003, pp 13-28.)*

phosphatase (TRAP), calcitonin receptor, and cathepsin-K.

b. Differentiation—Osteoclasts are hematopoietic cells, members of the monocyte/macrophage lineage. The multinuclear osteoclast polykaryons form by fusion of mononuclear precursors, a process that requires receptor activator for nuclear factor κ B ligand (RANKL) and macrophage-colony stimulating factor (M-CSF).

c. Activity and important features—Mature osteoclasts attach to bone/mineral surfaces and form a sealing zone underneath the cells. The plasma membrane underneath the cell forms the resorptive domain of the cell, which features a highly convoluted ruffled border. Proteases and ions are secreted through this domain to dissolve both organic and nonorganic material.

e. Regulation—Differentiation and activity of osteoclasts is regulated primarily by RANKL and osteoprotegerin (OPG). RANKL binds to its cognate receptor, RANK, on the membrane of monocyte/macrophage. OPG is a decoy receptor (member of the tumor necrosis factor [TNF] receptor family) that binds to and sequesters RANKL, thus inhibiting osteoclast differentiation and activity (**Figure 5**).

E. Bone homeostasis—Balanced bone formation and resorption.

1. Remodeling

a. Bone is a dynamic tissue that is constantly un-

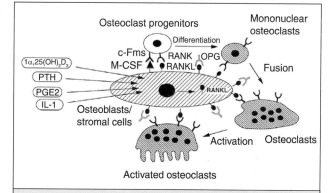

Figure 5 Schematic representation of osteoclast differentiation and function regulated by RANKL and M-CSF. Osteoclast progenitors and mature osteoclasts express RANK, the receptor for RANKL. Osteotropic factors such as $1\alpha,25(OH)_2D_3$, PTH, and IL-1 stimulate expression of RANKL in osteoblasts/stromal cells. Membrane- or matrix-associated forms of both M-CSF and RANKL expressed by osteoblasts/stromal cells are responsible for the induction of osteoclast differentiation in the coculture. RANKL also directly stimulates fusion and activation of osteoclasts. Mainly osteoblasts/stromal cells produce OPG, a soluble decoy receptor of RANKL. OPG strongly inhibits the entire differentiation, fusion, and activation processes of osteoclast induced by RANKL. *(Reproduced with permission from Takahashi N, Udagawa N, Takami M, Suda T: Osteoclast generation, in Bilezikian HP, Raisz LG, Rodan GA (eds): Principles of Bone Biology, ed 2. San Diego, CA, Academic Press, 2002, pp 109-126.)*

dergoing remodeling, primarily through osteoblasts (bone-forming cells) and osteoclasts (resorptive cells) (Figure 5).

1: Basic Science

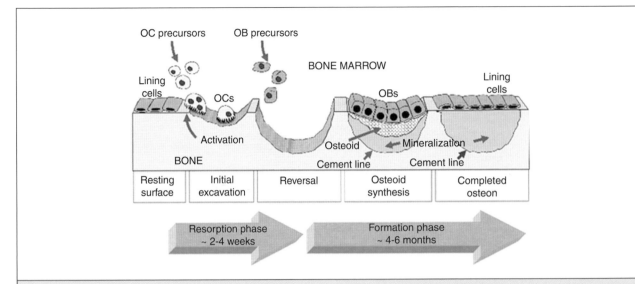

Figure 6 An illustration of a bone marrow unit showing the various stages of cellular activity that it passes through temporally from the resorption of old bone by osteoclasts and the subsequent formation of new bone by osteoblasts. For simplicity, the illustration shows remodeling in only two dimensions, whereas in vivo it occurs in three dimensions, with osteoclasts continuing to enlarge the cavity at one end and osteoblasts beginning to fill it in at the other end. OC = osteoclast, OB = osteoblast. *(Adapted with permission from Riggs BL, Parfitt AM: Drugs used to treat osteoporosis: The critical need for a uniform nomenclature based on their action on bone remodeling. J Bone Miner Res 2005;20:177-184.)*

b. The regulatory mechanisms of remodeling are critical to the understanding of bone homeostasis and disease states.

c. An individual's bone mass is "turned over" completely every 4 to 20 years, depending on age. At adulthood, the rate of turnover is 5% per year. This process of bone turnover replaces potentially compromised bone with structurally sound bone.

2. Trabecular bone remodeling (**Figure 6**)

   a. Osteoclastic activation leads to development of a resorption pit called a Howship lacuna.

   b. After pit formation, osteoclasts are replaced by osteoblasts that form new bone matrix.

   c. The cement line is the region where bone resorption stopped and new bone formation begins.

   d. After new bone formation is completed, bone lining cells cover the surface.

3. Cortical bone remodeling (**Figure 7**)

   a. Osteoclasts tunnel through bone to form a cutting cone of resorption.

   b. Blood vessel formation occurs in the cutting cone.

   c. Osteoblast recruitment and new bone formation occur in the resorbed space of the cutting cone.

d. This results in circumferential new bone formation around a blood vessel. This structure is called an osteon, and the vessel space is the haversian canal (**Figure 8**).

4. Mechanisms of osteoblast/osteoclast coupling

   a. The biologic activity of osteoblasts is closely associated with that of osteoclasts, and intercellular signaling mechanisms are being studied.

   b. Osteoblastic regulation of osteoclast function has been well documented. PTH is a pro-osteoclastogenic cytokine that acts through osteoblast cell-surface receptors. These receptors stimulate the synthesis of factors, including RANKL and M-CSF, that are critical to osteoclast development.

   c. In addition to secreting pro-osteoclastogenic RANKL, osteoblasts also can produce OPG, a potent anit-osteoclastogenic protein. Therefore, osteoblasts have positive and negative regulatory effects on osteoclast activity.

   d. Osteoclast activity is also regulated by systemic factors like serum calcium levels and circulating hormones.

      i. Vitamin D and PTH stimulate osteoclastic activity.

      ii. Calcitonin decreases osteoclastic activity.

   e. Osteoclast regulation of osteoblast differentiation and activity is less understood. One work-

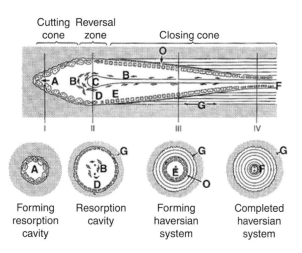

Figure 7 Diagram showing a longitudinal section through a cortical remodeling unit with corresponding transverse sections below. A—Multinucleated osteoclasts in Howship lacuna advancing longitudinally from right to left and radially to enlarge a resorption cavity. B—Perivascular spindle-shaped precursor cells. C—Capillary loop delivering osteoclast precursors and pericytes. D—Mononuclear cells (osteoblast progenitors) lining reversal zone. E—Osteoblasts apposing bone centripetally in radial closure and its perivascular precursor cells. F—Flattened cells lining the haversian canal of completed haversian system or osteon. Transverse sections at different stages of development: (I) resorptive cavities lined with osteoclasts; (II) completed resorption cavities lined by mononuclear cells, the reversal zone; (III) forming haversian sytem or osteons lined with osteoblasts that had recently apposed three lamellae; and (IV) completed haversian sytem or osteon with flattened bone cells lining canal. Cement line (G); osteoid (stippled) between osteoblast (O) and mineralized bone. *(Reproduced with permission from Parfitt AM: The actions of parathyroid hormone on bone: Relation to bone remodeling and turnover, calcium homeostasis, and metabolic bone diseases. II. PTH and bone cells: Bone turnover and plasma calcium regulation.* Metabolism *1976;25;909-955.)*

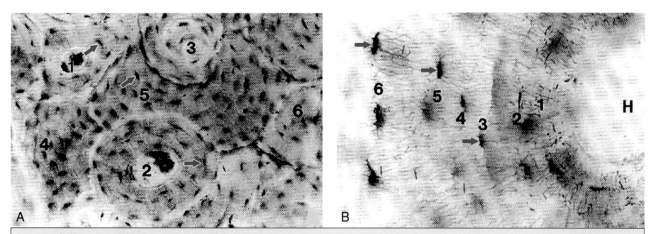

Figure 8 Electron photomicrographs of cortical bone. **A,** A thin-ground cross section of human cortical bone in which osteocyte lacunae (arrows) and canaliculi have been stained with India ink. Osteocytes are arranged around a central vascular channel to constitute haversian systems. Active haversian systems (1, 2, and 3) have concentric lamellae in this plane. Older haversian systems (4, 5, and 6) have had parts of their original territories invaded and remodeled. This is seen most clearly where 2 and 3 have invaded the territory originally occupied by 5. (Original magnification: X185.) **B,** Higher magnification of part of a haversian system showing the successive layering (numbers) of osteocytes (large arrows) from the central core (H) that contains the vasculature. Small arrows identify the canaliculi that connect osteocyte lacunae in different layers. (Original magnification: X718.) *(Adapted with permission from Marks SC, Odgren PR: Structure and development of the skeleton, in Bilezikian JP, Raisz LG, Rodan GA (eds):* Principles of Bone Biology, *ed 2. San Diego, CA, Academic Press, 2002, pp 3-15.)*

Table 1	
Characteristics of Various Disease States	
Disease	**Characteristics**
Osteoporosis	Decreased bone formation with age, leading to loss of bone mass
Osteopetrosis	Decreased bone resorption from loss of osteoclast function
Fibrodysplasia ossificans	Excess bone formation
Paget disease	Increased formation and resorption
Metastatic bone disease	Local tumor secretion of PTH and IL-1 stimulates osteoclast differentiation
Rheumatoid arthritis	Synovial fibroblasts secrete RANKL, which stimulates formation of periarticular erosions
Periprosthetic osteolysis	RANKL production in periprosthetic membrane stimulates local bone resorption

ing hypothesis is that osteoclastic bone resorption releases bioactive factors (BMP, TGF-β, IGF-1) that stimulate osteoblast differentiation and new bone formation.

f. The process of bone remodeling is abnormal in disease states (eg, osteoporosis and osteopetrosis), and therapies are directed at correcting the remodeling abnormalities.

F. Disease states

1. Characteristics (**Table 1**)

2. Therapies

a. Bisphosphonates—Inhibit osteoclastic bone resorption; used to treat osteoporosis, bone metastasis, and Paget disease.

b. Intermittent PTH dosing—Used to stimulate bone formation (continuous dosing stimulates bone resorption).

c. OPG and anti-RANKL antibodies—Potential use as antiresorptive agents for various bone loss disorders (not available for clinical use at press time).

d. Corticosteroids—Decrease bone formation and increase bone resorption. Osteopenia is a common side effect of chronic steroid use.

G. Injury and repair (fracture)

1. Injury

a. Bone injury can be caused by trauma or surgical osteotomy.

b. Injury disrupts the vascular supply to the affected tissue, leading to mechanical instability, hypoxia, depletion of nutrients, and elevated inflammatory response.

2. Repair

a. Unlike tissues that repair by the development of scar tissue, bone heals with the formation of new bone that is indistinguishable from the original tissue.

b. Motion at the fracture site (cast, external fixator, intramedullary rod) results in healing, primarily through endochondral ossification, whereas rigidity at the fracture site (plate fixation) enables direct intramembranous ossification. Most fractures heal with a combination of these bone repair processes.

3. Repair stages

a. Hematoma and inflammatory response—Macrophages and degranulating platelets infiltrate the fracture site and secrete various inflammatory cytokines, including platelet-derived growth factor (PDGF), TGF-β, IL-1 and IL-6, prostaglandin E2 (PGE2), and TNF-α. These factors impact a variety of cells in the fracture hematoma microenvironment.

b. Early postfracture

i. Periosteal preosteoblasts and local osteoblasts form new bone.

ii. Mesenchymal cells and fibroblasts proliferate and are associated with the expression of basic and acidic fibroblast growth factors. Primitive mesenchymal and osteoprogenitor cells are associated with expression of the BMPs and TGF-β family of proteins.

c. Fracture hematoma maturation

i. The fracture hematoma produces a collagenous matrix and network of new blood vessels. Neovascularization provides progenitor cells and growth factors for mesenchymal cell differentiation.

ii. Cartilage formation (endochondral ossification), identified by expression of collagen types I and II, stabilizes the fracture site. Chondrocytes proliferate, hypertrophy, and express factors that stimulate ossification.

d. Conversion of hypertrophic cartilage to bone—A complex process in which hypertrophic chondrocytes undergo terminal differentiation, cartilage calcifies, and new woven bone is formed.

i. A variety of factors are expressed as hypertrophic cartilage is replaced by bone. These include BMPs, TGF-β, IGFs, osteocalcin, and collagen I, V, and XI.

ii. Hypertrophic chondrocyte apoptosis and vascular invasion ensue.

e. Bone remodeling

i. The newly formed woven bone is remodeled through coordinated osteoblast and osteoclast functions.

ii. Mature bone is eventually established and is not distinguishable from the surrounding bone. Mature bone contains a host of growth factors, including TGF-β, BMPs, and IGFs.

II. Synovial Joints

A. Overview

1. Synovial joints are specialized structures that allow movement at bony articulations.

a. The structure is composed of a joint cavity lined by synovium and containing bones lined with articular cartilage.

b. Joints are stabilized by ligaments and motored by tendon attachments from adjacent musculature (**Figure 9**).

B. Formation—The formation and development of synovial joints is a poorly understood process.

1. Limb skeletogenesis starts with long uninterrupted condensations of mesenchymal tissue.

2. Condensations of mesenchymal cells form at specific locations. This appears to be controlled by the HOX family of genes.

3. Apoptosis then occurs within the so-called interzone, and the tissues separate through cavitation.

4. Joint-specific development then ensues through a control mechanism not yet understood.

C. Structure

1. Anatomy—The particular anatomy of each joint varies according to the location and demands of motion placed on the joint. Joint structure ranges from highly matched bony surfaces, such as the ball-and-socket hip joint, to the less congruent shoulder joint, which allows greater range of motion but provides less stability.

2. Structural components

a. Articular cartilage—Highly specialized tissue allowing low-friction movement.

b. Ligament—Collagenous structure connecting articulating bones; provides stability and restraint to nonphysiologic motion.

c. Joint capsule—Tough, fibrous tissue surrounding the joint cavity.

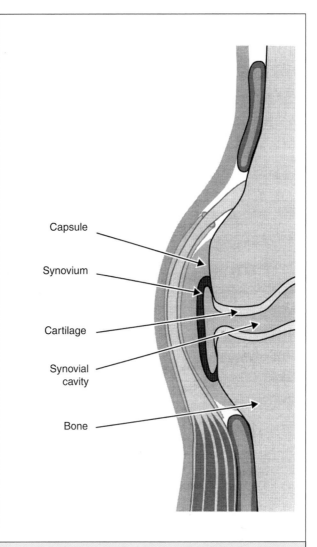

Figure 9 Schematic illustration of a synovial joint. (*Adapted from Recklies AD, Poole AR, Banerjee S, et al: Pathophysiologic aspects of inflammation in diarthrodial joints, in Buckwalter JA, Einhorn TA, Simon SR (eds):* Orthopaedic Basic Science: Biology and Biomechanics of the Musculoskeletal System, *ed 2. Rosemont, IL, American Academy of Orthopaedic Surgeons, 2000, p 490.*)

d. Synovium—This tissue, which lines the noncartilaginous portions of the joint cavity, is composed of two distinct layers, the intimal lining and the connective tissue sublining.

i. The intimal lining, which is only a few cells thick and is in direct contact with the joint cavity, produces the synovial fluid. The intimal layer functions as a porous barrier and lacks tight junctions between cells; it has no true basement membrane. This layer is composed of type A and type B cells. Type A cells, which make up only 10% to 20% of the synovial cells, derive from bone marrow precursors and function as tissue macrophages. Type B cells are from the fibroblast lineage. These cells produce hyaluronin and contain a unique enzyme, uridine diphosphoglucose dehydrogenase, which is critical in the pathway for synthesis of hyaluronin.

    ii. The sublining is relatively acellular and is composed of fibroblasts, fat, blood vessels, and lymphoid cells. A rich vascular network supplies the sublining and allows for the high solute and gas exchange that is needed to supply the cartilage with nutrition.

  e. Synovial fluid

    i. Produced and regulated by the synovium

    ii. This is an ultrafiltrate of plasma with a low albumin concentration (45% compared to plasma) and high concentration of hyaluronic acid and lubricin.

D. Sensory innervation—Composed of two systems.

  1. Fast-conducting myelinated type A fibers, found in the joint capsule and surrounding musculature, produce information on joint positions and motion.

  2. Slow-conducting unmyelinated type C fibers are found along blood vessels in the synovium and transmit diffuse pain sensations.

E. Function

  1. The synovial joint allows extremely low friction motion between articulating bones.

  2. Its function depends on the specific nature of the anatomic makeup of the joints, as well as the specific tissue characteristics of the tissue.

III. Nonsynovial Joints

A. Nonsynovial joints lack a synovial lining bordering the joint cavity and do not allow for low-friction or large-range movements. Different kinds of nonsynovial joints are found throughout the body, including symphyses, syndchondroses, and syndesmoses.

B. Symphyses

  1. In this type of joint, bone ends are separated by a fibrocartilaginous disk and are attached with well-developed ligamentous structures that control movement.

  2. Intervertebral disks form a symphysis between vertebral bodies.

  3. The pubic symphysis occurs at the anterior articulation between each hemipelvis and is composed of articular cartilage–covered rami separated by a fibrocartilage disk with firm ligamentous support. This joint is optimized for stability and load transmission but allows only limited motion.

C. Synchondroses

  1. In this type of joint, bone ends are covered with articular cartilage but no synovium is present and no significant motion occurs.

  2. Examples include the sternomanubrial joint, rib costal cartilage, and several articulations within the skull base.

D. Syndesmoses

  1. This type of joint consists of two bones that articulate without a cartilaginous interface and have strong ligamentous restraints that allow limited motion.

  2. The distal tibia-fibula syndesmosis is the only extracranial syndesmosis.

Bibliography

Gamble JG, Simmons SC, Freedman M: The symphysis pubis. *Clin Orthop Relat Res* 1986;203:261-272.

Miller JD, McCreadie BR, Alford AI, Hankenson KD, Goldstein SA: Form and function of bone, in Einhorn TA, O'Keefe RJ, Buckwalter JA (eds): *Orthopaedic Basic Science*, ed 3. Rosemont, IL, American Academy of Orthopaedic Surgeons, 2007, pp 129-160.

Pacifici M, Koyama E, Iwamoto M: Mechanisms of synovial joint and articular cartilage formation: Recent advances, but many lingering mysteries. *Birth Defects Research* 2005;75: 237-248.

Top Testing Facts

1. Endochondral bone formation (long and short bones) occurs through a cartilage model; intramembranous bone formation (flat bones) results from condensations of mesenchymal tissue.

2. The inner two thirds of cortical bone is vascularized by nutrient arteries that pass through the diaphyseal cortex and enter the intramedullary canal and are at risk during intramedullary reaming. The outer one third of the cortical bone derives blood supply from the periosteal membrane vessels. These vessels are at risk with periosteal stripping during surgical procedures.

3. The extracellular matrix of bone is composed of 60% to 70% mineral components and 20% to 25% organic components. The organic matrix is 90% type I collagen and 5% noncollagenous proteins.

4. Type I collagen is fibril-forming and has a triple helical structure (three α chains). The fibrils are intrinsically stable because of noncovalent interconnections and covalent cross-links between lysine residues.

5. Mature osteoblast marker proteins include alkaline phosphatase, osteocalcin, osteonectin, and osteopontin. The potential fates of a mature osteoblast include differentiation into an osteocyte or bone lining cell, or apoptosis.

6. The marker proteins for osteoclasts include TRAP, calcitonin receptor, and cathepsin-K. Osteoclast differentiation and activity are regulated in large part by the bioactive factors RANKL (positive regulator) and OPG (negative regulator).

7. Osteoblast and osteoclast functions are coupled via various systemic and local factors. Regulatory proteins (RANKL and OPG) secreted by osteoblasts provide direct coupling in bone remodeling.

8. Fractures commonly heal with a combination of endochondral and intramembranous bone formation. Motion at the fracture site results in healing primarily through endochondral ossification, whereas stability at the fracture site enables direct intramembranous ossification.

9. Fracture healing includes a sequence of biologic stages including injury, inflammation, hematoma maturation, hypertrophic cartilage formation, new bone formation, and remodeling to mature bone.

10. Articular joint synovium is composed of two layers—the intimal lining, which contains tissue macrophage-like cells and fibroblast-like cells that produce hyaluronin, and the connective tissue sublining.

1: Basic Science

Chapter 6
Articular Cartilage

Debdut Biswas, BA   Jesse E. Bible, BS   Jonathan N. Grauer, MD

I. Composition

A. Overview

1. Articular cartilage consists mainly of extracellular matrix (ECM) (95%) and a sparse population of chondrocytes (5%) that maintain the ECM throughout life.

2. The major components of the ECM are water, collagen, and proteoglycans.

B. Water

1. Water makes up 65% to 80% of articular cartilage.

2. The distribution is 80% at the superficial layers and 65% at the deep layers.

3. Most water is contained within the ECM and moved through the matrix by applying a pressure gradient across the tissue.

4. The frictional resistance of the water through the pores of the ECM and the pressurization of the water within the ECM are the basic mechanisms from which articular cartilage derives its ability to support very high joint loads.

5. Alteration of the water content affects the cartilage's permeability, strength, and Young modulus of elasticity.

6. The flow of water through the tissue also promotes the transport of nutrients and other factors through cartilage.

C. Collagen

1. Collagen makes up more than 50% of the dry weight of articular cartilage and 10% to 20% the of wet weight.

2. It provides shear and tensile strength.

3. Type II collagen comprises 90% to 95% of the total collagen weight in hyaline cartilage.

   a. Other minor types of collagen in articular cartilage include types V, VI, IX, X, and XI (Table 1).

   b. Type VI—Significant increase seen in early stages of osteoarthritis (OA).

   c. Type X—Produced only in endochondral ossification by hypertrophic chondrocytes; is associated with cartilage calcification. Examples include the growth plates, fracture sites, calcifying cartilage tumors, and the calcified deep zone of cartilage.

4. The specialized amino acid composition of increased amounts of glycine, proline, hydroxyproline, and hydroxylysine help form the triple helix collagen molecules, which line up in a staggered fashion resulting in banded fibrils (Figure 1).

   a. Intra- and intermolecular covalent cross-linking occurs between fibrils to help provide

Table 1	
Types of Collagen	
Type	**Location**
I	Bone Skin Tendon Anulus of intervertebral disk Meniscus
II	Articular cartilage Nucleus pulposus of intervertebral disk
III	Skin Blood vessels
IV	Basement membrane (basal lamina)
V	Articular cartilage with type I (in small amounts)
VI	Articular cartilage (in small amounts) Tethers the chondrocyte to pericellular matrix
VII	Basement membrane (epithelial, endothelial)
VIII	Basement membrane (epithelial)
IX	Articular cartilage with type II (in small amounts)
X	Hypertrophic cartilage Associated with calcification of cartilage (matrix mineralization)
XI	Articular cartilage with type II (in small amounts)
XII	Tendon
XIII	Endothelial cells

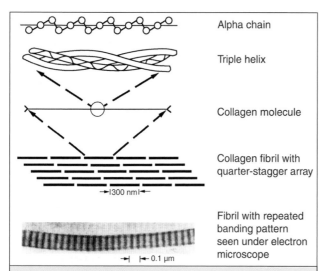

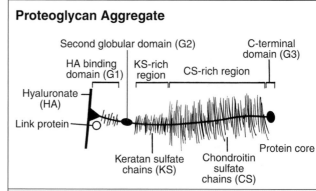

Figure 1 A scheme for the formation of collagen fibrils. The triple helix is made from three α chains, forming a procollagen molecule. Outside the cell the N- and C-terminal globular domains of the α chains are cleaved off to allow fibril formation, which occurs in a specific quarter-stagger array that ultimately results in the typical banded fibrils seen under electron microscopy. *(Reproduced with permission from Mow VC, Zhu W, Ratcliffe A: Structure and function of articular cartilage and meniscus, in Mow VC, Hayes WC (eds): Basic Orthopaedic Biomechanics. New York, NY, Raven Press, 1991, pp 143-198.)*

Figure 2 A schematic diagram of the aggrecan molecule and its binding to hyaluronate. The protein core has several globular domains (G1, G2, and G3), with other regions containing the keratin sulfate and chondroitin sulfate glycosaminoglycan chains. The N-terminal G1 domain is able to bind specifically to hyaluronate. This binding is stabilized by link protein. *(Reproduced from Buckwalter JA, Einhorn TA, Simon SR (eds): Orthopaedic Basic Science, ed. 2. Rosemont, IL, American Academy of Orthopaedic Surgeons, 2000, p 449.)*

strength and form the resulting collagen fiber.

  b. Types V, XI, and XI help mediate collagen-collagen and collagen-proteoglycan interactions.

  5. Cartilage disorders linked to defects or deficiencies in type II collagen

  a. Achondrogenesis

  b. Type II achondrogenesis-hypochondrogenesis

  c. Spondyloepiphyseal dysplasia

  d. Kniest dysplasia

D. Proteoglycans

  1. Represent 10% to 15% of dry weight.

  2. Provide compression strength to cartilage.

  3. Proteoglycans are produced and secreted into the ECM by chondrocytes.

  4. They are made up of repeating disaccharide subunits, glycosaminoglycans (GAG). Two subtypes are found in cartilage: chondroitin sulfate and keratan sulfate.

  a. Chondroitin sulfate is the most prevalent GAG. With increasing age, chondroitin-4-sulfate decreases and chondroitin-6-sulfate remains constant.

  b. Keratan sulfate increases with age.

  5. Sugar bonds link GAG to a long protein core to form a proteoglycan aggrecan molecule (**Figure 2**).

  6. Aggrecan molecules bind to hyaluronic acid molecules via link proteins to form a macromolecule complex known as a proteoglycan aggregate (**Figure 3**).

  7. Proteoglycans entangle between collagen fibers to create the fiber-reinforced solid matrix that helps determine the movement of water in the ECM (**Figure 4**).

  8. Proteoglycans also help trap water in the ECM by way of their negative charge.

E. Chondrocytes

  1. Represent 5% of dry weight.

  2. Chondrocytes are the only cells found in articular cartilage and are responsible for the production, organization, and maintenance of the ECM.

  3. Mesenchymal cells aggregate and differentiate into chondroblasts, which remain in lacunae to become chondrocytes.

  4. Chondrocytes produce collagen, proteoglycans, and other proteins found in the ECM.

  5. Compared to the more superficial levels of cartilage, chondrocytes in the deeper levels are less active and contain less rough endoplasmic reticulum and more intracellular degenerative products.

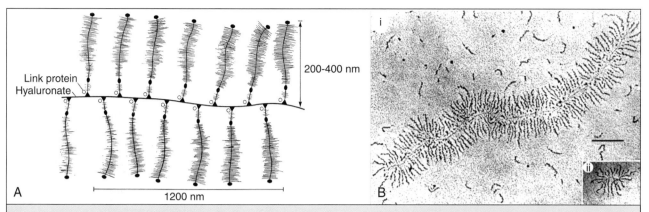

Figure 3   **A,** A diagram of the aggrecan molecules arranged as a proteoglycan aggregate. Many aggrecan molecules can bind to a chain of hyaluronate, forming macromolecular complexes that effectively are immobilized within the collagen network. **B,** Electron micrographs of bovine articular cartilage proteoglycan aggregates from (i) skeletally immature calf and (ii) skeletally mature steer. These show the aggregates to consist of a central hyaluronic acid filament and multiple attached monomers (bar = 500 μm). *(Reproduced with permission from Buckwalter JA, Kuettner KE, Thonar EJ: Age-related changes in articular cartilage proteoglycans: Electron microscopic studies. J Orthop Res 1985;3:251-257.)*

F.   Other matrix molecules

   1. Noncollagenous proteins

      a. These molecules play a role in the interactions between the ECM and chondrocytes.

      b. They include chondronectin, fibronectin, and anchorin.

   2. Lipids and phospholipids

II. Structure

A. Overview

   1. Articular cartilage can be divided into different layers, or zones, at various depths.

   2. Division is based on descriptive information such as collagen orientation, chondrocyte organization, and proteoglycan distribution.

B. Layers/zones (**Figures 5 and 6**)

   1. Superficial (tangential, or zone I)

      a. Lies adjacent to the joint cavity.

      b. Forms the gliding surface.

      c. Characterized by collagen fibers and disk-shaped chondrocytes uniformly aligned parallel to the articular surface along with a low proteoglycan concentration.

      d. High collagen and water concentrations are found in this zone.

   2. Middle (transitional, or zone II)

      a. Characterized by thicker, obliquely oriented collagen fibers, round chondrocytes, and

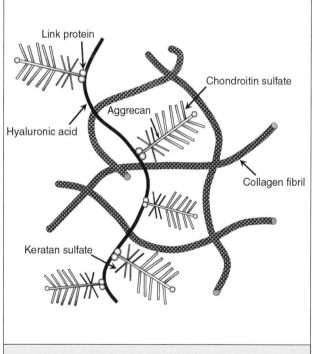

Figure 4   Diagram of aggrecan, collagen. (Courtesy of Dr. Andrew Thompson.)

marked proteoglycan content.

      b. Constitutes most of the cartilage depth.

   3. Deep (radial, or zone III)—Characterized by collagen fibers oriented perpendicular to the articular surface, round chondrocytes arranged in columns, and a high proteoglycan content.

   4. Calcified cartilage (zone IV)

      a. Characterized by radially aligned collagen fi-

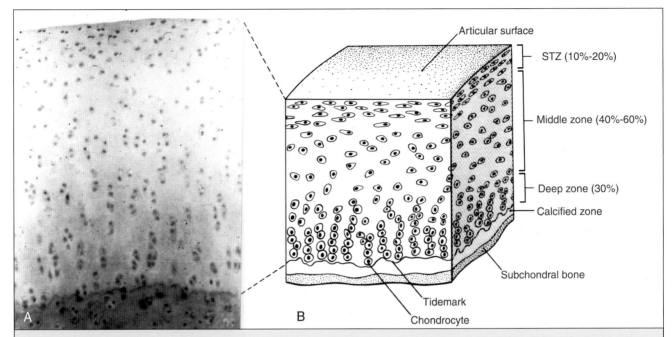

Figure 5 **A,** Histologic section of normal adult articular cartilage showing even Safranin 0 staining and distribution of chondrocytes. **B,** Schematic diagram of chondrocyte organization in the three major zones of the uncalcified cartilage, the tidemark, and the subchondral bone. STZ = superficial tangential zone. *(Reproduced with permission from Mow VC, Proctor CS, Kelly MA: Biomechanics of articular cartilage, in Nordin M, Frankel VH (eds): Basic Biomechanics of the Musculoskeletal System, ed 2. Philadelphia, PA, Lea & Febiger, 1989, pp 31-57.)*

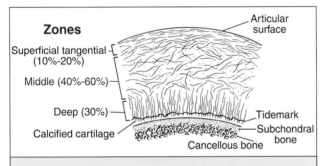

Figure 6 Diagram of collagen fiber architecture in a sagittal cross section showing the three salient zones of articular cartilage. *(Reproduced with permission from Mow VC, Proctor CS, Kelly MA: Biomechanics of articular cartilage, in Nordin M, Frankel VH (eds): Basic Biomechanics of the Musculoskeletal System, ed 2. Philadelphia, PA, Lea & Febiger, 1989, pp 31-57.)*

bers and round chondrocytes buried in a calcified matrix that has a high concentration of calcium salts and very low concentration of proteoglycans.

    b. Hypertrophic chondrocytes in this layer produce type X collagen and alkaline phosphatase, helping to mineralize the extracellular matrix.

    c. The borders of the calcified cartilage layer include the tidemark as the upper border and the cement line, which formed during growth plate

ossification at skeletal maturity, as the lower border.

C. Extracellular matrix

  1. The ECM can also be characterized based on its proximity to the surrounding chondrocytes.

  2. Each region has a different biochemical composition.

    a. Pericellular matrix—Thin layer that completely surrounds chondrocyte and helps control cell matrix interactions.

    b. Territorial matrix—Thin layer of collagen fibrils surrounding pericellular matrix.

    c. Interterritorial matrix

      i. Largest region

      ii. Contains larger collagen fibrils and a large content of proteoglycans.

III. Metabolism

A. Nutrition

  1. Cartilage is an avascular structure in the adult.

  2. It is believed that nutrients diffuse through the matrix from the surrounding synovial fluid, from the synovium, or from the underlying bone.

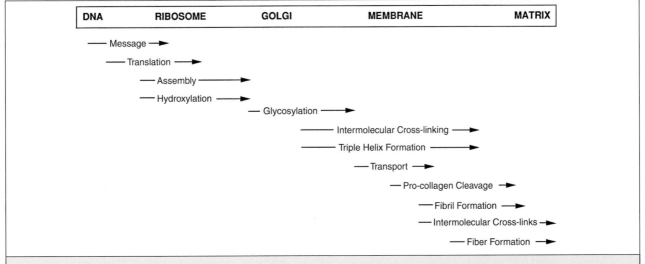

Figure 7 The events involved in the synthesis of collagen, showing the intracellular sites that are used for each procedure. *(Reproduced with permission from Mankin HJ, Brandt KD: Biochemistry and metabolism of articular cartilage in osteoarthritis, in Moskowitz RW, Howell DS, Goldberg VM, et al (eds): Osteoarthritis: Diagnosis and Medical/Surgical Management, ed 2. Philadelphia, PA, WB Saunders, 1992, pp 109-154.)*

B. Chondrocytes

1. Chondrocytes synthesize and assemble cartilaginous matrix components and direct their distribution within tissue.

2. The processes include the synthesis of matrix proteins and GAG chains, and their secretion into the ECM.

3. Each chondrocyte is responsible for the metabolism and maintenance of the ECM under avascular and at times anaerobic conditions.

4. The maintenance of the ECM is dependent on the proper incorporation of components into the matrix as well as the balance between synthesis and degradation of matrix components.

5. Chondrocytes respond to both their chemical and physical environments.

   a. Chemical (growth factors, cytokines)

   b. Physical (mechanical load, hydrostatic pressure changes)

C. Collagen

1. Collagen synthesis (**Figure 7**)

   a. Most knowledge about collagen synthesis has originated from studies of major fibrillar types (ie, types I through III).

   b. Hydroxylation requires vitamin C; deficiencies (eg, scurvy) can result in altered collagen synthesis.

2. Collagen catabolism

   a. The exact mechanism is unclear.

b. Breakdown occurs at a slow rate in normal cartilage.

c. In degenerative cartilage and cartilage undergoing repair (eg, during skeletal growth), there is evidence of accelerated breakdown.

d. Enzymatic processes have been proposed, such as the cleaving of metalloproteinases to the triple helix.

D. Proteoglycan

1. Proteoglycan synthesis

   a. A series of molecular events—beginning with gene expression, messenger RNA transcription, translation, and aggregate formation—are involved in proteoglycan synthesis (**Figure 8**).

   b. The chondrocyte is responsible for the synthesis, assembly, and sulfation of the proteoglycan molecule.

   c. The addition of GAG and other posttranslational modifications can result in tremendous variation in the final molecule.

   d. The control mechanisms for proteoglycan synthesis are very sensitive to biochemical, mechanical, and physical stimuli (eg, lacerative injury, OA, nonsteroidal anti-inflammatory drugs).

2. Proteoglycan catabolism (**Figure 9**)

   a. Proteoglycans are continually being broken down; this is a normal event in the maintenance of cartilage.

   b. Catabolism occurs during remodeling in repair

1: Basic Science

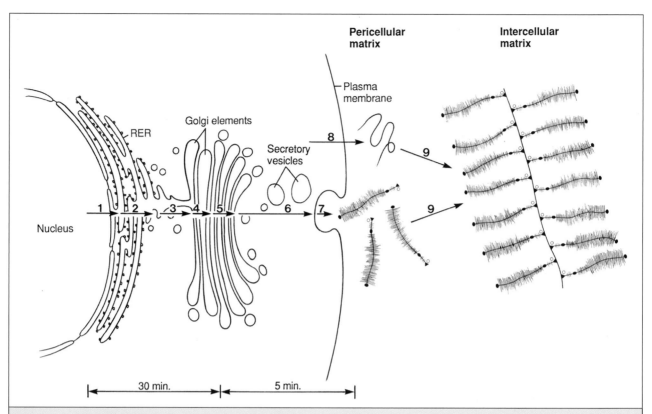

Figure 8 Diagram depicting the various stages involved in the synthesis and secretion of aggrecan and link protein by a chondrocyte. (1) The transcription of the aggrecan and link protein genes to mRNA. (2) The translation of the mRNA in the rough endoplasmic reticulum (RER) to form the protein core of the aggrecan. (3) The newly formed protein is transported from the RER to the (4) cis and (5) medial trans-Golgi compartments, where the glycosaminoglycan chains are added to the protein core. (6) On completion of the glycosylation and sulfation, the molecules are transported via secretory vesicles to the plasma membrane, where (7) they are released into the extracellular matrix. (8) Hyaluronate is synthesized separately at the plasma membrane. (9) Only in the extracellular matrix can aggrecan, link protein, and hyaluronate come together to form proteoglycan aggregates. *(Reproduced from Buckwalter JA, Einhorn TA, Simon SR (eds): Orthopaedic Basic Science, ed 2. Rosemont, IL, American Academy of Orthopaedic Surgeons, 2000, p 452.)*

processes and appears to be accelerated during degenerative processes.

   c. Catabolism can be affected by soluble mediators (interleukin [IL]-1) and joint loading (loss of proteoglycans during joint immobilization).

   d. GAG chains and other proteoglycan chains are released into synovial fluid during degradation. These may be quantified and could provide a diagnostic measure of catabolic activity in the joint.

E. Growth factors

   1. Polypeptide growth factors regulate synthetic processes in normal cartilage and have been implicated in the development of OA.

   2. Platelet-derived growth factor (PDGF)—In OA, and especially in lacerative injury, PDGF may play an increased role in healing.

   3. Basic fibroblast growth factor (bFGF)

      a. bFGF is a powerful stimulator of DNA synthe-

sis in adult articular chondrocytes and is a potent mitogen.

      b. bFGF may play a role in the cartilage repair process.

   4. Transforming growth factor-beta (TGF-β)

      a. TGF-β appears to potentiate DNA synthesis stimulated by bFGF, epidermal growth factor, and insulin-like growth factor (IGF)-1.

      b. TGF-β also appears to suppress type II collagen synthesis.

      c. TGF-β stimulates the formation of plasminogen activator inhibitor-1 and tissue inhibitor of metalloproteinase (TIMP), preventing the degradative action of these enzymes.

   5. Insulin-like growth factors (IGF-1 and IGF-2)— IGF-1 has been demonstrated to stimulate DNA and matrix synthesis in the immature cartilage of the growth plate as well as adult articular cartilage.

F. Degradation

1. The breakdown of the cartilage matrix in normal turnover and in degeneration appears to be by the action of proteolytic enzymes (proteinases).

2. The overactivity of proteinases may play a role in the pathogenesis of OA.

3. Metalloproteinases

   a. These proteinases include collagenase, stromelysin, and gelatinase.

   b. They are synthesized as latent enzymes (proenzymes) and require activation via enzymatic activation.

   c. The active enzymes can be inhibited irreversibly by TIMP. The molar ratios of metalloproteinases and TIMP determine if there is net metalloproteinase activity.

G. Aging and articular cartilage (**Table 2**)

   a. Immature articular cartilage varies considerably from adult articular cartilage.

   b. With aging, chondrocytes become larger, acquire increased lysosomal enzymes, and no longer reproduce.

   c. Cartilage becomes relatively hypocellular in comparison with immature articular cartilage.

   d. Proteoglycan mass and size decrease with aging in articular cartilage, with decreased concentrations of chondroitin sulfate and increased concentration of keratin sulfate.

   e. Water and proteoglycan content decrease with aging.

   f. As age advances, cartilage loses its elasticity, developing increased stiffness and decreased solubility.

IV. Lubrication and Wear

A. Synovium

1. Synovial tissue is vascularized tissue that mediates the diffusion of nutrients between blood and synovial fluid.

2. Synovium is composed of two cell types.

   a. Type A is important in phagocytosis.

   b. Type B comprises fibroblast-like cells that produce synovial fluid

3. Synovial fluid lubricates articular cartilage.

   a. Synovial fluid is composed of an ultrafiltrate of blood plasma and fluid produced by the synovial membrane.

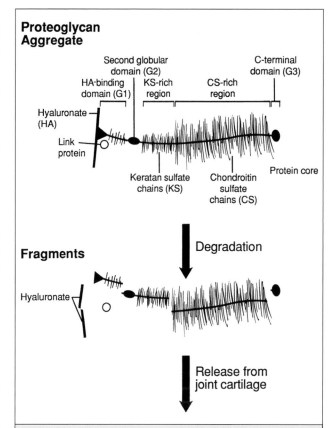

Figure 9 Representation of the mechanism of degradation of proteoglycan aggregates in articular cartilage. The major proteolytic cleavage site is between the G1 and G2 domains, making the glycosaminoglycan-containing portion of the aggrecan molecule nonaggregating. This fragment can now be released from the cartilage. Other proteolytic events also can cause the G1 domain and link protein to disaggregate and leave the cartilage. *(Reproduced from Buckwalter JA, Einhorn TA, Simon SR (eds): Orthopaedic Basic Science, ed 2. Rosemont, IL, American Academy of Orthopaedic Surgeons, 2000, p 454.)*

b. Synovial fluid is composed of hyaluronic acid, lubricin, proteinase, collagenases, and prostaglandins. Lubricin is the key lubricant of synovial fluid.

c. The viscosity coefficient of synovial fluid is not a constant; its viscosity increases as the shear rate decreases.

d. Hyaluronic acid molecules behave like an elastic solid during high-strain activities.

e. Synovial fluid contains no red blood cells, hemoglobin, or clotting factors.

B. Elastohydrodynamic lubrication is the major mode of lubrication of articular cartilage.

C. The coefficient of friction of human joints is 0.002 to 0.04.

1: Basic Science

Table 2		

Changes in Articular Cartilage Properties With Aging and Osteoarthritis

Property	Aging	Osteoarthritis
Water content (hydration, permeability)	↓	↑
Collagen	Remains relatively unchanged	Relative concentration ↑
	(some increase in type VI)	Content ↓ in severe OA
		Matrix becomes disordered
Proteoglycan content (concentration)	↓	↓
Proteoglycan synthesis	Unchanged	↑
Proteoglycan degradation	↓	↑
Total chondroitin sulfate concentration	↓	↑
Chondroitin-4-sulfate concentration	↓	↑
Keratan sulfate concentration	↑	↓
Chondrocyte size	↑	Unchanged
Chondrocyte number	↓	Unchanged
Modulus of elasticity	↑	↓

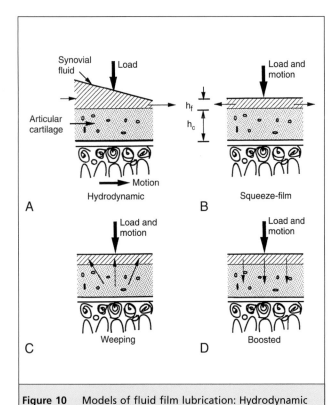

Figure 10 Models of fluid film lubrication: Hydrodynamic **(A)**, squeeze-film **(B)**, weeping **(C)**, and boosted **(D)**. *(Reproduced with permission from Mow VC, Soslowsky LJ: Friction, lubrication and wear of diarthrodial joints, in Mow VC, Hayes WC (eds): Basic Orthopaedic Biomechanics. New York, Raven Press, 1991, pp 245-292.)*

1. Fluid film formation, elastic deformation of articular cartilage, and synovial fluid decrease friction.

2. Fibrillation of articular cartilage increases friction.

D. Two forms of movement occur during joint range of motion: rolling and sliding. Almost all joints undergo both types of movement during range of motion.

1. Pure rolling—Instant center of rotation is at rolling surfaces.

2. Pure sliding—Pure translational movement without an instant center of rotation.

E. Types of lubrication (**Figure 10**)

1. Elastohydrodynamic

a. This is the major mode of lubrication during dynamic joint motion.

b. Deformation of articular surfaces and thin films of joint lubricant separate surfaces.

2. Boundary—also known as "slippery surfaces"

a. The load-bearing surface is largely nondeformable.

b. The lubricant only partially separates articular surfaces.

3. Boosted

a. Lubricating fluid pools in regions contained by articular surfaces in contact with one another.

b. The coefficient of friction is generally higher than in elastohydrodynamic lubrication.

4. Hydrodynamic—Fluid separates the articular surfaces.

5. Weeping—Lubricating fluid shifts toward load-bearing regions of the articular surface.

V. Mechanisms of Cartilage Repair

A. The repair of significant defects in articular cartilage is limited by a lack of vascularity and a lack of cells that can migrate to injured sites.

B. Cartilage also lacks undifferentiated cells that can migrate, proliferate, and participate in the repair response.

C. Repair of superficial lacerations

1. Superficial lacerations that do not cross the tidemark, the region between uncalcified and calcified cartilage, generally do not heal.

2. Chondrocytes proliferate near the site of injury and may synthesize new matrix, but they do not migrate toward the lesion and do not repair the defects.

3. The poor healing response is believed to be partly due to the lack of hemorrhage and the lack of an inflammatory response necessary for proper healing.

D. Repair of deep lacerations

1. Cartilage defects that penetrate past the tidemark into underlying subchondral bone may heal with fibrocartilage.

2. Fibrocartilage is produced by undifferentiated marrow mesenchymal stem cells that later differentiate into cells capable of producing fibrocartilage.

3. In most situations, the repair tissue does not resemble the normal structure, composition, or mechanical properties of an articular surface and is not as durable as hyaline cartilage.

E. Factors affecting cartilage repair

1. Continuous passive motion is believed to have a beneficial effect on cartilage healing; immobilization of a joint leads to atrophy and/or degeneration.

2. Joint instability (eg, anterior cruciate ligament transection) leads to an initial decrease in the ratio of proteoglycan to collagen (at 4 weeks) but a late (12 weeks) elevation in the ratio of proteoglycan to collagen and an increase in hydration.

3. Joint instability leads to a marked decrease in hyaluronan, but disuse does not.

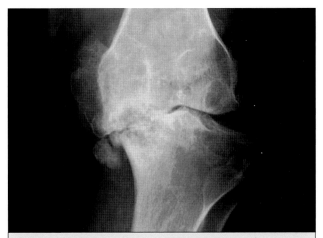

Figure 11 Osteoarthritic changes seen on a knee radiograph illustrating extensive loss of articular cartilage in the medial and patellofemoral compartments. Prominent osteophytes and subchondral cysts are also present.

VI. Osteoarthritis

A. Overview

1. OA, which eventually leads to destruction and loss of articular cartilage, is the most prevalent disorder of the musculoskeletal system.

2. The disease process leads to limitation of joint movement, joint deformity, tenderness, inflammation, and severe pain.

B. Radiographic findings (**Figure 11**)

1. Joint space narrowing

2. Subchondral sclerosis and cyst formation

3. Osteophyte formation

C. Macroscopic findings

1. Articular cartilage may show areas of softening (chondromalacia), fibrillation, and erosions.

2. With severe degeneration, there may be focal areas of ulceration with exposure of sclerotic, eburnated subchondral bone.

D. Histologic findings (**Figure 12**)

1. Early alterations include surface erosion and irregularities.

2. Other changes include replication and deterioration of the tidemark, fissuring, and cartilage destruction with eburnation of subchondral bone.

E. Biochemical changes

1. OA is directly linked to a loss of proteoglycan content and composition with increased water content.

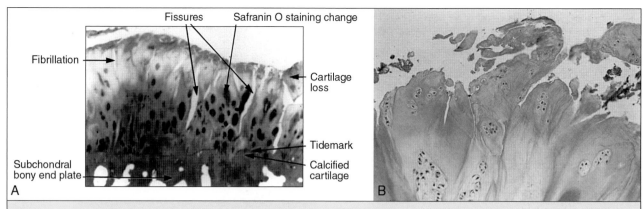

Figure 12 **A,** Low-power magnification of a section of a glenohumeral head of osteoarthritic cartilage removed at surgery for total shoulder replacement. Note the significant fibrillation, vertical cleft formation, the tidemark, and the subchondral bony end plate. **B,** A higher power magnification of surface fibrillation showing vertical cleft formation and widespread large necrotic regions of the tissue devoid of cells. Clusters of cells, common in osteoarthritic tissues, also are seen. *(Reproduced from Buckwalter JA, Einhorn TA, Simon SR (eds): Orthopaedic Basic Science, ed 2. Rosemont, IL, American Academy of Orthopaedic Surgeons, 2000, p 478.)*

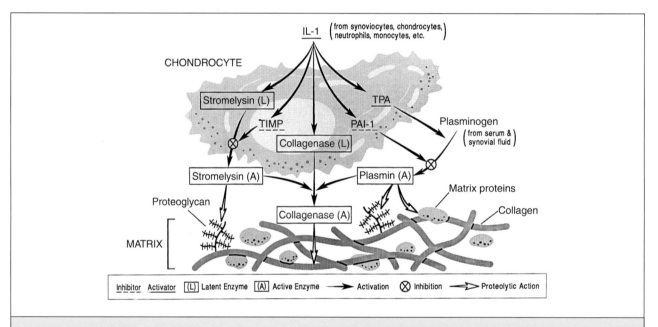

Figure 13 The cascade of enzymes and their activators and inhibitors involved in interleukin-1–stimulated degradation of articular cartilage. *(Reproduced from Buckwalter JA, Einhorn TA, Simon SR (eds): Orthopaedic Basic Science, ed 2. Rosemont, IL, American Academy of Orthopaedic Surgeons, 2000, p 486.)*

2. Proteoglycans exist in shorter chains with an increased chondroitin/keratin sulfate ratio.

3. Proteoglycans are largely unbound to hyaluronic acid because of proteolytic enzymes and decreased number of link proteins.

4. Collagen content is maintained, but its organization and orientation are severely disturbed, presumably due to collagenase.

F. Molecular mechanisms of OA (**Figure 13**)

1. Levels of proteolytic enzymes are found to be elevated in OA cartilage.

a. Metalloproteinases (collagenase, gelatinase, stromelysin)

b. Cathepsins B and D

2. Inflammatory cytokines may exacerbate degeneration seen in OA.

3. IL-1 and other cytokines may further disrupt cartilage homeostasis and amplify the destructive actions of proteolytic enzymes.

Top Testing Facts

1. Articular cartilage consists mainly of extracellular matrix (ECM), with only a small percentage of chondrocytes, which are responsible for the synthesis, maintenance, and homeostasis of cartilage.

2. The major components of the ECM are water, proteoglycans, and collagen.

3. Articular cartilage is classified into four layers (superficial, middle, deep, and calcified) according to collagen orientation, chondrocyte organization, and proteoglycan distribution.

4. Cartilage is an avascular structure in the adult; this has implications for repair and healing.

5. The breakdown of the cartilage matrix in normal turnover and in degeneration appears to be the action of proteinases; their overactivity is implicated in OA.

6. The water content of cartilage decreases with aging and increases in OA.

7. Proteoglycan content and keratan sulfate concentrations decrease with OA; proteoglycan degradation and chondroitin-4-sulfate concentration increase.

8. Elastohydrodynamic lubrication is the principal mode of lubrication of articular cartilage.

9. Superficial lacerations to cartilage rarely heal; deeper lacerations may heal with fibrocartilage.

10. Inflammatory cytokine and metalloproteinases are responsible for macroscopic and histologic changes seen in OA.

Bibliography

Buckwalter JA, Mankin HJ, Grodzinsky AJ: Articular cartilage and osteoarthritis. *Instr Course Lect* 2005;54:465-480.

Carter DR, Beaupré GS, Wong M, Smith RL, Andriacchi TP, Schurman DJ: The mechanobiology of articular cartilage development and degeneration. *Clin Orthop Relat Res* 2004;(427 Suppl):S69-S77.

Mankin HJ, Grodzinsky AJ, Buckwalter JA: Articular cartilage and osteoarthritis, in Einhorn TA, O'Keefe RJ, Buckwalter JA (eds): Orthopaedic Basic Science, ed 3. Rosemont, IL, American Academy of Orthopaedic Surgeons, 2007, pp 161-174.

Pearle AD, Warren RF, Rodeo SA: Basic science of articular cartilage and osteoarthritis. *Clin Sports Med* 2005;24:1-12.

Shojania K, Esdaile JM, Greidanus N: Arthritis, in Vaccaro AR (ed): *Orthopaedic Knowledge Update 8*. Rosemont, IL, American Academy of Orthopaedic Surgeons, 2005, pp 229-234.

Ulrich-Vinther M, Maloney MD, Schwarz EM, Rosier R, O'Keefe RJ: Articular cartilage biology. *J Am Acad Orthop Surg* 2003;11:421-430.

1: Basic Science

Chapter 7
Tendons and Ligaments

Stavros Thomopoulos, PhD

1: Basic Science

I. Tendons

A. Anatomy and function

1. Function—To transfer force from muscle to bone to produce joint motion.

2. Composition and structure

   a. Tendon is made up of collagen fibers embedded in water and a proteoglycan matrix. The tissue is relatively acellular.

   b. The fibroblast is the predominant cell type in tendon. In longitudinal histologic sections, fibroblasts appear spindle shaped, with the preferred orientation in the direction of muscle loading. In cross section, fibroblasts are star shaped, with long cytoplasmic processes.

   c. Tendon has a clearly defined hierarchical structure (**Figure 1**). Collections of collagen molecules are arranged in quarter-stagger arrays, forming ordered units of microfibrils, which combine to form subfibrils, which further combine to form fibrils. Fibril units then form highly ordered parallel bundles oriented in the direction of muscle force. Fibrils accumulate to form fascicle units, which in turn combine to form the tendon.

   d. Type I collagen is the major constituent of tendon (86% of the dry weight). The primary structure of collagen consists of glycine (33%), proline (15%), and hydroxyproline (15%). The collagen molecule is fibrillar in structure, with a length of 300 nm and a diameter of 1.5 nm.

   e. Proteoglycans make up from 1% to 5% of the dry weight of a tendon. Proteoglycans are highly hydrophilic and therefore bind tightly to water.

   f. Decorin is the predominant proteoglycan in tendon.

      i. The role of decorin during development and healing is to regulate collagen fiber diameter. The presence of decorin inhibits lateral fusion of collagen fibers.

      ii. The role of decorin during normal function is to transfer loads between collagen fibers. Decorin molecules form cross-links between collagen fibers and can therefore increase the stiffness of the fibrils.

   g. Aggrecan (a proteoglycan abundant in articular cartilage) is found in areas of tendon that are under compression (eg, regions of hand flexor tendons that wrap around bone).

   h. The vascularity of tendon varies. Sheathed tendons (eg, flexor tendons of the hand) have regions that are relatively avascular. These regions get nutrition through diffusion from the synovium. Tendons not enclosed by a sheath receive their blood supply from vessels entering from the tendon surface or from the tendon-to-bone insertion.

3. Biomechanics

   a. Tendons have high tensile properties and buckle under compression (ie, they behave like ropes). A typical load-elongation curve for tendon includes a toe region, a linear region, and a failure region (**Figure 2**).

   b. Tendon biomechanics can be characterized by either structural properties (load-elongation behavior) or material properties (stress-strain behavior, where stress is calculated by dividing

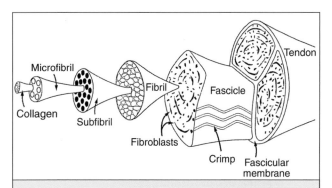

Figure 1   Tendon tissue has a highly ordered hierarchical structure. (*Adapted with permission from Kastelic J, Baer E: Deformation in tendon collagen, in Vincent JFV, Currey JD (eds): The Mechanical Properties of Biologic Materials. Cambridge, England, Cambridge University Press, 1980, pp 397-435.*)

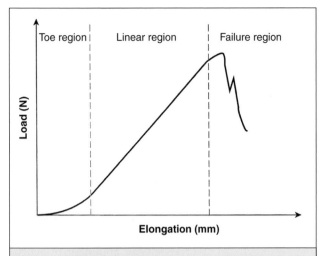

Figure 2   The tensile behavior of tendon and ligament tissue includes a nonlinear toe region at low loads, a linear region at intermediate loads, and a failure region at high loads.

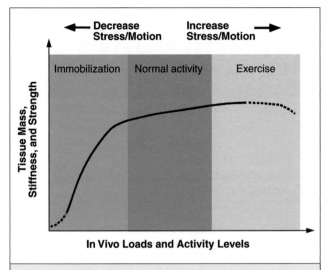

Figure 3   Immobilization leads to a dramatic drop in mechanical properties, and exercise has a positive effect on mechanical properties. (*Reproduced with permission from Woo SL-Y, Chan SS, Yamaji T: Biomechanics of knee ligament healing, repair and reconstruction.* J Biomechanics *1997;30:431-439.*)

load by cross-sectional area and strain is calculated by dividing change in elongation by initial length).

   i. Structural properties describe the overall load-bearing capacity of the tissue and include the contribution of the muscle and bone attachments as well as the geometry of the tissue (cross-sectional area and length). Structural properties include stiffness (the slope of the linear portion of the curve in Figure 2) and failure load.

   ii. Material properties (also referred to as mechanical properties) describe the quality of the tissue by normalizing for tissue geometry. Material properties include the modulus of elasticity (the slope of the linear portion of the stress-strain curve) and failure stress.

c. Tendons exhibit viscoelastic behavior; the mechanical properties of the tissue are dependent on loading history and time. Time dependence is best illustrated by the phenomena of creep and stress relaxation.

   i. Stress relaxation—The decrease in load/stress for a constant elongation/strain.

   ii. Creep—The increase in elongation/strain for a constant applied load/stress.

d. Several factors influence the biomechanical properties of tendons.

   i. Anatomic location—Tendons from different locations have different structural properties; eg, digital flexor tendons have twice the ultimate strength of digital extensor tendons.

   ii. Exercise and immobilization—Exercise has a

positive effect and immobilization has a detrimental effect on the biomechanical properties of tendons (**Figure 3**).

   iii. Age—Material and structural properties of tendons increase from birth through maturity. The properties then decrease from maturity through old age.

   iv. Laser/heat treatment causes tendons to shrink. Long-term effects are unclear, but early evidence suggests that laser/heat treatment has a detrimental effect on the biomechanical properties of the tissue.

e. Factors to consider when mechanically testing tendons:

   i. The mechanical properties of tendons vary with hydration, temperature, and pH, so tendons should be tested under physiologically relevant hydration, temperature, and pH conditions.

   ii. The high strength of tendons leads to difficulty in gripping the tissue during mechanical testing. Specialized grips (eg, freeze clamps) are often necessary to prevent the tendon from slipping out of the grip.

   iii. Knowledge of tissue cross-sectional area is necessary for the calculation of stress (recall that stress = load/cross-sectional area). Care must be taken when measuring the cross-sectional area of tendon because the tissue will deform if contact methods are used (eg, calipers).

iv. Because tendons are viscoelastic (their properties are time dependent), the rate at which the tendon is pulled can influence the mechanical properties. Higher strain rates result in a higher elastic modulus.

v. Specimens should be stored frozen and properly hydrated. Improper storage may affect tendon mechanical properties.

vi. The orientation of a tendon during testing will influence the mechanical properties measured; eg, the structural properties of the supraspinatus tendon depends on the angle of the humeral head relative to the glenoid.

B. Injury, repair, and healing

1. Tendon injury occurs because of direct trauma (eg, laceration of a flexor tendon) or indirect tensile overload (eg, Achilles tendon rupture).

2. Three phases of healing:

   a. Hemostasis/inflammation—After injury, the wound site is infiltrated by inflammatory cells. Platelets aggregate at the wound and create a fibrin clot to stabilize the torn tendon edges. The length of this phase is on the order of days.

   b. Matrix and cell proliferation—Fibroblasts infiltrate the wound site and proliferate. They produce extracellular matrix, including large amounts of type III collagen. The injury response in adult tendon is scar mediated (ie, large amounts of disorganized collagen are deposited at the repair site). The length of this phase is on the order of weeks.

   c. Remodeling/maturation—Matrix metalloproteinases degrade the collagen matrix, replacing type III collagen with type I collagen. Collagen fibers are reorganized so that they are aligned in the direction of muscle loading. The length of this phase is on the order of months or years.

3. Long-term effects—The structural properties of repaired tendons typically reach only two thirds of normal, even years after repair. Material property differences are even more dramatic.

4. Sheathed tendons—Often injured through direct trauma (eg, laceration of a flexor tendon). The two critical considerations for sheathed tendon healing are prevention of adhesion formation and accrual of mechanical strength (**Figure 4**).

5. Tendons not enclosed in sheaths fail because of trauma (eg, an acute sports injury) or preexisting pathology (eg, a rotator cuff tear after years of chronic tendon degeneration). Injury often occurs at the attachments of the tendon (ie, at the musculotendinous junction or at the tendon-to-bone insertion).

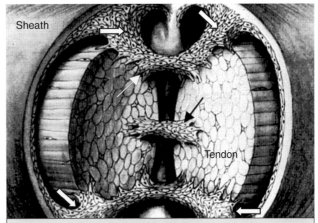

Figure 4   Sheathed tendons heal primarily through infiltration of fibroblasts from the outer and inner surfaces of the tendon (black arrows). Adhesions between the outer surface of the tendon and the sheath (white arrows) can be prevented with passive motion rehabilitation. (*Courtesy of Dr. R.H. Gelberman, Boston.*)

6. The role of the mechanical environment in healing is complex.

   a. Protective immobilization in the early period after tendon repair is beneficial in many scenarios (eg, after rotator cuff repair).

   b. Exercise can be detrimental if started too early in the rehabilitation period, but it is beneficial during the remodeling phase of healing.

   c. Early passive motion is beneficial for flexor tendon healing. Early motion suppresses adhesion formation between the tendon and the sheath, preventing the typical range of motion losses seen with immobilized tendons.

II. Ligaments

A. Anatomy and function

1. The function of ligaments is to restrict joint motion (ie, to stabilize joints).

2. Composition and structure

   a. Ligaments are composed of dense connective tissue.

   b. Ligaments are similar in composition and structure to tendons, but there are several important differences (**Figure 5**).

      i. Ligaments are shorter and wider.

      ii. Ligaments have a lower percentage of collagen and a higher percentage of proteoglycans and water.

1: Basic Science

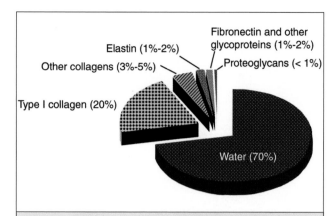

Figure 5 The biochemical composition of a typical ligament. (*Reproduced with permission from Frank CB: Ligament injuries: Pathophysiology and healing, in Zachazewski JE, Magee DJ, Quillen WS (eds): Athletic Injuries and Rehabilitation. Philadelphia, PA, WB Saunders, 1996, p 15.*)

iii. Collagen fibers are less organized in ligaments.

c. Ligaments have a highly ordered hierarchical structure, similar to tendons.

d. Type I collagen makes up 70% of the dry weight of ligaments.

e. Like tendons, the main cell type in ligaments is the fibroblast, but ligament fibroblasts appear rounder than tendon fibroblasts.

f. Ligaments have relatively low vascularity and cellularity.

3. Biomechanics

a. The biomechanical properties of ligaments are expressed as either the structural properties of the bone-ligament-bone complex or the material properties of the ligament midsubstance itself.

b. Ligaments exhibit viscoelastic behavior similar to that of tendons.

c. Several factors that influence the mechanical properties of ligaments are the same as those described earlier for tendon (I.A.3.d).

d. Factors that must be considered when mechanically testing ligaments are the same as those listed earlier for tendon (I.A.3.e).

B. Injury, repair, and healing

1. Ligament injuries are generally classified into three grades (I, II, and III). Grade I corresponds to a mild sprain, grade II corresponds to a moderate sprain/partial tear, and grade III corresponds to a complete ligament tear. An additional type of injury is avulsion of the ligament from its bony insertion.

2. Ligament healing occurs through the same phases as tendon healing (hemostasis/inflammation, matrix and cell proliferation, remodeling/maturation).

3. Extra-articular ligaments (eg, the medial collateral ligament (MCL) of the knee) have a greater capacity to heal than do intra-articular ligaments (eg, ACL of the knee).

a. MCL of the knee

i. Grade I and II injuries to the MCL heal without surgical treatment.

ii. The optimal treatment of grade III MCL injuries is controversial. Up to 25% of patients with these injuries continue to have clinical problems whether or not the tear is surgically repaired.

b. Anterior cruciate ligament (ACL) of the knee—Midsubstance ACL injuries typically do not heal. Surgical reconstruction of the ACL often is necessary to restore stability in the injured knee. Several graft materials have been used to reconstruct the ACL, including both autograft and allograft.

i. Autografts, including bone–patellar tendon–bone, semitendinosus, quadriceps, and gracilis—are commonly used. The structural properties of the reconstructed graft reach only 50% of normal properties at the longest follow-up studied. The major disadvantage of autograft is donor site morbidity.

ii. ACL allografts (taken from cadavers) are also used for ACL reconstruction. Disadvantages of these grafts include the potential for disease transmission and the loss of mechanical properties because of graft sterilization.

iii. A process described as "ligamentization" occurs in both auto- and allografts after reconstruction when a tendon is used to replace the function of a ligament. Autograft fibroblasts die soon after reconstruction and are replaced by local fibroblasts. Similarly, allografts are infiltrated by local fibroblasts in the early period after implantation.

III. Enthesis (Tendon/Ligament–Bone Junction)

A. Anatomy and function

1. Tendons and ligaments insert into bone across a complex transitional tissue, the enthesis.

2. Composition and structure

a. Indirect insertions (eg, the femoral insertion of the MCL)—The superficial layer connects with the periosteum and the deep layer anchors to bone via Sharpey fibers.

b. Direct insertions (eg, the supraspinatus insertion of the rotator cuff) have classically been categorized into four zones.

   i. First zone: tendon proper; properties similar to those found at the tendon midsubstance. Consists of well-aligned type I collagen fibers with small amounts of the proteoglycan decorin.

   ii. Second zone: fibrocartilage; marks the beginning of the transition from tendinous material to bony material. Composed of types II and III collagen, with small amounts of types I, IX, and X collagen, and small amounts of the proteoglycans aggrecan and decorin.

   iii. Third zone: mineralized fibrocartilage, indicating a marked transition toward bony tissue. Predominant collagen is type II, with significant amounts of type X collagen and aggrecan.

   iv. Zone four: bone, which is made up predominantly of type I collagen with a high mineral content.

c. Although the insertion site is typically categorized into four zones, changes in the tissue are gradual and continuous. This continuous change in tissue composition is presumed to aid in the efficient transfer of load between two very different materials.

3. Biomechanics

a. A fibrocartilaginous transition is necessary to reduce stress concentrations that would otherwise arise at the interface of two very different materials (tendon/ligament and bone).

b. The enthesis typically has lower mechanical properties in tension than does the tendon or ligament midsubstance.

B. Injury, repair, and healing

1. Tendon-to-bone and ligament-to-bone healing is necessary in several scenarios.

a. Rotator cuff injuries, which represent most soft-tissue injuries to the upper extremities, commonly require surgical repair to the humeral head.

b. Typical ACL reconstruction techniques use tendon grafts that must heal in tibial and femoral bone tunnels.

c. Avulsion injuries to the flexor tendons of the hand require tendon-to-bone repair.

2. In most cases of tendon-to-bone healing, clinical outcomes have been disappointing. The most dramatic feature of the failed healing response is the lack of a transition zone between the healing tendon and bone. Regeneration of the natural transitional tissue between tendon and bone is critical for the restoration of joint function and for the prevention of reinjury.

IV. Tissue Engineering

A. General

1. Definition—Tissue engineering is the regeneration of injured tissue through the merging of three areas: scaffold microenvironment, responding cells, and signaling biofactors.

2. Tissue engineering holds great promise for improving tendon and ligament repair.

B. Scaffold

1. Can serve as a delivery system for biofactors, an environment to attract or immobilize cells, and/or a mechanical stabilizer.

2. Scaffold matrices commonly are made of collagen, fibrin, polymer, or silk.

C. Responding cells

1. Tendon/ligament fibroblasts, mesenchymal stem cells

2. May either be seeded onto the scaffold before implantation or may infiltrate the acellular scaffold after it is implanted.

D. Signaling biofactors

1. Growth factors

a. Platelet-derived growth factor-BB (PDGF-BB) promotes cell proliferation and matrix synthesis.

b. Transforming growth factor-beta (TGF-β) promotes matrix synthesis.

c. Basic fibroblast growth factor (bFGF) promotes cell proliferation and matrix synthesis.

2. Mechanical signals

a. Cyclic tensile loads promote matrix synthesis.

b. Compressive loads promote proteoglycan production.

1: Basic Science

Top Testing Facts

1. Tendons and ligaments are materials with highly ordered hierarchical structure.

2. The composition of tendons and ligaments is primarily type I collagen, aligned in the direction of loading (anisotropic).

3. Structural properties describe the capacity of the tissue to bear load; material properties describe the quality of the tissue.

4. Tendons and ligaments are viscoelastic (their properties are time dependent).

5. Several biologic (eg, age) and environmental (eg, temperature) factors influence the mechanical properties of tendons and ligaments.

6. Tendon/ligament healing progresses through clearly defined phases: hemostasis/inflammation, matrix and cell proliferation, and remodeling/maturation.

7. Nonsheathed tendons and extra-articular ligaments have a greater capacity to heal than do sheathed tendons and intra-articular ligaments.

8. For tendon and ligament healing, increased loading can be either beneficial or detrimental, depending on the anatomic location and type of injury.

9. The physical environment influences tissue maintenance: immobilization is detrimental and exercise is beneficial to the biomechanical properties of these tissues (tendon and ligament).

10. The tendon/ligament enthesis is a specialized tissue that is necessary to minimize stress concentrations at the interface between two very different materials (tendon/ligament and bone).

Bibliography

Amiel D, Kleiner JB, Roux RD, Harwood FL, Akeson WH: The phenomenon of "ligamentization": Anterior cruciate ligament reconstruction with autogenous patellar tendon. *J Orthop Res* 1986;4:162-172.

Frank CB, Shrive NG, Lo IK, Hart DA: Form and function of tendon and ligament, in Einhorn TA, O'Keefe RJ, Buckwalter IA (eds): *Orthopaedic Basic Science*, ed 3. American Academy of Orthopaedic Surgeons, 2007, pp 191-222.

Gelberman RH, Woo SL, Lothringer K, Akeson WH, Amiel D: Effects of early intermittent passive mobilization on healing canine flexor tendons. J Hand Surg Am 1982;7:170-175.

Lin TW, Cardenas L, Soslowsky LJ: Biomechanics of tendon injury and repair. *J Biomech* 2004;37:865-877.

Molloy T, Wang Y, Murrell G: The roles of growth factors in tendon and ligament healing. *Sports Med* 2003;33:381-394.

Thomopoulos S, Williams GR, Soslowsky LJ: Tendon to bone healing: Differences in biomechanical, structural, and compositional properties due to a range of activity levels. *J Biomech Eng* 2003;125:106-113.

1: Basic Science

Chapter 8

Peripheral Nervous System
Seth D. Dodds, MD

I. General Information

A. Peripheral nerves connect the central nervous system (CNS) to tissues such as bone, joints, muscles, tendons, and skin.

B. Nerves that supply the musculoskeletal system provide both motor and sensory function.

II. Histology

A. Cell body

1. Each neuron contains a cell body, which is the metabolic center that gives rise to two different processes: dendrites and axons (**Figure 1,** *A*).

   a. Dendrites are thin nerve processes that receive input from other nerves.

   b. The axon is the primary distal offshoot of the cell body.

      i. The axon is the primary route of conduction for the cell body to convey messages to tissues via action potentials.

      ii. Axons typically measure 0.2 to 20 μm in diameter and arise from an axon hillock, which is responsible for the initiation of the action potential.

   c. Myelin is a fatty insulating sheath formed by neighboring glial cells (specifically Schwann cells in the peripheral nervous system); it surrounds larger axons to speed the conduction of action potentials.

   d. In unmyelinated nerves, a single Schwann cell envelops multiple axons, and conduction proceeds more slowly. In myelinated nerves, each axon is circumferentially laminated by a single Schwann cell.

   e. Nodes of Ranvier are interruptions or gaps between Schwann cell segments of myelin sheath that allow for propagation of the action potential.

   f. As an axon reaches its end organ, it divides into fine terminal branches with specialized endings called presynaptic terminals, which are responsible for transmitting a signal to postsynaptic receptors.

B. Nerve fibers

1. Nerve fibers are collections of axons with the Schwann cell sheaths surrounding them.

2. Afferent nerve fibers convey information from sensory receptors to the CNS.

3. Efferent nerve fibers transmit signals from the CNS to the periphery.

4. Nerve fibers have been classified based on their size and conduction velocity into three types—A, B, and C (Table 1).

C. Nerve metabolism

1. Axoplasmic transport is made possible by the polarization of the neuron.

2. Proteins, which are created only in the cell body, travel via antegrade transport to support neural functions such as action potential propagation and neurotransmitter release.

3. Degradation products travel back to the cell body by retrograde transport.

4. The rate of axonal transport is slowed by decreasing temperature and by anoxia.

5. Several other factors also travel to the cell body in a retrograde fashion, including nerve growth factors, some viruses (eg, herpes simplex, rabies, and polio), tetanus toxin, and horseradish peroxidase (used in the laboratory to identify the location of a cell body in a dorsal root ganglion or in the spinal cord).

III. Nerve Physiology

A. Axon membrane—Made up of a selectively permeable lipid bilayer with sodium/potassium ATP-dependent pumps and gated ion channels. The sodium/potassium ATP-dependent pumps are responsible for an accumulation of sodium ions outside the membrane and the negative resting membrane potential within the axon membrane. When a

1: Basic Science

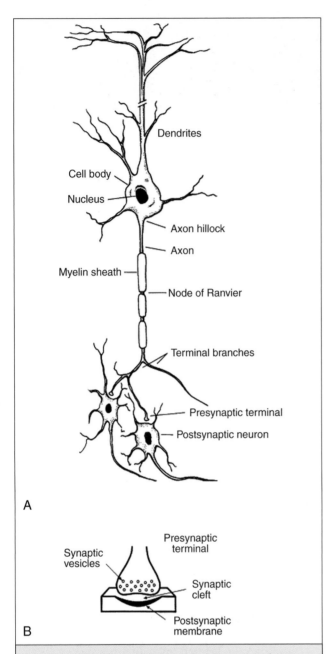

Figure 1 **A,** The primary morphologic features of a peripheral nerve cell are the dendrites, cell body, axon, and presynaptic terminals. **B,** Communication between the terminal end of a nerve axon and an end organ occurs by synaptic vesicle release from the presynaptic terminal. (*Reproduced from Bodine SC, Lieber RL: Peripheral nerve physiology, anatomy, and pathology, in Buckwalter JA, Einhorn TA, Simon SR (eds): Orthopaedic Basic Science, ed. 2. Rosemont, IL, American Academy of Orthopaedic Surgeons, 2000, p 618.*)

membrane is depolarized beyond a critical threshold. The control of gated ion channels (Na^+ and K^+) is governed primarily by electrical, chemical, and mechanical stimuli.

2. The rate at which an action potential is conducted along an axon depends on the size of the axon (larger axon = faster) and the presence of myelin (myelin present = faster).

3. Within the nodes of Ranvier along the axon, dense collections of sodium channels propagate the action potential, allowing for saltatory conduction from node to node.

4. Most motor and sensory peripheral nerves are myelinated, with efferent motor axons being the most heavily myelinated. Autonomic fibers and slow pain fibers are examples of unmyelinated nerves.

5. Multiple sclerosis and Guillain-Barré syndrome are examples of nervous system diseases that lead to demyelination and slowed conduction velocities.

   a. Multiple sclerosis is a chronic (and occasionally remitting) neurologic disorder characterized by perivascular infiltration of inflammatory cells followed by damage of the myelin sheath as well as nerve fibers. Patients develop problems with motor control (vision, strength, balance) and cognition.

   b. Guillain-Barré syndrome is an acute inflammatory polyradiculoneuropathy. It is presumed to be an autoimmune disease (typically triggered by a viral or bacterial infection) that causes the production of antibodies that attack the myelin sheath. The loss of myelin leads to an acute impairment of sensory and motor nerve function ranging in severity from paresthesias and weakness to complete loss of sensation and paralysis.

B. Neuromuscular junction—This is the highly specialized region between the distal nerve terminal and a skeletal muscle fiber. It consists of the presynaptic terminal (the distalmost end of a nerve fiber), a synaptic cleft (the space into which neurotransmitters are released), and a postsynaptic membrane (the tissue responding to the nerve signal) (Figure 1, B).

1. The arrival of an action potential at the presynaptic terminal triggers the vesicular release of acetylcholine.

2. Acetylcholine travels across the synaptic cleft and, once bound to receptors on the postsynaptic membrane, causes depolarization of the motor end plate and stimulation of the muscle fiber.

stimulus causes the gated ion channels to open, sodium flows rapidly into the axon, causing depolarization.

1. Conduction of signals along an axon begins with action potentials, which are generated when the

Table 1

Classification of Peripheral Nerve Fibers

Fiber Type	Example of Function	Fiber Characteristic	Fiber Diameter (μm)	Conduction Velocity (m/s)
Aα	Motor axon	Myelinated—Large	12-20	72-120
Aβ	Cutaneous touch and pressure	Myelinated—Medium	6-12	36-72
Aδ	Pain and temperature	Myelinated—Small	1-6	4-36
B	Sympathetic preganglionic	Myelinated—Small	1-6	3-15
C	Cutaneous pain, sympathetic postganglionic	Unmyelinated	0.2-1.5	0.4-2

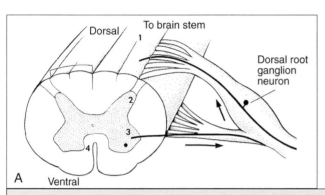 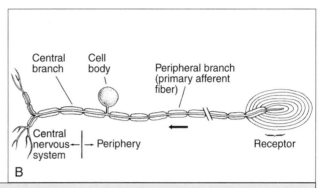

Figure 2   The cell body of a sensory nerve resides in the dorsal root ganglion, far from its distal nerve ending. The dorsal root ganglion is located proximally, near the spinal cord where the spinal nerve enters the thecal sac. **A,** Projections of the central branch. **B,** Morphology of a dorsal root ganglion cell. (*Adapted with permission from Kandel ER, Schwartz JH, Jessell TM:* Principles of Neural Science, *ed 3. Norwalk, CT, Appleton & Lange, 1991, pp 287-342.*)

IV. Embryology and Nerve Growth

A. Nervous system

1. The nervous system (and skin) is formed by the ectoderm (one of the three germ layers: ectoderm, mesoderm, and endoderm).

2. The ectoderm divides to form the neural tube (brain, spinal cord, and motor neurons), the neural crest (afferent neurons), and the epidermis.

3. The peripheral nervous system itself is divided into a purely motor visceral system (autonomic) and a mixed sensory and motor somatic system, which helps control voluntary motion.

B. Spinal nerves

1. Spinal nerves are collections of axons that exit the spinal cord at distinct levels. There are 8 cervical, 12 thoracic, 5 lumbar, 5 sacral, and 1 coccygeal spinal nerves.

2. The efferent ventral root transmits information from brain to muscle; the afferent dorsal root carries signals from the periphery back to the CNS (**Figure 2**).

a. The cell bodies for afferent sensory nerves are located in the dorsal root ganglion, which lies near the entry of the spinal nerve into the thecal sac.

b. The cell bodies for efferent motor nerves reside in the anterior horn of the spinal cord.

3. Spinal nerves frequently collect into plexuses (cervical, brachial, and lumbar) before branching.

C. Axonal growth and development—Initially guided by different nerve growth factors.

1. N-cadherin and neural cell adhesion molecule are adhesive membrane glycoproteins that are expressed on neural ectoderm and help guide growing axons.

2. Laminin and fibronectin are extracellular matrix glycoproteins that promote directional nerve fiber outgrowth.

3. Other factors believed to enhance nerve regeneration include nerve growth factor, fibroblastic growth factor, ciliary neuronotrophic factor, and insulin-like growth factor.

1: Basic Science

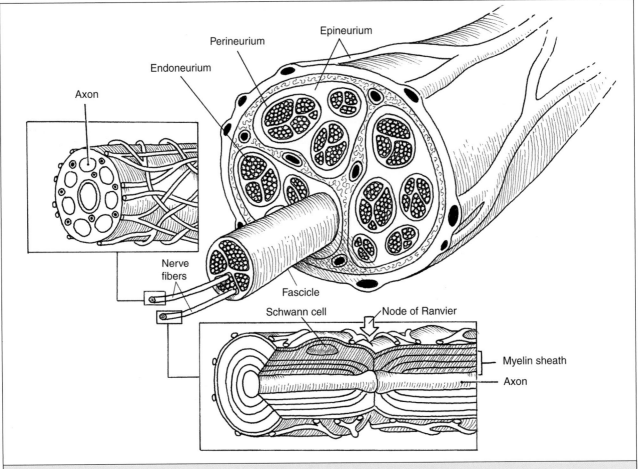

Figure 3 The anatomy of a peripheral nerve. (*Reproduced with permission from Lundborg G:* Nerve Injury and Repair. *New York, NY, Churchill Livingstone, 1988, p 33.*)

V. Peripheral Nerve Anatomy and Biomechanics

A. Composition—Each nerve is composed of collections of nerve fibers called fascicles and neural connective tissue, which both surrounds and lies within each fascicle (Figure 3).

1. Axons within each fascicle are surrounded by a connective tissue layer referred to as endoneurium. Endoneurium is primarily composed of a collagenous matrix with fibroblasts, mast cells, and capillaries and forms a bilaminar sheath around the axon, Schwann cell, and myelin of each nerve fiber.

2. Perineurium is a thin, dense connective tissue layer that surrounds the fascicles.

    a. It has a high tensile strength and maintains interfascicular pressure, providing a perineurial diffusion barrier. This barrier limits injury to nerve fibers by limiting the diffusion of epineurial edema, which occurs in stretch and compression type injuries. It also limits the diffusion of endoneurial edema that can occur

when a nerve is compressed.

    b. Spinal nerve roots have less perineurium than peripheral nerves and are more susceptible to stretch and compression injury.

3. Epineurium is the supportive sheath that contains the multiple groups of fascicles. It contains a well-developed network of extrinsic, interconnected blood vessels that run parallel with the nerve.

4. The structural organization of fascicles changes throughout the length of the nerve. Fascicles do not run as isolated, parallel strands from spinal cord to the presynaptic terminal or end organ. The number and size of fascicles changes as fascicular plexuses unite and divide within the nerve (Figure 4).

    a. At the joint level, fascicles are numerous and of smaller size to accommodate nerve deformation as the joint goes through a range of motion; eg, in the ulnar nerve at the elbow are many small fascicles, which minimize injury with elbow flexion and extension.

b. In contrast, at the level of the spiral groove, the radial nerve has a low number of large fascicles, which do not tolerate stretch very well. This level-specific internal anatomy places the radial nerve at higher risk for neurapraxia when it is mobilized and retracted from the spiral groove.

B. Blood supply—A peripheral nerve has both intrinsic and extrinsic vessels with multiple anastomoses throughout the length of the nerve.

1. At the epineurial level, there is no blood-nerve barrier.

2. At the capillary level within the endoneurium, however, there is a blood-nerve barrier, similar to the blood-brain barrier, which prevents diffusion of many macromolecules to maintain neural integrity. The blood-nerve diffusion barrier can be injured by infection, radiation, or metabolic disease.

C. Nerve endings—Afferent nerve fibers use specific primary receptors to collect sensory information from the periphery. There are three modalities and four attributes of sensory information that is conveyed.

1. Modalities

   a. Mechanical stimulation (touch, proprioception, and pressure)

   b. Painful stimulation (noxious, tissue-damaging stimulus)

   c. Thermal stimulation (hot and cold)

2. Attributes: location, intensity, quality, and duration.

3. Nociceptors and thermoceptors consist of bare nerve endings (Table 2).

4. Mechanoreceptors—Two types

   a. Superficial skin mechanoreceptors: (small)

      i. Meissner corpuscle, a rapidly adapting sensory receptor that is very sensitive to touch.

      ii. Merkel disk receptors, which adapt slowly and sense sustained pressure, texture, and low-frequency vibrations.

   b. Subcutaneous mechanoreceptors: (larger and fewer in number)

      i. Pacini, or pacinian, corpuscles are ovoid in shape, measuring approximately 1 mm in

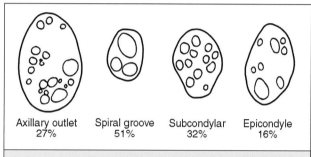

Axillary outlet 27%   Spiral groove 51%   Subcondylar 32%   Epicondyle 16%

Figure 4   The size, number, and arrangement of fascicles within a nerve vary along the course of the nerve. This figure depicts the percentage of cross-sectional area of the nerve devoted to fasciculi (given as a percentage of total cross-sectional area) in the radial nerve from the shoulder to elbow. (*Reproduced with permission from Lundborg G:* Nerve Injury and Repair. *New York, NY, Churchill Livingstone, 1988, p 198.*)

Table 2

Types of Receptors

	Receptor Type	Quality	Fiber Type
Nociceptors	Mechanical	Sharp, pricking pain	Aδ
	Polymodal	Slow, burning pain	C
Cutaneous mechanoreceptors	Meissner corpuscle	Touch	Aβ
	Merkel receptor	Steady skin indentation	Aβ
Subcutaneous mechanoreceptors	Pacini corpuscle	Vibration	Aβ
	Ruffini corpuscle	Skin stretch	Aβ
Muscle and skeletal mechanoreceptors	Muscle spindle primary	Limb proprioception	Aα
	Muscle spindle secondary	Limb proprioception	Aβ
	Golgi tendon organ	Limb proprioception	Aα
	Joint capsule mechanoreceptor	Limb proprioception	Aβ

(*From Kandel ER, Schwartz JH, Jessel TM (eds):* Principles of Neural Science, *ed 3, Norwalk, CT, Appleton & Lange, 1991, p 342.*)

Table 3

Nerve Injury Classification

Seddon	Sunderland	Pathoanatomy	Prognosis
Neurapraxia	Type 1	Temporary conduction block with local myelin damage	Typically full recovery
Axonotmesis	Type 2	Axons disrupted; endoneurium, perineurium, and epineurium intact	Reasonable recovery of function
	Type 3	Axons and endoneurium disrupted; perineurium and epineurium intact	Incomplete recovery due to intrafascicular fibrosis
	Type 4	Axons, endoneurium, and perineurium disrupted; epineurium intact	Negligible recovery due to axonal misdirection
Neurotmesis	Type 5	Complete disruption of nerve	No spontaneous recovery

(Adapted from Lee SK, Wolfe SW, Peripheral nerve injury and repair. J Am Acad Orthop Surg 2000;8:245.)

length. They react to high-frequency vibration and rapid indentations of the skin.

    ii. Ruffini corpuscles are slowly adapting receptors that respond to stretching of the skin, such as occurs with finger motion.

D. Biomechanics

1. Nerves are viscoelastic structures demonstrating nonlinear responses to stretch.

2. When a nerve is stretched, it becomes ischemic before disrupting; for example, a nerve may undergo ischemia at 15% strain and rupture at 20% strain.

3. The ultimate strain of a nerve ranges from 20% to 60%.

VI. Peripheral Nerve Injury

A. Response to injury

1. Peripheral nerves respond to trauma with an initial inflammatory response.

    a. This typically leads to increased epineurial permeability and edema, as the vessels within the epineurium lack a blood-nerve barrier.

    b. If the injury involves disruption (crush or transection) that exposes the endoneurium, then the blood-nerve barrier is disrupted and the permeability of the endoneurial capillaries increases.

2. Injury from ischemia and compression can cause increased endoneurial pressure, fluid edema, and capillary permeability while the perineurial vascular system remains unaffected.

    a. In these cases, the positive fluid pressure inside the endoneurium affects blood flow (decreased

nutrition and oxygen delivery) and the removal of waste products.

    b. When persistent, intraneural edema can diminish nerve function as seen in chronic compressive neuropathies.

B. Seddon's classification of nerve injury (**Table 3**)

1. Neurapraxia

    a. Neurapraxia is an immediate, localized conduction block with normal conduction above and below the injury site.

    b. Neurapraxias are typically reversible. Axon continuity is maintained, but local demyelination and ischemia occur.

    c. Mechanisms of injury include compression, traction, and contusion.

2. Axonotmesis

    a. Axonotmesis involves axon disruption, but some degree of the surrounding neural connective tissue is preserved. The axon distal to the point of injury degenerates (Wallerian degeneration).

    b. Some nerve function may be recovered as nerve fiber regeneration is guided by an intact neural connective tissue layer (eg, intact endoneurium).

    c. Mechanisms of injury include crush and forceful stretch.

3. Neurotmesis

    a. Neurotmesis is complete disruption of nerve.

    b. No spontaneous recovery of the affected nerve can be expected.

    c. Mechanisms of injury include open crush, violent stretch, and laceration.

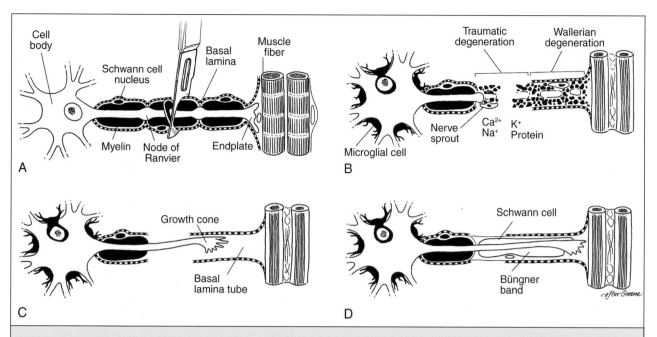

Figure 5 Peripheral nerve injury, degeneration, and regeneration. **A,** Laceration of the nerve fiber. **B,** Degeneration of the proximal stump to the closest node of Ranvier and Wallerian degeneration of the distal stump. **C,** Axonal sprouting of the growth cone into a basal lamina tube. **D,** The Schwann cell forms a column (Büngner band) to assist directed axonal growth. *(Adapted from Seckel BR: Enhancement of peripheral nerve regeneration.* Muscle Nerve *1990;13:785-800.)*

4. Sunderland revised Seddon's classification by defining three subtypes of axonotmesis.

C.   Pathoanatomy of injury

1. Laceration (Figure 5, *A* and *B*)

   a. When the continuity of a nerve is disrupted, the two nerve ends retract, the cell body swells, the nucleus is displaced peripherally, and chromatolysis (dispersion of basophilic Nissl granules with relative eosinophilia of the cell body) occurs.

   b. The nerve cell stops producing neurotransmitters and starts synthesizing proteins required for axonal regeneration.

   c. Wallerian degeneration distal to the site of the injury begins within hours of injury and is characterized by axonal disorganization from proteolysis, followed by the breakdown of myelin.

   d. Schwann cells become active in clearing myelin and axonal debris.

2. Compression

   a. When a nerve is compressed, nerve fibers are deformed, local ischemia occurs, and vascular permeability is increased.

   b. Edema then affects the endoneurial environment, leading to poor axonal transport and nerve dysfunction.

   c. If compression continues, the edema and dysfunction persist and fibroblasts invade, producing scar tissue, which impairs fascicular gliding.

   d. Tissue pressures up to 30 mm Hg can cause paresthesias and increased nerve conduction latencies. A tissue pressure of 60 mm Hg can cause a complete block of nerve conduction.

3. Ischemia

   a. After 15 minutes of anoxia, axonal transport stops.

   b. It can recover if reperfusion occurs within 12 to 24 hours.

D.   Nerve regeneration after injury

1. With or without suture reapproximation of the disrupted nerve ends, nerve regeneration begins with axonal elongation across the zone of injury (Figure 5, *C* and *D*).

   a. The zone of injury undergoes an ingrowth of capillaries as well as Schwann cells.

   b. The Schwann cells migrate into the gap from both proximal and distal stumps and attempt to form columns (Büngner bands) to guide the tip or growth cone of the sprouting axons.

   c. The growth cone is sensitive to neurotrophic growth factors, such as nerve growth factor, and neurite promoting factors such as laminin.

1: Basic Science

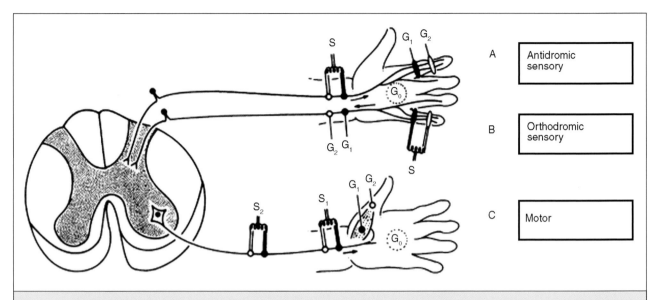

Figure 6 Illustration of electrode placement for three types of nerve conduction studies: antidromic sensory study **(A)**, orthodromic sensory study **(B)**, and motor nerve conduction study **(C)**. G1 = active recording electrode; G2 = reference recording electrode; G0 = ground electrode; S = stimulating electrode; S1 = distal stimulation site; S2 = proximal stimulation site. The cathode is black and the anode is white. (*Reproduced with permission from Sethi RD, Thompson LL: The Electromyographer's Handbook, ed 2. Boston, MA, Little, Brown and Co, 1989, p 4.*)

2. Distal reinnervation of muscle will be successful only if the muscle has viable motor end plates for the regenerating nerve to stimulate.

   a. In the acute period after a nerve injury, the muscle increases the number of motor end plates, seeking nerve stimulus.

   b. As fibrosis sets in over time, the number of motor end plates diminishes.

   c. Typically, after 12 months, a muscle is no longer receptive to reinnervation.

VII. Diagnostic Studies

A. Overview

1. The primary tests used to evaluate the integrity of the peripheral nervous system are nerve conduction velocity studies and EMG.

2. These tests assess the function of sensory nerves, motor nerves, and muscles to confirm the diagnosis of neuropathies and myopathies.

3. They also can differentiate causes of weakness, identify the level and severity of nerve injury or conduction abnormality, and demonstrate the existence of denervated muscle and its reinnervation.

B. Nerve conduction velocity studies

1. Sensation

   a. A stimulation recording from a mixed (motor and sensory) nerve is called a compound nerve action potential.

   b. A sensory-specific recording is called a sensory nerve action potential (SNAP).

   c. The nerve can be stimulated in an antidromic (from proximal to distal) or orthodromic (from distal to proximal) fashion (Figure 6). The speed of conduction is similar in either direction.

   d. The distance (in millimeters) and time (in milliseconds) an action potential travels between electrodes must be known to quantify the speed of conduction.

   e. Nerve conduction velocity (distance/time) or latency (time between the stimulus and the onset of the action potential) are typically recorded (Figure 7). These values are negatively impacted by temperature, age, demyelination, and loss of axons.

   f. The amplitude of the action potential can also be measured. Cold temperature increases SNAP amplitude, whereas age decreases it.

2. Motor nerve function

   a. A motor nerve action potential is recorded from a muscle, where multiple muscle fibers are innervated by a single nerve. Thus, the information recorded is a compound muscle action potential (CMAP).

   b. The CMAP measures not only the speed of a stimulus over the course of a nerve but also the transmission over the neuromuscular junction and muscle fiber conduction.

  c. An F-wave is a late response recording from distal muscles during CMAP testing.

    i. When a stimulus is applied, the signal travels in the typical proximal-to-distal fashion. However, a separate signal also may be sent distal-to-proximal along the nerve to the spinal cord anterior horn cells.

    ii. With sufficient anterior horn cell stimulation, these cells may discharge another proximal-to-distal stimulus called an F-wave, which will be recorded after the initial CMAP.

C. Electromyography

  1. EMG studies the entire motor unit (anterior horn cell, motor neuron, and muscle) and involves measuring insertional activity, spontaneous activity, motor unit action potentials (MUAPs), and recruitment (but not sensory information).

  2. Insertional activity is measured as the needle is passed into the muscle belly.

    a. Decreased insertional activity occurs from poor muscle viability, muscle fibrosis, or muscle atrophy.

    b. Increased insertional activity may be a sign of denervation or a primary muscle disorder (eg, polymyositis or myopathy).

  3. Spontaneous activity involves electrical discharges that occur without muscle contraction and without movement of the testing needle.

    a. Fibrillations are an example of abnormal spontaneous activity; they occur in denervated muscle fibers and some myopathies. The density of fibrillations is graded from 1+ to 4+, but it is the amplitude that is helpful in understanding the timing of denervation. Large-amplitude fibrillations frequently occur acutely (within 3 to 12 months), and smaller amplitude fibrillations occur later in the process of denervation (after the muscle has atrophied).

    b. Positive sharp waves are abnormal single muscle fiber discharges and can be seen in association with fibrillations. They can be seen without fibrillations when the muscle is traumatized but not denervated. Fibrillations and positive sharp waves typically appear 2 to 3 weeks after the onset of denervation.

    c. Fasciculations are spontaneous discharges of a single motor unit and can be seen clinically on the skin. Fasciculations occur in various neuromuscular disorders (the syndrome of benign fasciculations, chronic radiculopathies, peripheral polyneuropathies, thyrotoxicosis, and

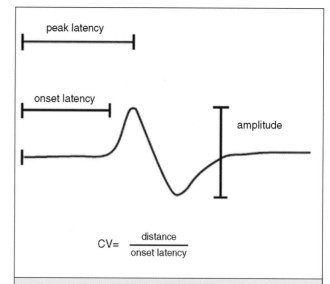

Figure 7 Conduction velocity (CV) is the distance from the stimulating electrode to the receiving electrode divided by the time from the stimulus to either the onset of the action potential (onset latency) or the peak of the action potential (peak latency). (*Reproduced from Robinson LR, Role of neurophysiologic evaluation in diagnosis. J Am Acad Orthop Surg 2000;8:191.*)

overdose of anticholinesterase medications).

  4. MUAPs can measure voluntary muscle activity and are characterized by the duration, amplitude, and shape of the action potential.

    a. The amplitude characterizes the density of the muscle fibers within the motor unit.

    b. The duration and shape of the wave produced by the MUAP are affected by the quality of conduction. For example, as a partially denervated motor unit is reinnervated with axonal sprouting, the MUAP will be prolonged in duration and polyphasic in shape. If no reinnervation occurs, no MUAP will be generated.

  5. Recruitment is also measured by MUAPs and can be used to understand whether muscle weakness is the result of a decrease in the peripheral motor neurons and motor units or a central recruitment problem from a CNS lesion, pain, or poor voluntary effort.

D. Magnetic resonance imaging

  1. MRI can be a useful adjunct to electrodiagnostic studies for assessing various disorders of the peripheral nervous system.

  2. MRI can show changes in muscle from denervation. For example, chronic denervation will show evidence of fatty atrophy.

  3. High-resolution images with sufficient contrast are required to emphasize the underlying periph-

eral nerve anatomy and nerve morphology.

4. These scans take advantage of signal differences between distinct intraneural tissues, specifically differences in the water content and physical structure of fascicles, perineurium, and epineurium.

VIII. Peripheral Nerve Pharmacology

A. Local anesthetics

1. Create a sensorimotor nerve block, causing transient numbness and paralysis by temporarily disrupting the transmission of action potentials along the course of axons.

2. Lidocaine, mepivacaine, and bupivacaine (all amide-type) have different durations of action based on their specific biochemistry, with lidocaine the shortest duration of action and bupivacaine the longest.

3. C-type nerve fibers (cutaneous pain fibers) are most susceptible to local anesthetics, and A-type fibers (motor axons and deep pressure sense) are the least susceptible.

4. Local anesthetics (amide type) are processed by the liver (P450 enzyme) into more water-soluble metabolites, which are then excreted in the urine.

5. Epinephrine may be combined with these anesthetics for vasoconstriction.

   a. This reduces systemic absorption of local anesthetics from the injection site by decreasing blood flow in these areas.

   b. Systemic blood levels are lowered up to 30%.

   c. Local neuronal uptake is increased in the region of drug administration as local vasoconstriction causes less of the drug to be absorbed systemically.

B. Botulinum toxin

1. Botulinum toxin can be injected into muscle to treat muscular spasticity.

2. The bacterium *Clostridium botulinum* produces botulinum toxin.

3. The toxin works at the level of the neuromuscular junction, blocking vesicular release of acetylcholine at the presynaptic clefts and leading to chemical denervation (paralysis) when injected into muscle.

4. The beneficial effect begins at approximately 7 to 14 days and typically lasts 3 months.

IX. Treatment of Peripheral Nerve Injuries

A. Nonsurgical treatment

1. Nonsurgical treatment is appropriate for all neurapraxias and most axonotmeses.

2. While awaiting nerve recovery, great care should be taken to maintain limb functionality and viability. Specifically, distal joints should be mobilized and distal muscle groups stretched or protectively splinted to avoid contractures.

3. Osteopenia, joint stiffness, and muscle atrophy can occur if the affected limb is ignored.

B. Recovery of an injured sensory nerve occurs in the following sequence:

1. Pressure sense

2. Protective pain

3. Moving touch

4. Moving 2-point discrimination

5. Static 2-point discrimination

6. Threshold sensation (Semmes-Weinstein monofilament and vibration).

C. Surgical repair

1. Prerequisites to nerve repair (neurorrhaphy) include a clean wound, a well-vascularized repair bed, skeletal stability, and viable soft-tissue coverage.

2. Nerve ends are sharply débrided of injured or devitalized nerve, scar, and fibrosis to expose healthy nerve fascicles.

3. A repair should occur urgently, within the first few days after injury, because disrupted nerves retract and scar tissue and neuromas form quickly.

4. Postoperatively, limited immobilization for 2 to 3 weeks prevents stress at the repair site.

5. Currently the most effective repair technique is an epineurial repair (suturing repair of the epineurium only) performed with a fine monofilament nylon suture (eg, No. 9-0) using microsurgical instrumentation and technique.

   a. In reapproximating the nerve ends with an epineurial repair, care should be taken to orient the nerve ends to match fascicles as accurately as possible. This technique typically minimizes scar formation.

   b. It can be performed with suture or with fibrin glue.

   c. The repair should be done under minimal tension.

6. A group fascicular repair involves reapproximating fascicular groups by perineurial repair. This technique is more precise than epineurial repair, but it typically requires intraneural dissection, which leads to more scar tissue formation and intraneural fibrosis.

7. Muscular neurotization involves implanting the nerve end directly into the muscle belly.

8. Nerve grafting is used when segmental defects in a nerve exist that cannot be overcome with joint flexion or nerve transposition.

   a. Autografts are inset in the same manner as a primary repair, although it is recommended to reverse the graft to decrease axonal dispersion through the nerve graft.

   b. The sural nerve is a common autograft that can be cut into parallel sections to create a cable graft of greater diameter.

   c. Fresh allografts require immunosuppression and are infrequently used.

   d. In lieu of an autograft, nerve gaps can be bridged with either biologic (vein graft) or bioabsorbable nerve conduits (polyglycolic acid or collagen).

9. Results of peripheral nerve repair vary.

   a. Young patients with early repairs of distal single-function nerves using short nerve grafts or direct repair do better than older patients with late repairs of proximal, mixed nerves using long nerve grafts.

   b. The rate of nerve regeneration after repair also varies and has been historically estimated to be 1 to 2 mm per day in humans, which is approximately equal to the rate of axonal transport of neurofilament proteins essential to nerve growth.

Top Testing Facts

1. Schwann cell myelination speeds transmission of action potentials by saltatory conduction occurring at nodes of Ranvier.

2. Most motor and sensory nerves are myelinated except for autonomic and slow pain fibers.

3. Nerve fibers (axons) are surrounded by endoneurium, collections of nerve fibers (fascicles) by perineurium, and collections of fascicles by epineurium.

4. Nerve injury causes loss of distal function in the following sequence: motor, proprioception, touch, temperature, pain, and sympathetics. Nerves recover in the inverse order.

5. Neurapraxia is a reversible conduction block (traction or compression); axonotmesis involves axon disruption with preserved neural connective tissue (stretch or crush); neurotmesis is complete disruption of a nerve (open crush or laceration).

6. Tissue pressures up to 30 mm Hg can cause paresthesias and increased nerve conduction latencies.

7. Temperature, age, demyelination, and loss of axons decrease rate of transmission.

8. Fibrillations are an EMG finding of abnormal spontaneous activity that occur in muscle fibers 2 to 3 weeks after denervation (transient or complete).

9. Nerve repair (neurorrhaphy) involves reapproximation of the nerve ends with fascicles appropriately oriented under minimal tension using a fine monofilament epineurial suture. Group fascicular repair increases scarring at the repair site.

10. Nerve grafts may be cabled to increase diameter; they should also be reversed to minimize early arborization of regenerating nerve fibers.

Bibliography

Gupta R, Mozaffar T: Form and function of the peripheral nerves and spinal cord, in Einhorn TA, O'Keefe RJ, Buckwalter JA (eds): Orthopaedic Basic Science, ed 3. Rosemont, IL, American Academic of Orthopaedic Surgeons, 2007, pp 245-258.

Lee SK, Wolfe SW: Peripheral nerve injury and repair. J Am Acad Orthop Surg 2000;8:243-252.

Lundborg G: A 25-year perspective of peripheral nerve surgery: Evolving neuroscientific concepts and clinical significance. J Hand Surg Am 2000;25:391-414.

Robinson LR: Role of neurophysiologic evaluation in diagnosis. J Am Acad Orthop Surg 2000;8:190-199.

1: Basic Science

Chapter 9
Skeletal Muscle

Michael J. Medvecky, MD

1: Basic Science

I. General Information

A. Skeletal muscles receive innervation from the peripheral nervous system.

B. They affect volitional control of the axial and appendicular skeleton.

II. Muscle Structure and Function

A. Muscle structure

 1. Skeletal muscle fibers are highly specialized multinucleated cells characterized by a collection of contractile filaments called myofilaments (**Figure 1**). Filaments are organized in a defined hierarchy, with the basic functional unit of muscle contraction being the sarcomere.

 2. The largest functional unit is the myofibril, which is a string of sarcomeres arranged in series. Adjacent myofibrils are connected by a set of specialized proteins called intermediate filaments. These allow for mechanical coupling between myofibrils.

 3. Endomysium is the connective tissue surrounding individual fibers.

 4. Perimysium is the connective tissue surrounding collections of muscle fibers, or fascicles.

 5. Epimysium is the connective tissue covering of the entire muscle.

B. Cell membrane systems

 1. A specially designed membrane system exists within the cell that assists in activating the contractile properties of the muscle cell. The system consists of two main components: the transverse tubular system and the sarcoplasmic reticulum (**Figure 2**).

  a. The transverse tubular system begins as invaginations of the cell membrane and extends into the cell, perpendicular to its long axis. It functions to relay the activation signal from the motor neuron to the myofibrils.

  b. The sarcoplasmic reticulum is a system of membrane-bound sacs that function to collect,

release, and re-uptake calcium stores to regulate the muscle contractile process.

  i. Calcium channels and pumps are contained within the sarcoplasmic reticulum and are regulated by a complex enzymatic system.

  ii. The portion of the sarcoplasmic reticulum that abuts the transverse tubules is called the junctional sarcoplasmic reticulum.

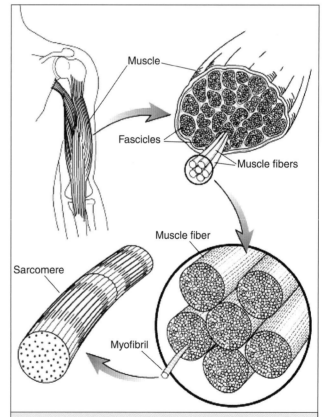

Figure 1 Structural hierarchy of skeletal muscle. Whole skeletal muscles are composed of numerous fascicles of muscle fibers. Muscle fibers are composed of myofibrils arranged in parallel. Myofibrils are composed of sarcomeres arranged in series. Sarcomeres are composed of interdigitating actin and myosin filaments. (*Reproduced with permission from Lieber R (ed): Skeletal Muscle Structure, Function, and Plasticity: The Physiological Basis of Rehabilitation, ed 2. Philadelphia, PA, Lippincott Williams & Wilkins, 2002, p 18.*)

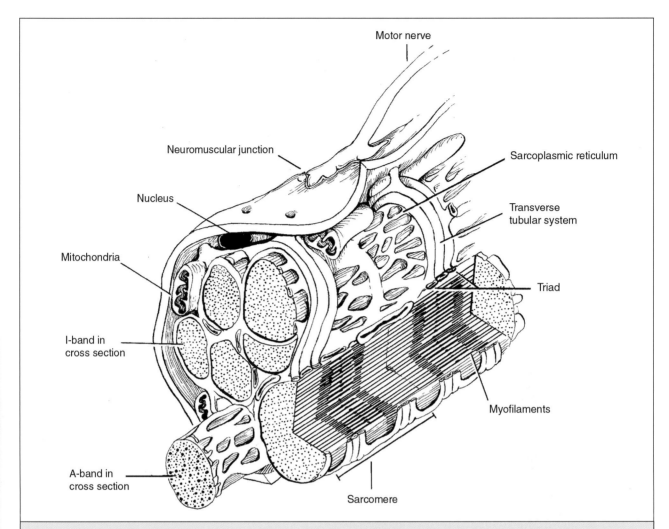

Figure 2 Schematic representation of the muscle cell. The muscle cell, which is specialized for the production of force and movement, contains an array of filamentous proteins as well as other subcellular organelles such as mitochondria, nuclei, satellite cells, sarcoplasmic reticulum, and the transverse tubular system. Note the formation of "triads," which represent the T-tubules flanked by the terminal cisternae of the sarcoplasmic reticulum. Also note that when the myofilaments are sectioned longitudinally, the stereotypic striated appearance is seen. When myofilaments are sectioned transversely at the level of the A- or I-bands, the hexagonal array of the appropriate filaments is seen. *(Reproduced with permission from Lieber R (ed): Skeletal Muscle Structure, Function, and Plasticity: The Physiological Basis of Rehabilitation, ed 2. Philadelphia, PA, Lippincott Williams & Wilkins, 2002, p 15.)*

iii. The transverse tubule and the two adjacent sacs of the junctional reticulum together is called a triad.

C. Sarcomere composition

1. Sarcomeres are composed of two major types of contractile filaments:

a. Myosin (thick filaments)

b. Actin (thin filaments)

2. The two sets of filaments interdigitate, and it is the active interdigitation of these filaments that produces muscle contraction via a shortening translation of the filaments.

3. The arrangement of these filaments also creates the characteristic pattern of alternating bands of light and dark seen with microscopy.

a. Tropomyosin, another protein, is situated between two actin strands in its double-helix configuration. In the resting state, tropomyosin blocks the myosin binding sites on actin (**Figure 3**).

b. Troponin is a complex of three separate proteins that is intimately associated with tropomyosin.

i. When troponin binds calcium, a conformational change in the troponin complex ensues.

ii. This in turn results in a conformational change of tropomyosin, exposing the myosin-binding sites on actin.

    iii. A resultant contractile protein interaction occurs, and muscle contraction is initiated.

D. Sarcomere organization

  1. The structure of the sarcomere is shown in **Figure 4**.

    a. The A-band is composed of both actin and myosin.

    b. The M-line is a central set of interconnecting filaments for myosin.

    c. The H-band contains only myosin.

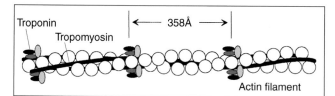

Figure 3   Features of regulation of muscle contraction. Structure of actin is represented by two chains of beads in a double helix. The troponin complex consists of calcium-binding protein (TN-C, black); inhibitory protein (TN-I, red); and protein binding to tropomyosin (TN-T, yellow). The tropomyosin (dark line) lies in each groove of the actin filament. (*Reproduced from Garrett WE Jr, Best TM: Anatomy, physiology, and mechanics of skeletal muscle, in Buckwalter JA, Einhorn TA, Simon SR (eds): Orthopaedic Basic Science: Biology and Biomechanics of the Musculoskeletal System, ed 2. Rosemont, IL, American Academy of Orthopaedic Surgeons, 2000, p 690.*)

    d. The I-band is composed of actin filaments only, which are joined together at the interconnecting Z-line.

  2. During muscle contraction, the sarcomere length decreases but the length of individual thick and thin filaments remains the same. During contraction, the thick and thin filaments bypass one another, resulting in increased overlap.

E. Nerve-muscle interaction

  1. A motor unit consists of a single motor neuron and all of the muscle fibers it contacts.

    a. Every muscle fiber is contacted by a single nerve terminal at a site called the motor end plate (**Figure 5**).

    b. The number of muscle fibers within a motor unit varies widely.

  2. Chemical transmission of the electrical impulse passing down the cell membrane of the axon occurs at the motor end plate or neuromuscular junction (NMJ). The primary and secondary synaptic folds or invaginations of the cell membrane increase the surface area for communication.

  3. Acetylcholine (ACh) is the neurotransmitter released into the synaptic cleft.

    a. The electrical impulse reaches the terminal axon, and calcium ions are allowed to flow into the neural cell.

    b. This increase in intracellular calcium causes the neurotransmitter vesicles to fuse with the axon membrane, and the ACh is released into the synaptic cleft.

1: Basic Science

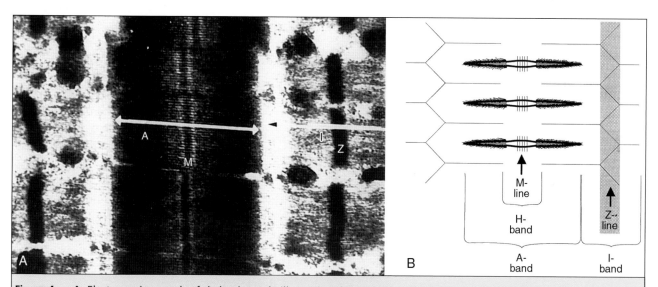

Figure 4   **A,** Electron micrograph of skeletal muscle illustrating the striated, banded appearance. A = A-band; M = M-line; I = I-band; Z = Z-line. **B,** The basic functional unit of skeletal muscle, the sarcomere. (*Reproduced from Garrett WE, Best TM: Anatomy, physiology, and mechanics of skeletal muscle, in Buckwalter JA, Einhorn TA, Simon SR (eds): Orthopaedic Basic Science: Biology and Biomechanics of the Musculoskeletal System, ed 2. Rosemont, IL, American Academy of Orthopaedic Surgeons, 2000, p 688.*)

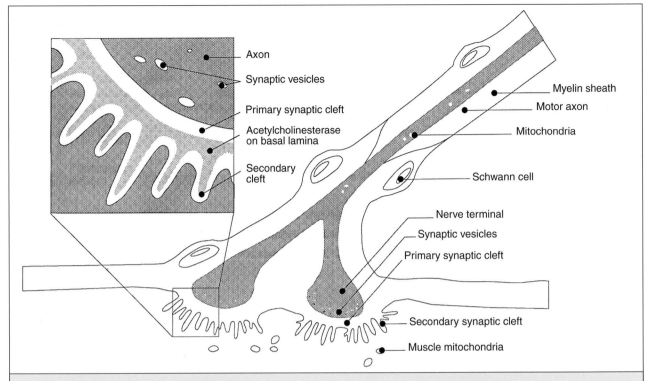

Figure 5 Schematic representation of the motor end plate. (*Reproduced from Garrett WE, Best TM: Anatomy, physiology, and mechanics of skeletal muscle, in Buckwalter JA, Einhorn TA, Simon SR (eds):* Orthopaedic Basic Science: Biology and Biomechanics of the Musculoskeletal System, *ed 2. Rosemont, IL, American Academy of Orthopaedic Surgeons, 2000, p 686.*)

c. ACh then binds to receptors on the muscle membrane, triggering depolarization of the cell, which in turn triggers an action potential.

d. This action potential is passed along through the sarcoplasmatic reticulum network.

e. The ACh is enzymatically deactivated by acetylcholinesterase located within the extracellular space.

4. Pharmacologic and physiologic alteration of neuromuscular transmission

a. Myasthenia gravis is a disorder resulting in a shortage of ACh receptors; it is characterized by severe muscle weakness.

b. Nondepolarizing drugs (eg, pancuronium, vecuronium, and curare)

i. Competitively bind to ACh receptor, blocking transmission.

ii. Site of action is the NMJ.

c. Polarizing drugs (eg, succinylcholine)

i. Bind to ACh receptor, causing temporary depolarization followed by failure of the impulse transmission.

ii. Site of action is the NMJ.

d. Reversible acetylcholinesterase inhibitors (eg, neostigmine, edrophonium)

i. Prevent breakdown of ACh.

ii. Allow for prolonged interaction with ACh receptor.

e. Irreversible acetylcholinesterase inhibitors (eg, nerve gases and certain insecticides)

i. Similarly prevent breakdown of ACh.

ii. Result in sustained muscle contraction.

III. Muscle Function

A. Nerve activation of muscle contraction

1. A muscle twitch (**Figure 6**, *A*) is the muscle tension response to a single nerve stimulus.

a. If a second nerve stimulus arrives after the muscle tension has returned to baseline resting tension, there is no increase in muscle tension development.

b. Absolute refractory period—The time period during which no stimulus will produce a muscle contraction.

c. Relative refractory period—The time period during which the stimulus required for muscle activation is greater than the typical threshold stimulus level.

2. Paired twitch (**Figure 6**, *B*)—If a successive nerve stimulus arrives before the resting tension reaches baseline, the tension rises above the level of a single twitch.

   a. This phenomenon is called summation (wave summation or temporal summation).

   b. As the frequency of gross muscle stimulation increases, higher peak tensions develop (**Figure 6**, *C*).

   c. A plateau of maximal tension eventually is reached (**Figure 6**, *D*) where there is no relaxation of muscle tension between successive stimuli (tetany).

B. Skeletal muscle can develop varying levels of muscle force, even though each individual motor unit contracts in an all-or-none fashion. This graded response is controlled by different mechanisms.

   1. Spatial summation—Different motor units have different thresholds of stimulation, and therefore more motor units are activated with increased stimulus intensity.

   2. Temporal summation—Increasing stimulus frequency results in increased tension development by each individual motor unit (eg, tetany).

   3. Maximal force production is proportional to muscle physiologic cross-sectional area (PCSA); however, force production is not directly related to anatomic cross-sectional area.

      a. Other factors that contribute to PCSA are surface pennation angle (fiber angle relative to the force-generating axis of the muscle), muscle density, and fiber length.

      b. Longer fiber lengths allow for long excursions with less force production.

C. Types of muscle contraction

   1. Isotonic—Muscle shortens against a constant load. Muscle tension remains constant.

   2. Isokinetic—Muscle contracts at a constant velocity.

   3. Isometric—Muscle length remains static as tension is generated.

   4. Concentric—Muscular contraction that results in decrease in muscle length. This occurs when the resisting load is less than the muscle force generated.

   5. Eccentric—Muscular contraction that accommodates an increase in muscle length. This occurs when the resisting load is greater than the muscle force generated.

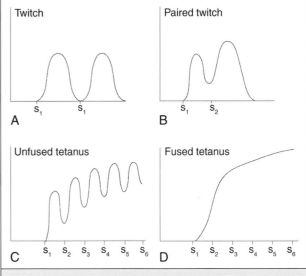

Figure 6   Twitch (**A** and **B**) and tetanus (**C** and **D**). As the frequency of stimulation is increased, muscle force rises to an eventual plateau level known as fused tetanus. (*Reproduced from Garrett WE, Best TM: Anatomy, physiology, and mechanics of skeletal muscle, in Buckwalter JA, Einhorn TA, Simon SR (eds):* Orthopaedic Basic Science: Biology and Biomechanics of the Musculoskeletal System, *ed 2. Rosemont, IL, American Academy of Orthopaedic Surgeons, 2000, p 691.*)

   6. Isotonic and isokinetic contractions can demonstrate either concentric action or eccentric action. However, isometric contractions do not fit the definition of either concentric or eccentric action.

D. Force-velocity relationship (**Figure 7**)—Under experimental conditions, a load is applied to a contracting muscle until no change in length is seen (isometric length). As higher external load is applied, the muscle begins to lengthen and tension increases rapidly (eccentric contraction). If load is decreased from the isometrically contracting muscle, the muscle force will rapidly decrease and the muscle will shorten in length (concentric contraction). Progressively decreased loads result in increased contraction.

   1. Concentric contractions—The force generated by the muscle is always less than the muscle's maximum force. As seen from the force-velocity curve, the force drops off rapidly as velocity increases. For example, when the muscle velocity increases to only 17% of maximum, the muscle force has decreased to 50% of maximum.

   2. Eccentric contractions—The absolute tension quickly becomes very high relative to the maximum isometric tension. Eccentric generates the highest tension and greatest risk for musculotendinous injury. The absolute tension is relatively independent of the velocity.

1: Basic Science

E. Fiber types

1. The muscle fibers of each motor unit share the same contractile and metabolic properties.

2. These muscle fibers may be one of three primary types (types I, IIA, or IIB), characterized according to their structural, biochemical, and physiologic characteristics (**Table 1**).

   a. Type I fibers (slow-contracting, oxidative)

      i. High aerobic capacity

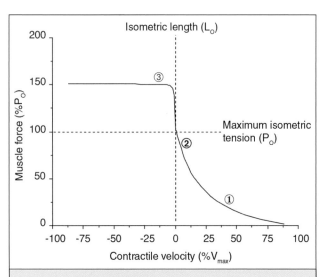

Figure 7   The muscle force-velocity curve for skeletal muscle obtain using sequential isotonic contractions. Note that force increases dramatically upon forced muscle lengthening and drops precipitously upon muscle shortening. (*Reproduced with permission from Lieber R (ed):* Skeletal Muscle Structure, Function, and Plasticity: The Physiological Basis of Rehabilitation, *ed 2. Philadelphia, PA, Lippincott Williams & Wilkins, 2002, p. 62.*)

      ii. Resistant to fatigue

      iii. Contain more mitochondria and more capillaries per fiber than other types

      iv. Slower contraction and relaxation times than other fiber types

   b. Type IIA (fast-contracting and oxidative and glycolytic)—Intermediate fiber type between the slow oxidative type I fiber and the fast glycolytic type IIB fiber.

   c. Type IIB (fast-contracting, glycolytic)

      i. Primarily anaerobic

      ii. Least resistant to fatigue

      iii. Most rapid contraction time

      iv. Largest motor unit size

   d. Strength training may result in an increased percentage of type IIB fibers, whereas endurance training may increase the percentage of type IIA fibers.

IV. Energetics

A. Three main energy systems provide fuel for muscular contractions.

   1. The phosphagen system (**Figure 8**)

      a. The adenosine triphosphate (ATP) molecule is hydrolyzed and converted directly to adenosine diphosphate (ADP), inorganic phosphate, and energy. ADP may also be further hydrolyzed to create adenosine monophosphate (AMP), again releasing inorganic phosphate and energy.

Table 1

Characteristics of Human Skeletal Muscle Fiber Types

	Type I	Type IIA	Type IIB
Other Names	Red, slow twitch (ST) Slow oxidative (SO)	White, fast twitch (FT) Fast oxidative glycolytic (FOG)	Fast glycolytic (FG)
Speed of contraction	Slow	Fast	Fast
Strength of contraction	Low	High	High
Fatigability	Fatigue-resistant	Fatigable	Most fatigable
Aerobic capacity	High	Medium	Low
Anaerobic capacity	Low	Medium	High
Motor unit size	Small	Larger	Largest
Capillary density	High	High	Low

(*Reproduced from Garrett WE, Best TM: Anatomy, physiology, and mechanics of skeletal muscle, in Buckwalter JA, Einhorn TA, Simon SR (eds):* Orthopaedic Basic Science: Biology and Biomechanics of the Musculoskeletal System, *ed 2. Rosemont, IL, American Academy of Orthopaedic Surgeons, 2000, p 692.*)

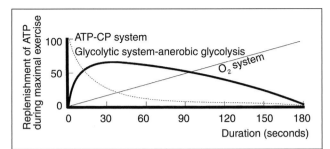

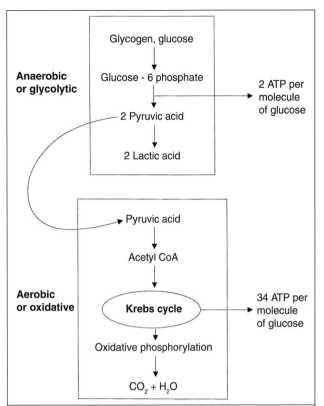

Figure 8 Energy sources for anaerobic activity. (*Reproduced from Garrett WE, Best TM: Anatomy, physiology, and mechanics of skeletal muscle, in Buckwalter JA, Einhorn TA, Simon SR (eds):* Orthopaedic Basic Science: Biology and Biomechanics of the Musculoskeletal System, *ed 2. Rosemont, IL, American Academy of Orthopaedic Surgeons, 2000, p 694.*)

Figure 9 Diagram summarizing ATP yield in the anaerobic and aerobic breakdown of carbohydrates. Glycolysis and anaerobic metabolism occur in the cytoplasm; oxidative phosphorylation occurs in the mitochondria. (*Reproduced from Garrett WE, Best TM: Anatomy, physiology, and mechanics of skeletal muscle, in Buckwalter JA, Einhorn TA, Simon SR (eds):* Orthopaedic Basic Science: Biology and Biomechanics of the Musculoskeletal System, *ed 2. Rosemont, IL, American Academy of Orthopaedic Surgeons, 2000, p 696.*)

b. Creatine phosphate is another source of high-energy phosphate bonds. However, its high-energy phosphate bond is used by creatine kinase to synthesize ATP from ADP.

c. Myokinase is used to combine two ADP molecules to create one ATP molecule and one AMP molecule.

d. Total energy from the entire phosphagen system is enough to fuel the body to run approximately 200 yards.

e. No lactate is produced via this pathway; also, no oxygen is used.

2. Anaerobic metabolism (glycolytic or lactic acid metabolism) (**Figure 9**)

a. Glucose is transformed into two molecules of lactic acid, creating enough energy to convert two molecules of ADP to ATP.

b. This system provides metabolic energy for approximately 20 to 120 seconds of intense activity.

c. Oxygen is not used in this pathway.

3. Aerobic metabolism (**Figure 10**)

a. Glucose is broken into two molecules of pyruvic acid, which then enter the Krebs cycle, resulting in a net gain of 34 ATP per glucose molecule.

b. Glucose exists in the cell in a limited quantity of glucose-6-phosphate. Additional sources of energy include stored muscle glycogen.

c. Fats and proteins also can be converted to energy via aerobic metabolism.

d. Oxygen is used in this pathway.

B. Training effects on muscle

1. Strength training usually consists of high-load, low-repetition exercise and results in increased muscle cross-sectional area. This is more likely due to muscle hypertrophy (increased size of muscle fibers) rather than hyperplasia (increased number of muscle fibers).

a. Increased motor unit recruitment or improved synchronization of muscle activation is another way weight training contributes to strength gains.

b. Strength training results in adaptation of all fiber types.

c. Little evidence exists at a microscopic, cellular level that muscle cell injury is required to generate muscle strengthening or hypertrophy.

2. Endurance training

a. Aerobic training results in changes in both central and peripheral circulation as well as muscle metabolism. Energy efficiency is the primary adaptation seen in contractile muscle.

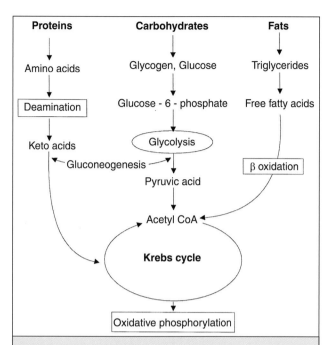

Figure 10 Foodstuffs (fats, carbohydrates, proteins) containing carbon and hydrogen for glycolysis, fatty acid oxidation, and the Krebs cycle in a muscle cell. (*Reproduced from Garrett WE, Best TM: Anatomy, physiology, and mechanics of skeletal muscle, in Buckwalter JA, Einhorn TA, Simon SR (eds):* Orthopaedic Basic Science: Biology and Biomechanics of the Musculoskeletal System, *ed 2. Rosemont, IL, American Academy of Orthopaedic Surgeons, 2000, p 695.*)

b. Mitochondrial size, number, and density increase. Enzyme systems of the Krebs cycle, respiratory chain, and those involved with the supply and processing of fatty acids by mitochondria all increase markedly.

c. Metabolic adaptations occur that result in an increased use of fatty acids rather than glycogen.

d. The oxidative capacity of all three fiber types increases. In addition, the percentage of the more highly oxygenated type IIA fibers increases.

V. Muscle Injury and Repair

A. Cytokines and growth factors regulate the repair processes after muscle injury. Sources of cytokines include infiltrating neutrophils, monocytes, and macrophages; activated fibroblasts; and stimulated endothelial cells.

1. Necrotic muscle fibers are removed by macrophages. New muscle cells are thought to arise from satellite cells, which are undifferentiated cells that exist in a quiescent state until needed for a reparative response.

2. The simultaneous formation of fibrotic connective tissue or scar may interfere with a full recovery of muscle tissue after injury.

B. Delayed-onset muscle soreness (DOMS) is muscle ache and pain that typically occurs 24 to 72 hours after intense exercise.

1. DOMS is primarily associated with eccentric loading–type exercise.

2. Several theories have been proposed to explain DOMS, the most popular being that structural muscle injury occurs and leads to progressive edema formation and resultant increased intramuscular pressure.

3. These changes seem to occur primarily in type IIB fibers.

C. Muscle contusion is a nonpenetrating blunt injury to muscle resulting in hematoma and inflammation. Characteristics include:

1. Later development of scar formation and variable amount of muscle regeneration.

2. New synthesis of extracellular connective tissue within 2 days of the injury, with peak at 5 to 21 days.

3. Myositis ossificans (bone formation within muscle) secondary to blunt trauma. This sometimes mimics osteogenic sarcoma on radiographs and biopsy. Myositis ossificans becomes apparent approximately 2 to 4 weeks post-injury.

4. Muscle strain

a. Both complete and incomplete muscle tears usually occur by passive stretch of an activated muscle.

b. Muscles at greatest risk are those that cross two joints, eg, the rectus femoris and gastrocnemius.

c. Incomplete muscle tears also typically occur at the myotendinous junction, with hemorrhage and fiber disruption. A cellular inflammatory response occurs for the first few days, with the muscle demonstrating decreased ability to generate active tension. In an animal model, force production normalized after 7 days.

d. Complete muscle tears typically occur near the myotendinous junction. They are characterized by muscle contour abnormality.

5. Muscle laceration

a. After complete laceration of muscle, fragments heal by dense connective scar tissue. Regeneration of muscle tissue across the laceration or reinnervation is not predictable, and only partial recovery is likely.

b. Muscle activation does not cross the scar.

c. Unstimulated muscle segment shows histologic characteristics of denervated muscle.

D. Immobilization and disuse

1. Immobilization and disuse results in muscle atrophy with associated loss of strength and increased fatigability.

2. A nonlinear rate of atrophy occurs, with changes occurring primarily during initial days. Atrophy is seen at a cellular level, with loss of myofibrils within the muscle fibers.

3. Atrophic changes are related to the length at which muscle is immobilized. Atrophy and strength loss are more prominent when muscle is immobilized under no tension; eg, when the knee is immobilized in extension, quadriceps atrophy is greater than hamstring atrophy.

4. Muscle fiber held under stretch creates new contractile proteins with sarcomeres added onto existing fibrils. This slightly offsets the atrophy of cross-sectional muscle mass.

Top Testing Facts

1. Muscle fiber is a collection of myofibrils.

2. Fascicles are collections of muscle fibers.

3. Actin's binding sites for myosin are blocked by tropomyosin.

4. Know all bands and lines of sarcomere organization—A, I, H, M, and Z. (See section II.D and Figure 4.)

5. Site of action of both depolarizing and non-depolarizing drugs is the NMJ.

6. Maximal force production is proportional to muscle physiologic cross-sectional area (PCSA).

7. Phosphagen energy system has enough ATP for approximately 20 seconds of activity.

8. DOMS peaks at 24 to 72 hours post-exercise, is most common in type IIB fibers, and is associated primarily with eccentric exercise.

9. Eccentric contraction generates the highest tension and greatest risk for musculotendinous injury.

10. Muscle strain is most likely in muscles that cross two joints.

Bibliography

Best TM, Kirkendall DT, Almekinders LC, Garrett WE Jr: Basic science of soft tissue, in DeLee J, Drez D, Miller MD (eds): *Orthopaedic Sports Medicine: Principles and Practice.* Philadelphia, PA, Saunders, 2002, vol 1, pp 1-19.

Garrett WE Jr, Best TM: Anatomy, physiology, and mechanics of skeletal muscle, in Buckwalter JA, Einhorn TA, Simon SR (eds): *Orthopaedic Basic Science: Biology and Biomechanics of the Musculoskeletal System.* Rosemont, IL, American Academy of Orthopaedic Surgeons, 2000, pp 683-716.

Lieber RL: Form and function of skeletal muscle, in Einhorn TA, O'Keefe RJ, Buckwalter JA (eds): *Orthopaedic Basic Science: Biology and Biomechanics of the Musculoskeletal System,* ed 3. Rosemont, IL, American Academy of Orthopaedic Surgeons, 2007, pp 223-242.

1: Basic Science

Chapter 10
Intervertebral Disk

S. Tim Yoon, MD, PhD

I. Function

A. The intervertebral disk connects adjacent vertebral bodies.

B. The disk and the facet joints constitute the functional spinal unit that provides mechanical stability and allows physiologic motion.

II. Anatomy

A. Nucleus pulposus (**Figure 1**)

1. The nucleus pulposus is the central portion of the disk.

2. The hydrophilic matrix of the nucleus pulposus provides the swelling pressure that contributes to the normal height of the disk.

3. The matrix is viscoelastic and therefore dampens and distributes forces evenly across the end plate and anulus fibrosus.

4. The nucleus pulposus is hypoxic and relatively acidic. Nucleus pulposus cells are more synthetically active in this type of environment.

5. The nucleus pulposus has primarily type II collagen.

B. Anulus fibrosus

1. The anulus fibrosus surrounds and contains the centrally located nucleus pulposus.

2. The anulus fibrosus has high tensile strength and resists intervertebral distraction, but it is flexible enough to deform and allow intervertebral motion.

3. As the nucleus pulposus degenerates, the anulus fibrosus takes proportionately more axial load.

4. The annulus has primarily type I collagen.

C. End plates

1. The end plates form the interface between the vertebra and the disk and define the upper and lower boundaries of the disk.

2. The central portion of the end plate provides a major pathway for nutrients from the vertebral bodies to diffuse into the disk.

D. Vascular supply

1. In the adult, the disk is avascular. The blood supply ends at the bony end plate of the vertebral body and the outer anulus fibrosus. Thus most of the disk is considered immunologically isolated.

2. Because of this avascularity, the nutritional supply to the disk cells is primarily though diffusion (**Figure 2**). As the disk gets larger, the distances nutrition must diffuse across become larger, further impeding nutritional supply to the disk cells.

E. Innervation

1. The disk is minimally innervated. The sinuvertebral nerve (which arises from the dorsal root ganglion) innervates the outer anulus fibrosus. Nerve fibers do not penetrate beyond this superficial

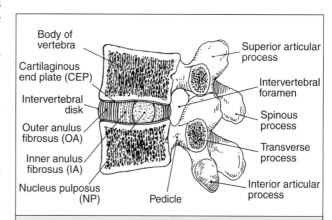

Figure 1   Sagittal section view of a motion segment comprising two vertebral bodies and an intervertebral disk forming a strong connection between the bones. The four regions of the disk are shown: cartilaginous end plate, outer anulus fibrosus, inner anulus fibrosus, and nucleus pulposus. The posterior articular and spinous processes and the articular surface of a facet joint are also shown. (*Reproduced with permission from Ashton-Miller JA, Schultz AB: Biomechanics of the human spine, in Mow VC, Hayes WC (eds): Basic Orthopaedic Biomechanics. Philadelphia, PA, Lippincott Williams & Wilkins, 1997, pp 353-393.*)

1: Basic Science

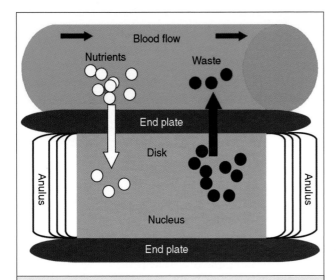

Figure 2 Disk nutrition. The blood supply reaches the bony end plate but does not cross into the disk. The nutrients diffuse across the end plate to reach disk cells. The metabolic waste products leave the disk tissue by diffusing across the end plate and are carried away by blood flow.

zone; therefore, most of the disk is not innervated.

2. Pain sensation from the disk arises only from the anulus fibrosus, but the nucleus pulposus can generate pain molecules that can stimulate the nerves found in the anulus fibrosus.

III. Biologic Activity

A. Homeostasis

1. Disk cells are metabolically active, synthesizing disk matrix, catabolic enzymes, and growth factors (BMP-2, BMP-7, TGF-β, etc). Although disk cells constitute only a small proportion of the volume of the adult disk, they are responsible for maintaining the volume and composition of the disk matrix.

2. The normal turnover rate of the disk matrix is slow, but even a small deviation in the balance of disk homeostasis can result in disk degeneration over a period of years.

B. Cell characteristics by region

1. Nucleus pulposus cells are chondrocyte-like.

a. They exist in a hypoxic environment.

b. They characteristically synthesize proteoglycans (aggrecan, versican, and small leucine-rich proteoglycans [SLRPs]), collagen type II, and other matrix molecules.

2. Anulus fibrosus cells are fibroblast-like.

a. They characteristically produce type I collagen but also produce other matrix molecules, including proteoglycans.

b. The inner anulus cells produce relatively more proteoglycans than the outer anulus cells.

IV. Disease

A. Aging

1. Disks undergo a natural degenerative process during aging that does not implicate a disease process.

2. In the young individual, the disk is tall, the nucleus pulposus is very watery, and the anulus fibrosus is intact. In the young child, the nucleus pulposus cells are mostly notochordal cells.

3. By age 10 years, notochordal cells have disappeared and are replaced by chondrocyte-like cells.

4. With increasing age, the disk cells produce less aggrecan and type II collagen, leading to decreases in proteoglycan and water content. As the nucleus pulposus desiccates, disk height is lost and the anulus fibrosus develops fissures.

5. 90% of asymptomatic individuals older than 60 years have MRI evidence of disk degeneration.

B. Genetics

1. Strong evidence suggests that genetics plays an important role in disk degeneration. Twins studies have indicated that genetic factors are more important determinants of disk degeneration than factors such as lifetime occupation and leisure activities.

2. Mutations in the vitamin D receptor and COL9A2 genes have been implicated in disk degeneration.

3. A mutation in the cartilage intermediate layer protein (CILP) has been associated with an increased need for surgery to treat sciatica resulting from lumbar disk herniation.

C. Pain

1. Disk degeneration has been statistically associated with a higher incidence of low back pain, but the presence of one or more degenerated disks does not directly correlate with low back pain.

2. Despite improvements in imaging modalities such as MRI and CT, imaging studies remain unreliable in identifying a painful disk.

3. Diskography assesses disk morphology and may be helpful in identifying a painful disk (pain generator).

a. Diskography involves introducing a needle into the disk and injecting fluid under pressure.

b. Elicitation of the familiar, or concordant, pain is considered a positive test.

c. Diskography has been shown to have a high false-positive rate, especially in patients with chronic pain and abnormal psychometric testing results. There is a low predictive power for good results after fusion surgery.

V. Repair

A. Natural repair process—Perhaps because the disk is avascular, spontaneous biologic repair processes are quite limited and are thought to be ineffective.

B. Biologic therapy—Disk repair has been successful in some small animal experiments, but as of yet no credible report of success in humans has been published.

Top Testing Facts

1. The disk allows motion and provides mechanical stability of the functional spinal unit.

2. The disk is mostly avascular and depends on diffusion through pores in the end plate to provide nutrition to the disk cells.

3. Nucleus pulposus cells are more synthetically active in a hypoxic environment.

4. The nucleus pulposus is normally rich in aggregating proteoglycans (aggrecan and versican), which attract water and help maintain disk height. The nucleus pulposus has a higher concentration of type II collagen than the anulus fibrosus.

5. The anulus fibrosus is a well-organized laminated fibrous tissue composed primarily of type I collagen.

6. With increasing age, the disk cells produce less aggrecan and type II collagen, leading to decreases in proteoglycan and water content. As the nucleus pulposus desiccates, disk height is lost and the anulus fibrosus develops fissures.

7. Ninety percent of asymptomatic individuals older than 60 years have MRI evidence of disk degeneration.

8. Genetics plays a strong role in disk degeneration, but this seems to involve a multifactorial process that does not fit a Mendelian pattern.

9. Disk degeneration is not necessarily a painful condition.

10. Diskography has a high false-positive rate in patients with abnormal psychometric testing results.

1: Basic Science

Bibliography

Anderson DG, Tannoury C: Molecular pathogenic factors in symptomatic disc degeneration. *Spine J* 2005;5:260S-266S.

Battie MC, Videman T: Lumbar disc degeneration: Epidemiology and genetics. *J Bone Joint Surg Am* 2006;88(suppl 2): 3-9.

Park AE, Boden SD: Form and function of the intervertebral disk, in Einhorn TA, O'Keefe RJ, Buckwalter JA (eds): *Orthopaedic Basic Science: Foundations of Clinical Practice*, ed 3. Rosemont, IL, American Academy of Orthopaedic Surgeons, 2007, pp 259-264.

Chapter 11
Musculoskeletal Infections and Microbiology

R. Stephen J. Burnett, MD, FRCSC   Nikos Pavlides, MD

I. Introduction

A. Infections may involve bone (osteomyelitis), joint spaces (septic arthritis), soft tissues (muscle, fascia, subcutaneous tissues, skin), or the disks and spinal column, and may present with either an acute or an indolent/chronic clinical course.

B. Infections may occur de novo or at a previous surgical site.

C. Infectious agents include bacterial, viral, fungal, or other microorganisms.

II. Clinical Presentation

A. History and physical examination

1. The most common symptom is pain localized to the site of infection; it is rare for patients to not report pain as a presenting symptom.

2. History of previous trauma in the region of the symptoms: a penetrating injury, break in the skin, or laceration.

3. Intermittent fevers, chills, sweats (night sweats with chronic infections), general malaise, reduced appetite, and weight loss (chronic infection).

4. Localized soft-tissue swelling and/or warmth, redness or skin discoloration, or fluctuance in the vicinity of the pain.

5. Symptoms of untreated infection may progress rapidly, leading to hypotension, shock, coma, or death.

B. Septic arthritis

1. In addition to the general symptoms described earlier, recent loss of and unwillingness to perform range of joint motion is suggestive of acute septic arthritis.

2. *Neisseria gonorrhea* is historically a common causative organism in young males with isolated monoarticular septic arthritis of the knee.

a. Migratory polyarthritis, rash, and tenosynovitis of the dorsal wrist and hand may occur.

b. The knee joint is most commonly involved.

3. *Staphylococcus aureus* is the second most common pathogen causing adult septic arthritis.

4. In children, involvement of the hip produces a flexed, abducted, externally rotated position to accommodate the increased joint volume.

C. Adult osteomyelitis

1. Chronic draining sinuses are commonly present in chronic osteomyelitis. A history of acute purulent drainage from the skin, preceded by fever, pain, localized swelling, tenderness, and systemic symptoms is suggestive of a draining sinus associated with osteomyelitis. Such sinuses are complicated by malignant squamous cell carcinoma transformation in 1% of cases.

2. *S aureus* is the most common causative organism, although other microorganisms can be involved (**Table 1**).

3. The ability of the host to respond to any type of clinical infection has been classified by Cierny (**Table 2**).

4. The tibia is the most common site.

5. Hematogenous osteomyelitis may occur in IV drug users.

6. Two types of pediatric osteomyelitis have been identified: acute hematogenous (AHO) and subacute hematogenous (SHO).

7. Chronic pediatric recurrent multifocal osteomyelitis is usually bilateral and symmetric. It is often associated with intermittent symptoms and a pustular rash on the palms.

D. Necrotizing infections

1. Necrotizing fasciitis

a. Necrotizing fasciitis is any necrotizing soft-tissue infection spreading along fascial planes, with or without overlying cellulitis. The edema

---

Table 1

Microoganisms Isolated From Patients With Bacterial Osteomyelitis

Microorganism	Most Common Clinical Association
S aureus (susceptible or resistant to methicillin)	Most frequent microorganism in any type of osteomyelitis
Coagulase-negative staphylococci or propionibacterium	Foreign-body–associated infection
Enterobacteriaceae or *Pseudomonas aeruginosa*	Common in nosocomial infections
Streptococci or anaerobic bacteria	Associated with bites, clenched-fist injury caused by contact with another person's mouth, diabetic foot lesions, and decubitus ulcers
Salmonella or *Streptococcus pneumoniae*	Sickle cell disease
Bartonella henselae	Human immunodeficiency virus infection
Pasteurella multocida or *Eikenella corrodens*	Human or animal bites
Aspergillus, *Mycobacterium avium* complex, or *Candida albicans*	Immunocompromised patients
Mycobacterium tuberculosis	Populations in which tuberculosis is prevalent
Brucella, *Coxiella burnetii* (chronic Q fever), or other fungi found in specific geographic areas	Populations in which these pathogens are endemic

(*Adapted from Gross JM, Schwarz EM: Infections in Orthopaedics, in Einhorn TA, O'Keefe RJ, Buckwalter JA (eds): Orthopaedic Basic Science, ed 3. Rosemont, IL, American Academy of Orthopaedic Surgeons, 2007, pp 299-314.*)

Table 2

Cierny Classification of Host Response to Infection

Class	Response
A	Normal response to infection and surgery
B	Compromised, with local, systemic, or combined deficiencies in wound healing
C	Development of a condition that is potentially more compromising than the presenting infection

and induration extend beyond the area of erythema.

b. Either of the well-defined bacterial groups responsible for necrotizing fasciitis infections may be introduced into the soft tissues in contaminated environments, including IV drug use, hypodermic therapeutic injections, insect bites, or skin abrasions.

c. Clinical signs

    i. Severe pain, hyperpyrexia, and chills

    ii. The infection typically begins as a localized abscess, particularly among at-risk groups such as IV drug users, patients with diabetes mellitus, alcoholics, post-abdominal surgery patients, obese patients, or patients with ei-

ther perineal infections or peripheral vascular disease.

    iii. The initial findings are localized pain and minimal swelling, often with no visible trauma or discoloration of the skin.

    iv. Dermal induration and erythema eventually become evident; blistering of the epidermis is a late finding. Necrotizing fasciitis may be caused by a single organism (*Streptococci pyogenes* or *Streptococci vibrio*) or a combination of organisms. Anaerobic or microaerophilic streptococci are believed to be the usual cause, but these microorganisms are difficult to culture.

    v. The diagnosis may be missed initially in a patient presenting with mild symptoms such as pain, edema, tachycardia, and fear because signs such as skin bullae and subcutaneous gas have not yet developed.

    vi. The underlying tissue destruction initially manifests itself in the skin with painful ischemic patches and overlying blisters that consolidate over the course of 3 to 5 days to form cutaneous gangrene. The tissue becomes less painful due to small vessel thrombosis, neurotoxin production, and necrosis. The anesthesia may precede obvious skin necrosis and can aid in the early differential diagnosis of necrotizing fasciitis from simple cellulitis.

vii. High elevations of body temperature can help differentiate systemic necrotizing fasciitis from anaerobic cellulitis and clostridial myonecrosis, which produce modest, if any, changes in temperature.

2. Clostridial myonecrosis (gas gangrene)

   a. Triad of symptoms strongly suggests Clostridial myonecrosis:

      i. Progressively severe pain out of proportion to obvious injury

      ii. Tachycardia not explained by fever

      iii. Crepitus

   b. The buttocks, thighs, and perineum are common sites of infection.

   c. *Clostridium perfringens* and other clostridial species are common pathogens, but the condition can also develop from gram-negative and gram-positive (streptococcal) infections.

   d. Clinical presentation usually includes progressive pain; edema (distant from wound); foul-smelling, serosanguinous discharge; and feeling of impending doom. Other findings include ecchymosis, necrosis, edematous skin, dark red serous fluid, and numerous gas-filled vesicles and bullae.

   e. Intense pain out of proportion to the wound is characteristic; within hours, signs of systemic toxicity appear, including confusion, tachycardia, and diaphoresis.

   f. This infection may be associated with bowel cancer.

   g. Radiographs typically show widespread gas in tissues.

   h. Treatment is high-dose penicillin (and aminoglycoside and cephalosporin), hyperbaric oxygen (inhibits toxins), and surgical irrigation and débridement.

III. Diagnostic Evaluation

A. Radiographic findings

   1. Swelling and loss of tissue planes are evident at an early stage of osteomyelitis.

   2. Bone changes will not be present until 1 to 2 weeks of established infection.

   3. Bone loss of 30% to 40% is required before the classic signs of osteomyelitis are seen: bone resorption, destruction, periosteal elevation.

   4. New periosteal bone forms parallel to the cortex, tapering to the cortex farther from the nidus of

infection. The elevated periosteum lays down new bone initially (involucrum) around the shell of old bone, and the dead medullary or cortical bone becomes a sequestrum by occlusion of the nutrient vessels caused by infection.

B. Nuclear medicine imaging

   1. Three-phase technetium Tc 99m bone scan

      a. Bone infection is strongly suspected when the radioactive material localizes in the bone after 3 hours.

      b. Measures osteoblastic activity. Sensitive for detecting AHO and septic arthritis.

      c. False-negative "cold" bone scans sometimes occur in neonates. False-positive results may be seen with other disease processes, including fractures, tumors, and sickle cell disease.

      d. Technetium scans may be positive for up to 2 years after total joint arthroplasty (TJA).

   2. Leukocyte-labeled indium In 111 scan

      a. Delayed-imaging process obtained at 48 hours after injection.

      b. Reinjected white blood cells (WBCs) accumulate at the sites of inflammation and help distinguish between an infectious and noninfectious etiology (85% sensitivity; 75% to 94% specificity).

      c. Combining these two radioisotope scans (Tc 99m and In 111) produces a 90% to 93% sensitivity and 85% to 89% specificity for infection.

   3. Positron-emission tomography (PET) scans have 100% sensitivity and 88% specificity in the diagnosis of chronic musculoskeletal infection.

C. CT scans

   1. CT may be useful to localize a nidus of infection within an area of focal osteomyelitis.

   2. Reconstructed images provide anatomic bone images helpful for localizing infection and surgical planning.

   3. CT findings may include interosseous gas, decreased density of infected bone, and soft-tissue masses.

D. MRI

   1. MRI is superior to CT for the evaluation of soft tissues and bone marrow. It will detect subtle marrow changes associated with very early stage osteomyelitis with nearly 100% sensitivity.

   2. Classic findings

      a. Signal change due to the increased edema and water content in bone.

1: Basic Science

b. Reduction in T1 marrow signal and an increase in T2 signal. T2 images have an increased signal because the fatty marrow has been replaced by inflammation.

3. Also useful for localizing sequestra, areas of focal infection/abscess, and sinus tracts.

E. Blood tests

1. C-reactive protein (CRP) and erythrocyte sedimentation rate (ESR) measure acute-phase response markers that are elevated in the presence of infection and/or inflammation.

2. CRP (elevated in 98% of pediatric patients with osteomyelitis) rises within a few hours of infection, reaching values up to 400 mg/L within 36 to 50 hours. It may normalize within 1 week of treatment of the infection.

3. ESR (elevated in 92% of pediatric patients with osteomyelitis) rises within 2 days of the onset of infection and continues to rise for 3 to 5 days after appropriate antibiotic treatment is instituted. The ESR returns to normal after 3 to 4 weeks. Surgical treatment prolongs both the peak time and normalization time of the ESR and CRP.

4. Normal values may vary between laboratories; however, an ESR value of 30 and a CRP of 5 are commonly considered upper limits of normal.

5. Elevated peripheral WBC count with increased number and percentage of polymorphonuclear leukocytes (PMNs) is indicative of infection, but these values are elevated in less than 50% of patients with septic arthritis. Therefore, the absence of this finding does not rule out infection, and this value alone should not be used to diagnose infection.

F. Infection site cultures

1. The use of tissue or fluid cultures from the site of infection is the gold standard for treatment and allows directed antimicrobial therapy.

2. A WBC count >50,000/mm^3 is found in the synovial fluid aspirate of 50% of patients with septic arthritis.

3. Gram stain may identify the infecting organism in one third of patients with septic arthritis. Despite this low yield, initial antibiotic therapy may be directed if organisms are visualized.

4. Obtaining multiple cultures to test for anaerobic and aerobic organisms, tuberculosis, and fungal infection is mandatory.

5. Prior or concurrent administration of antibiotics, aspiration in a joint containing antibiotic-impregnated bone cement, sampling error during aspiration or biopsy, or improper handling or processing of specimens may produce inaccurate results.

G. Periprosthetic TJA infections

1. Synovial fluid WBC count >2,500/mm^3 or >90% PMN is strongly indicative of infection in a total knee arthroplasty (TKA). Synovial fluid with a majority of neutrophils is suggestive of an infection in a TKA or total hip arthroplasty (THA).

2. The use of antibiotics before aspiration is a major cause of false-negative results.

3. If the TJA patient has recently received antibiotics, a 4- to 6-week delay before aspiration is recommended.

4. For periprosthetic THA infections, Gram staining has 19% sensitivity and 98% specificity.

5. Intraoperative frozen sections using >5 PMN/hpf improves the sensitivity and specificity to 80% and 94%, respectively, in THA infection.

IV. Pathophysiology of Bacterial Musculoskeletal Infections

A. Pathogenesis—Several complex interactions must take place before musculoskeletal infection can develop. This process involves the inoculation of the microorganism, interaction with the host soft tissues, virulence, release of toxins and creation of an inflammatory reaction, and local and systemic host factors that influence the infection.

1. Inoculation of the microorganism

a. S aureus is the most common organism responsible for musculoskeletal infections.

b. The ability of any organism to enter the host system depends on the mode of entry or inoculation and the host environment. The four most common forms of entry of microorganisms into the host system are:

i. Surgical procedures

ii. Trauma or injury to the musculoskeletal system (bone and soft tissues)

iii. Hematogenous spread

iv. Spread from a contiguous source

2. Possible interactions of the bacteria with the host:

a. Destroyed by the host

b. Live symbiotically with the host

c. Flourish and cause host sepsis

3. Virulence—Ability of the microorganism to overcome the host defenses and cause clinical infection.

Table 3			
Classification of Periprosthetic TKA and THA Infections			
	Timing	**Definition**	**Treatment**
Type 1	Positive intraoperative culture	≥ 2 positive cultures	Antibiotics
Type 2	Early postoperative infection	< 4 weeks postoperative	Irrigation and débridement plus component retention; IV antibiotics for 6 weeks; 2-stage revision often necessary
Type 3	Acute hematogenous infection	Acute hematogenous seeding from a distant source of a previously well-functioning prosthetic joint	Irrigation and débridement plus component retention. 2-stage revision if this fails. IV antibiotics for 6 weeks
Type 4	Late (chronic) Infection	Chronic indolent course; infection present > 1 month or chronic sinus drainage	Removal of implant with 2-stage reimplantation; IV antibiotics for 6 weeks; consider longer oral antibiotic treatment postoperatively; consider reimplantation once infection is eradicated

a. The virulence of an organism varies among and within species.

b. The virulence of *S aureus* is multifactorial, allowing this organism to survive and perpetuate infection.

c. *S aureus* is protected from host immune defenses by three mechanisms:

   i. Excretion of protein A, which inactivates IgG.

   ii. Production of a capsular polysaccharide, which reduces opsonization and phagocytosis of the organism.

   iii. Formation of a biofilm (a "slime" containing an aggregation of microbial colonies embedded within a glycocalyx matrix that most commonly develops on TJA implants or a devitalized bone surface), which also secludes the organism from host defense mechanisms.

4. Local host factors that increase the likelihood of infection:

   a. Reduced host vascularity

   b. Neuropathy

   c. Trauma

   d. Presence of prosthetic implants

B. Periprosthetic infections

1. *S aureus* and *Staphylococcus epidermidis* most common

2. Classification of periprosthetic THA and TKA infections—**Table 3** lists types of these infections and their treatment. Two-stage reimplantation is the gold standard for management of infected THAs and TKAs.

C. Immune response to microorganisms

1. Systemic factors such as renal or hepatic disease, malignancy, or malnutrition may reduce the ability of the host immune system to respond to the microorganism.

2. The immune response to bacterial infection comprises both cell-mediated and humoral components.

3. When PMNs attack the microorganism, damage to the bacteria releases additional chemotactic molecules, attracting larger numbers of PMNs. Bacteria in proximity to PMNs may be phagocytosed; for this to occur, opsonins or components in the serum must coat the bacteria, making them more attractive for the macrophages.

4. Nonspecific immune responses may be affected by medications such as NSAIDs, steroids, and aspirin.

5. Steroids have been implicated in reduced chemotaxis in PMNs in a tibial osteomyelitis model.

D. Infection in joints with intra-articular metaphysis

1. May result in contiguous septic arthritis.

2. Occurs most classically in the proximal femur in the child.

3. Alternatively, as the metaphyseal infection exits the bone, it may form a sinus tract to the skin.

E. Etiology of bacterial infections

1. Pathogen depends on the circumstances of the infection, patient age, and host immune response.

2. The most common pathogens and suggested empiric antibiotic therapies in musculoskeletal infections are outlined in **Table 4**.

1: Basic Science

Table 4

Most Common Pathogens and Suggested Empiric Antibiotic Therapy in Musculoskeletal Infections

Infection and Clinical Setting	Most Common Pathogens	Empiric Antibiotic Therapy
Osteomyelitis and septic arthritis		
Infant	S aureus S pyogenes S pneumoniae Gram-negative organisms	Penicillinase-resistant penicillin and aminoglycoside or ceftriaxone
Child < 3 years	S aureus S pneumoniae H influenzae (if nonimmunized)	Ceftriaxone
Older child	S aureus	Cefazolin or penicillinase-resistant penicillin
Child with sickle cell disease	Salmonella species S aureus	Ceftriaxone
Adult	S aureus Suspected MRSA	Penicillinase-resistant penicillin Vancomycin or clindamycin
Immunocompromised adult or child	Gram-positive cocci Gram-negative organisms	Penicillinase-resistant penicillin and aminoglycoside
Septic arthritis in sexually active patients	S aureus N gonorrhoeae	Ceftriaxone
Diskitis	S aureus	Penicillinase-resistant penicillin
Lyme disease	B burgdorferi	Amoxicillin-doxycycline
Clenched-fist bite wounds	E corrodens P multocida Anaerobes	Ampicillin-sulbactam or piperacillin-tazobactam
Nail puncture wounds	S aureus P aeruginosa	Penicillinase-resistant penicillin and aminoglycoside or piperacillin-tazobactam
Necrotizing fasciitis	Streptococcus group A beta-hemolytic Gram-positive cocci, anaerobes ± gram-negative organisms	Penicillin and clindamycin ± aminoglycoside

MRSA = methicillin resistant *Staphylococcus aureus*
(Reproduced from Patzakis MJ, Zalavras C: Infection, in Vaccaro AR (ed): Orthopaedic Knowledge Update 8. Rosemont, IL, American Academy of Orthopaedic Surgeons, 2005, pp 217-228.)

F. Cartilage injury

1. Septic arthritis with bacterial infection has the potential for irreversible cartilage destruction in an involved joint.

2. Initially, this occurs by dissolution of the glycosaminoglycan (GAG) units of cartilage. GAG units function as subunits of the proteoglycan molecule, in part giving rise to its physical properties of fluid retention or swelling pressure of the cartilage.

3. Following the destruction of the GAG units, collagen breakdown occurs and is evident by gross alteration in the cartilage. Subsequent rapid degenerative osteoarthritis may develop in association with this septic process.

V. Antibiotic Prophylaxis for Orthopaedic Surgery

A. Surgical prophylaxis is the administration of antibiotics to patients without clinical evidence of infection in the surgical field.

B. 25% to 50% of all antimicrobial usage is for the prevention rather than the treatment of infection.

C. Routine administration of prophylactic antibiotics to patients who will have a foreign body implanted, a bone graft procedure, or extensive dissection resulting in a potential residual dead space or subsequent hematoma is well accepted.

D. Routine use of prophylactic antibiotics in soft-tissue procedures or diagnostic arthroscopy is not well studied and continues to be controversial. Use of prophylaxis in these instances, especially in high-risk or immunocompromised patients, is at the discretion of the surgeon.

E. The most likely pathogens to cause infection in elective musculoskeletal procedures include *S aureus*, *S epidermidis*, aerobic streptococci, and anaerobic cocci.

F. Prophylaxis is indicated when the risk of infection is low but the development of an infection would have devastating results. Procedures with a high inherent infection rate are ideally suited for prophylaxis.

G. Open fractures

  1. Patients sustaining open fractures or traumatic open arthrotomy wounds should receive prophylactic antibiotics, and their tetanus status should be updated.

  2. All patients with open fractures should receive a first-generation cephalosporin. A randomized trial showed a reduction in open grade II infection rates from 29% to 9% when an aminoglycoside plus cephalosporin was used, compared to a cephalosporin alone. Alternatively, a second-generation cephalosporin is effective.

  3. In open fracture wounds with a high level of contamination, an additional agent may be required. Patients with open farmyard fractures should be treated with penicillin to prevent *C perfringens* infection; soil injuries require anaerobic coverage with either metronidazole or clindamycin. Open fracture wounds exposed to freshwater are at risk for contamination with *Pseudomonas* and require additional coverage with a third-generation cephalosporin or a fluoroquinolone. Coverage should include an aminoglycoside and penicillin to cover gram-negative and anaerobic organisms, respectively, in addition to a first-generation cephalosporin.

H. Hip fracture surgery and TJA

  1. Decreased incidence of postoperative surgical site infections (SSIs) has been reported when perioperative prophylactic antibiotics are used.

  2. A single preoperative IV dose followed by two postoperative doses of IV antibiotics is effective for prophylactic treatment. In TJA, a single preoperative dose of cefazolin was as effective as continuation for 48 hours postoperatively. More prolonged therapy is therefore not indicated in routine surgery. More prolonged postoperative therapy may be considered in certain situations, including compromised host, immune deficiency, periprosthetic infection surgery, second-stage reimplantation joint arthroplasty surgery, and surgery on a contaminated wound.

Table 5

Patients at Increased Risk of Hematogenous TJA Infection

All patients during the first 2 years after prosthetic joint replacement
Immunocompromised/immunosuppressed patients
Inflammatory arthropathies (rheumatoid arthritis, systemic lupus erythematosus)
Drug-induced immunosuppression
Radiation-induced immunosuppression
Patients with comorbidities such as previous prosthetic joint infections, malnourishment, hemophilia, human immunodeficiency virus infection, insulin-dependent (type 1) diabetes, malignancy

(Reproduced from Clark CR: Perioperative medical management, in Barrack RL, Booth RE Jr, Lonner JH, McCarthy JC, Mont MA, Rubash HE (eds): Orthopaedic Knowledge Update: Hip and Knee Reconstruction 3. Rosemont, IL, American Academy of Orthopaedic Surgeons, 2006, pp 205-216.)

I. Timing of antibiotic prophylaxis

  1. Preoperative IV antibiotics should be administered such that the antibiotics are in the system within 1 hour before the time of incision.

  2. When these agents are started after the surgical procedure is completed, infection rates are not significantly affected.

  3. Prophylaxis given several hours before surgery has a reduced efficacy.

  4. Administration 1 or more days in advance of surgery, altering the patient's normal host bacterial flora, may be detrimental.

J. Selection of antibiotic prophylaxis

  1. Cephalosporins are the perioperative prophylactic antibiotic of choice in most centers. These agents provide coverage against most bacteria associated with musculoskeletal SSIs, are relatively nontoxic (hypersensitivity is rare; they have <10% cross-reactivity with penicillin allergy), and they are relatively inexpensive.

  2. With the emergence of antimicrobial-resistant microorganisms, the incidence of methicillin-resistant *S aureus* infections (MRSAs) in association with SSIs has increased significantly.

  3. The SSI profile in individual hospitals varies; communication with the infection control representative will aid in the selection of preoperative antibiotic prophylaxis.

  4. Currently, in institutions where the incidence of MRSA SSIs is significant, vancomycin is used, either alone or in addition to a cephalosporin.

1: Basic Science

K. Antibiotic prophylaxis in dental patients with a TJA

1. The American Academy of Orthopaedic Surgeons and the American Dental Association have published an advisory statement regarding antibiotic prophylaxis in dental patients with a TJA.

2. Antibiotic prophylaxis is indicated in TJA patients at increased risk for hematogenous seeding (**Table 5**). Bacteremia may lead to hematogenous seeding even years following the TJA, with the highest risk within the first 2 years.

3. Antibiotics are not indicated for most dental patients with a TJA.

L. Antibiotic prophylaxis in urologic surgery patients with a TJA

1. Recommendations are similar to those for dental patients.

2. The only difference is that all patients with diabetes mellitus (types 1 and 2) are considered at risk and should receive antibiotic prophylaxis.

VI. Antibiotics—Mechanism of Action

A. The mechanism of action, ribosomal subunit binding, clinical use, side effect profiles, and pertinent pearls for the antibiotics most frequently prescribed to treat musculoskeletal infections are summarized in **Table 6**.

B. Mechanisms of antibiotic resistance are outlined in **Table 7**.

VII. Nonbacterial Infections

A. Tuberculosis

1. Tuberculosis infections are encountered in the United States. From 1985 through 1993 there was a 14% increase in morbidity in the United States. The correlated rise of HIV during that decade is the leading known risk factor for reactivation of latent infections and progression of active disease; an aging population and development of drug-resistant strains of *Mycobacterium tuberculosis* also have contributed to the increased rate.

2. The orthopaedic manifestation of tuberculosis infection may involve the entire skeletal system. The spine is the major site of infection, being involved in 50% of cases, half thoracic and one fourth in the cervical and lumbar spine.

3. Clinical presentation—Localized pain with fever and weight loss; when the spine is involved,

rigidity, paravertebral swelling, and possible neurologic findings.

4. Radiographic evaluation

a. Radiographic changes are limited early in the disease process, with 50% bone mass loss needed for significant changes to be apparent.

b. Common findings—Cystic formation and subchondral erosions around joints, soft-tissue swelling, and mild periosteal reactions; with spine involvement, skip lesions, thinning of end plates, loss of disk height, and possible collapse and late fusion.

5. MRI is useful to identify earlier stages of the disease and also assess bone elements for abscess formation, which may differentiate from malignancies.

6. Biopsy and culture for definitive diagnosis is recommended. *M tuberculosis*, which stains when the Ziehl-Neelsen technique is used and therefore is considered an acid-fast bacillus, requires an egg-based medium and may take up to 2 to 4 weeks to grow. Therefore, empiric treatment is started at the initiation of biopsy.

7. Treatment

a. Management of these infections is primarily medical.

b. Extended triple drug therapy of isoniazid, rifampin, and pyrazinamide for 6 to 12 months has been shown to be effective with osseous involvement.

c. Joints—Irrigation and débridement in large joints is only necessary for abscess drainage.

d. Spine—The only absolute indications for surgical intervention of the spine are marked neurologic involvement related to a kyphotic deformity or herniation, worsening neurologic condition despite chemotherapy, an abscess with respiratory obstruction, and worsening kyphosis with instability. Anterior column involvement is most common: anterior decompression, débridement, and stabilization should be performed. A posterior approach should be reserved for specific situations involving posterior stabilization or débridement.

B. HIV/AIDS

1. Prevalence—0.5% of the US population; as high as 10% reported in trauma centers located in high-prevalence areas. The need for orthopaedic care for HIV-positive patients is becoming increasingly common.

2. The risks of occupational transmission have been shown to be extremely low, with only 49 well-documented seroconversions among health care

Table 6

Summary of Antimicrobial Agents and Mechanism of Action

Antibiotic	Category	Mode of Action	Clinical Use	Side Effects/Toxicity	Notes of Interest
Penicillins	Bactericidal	Inhibition of cell wall synthesis by blocking cross-linking	DOC for gram-positive bacteria, *S pyogenes*, *Streptococcus agalactiae*, and *C perfringens*. Ampicillin/amoxicillin: DOC for *Escherichia faecalis*, *E coli*. Ticarcillin: DOC-antipseudomonal	Hypersensitivity reaction, hemolytic anemia Nafcillin/oxacillin can cause interstitial nephritis	Probenecid inhibits renal tubular secretion of penicillin, carboxy-penicillins, and ureidopenicillins, inactive aminoglycosides
Beta-lactamase inhibitors (clavulanic acid, sulbactam, tazobactam)	Bactericidal	Inhibition of cell wall synthesis by blocking cross-linking	DOC against gram-positive (*S aureus*, *S epidermidis*) and gram-negative (*E coli*, *Klebsiella*) bacteria	Hypersensitivity, hemolytic anemia	
Cephalosporins First-generation (cephalothin, cephapirin, cefazolin) Second-generation (cefoxitin, cefotetan) Third-generation (cefotaxime, ceftriaxone, ceftazidime) Fourth-generation (cefepime)	Bactericidal	Inhibition of cell wall sythesis by blocking cross-linking	Effective against *S aureus*, *S epidermidis*, and some gram-negative activity (*E coli*, *Klebsiella*, *Proteus mirabilis*) More active against gram-positive bacteria Less active against gram-positive bacteria, but more active against Enterobacteriaceae. Ceftazidime highly effective against *Pseudomonas* High activity against gram-positive bacteria	Allergic reactions (3% to 7% cross-reactivity with penicillin. Coombs-positive anemia in 3%. Second- and third-generation drugs may cause a disulfiram reaction with alcohol	Cefazolin has the longest half-life of the first-generation cephalosporins. No activity against *Enterococcus*.
Vancomycin	Bactericidal	Inhibition of cell wall synthesis. Disrupts peptioglycan cross-linkage	DOC for MRSA. DOC for patients with penicillin and cephalosporin allergies. Excellent activity against *S aureus*, *S epidermidis*	Red man syndrome (5% to 13% of patients), nephrotoxicity/ototoxicity, neutropenia, thrombocytopenia	
Aminoglycosides (gentamicin, tobramycin, streptomycin, amikacin)	Bactericidal	Inhibition of protein synthesis, irreversibly binding to 30S ribosomal subunit	Effective against aerobic gram-negative organisms and Enterobacteriaceae, *Pseudomonas*	Nephrotoxicity/ototoxicity increased with multiple drug interactions.	
Lincosamide (clindamycin)	Bacteriostatic	Inhibition of protein synthesis, binds 50S ribosomal subunit, inhibits peptidyl transferase by interfering with binding amino acyl-tRNA complex	Effective against *Bacteroides fragilis*, *S aureus*, coagulase-negative *Staphylococcus*, *Streptococcus*	Pseudomembranous colitis (*Clostridium difficile*), hypersensitivity reaction	Excellent penetration into bone. Potentiates neuromuscular blocking agents.

(continued on next page)

1: Basic Science

Table 6

Summary of Antimicrobial Agents and Mechanism of Action (continued)

Antibiotic	Category	Mode of Action	Clinical Use	Side Effects/Toxicity	Notes of Interest
Tetracycline	Bacteriostatic	Blocks tRNA binding to 50S ribosome	Effective against mycoplasma, rickettsia, Lyme disease, *S aureus*	Anorexia, nausea, diarrhea Interacts with divalent metal agents (antacids), inhibiting antibiotic absorption. May cause hepatotoxicity	Not used in children under 12 because of discoloration of teeth and impairment of bone growth
Macrolides (erythromycin, clarithromycin, azithromycin)	Bacteriostatic	Reversibly binds to 50S ribosomal subunit	Effective against *Streptococcus*, *Haemophilus influenzae*, *Moraxella catarrhalis*, *Mycoplasma pneumonia*, Legionella, Chlamydia	Nausea, vomiting. Drug interaction with coumadin and other drugs due to stimulated cytochrome P450	
Rifampin	Bactericidal	Binds to DNA-dependent RNA polymerase inhibition RNA transcription	Most active antistaphylococcal agent. Used in combination with semisynthetic penicillin. Effective against *Mycobacterium* species	Rust discoloration of body fluids, GI symptoms, hepatitis. Multiple drug interactions inducing hepatic microsomal pathway and altering drug metabolism. Interaction with INH can result in hepatotoxicity. Interaction with ketoconazole may decrease the effectiveness of both drugs.	Resistant organisms rapidly develop if used alone.
Fluoroquinolones Second-generation (ciprofloxacin, ofloxacin) Third-generation (levofloxin) Fourth-generation (trovafloxacin)	Bactericidal	Inhibit DNA gyrase, required for DNA synthesis	Effective against gram-negative *Streptococcus*, Mycoplasma, Legionella, Chlamydia. Aerobic gram-positive Anaerobic coverage	GI symptoms (nausea, vomiting), phototoxicity, tendinitis, predisposition to Achilles tendon rupture. Drug interactions	Poor *Enterococcus* coverage Later generation fluoroquinolones have better gram-positive coverage
Trimethoprim/ sulfamethoxazole	Bacteriostatic	Competitive inhibition with PABA Inhibit folic acid synthesis	Aerobic gram-negative, GI and UTI organisms. Some gram-positive, such as *Staphylococcus* and *Streptococcus*, in addition to *Enterobacter*, *Proteus*, *H influenzae*	GI, hemolytic anemia, agranulocytopenia, thrombocytopenia, urticaria, erythema nodosum. Serum sickness. Drug interactions	Not to be used in third trimester of pregnancy
Metronidazole (Flagyl)	Bactericidal	Metabolic by-products disrupt DNA	Anerobic organisms	Seizures, cerebellar dysfunction, disulfram reaction with alcohol	
Chloramphenicol	Bacteriostatic	Inhibits 50S ribosomal subunit/inhibits protein synthesis	*H influenzae*, bacterial meningitis, brain abscess	Aplastic anemia, gray baby syndrome	

DOC = drug of choice, PABA = p-aminobenzoic acid, GI = gastrointestinal, UTI = urinary tract infection workers, none of which involved needle sticks. In addition to exposure risks, patients' postoperative outcomes and complication rates have been a concern, with the potential for higher infection rates and longer healing times because of impaired cellular and humoral immunity.

3. Mechanisms that decrease host response to common pathogens and opportunistic infections include decreased absolute PMN count and function, platelet deficiency, and hypoalbuminemia.

4. The most common infecting organism is reported to be *S aureus*, followed by *Streptococcus pneumoniae* and *Escherichia coli*.

5. Studies comparing the infection rates of HIV-negative patients with asymptomatic HIV-positive patients have found no significant difference. Patients with CD4 counts <200, diagnostic for AIDS, were found to have a 10 times higher rate of infection than individuals without AIDS.

6. Recommendations for reducing the risk of infection during elective orthopaedic surgery include

   a. Absolute PMN count >1,000.

   b. Platelet count >60,000.

   c. Serum albumin >25 g/L.

   d. Reduction of viral loads to undetectable levels, which will in turn raise the lymphocyte count.

   e. Cessation of marrow-suppressing drugs (zidovudine, didanosine, and zalcitabine) a few days before surgery and held until after the first postoperative week.

   f. Drugs such as 3TC and D4T do not suppress the marrow and therefore should be maintained.

   g. Evaluation of the surgical risk-to-benefit ratio and patient understanding of potential complications.

C. Lyme disease

1. Multisystem spirochetal disorder caused by *Borrelia burgdorferi*; transmitted by the bite of an infected tick.

2. Geographic predominance: Northeast, Midwest, and Northwest United States.

3. Disease occurs in three clinical stages

   a. Early/localized disease—Pathognomonic skin lesion of erythema migrans.

   b. Early disseminated disease—Neurologic and cardiac manifestations.

   c. Late disease—Musculoskeletal symptoms (arthralgia, intermittent arthritis, and resultant chronic monoarthritis, most commonly in the knee) develop in 80% of untreated patients.

Table 7

Mechanisms of Antibiotic Resistance

Antibiotic Class and Type of Resistance	Specific Resistance Mechanism
Altered Target	
β-lactam antibiotics	Altered penicillin-binding proteins
Vancomycin	Altered peptidoglycan subunits
Aminoglycosides	Altered ribosomal proteins
Macrolides	Ribosomal RNA methylation
Quinolones	Altered DNA gyrase
Sulfonamides	Altered DNA dihydropteroate
Trimethoprim	Altered dihydrofolate reductase
Rifampin	Altered RNA polymerase
Detoxifying Enzymes	
Aminoglycosides	Phosphotransferase, acetylotransferase, nucleotidyltransferase
β-Lactam antibiotics	β-Lactamase
Chloramphenicol	The HIV virus inhibits chloramphenicol trans-acetylate, reducing the resistance of chloramphenicol in HIV.
Decreased Cellular Concentration	
β-lactam antibiotics	Diminished permeabililty
Tetracycline, fluoroquinolones, trimethoprim, erythromycin	Active efflux pumps

(Adapted with permission from the Centers for Disease Control and Prevention.)

4. Acute form of monoarthritis may resemble septic arthritis; however, the synovial fluid cell count (10,000 to 25,000 wbc/mm³) is typically lower than observed with bacterial septic arthritis, but still has a predominance of PMNs. Unlike chronic Lyme disease, acute monoarthritis is associated with HLA-DRB1*40, which suggests an autoimmune mechanism.

5. Diagnosis—Enzyme-linked immunosorbent assay (ELISA) testing will confirm the diagnosis.

6. Treatment—Oral amoxicillin or doxycycline for 4 weeks. IV ceftriaxone is recommended for patients with neurologic symptoms or recurrent episodes of arthritis. Prophylaxis may be administered using a

single 200-mg dose of doxycycline in the event of a tick bite occurring in an endemic region.

D.   Fungal infections

1.   The most common location of fungal infections is in the hand.

2.   Periprosthetic TJA infections may rarely be associated with fungal organisms.

a.   The most common infecting organism is *Candida albicans*.

b.   Deep periprosthetic infection with fungal organisms is rare and is associated with an immunocompromised host.

c.   Less favorable results with a two-stage exchange procedure for infected TJA have been described than for bacterial organisms, requiring a more prolonged antifungal treatment between stages.

d.   The use of amphotericin IV may be associated with renal toxicity and is often poorly tolerated by TJA patients.

e.   Amphotericin powder is effective as a local elution antifungal agent in antibiotic-impregnated cement spacers used between stages of treatment for an infected TJA.

f.   Adjuvant treatment of periprosthetic infections, in addition to IV amphotericin, may involve the use of oral fluconazole. Because of its mechanism of action, this agent requires periodic monitoring of hepatic enzymes.

3.   Onychomycosis or fungal nail bed infections are commonly caused by dermatophytes such as *Trichophyton rubrum*.

4.   Superficial skin infections are caused by dermatophytes and *C albicans* and may be treated successfully with topical antifungal agents, with conversion to oral agents if topical treatment is ineffective.

5.   Spinal infections are commonly hematogenous bacterial or fungal infections. The widespread use of broad-spectrum antibiotics and the increasing number of immunocompromised patients have led to spinal infections with unusual organisms. Biopsies should be sent for Gram stain, acid-fast stain, and aerobic, anaerobic, fungal, and tuberculosis cultures.

6.   Fungi such as *Coccidioides immitis* and *Blastomyces dermatitidis* are limited to specific geographic areas, whereas *Cryptococcus*, *Candida*, and *Aspergillus* are found worldwide. *Candida* and *Aspergillus* are normal commensals of the body and produce disease in susceptible organisms when they gain access to the vascular system through IV lines, during implantation of prosthetic devices, or during surgery.

7.   Coccidiomycosis is an infection caused by the fungus *C immitis*, a dimorphic fungus endemic to the southwestern United States, Central America, and parts of South America.

a.   Infection with *C immitis* primarily causes pulmonary disease, with extrapulmonary dissemination occurring in fewer than 1% of patients. When extrapulmonary dissemination occurs, the most common sites of infection are the skin, meninges, and skeletal system.

b.   Dissemination can occur in almost any organ system.

c.   Septic arthritis usually occurs secondary to direct extension from infected adjacent bone, but primary synovial coccidiomycosis also may occur. The knee is the most frequently involved joint.

d.   Most patients with musculoskeletal manifestations have pre-existing pulmonary coccidiomycosis or symptoms such as cough, dyspnea, and chest pain.

e.   Aggressive surgical and antibiotic treatment is required to eradicate this infection.

f.   Coccidiomycosis rarely should be considered in a differential diagnosis of patients with popliteal cysts without other obvious etiologies.

g.   Coccidiomycosis rarely causes cardiac disease. Constrictive pericarditis in the setting of disseminated coccidiomycosis can be fatal, despite antifungal therapy and pericardiectomy.

Top Testing Facts

1. The most common general infectious symptom is pain localized to the site of infection; it is rare for patients to not report pain as a presenting symptom.

2. Septic arthritis in adults is most commonly associated with *N gonorrhea* in otherwise healthy patients. *S aureus* is the second most common pathogen causing adult septic arthritis.

3. Triad of symptoms strongly suggesting Clostridial myonecrosis: (a) progressively severe pain out of proportion to obvious injury, (b) tachycardia not explained by fever, (c) crepitus.

4. Bone loss of 30% to 40% is required before the classic signs of osteomyelitis (bone resorption, destruction, periosteal elevation) can be seen on radiographs.

5. The most sensitive imaging tool for diagnosing osteomyelitis is MRI. The classic finding includes a signal change that is due to the increased edema and water content in bone, which is manifested as a reduction in T1 and an increase in T2 marrow signal. The increased signal intensity on T2 images results because the fatty marrow has been replaced by inflammation.

6. Synovial fluid WBC count >2,500/mm^3 or with >90% PMNs is strongly indicative of infection in a TKA.

7. *S aureus* is protected from host immune defenses by three mechanisms: (a) Excretion of protein A, which inactivates IgG; (b) production of a capsular polysaccharide, which reduces opsonization and phagocytosis of the organism; (c) formation of a biofilm (a "slime" containing an aggregation of microbial colonies embedded within a glycocalyx matrix that most commonly develops on THA/TKA implants or a devitalized bone surface), which also secludes the organism from host defense mechanisms.

8. Antibiotics have different modes of action (penicillin and cephalosporins—inhibition of cell wall synthesis; aminoglycoside—binds 30S ribosomal subunit; clindamycin—binds 50S ribosomal subunit).

9. Tuberculosis treatment—Extended triple drug therapy of isoniazid, rifampin, and pyrazinamide for 6 to 12 months has shown to be effective with osseous extrapulmonary involvement.

10. The treatment of choice for MRSA is vancomycin.

Bibliography

Barrack RL, Booth RE, Lonner JH, McCarthy JC, Mont MA, Rubash HE: *Orthopaedic Knowledge Update: Hip and Knee Reconstruction* ed 3. Rosemont, IL, American Academy of Orthopaedic Surgeons, 2006.

Barrack RL, Jennings RW, Wolfe MW, Bertot AJ: The Coventry Award: The value of preoperative aspiration before total knee revision. *Clin Orthop Relat Res* 1997;345:8-16.

Cierny G III, Dipasquale D: Treatment of chronic infection. *J Am Acad Orthop Surg* 2006;14(10 suppl):S105-S110.

Fontes RA Jr, Ogilvie CM, Miclau T: Necrotizing soft-tissue infections. *J Am Acad Orthop Surg* 2000;8:151-158.

Gross JM, Schwarz EM: Chapter 16: Infections in orthopaedics, in *Orthopaedic Basic Science*, ed 3. Rosemont, IL, American Academy of Orthopedic Surgeons, 2006.

Leone JM, Hanssen AD: Management of infection at the site of a total knee arthroplasty. *Instr Course Lect* 2006;55:449-461.

Luck JV, Logan LR, Benson DR, Glasser DB: Human Immunodeficiency Virus infection: Complications and outcome of orthopaedic surgery. *J Am Acad Orthop Surg* 1996;4:297-304.

Mahoney CR, Glesby MJ, DiCarlo EF, Peterson MG, Bostrom MP: Total hip arthroplasty in patients with human immunodeficiency virus infection: Pathologic findings and surgical outcomes. *Acta Orthop* 2005;76:198-203.

Parvizi J, Sullivan TA, Pagnano MW, Trousdale RT, Bolander ME: Total joint arthroplasty in human immunodeficiency virus-positive patients: An alarming rate of early failure. *J Arthroplasty* 2003;18:259-264.

Richards SB: *POSNA: Orthopaedic Knowledge Update Pediatrics*. Rosemont, IL, American Academy of Orthopaedic Surgeons, 1996.

Schmidt AH, Swiontkowski MF: Pathophysiology of infections after internal fixation of fractures. *J Am Acad Orthop Surg* 2000;8:285-291.

Segawa H, Tsukayama DT, Kyle RF, Becker DA, Gustilo RB: Infection after total knee arthroplasty: A retrospective study of the treatment of eighty-one infections. *J Bone Joint Surg Am* 1999;81:1434-1445.

Tsukayama DT, Estrada R, Gustilo RB: Infection after total hip arthroplasty: A study of the treatment of one hundred and six infections. *J Bone Joint Surg Am* 1996;78:512-523.

Vaccaro AR: *Orthopaedic Knowledge Update 8: Home Study Syllabus*. Rosemont, IL, American Academy of Orthopaedic Surgeons, 2005.

1: Basic Science

Chapter 12

Bone Grafting/Bone Graft Substitutes

*Hyun Bae, MD   Justin S. Field, MD

I. Bone Grafting

A. Bone graft may be considered for a number of different applications:

1. To facilitate healing of fractures, delayed unions, or nonunions.

2. To induce fusion of osseous structures that are normally independent (**Figure 1**).

3. To replace bone defects secondary to trauma, tumor, or wear.

B. Bone grafting properties—Bone grafts may be osteogenic, osteoinductive, or osteoconductive.

1. Osteogenic

    a. Osteogenic graft material directly provides cells, which go on to produce bone.

    b. Osteoprogenitor cells can proliferate and differentiate to osteoblasts and eventually to osteocytes. Mesenchymal stem cells have the potential to go down any differentiation route, including bone formation.

    c. Because cancellous bone has a larger surface area, it has a greater potential for forming new bone than does cortical bone.

    d. Bone marrow aspirate and autologous bone graft are osteogenic.

2. Osteoinductive

    a. Osteoinductive graft material has factors that induce progenitor cells down a bone-forming lineage.

    b. This is most commonly seen with a family of proteins known as bone morphogenetic proteins (BMPs).

3. Osteoconductive

    a. Osteoconductive bone graft serves as a scaffold onto which new bone can form.

    b. The three-dimensional configuration and building-block material will dictate the osteoconductive properties.

    c. Demineralized bone matrices (DBMs) are osteoconductive.

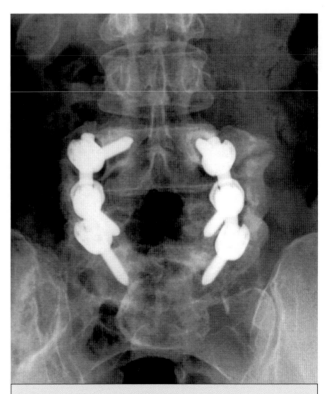

Figure 1   L4-S1 instrumented fusion with bone graft seen in the posterolateral gutters.

Hyun Bae, MD, or the department with which he is affiliated has received research or institutional support from Stryker, has received miscellaneous nonincome support, commercially-derived honoraria, or other nonresearch-related funding from Abbott, has received royalties from Biomet, holds stock or stock options in LDR, Spinal Restoration, and Paradigm, and is a consultant for or an employee of Stryker and Zimmer.

1: Basic Science

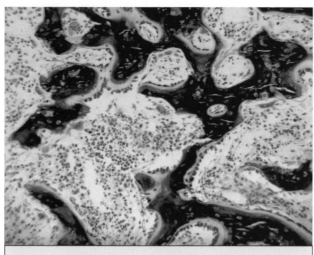

Figure 2 Reparative bone healing with osteoblasts lining new trabecular bone spicules.

II. Bone Healing

A. Bone formation involves three phases:

 1. Inflammation (early)

 a. Hematoma formation and inflammation occur rapidly in the early phases of bone repair.

 b. Surface osteocytes may survive and are important in synthesizing new bone during this initial phase.

 c. Infiltrate consists principally of small mononuclear cells.

 d. Capillary ingrowth is initiated.

 e. BMPs play an important role in inducing host mesenchymal stem cells to migrate into the repair site.

 2. Reparative (middle) (**Figure 2**)

 a. New bone formation takes the form of immature woven bone (soft callus).

Table 1				

Characteristics of Bone Grafts and Grafting Substitutes

Grafting Modality	Substance/ Implant	Osteogenic	Osteoinductive	Osteoconductive
Autografts	Cancellous bone Morcellized iliac crest Metaphyseal long bone	+++	++	+++
	Cortical bone Local bone Iliac crest Fibula	+	+/–	+/–
	Cellular Bone marrow aspirate	++	+/–	–
Allografts	Fresh	–	+/–	++
	Frozen	–	+/–	+
	Freeze-dried Cortical cancellous chips	–	+/–	+
	Demineralized bone matrix (DBM) Various preparations	–	+/–	+
Growth factors	rhBMP-2 rhBMP-7	–	+++	–
Ceramics	Hydroxyapatite Tricalcium phosphate (TCP)	–	–	+
Collagen	Absorbable collagen hemostatic sponge	–	–	–

1: Basic Science

b. Seams of osteoid surround the core of necrotic bone and form viable new bone (hard callus).

3. Remodeling (late)

   a. Coupled resorption and replacement occur.

   b. Remodeling is influenced by Wolff's law and is usually complete by 1 year.

B. Factors that impair bone healing

   1. Motion at the site of attempted union

   2. Lack of blood supply, which is generally associated with an anatomic site or stripping from injury or surgical dissection

   3. Nonsteroidal anti-inflammatory drugs

   4. Smoking

   5. Nonapposition of bone ends

III. Bone Graft Options (Table 1)

A. Autograft is tissue transferred from one site to another in the same individual and is commonly regarded as the gold standard bone graft material.

   1. Autograft is osteogenic, osteoinductive, and osteoconductive.

   2. Autograft may be cortical, cancellous, or corticocancellous; this may be nonvascular or vascularized.

      a. Cortical autograft has the advantage of being able to provide structural support.

      b. Cancellous autograft provides less structural support but greater osteoconduction and potentially greater osteogenesis and osteoinduction.

   3. The iliac crest is the most frequent autograft donor site (iliac crest bone graft [ICBG])

Characteristics of Bone Grafts and Grafting Substitutes

Donor-Site Morbidity	Immunogenicity	Absorption/ Remodeling rate	Immediate Structure/ Torque Strength	Typical Orthopaedic Applications
++++	–	+++	–	Lumbar spine Cervical spine Long bones
++++	–	++	++	Spine Tibial nonunion
+/–	–	–	–	Augmentation of other grafting materials Spine Long-bone fracture
–	++	+	++	Spine Long-bone fracture
–	+	–	++	Spine Long-bone fracture
–	+/–	–	+	Spine Long-bone fracture
–	+	–	–	Spine Long-bone fracture
–	–	–	–	Spine Long-bone fracture Nonunions
–	–	–	+/–	Spine Coating for fixation/ arthroplasty devices
–	+	–	+/–	Functions poorly alone but functions well coupled with BMPs

1: Basic Science

a. It has the potential to provide abundant cancellous and/or cortical graft.

b. Complications have been associated with ICBG in 2% to 36% of cases. These include hematoma formation, blood loss, injury to the lateral femoral cutaneous nerve or cluneal nerve, hernia formation, infection, fracture, cosmetic defects, and sometimes chronic pain at the donor site.

4. Other bone graft sources include the ribs, fibula, and tibial metaphysis. The fibula and rib are the most common potentially vascularized options considered.

B. Allograft is tissue harvested from a cadaver, processed, and then implanted into another individual of the same species.

1. Allograft is the most frequently chosen bone substitute in the United States.

2. Allograft can be cortical, cancellous, or cortico-cancellous.

3. Allograft lacks viable cells and therefore does not provide osteogenic properties, nor is it osteoinductive.

4. The extent of osteoconductive properties, as well as mechanical strength, depends in part on the method of graft processing (ie, fresh, frozen, or freeze-dried form) and whether it is cortical or cancellous.

5. The quoted rate of potential HIV disease transmission is 1 per million.

6. Several different types of allograft may be considered.

a. Fresh allograft

i. Rarely used because of immune response and potential disease transmission.

ii. Fresh allograft may be cleaned and processed to remove cells and reduce the host immune reaction. This has been shown to improve incorporation.

b. Frozen or freeze-dried allograft

i. Reduces immunogenicity

ii. Maintains the osteoconductive properties and potentially some limited osteoinductive capabilities

c. Demineralized bone matrix

i. DBM is allograft treated with a mild acid extraction to remove the mineral content of bone, but leaving behind the collagenous structure and noncollagenous proteins.

ii. The osteoinductive molecules are potentially preserved, but they have minimal or no osteoinductive activity.

iii. DBMs are osteoconductive and serve as a scaffold for new bone.

iv. These extracts are combined with carriers such as collagen, gelatin, hyaluronic acid, and glycerol.

v. Evidence has shown significant interproduct and interlot variability of DBM products.

7. The use of allograft has increased 15 fold over the past decade. Its increasing availability has made it possible to manufacture customized types, such as dowels, strips, chips, and powder. DBMs do not provide structural support.

8. The shelf life of fresh frozen bone stored at −20° C is 1 year; it is 5 years if stored at −70° C. The shelf life of freeze-dried bone is indefinite.

C. Collagen

1. Collagen contributes to mineral deposition, vascular ingrowth, and growth factor binding, providing a favorable environment for bone regeneration.

2. Collagen does not provide structural support and does carry immunogenic potential.

3. Collagen functions poorly alone, but it performs better when coupled with bone. It is considered a potential carrier for BMPs, DBMs, or other graft materials.

D. Bone marrow aspirate

1. Bone marrow aspirate is a potential source of osteogenic mesenchymal precursor cells.

2. It may be from the iliac crest, vertebral body, or other sources.

3. The number of cells varies depending on variables such as host age.

4. It has been suggested that the potency of marrow aspirates could be increased via selective precursor selection, centrifugation, or clonal expansion.

E. Ceramics

1. Ceramics are inorganic compounds consisting of metallic and nonmetallic elements held together by ionic or covalent bonds.

2. There are several classes of ceramic materials.

a. Hydroxyapatite (HA)

b. Beta tricalcium phosphate (β-TCP)

c. Other molecules, such as silicone (Si)

3. Alone, ceramics possess no osteogenic or osteoinductive properties, and they have variable immediate structural support secondary to resorption.

F. Bone morphogenetic proteins

1. BMPs are members of the transforming growth factor-β (TGF-β) superfamily

2. BMPs play a key role in normal development, but they also have increasingly appreciated osteoinductive potential.

3. Two recombinant human BMPs (rhBMPs) have been approved for clinical use: rhBMP-2 and rhBMP-7 (OP-1). Their FDA-approved applications are in the long bones and spine.

4. Potential adverse effects include underproduction or overproduction of bone, exuberant inflammatory responses, and early bone resorption.

IV. Other Modalities to Enhance Bone Healing

A. Electromagnetic stimulation (EMS)

1. Bone tissue has electrical potential, known as bioelectric potential.

    a. The bioelectric potential is electronegative in area of growth or healing. The area returns to neutral or electropositive as healing progresses.

    b. The bioelectric potential is electronegative in areas of compression and electropositive in areas of tension.

2. Direct current electrical stimulation (DCES)—Direct current delivered through implanted electrodes.

3. Pulsed electromagnetic field (PEMF)—Alternating current delivered through an external coil used intermittently during the treatment period.

4. Capacitively coupled electrical stimulation (CCES)—Current delivered between two plates that form a magnetic field and are used throughout the treatment period.

5. The mechanism of action of EMS has not been fully resolved and may be slightly different for each type of stimulation listed above.

B. Shock wave therapy

1. Shock wave therapy theoretically creates microfractures in hypertrophic nonunions, which leads to neovascularization and osteoinduction.

2. Reported results are controversial.

C. Low-intensity ultrasound also may affect bone healing.

Top Testing Facts

1. Bone grafts may be osteogenic, osteoinductive, or osteoconductive.

2. Bone healing progresses through three stages: early (inflammation), middle (reparative), and late (remodeling).

3. Bone healing may be affected by host and local factors.

4. Autograft is the gold standard bone graft material.

5. Allograft has a reported rate of potential HIV transmission of 1 per million.

6. DBMs have been shown to have significant interproduct and interlot variability. DBMs are predominantly osteoconductive.

7. Bone marrow aspirates provide potential access to osteogenic mesenchymal precursor cells.

8. Ceramics are inorganic compounds consisting of metallic and nonmetallic elements held together by ionic or covalent bonds.

9. BMPs are potent osteoinductive factors of the TGF-β superfamily.

10. Several forms of electromagnetic stimulation may facilitate bone healing.

Bibliography

Bauer TW, Muschler GF: Bone graft materials: An overview of the basic science. *Clin Orthop Relat Res* 2000;371:10-27.

Friedlaender GE, Mankin HJ, Goldberg VM (eds): *Bone Grafts and Bone Graft Substitutes*. Rosemont, IL, American Academy of Orthopaedic Surgeons, 2006.

Giannoudis PV, Dinopoulos H, Tsiridis E: Bone substitutes: An update. *Injury* 2005;36 (Suppl 3):S20-S27.

Miclau T III, Bozic KJ, Tay B, et al: Bone injury, regeneration, and repair, in Einhorn TA, O'Keefe RJ, Buckwalter JA (eds): *Orthopaedic Basic Science*, ed 3. Rosemont, IL, American Academy of Orthopaedic Surgeons, 2007, pp 331-348.

Watson JT: New horizons in orthopaedics: A rational discussion of biologics and bone graft substitutes. *Mo Med* 2005; 102:240-244.

1: Basic Science

Section 2

General Knowledge

Section Editor

Kevin J. Bozic, MD, MBA

Chapter 13

Medicolegal Issues

David A. Halsey, MD

I. Patient Safety and Medical Errors

A. Institute of Medicine (IOM) Effort—The IOM launched a concerted, ongoing effort focused on assessing and improving the nation's quality of care in 1996.

1. First phase (1996–1998)—Documented the serious and pervasive nature of the nation's overall quality problem, concluding that "the burden of harm conveyed by the collective impact of all of our health care quality problems is staggering."

2. Second phase (1999–2001)—The Committee on Quality of Health Care in America released two reports, establishing a vision for how the health care system and related policy environment must be radically transformed.

   a. *To Err Is Human: Building a Safer Health System* (1999) reported that tens of thousands of Americans die each year from medical errors. It highlighted the importance of patient safety and quality issues for public and private policymakers.

   b. *Crossing the Quality Chasm: A New Health System for the 21st Century* (2001) stressed broader quality issues and described six aims of care: safe, effective, patient-centered, timely, efficient, and equitable.

3. Third phase (2002–present)—Operationalized the vision of a future health system described in the *Quality Chasm* report.

   a. Identifies stakeholders in creating a more patient-responsive health system: clinicians/health care organizations, employers/consumers, research foundations, government agencies, quality organizations.

   b. Focuses reform at three levels: environmental, the health care organization, the interface between clinicians and patients.

B. Collaborative efforts

1. Agency for Healthcare Research and Quality (AHRQ)

   a. Research arm of the US Department of Health and Human Services (HHS) and sister agency to the National Institutes of Health (NIH).

   b. Home to specialized research centers in major areas of health care research. These centers focus on:

      i. Quality improvement in patient safety—Identifying factors that put patients at risk; using computer and other information technology to reduce and prevent errors; developing innovative approaches that reduce errors and produce safety in various health care settings and geographically diverse locations; disseminating research results; and improving patient safety education and training for clinicians and other providers.

      ii. Outcomes and effectiveness of care.

      iii. Clinical practice and technology assessment.

      iv. Health care organization and delivery systems.

      v. Primary care.

      vi. Health care costs and sources of payment.

   c. The AHRQ supports research on health disparities, drugs and other therapeutics, primary care practice, and integrated health care delivery systems.

   d. It focuses on evidence-based practice and the translation of research into clinical practice to improve patient care in diverse health care settings.

   e. It identifies strategies to improve health care access, foster appropriate use, and reduce unnecessary expenditures.

2. Joint Commission on Accreditation of Healthcare Organizations (JCAHO)

   a. The JCAHO is the major accrediting agency for hospitals.

   b. It developed a sentinel reporting policy in 1996 that encourages accredited health care organizations to voluntarily report "sentinel" events within 5 days and submit a root cause analysis within 45 days of discovery. A sentinel event is an unexpected occurrence involving death or serious physical or psychological injury, the risk for which a recurrence would carry a significant chance of a serious adverse outcome.

c. Based on root cause analyses, the JCAHO identified the need to establish national patient safety goals. The first National Patient Safety Goals were established in 2002. The JCAHO reevaluates goals annually and identifies steps annually to accomplish goals. It allows alternatives to specific recommendations as long as the alternative is as effective as the original recommendation in achieving the specific patient safety goal.

d. The JCAHO identified 15 National Patient Safety Goals; each year specific steps are identified to accomplish the overarching goals. Examples of goals or steps specific to orthopaedics:

   i. JCAHO 2006 National Patient Safety Goal #1: improve the accuracy of patient identification with the elimination of wrong site surgery. Uses the American Academy of Orthopaedic Surgeons' (AAOS) Sign Your Site program. Requires a preprocedure "time-out" to confirm the correct patient, procedure, and site using active communication techniques.

   ii. JCAHO 2006 National Patient Safety Goal #7: reduce the risk of health care-associated infections. Requires that health care organizations establish systems to ensure that the use of prophylactic antibiotic for total hip arthroplasty, total knee arthroplasty, and hip fracture management adhere to the best available evidence, including appropriate antibiotic selection, administration of the antibiotic within 60 minutes of the surgical incision, and discontinuation of prophylactic antibiotic therapy within 24 hours of the time of wound closure.

3. National Patient Safety Foundation (NPSF)

   a. Stakeholders include health care practitioners and institutions, manufacturers, educators, insurers, researchers, legal advisers, policymakers, and patients.

   b. Mission

      i. Identify a core body of knowledge.

      ii. Identify pathways to apply the knowledge.

      iii. Develop and enhance the culture of receptivity about patient safety.

      iv. Raise public awareness and foster communications about patient safety.

Table 1

Chronology of Stark Laws

1989: Stark (I) enacted.

1993: Broadened version (Stark II) enacted.

1995: Final regulations for enactment of Stark I.

1998: Regulations proposed for two-phase enactment of Stark II.

2001: Phase I rolled out.

2004: Phase II rolled out.

II. Compliance

A. Stark laws (see **Table 1**)

1. Rationale for prohibitions

   a. In some cases, excessive medical services were ordered for which the patient received unnecessary care, resulting in higher health care costs.

   b. Costs for patients covered by government programs were ultimately passed on to taxpayers.

2. Stark I (1989)

   a. Prohibits referral of Medicare patients who need clinical laboratory service to entities in which the physician has an ownership interest.

   b. Prohibits referral of Medicare and certain Medicaid patients for "designated health services" to entities in which the physician or an immediate family member has a financial interest, unless an exemption applies.

   c. Proscribes entities to which referrals are made from submitting payment claims to the government for specified services.

3. Stark II (1993)

   a. Expands the list of referral services that are prohibited from physician ownership.

   b. Expands the referral band to include patients covered by certain Medicaid managed care programs.

   c. Identifies circumstances under which referrals are permitted activities, known as exceptions.

4. Final regulations for enactment of Stark II (1998)

   a. Issued in 1995, but rolled out in two phases.

   b. Supersede the 1995 Stark I regulations.

   c. Consist of actual rules physicians must follow.

5. Penalties for violating Stark II phase (Phase I and II) regulations

a. Denial of payment

b. Mandatory refunding of payments that were made in error

c. Civil monetary penalties of $15,000 per claim

d. Prohibition from participation in Medicare and Medicaid programs

6. Phase II exceptions—Five are most important to orthopaedic surgeons.

   a. In-office ancillary service in a group practice or by a sole practitioner

   b. Bona fide employment

   c. Personal service arrangements

   d. Fair market value compensation

   e. Academic medical centers

B. Health Insurance Portability and Accountability Act (HIPAA; 1996)

1. Title I protects health insurance coverage for workers and their families when the workers change or lose their jobs.

2. Title II addresses "administrative simplification," as well as fraud, abuse, and medical liability reform.

3. Title III establishes medical savings accounts and health insurance deductions for the self-employed.

4. Title IV covers the enforcement of group health plan provisions.

5. Title V focuses on revenue offset provisions.

6. Privacy rules

   a. Create national standards to protect patient's medical records and other personal health information.

   b. Give patients more control over their health data.

   c. Limit the way health care providers may use the information and release it to third parties.

   d. Establish guidelines that must be followed to protect the privacy of patient's "protected health information."

   e. Hold health plans, health care clearinghouses, and health care providers accountable for violations.

C. Fraud

1. Centers for Medicare & Medicaid Services (CMS) definition (verbatim)

   a. Intentional deception or misrepresentation that an individual knows to be false (or does not

believe to be true) and he or she makes, knowing that the deception could result in some unauthorized benefit to himself or herself or some other person.

   b. Most commonly arises from a false statement or misrepresentation made, or caused to be made, that is material to entitlement or payment under the Medicare program.

2. Most common types of fraud in Medicare

   a. Billing for services not rendered

   b. Misrepresenting a diagnosis to justify payment

   c. Soliciting, offering, or receiving a kickback

   d. Unbundling

   e. Falsifying treatment plans and medical records to justify payment

   f. Up-coding

III. Medical Malpractice Claims

A. Elements that the patient must prove

1. Duty—Physician's obligation to care for the patient in a manner that is consistent with the quality of care provided by other physicians in treating a patient's particular condition.

2. Breach of duty

   a. Facts show that the physician failed to meet the standard of care in treating the patient.

   b. Poor outcome, whether permanent or not, or a predictable complication does not necessarily mean that the physician has deviated from the standard of care.

3. Causation—Proof that the violation caused the patient's injury.

4. Damage—Proof that the physician's deviation from the standard of care resulted in physical, emotional, or financial injury to the patient.

B. Informed consent

1. Requires that a physician obtain consent before any treatment is rendered or operation is performed, and before many diagnostic procedures can be performed.

2. Requires a patient to give permission before being "touched" by another; without permission, contact may be considered an "assault," a "battery," or a "trespass" upon the patient.

3. Without an informed consent, the orthopaedic physician may be held liable for violation of the patient's rights, regardless of whether the treatment was appropriate and rendered with due care.

4. Medical care cannot be provided without either expressed or implied permission for the physician to act.

IV. Patient Complaints

A. Factors that contribute to both the likelihood a patient will bring suit as well as the successful prosecution of medical malpractice claims

   1. Miscommunication

   2. Delay in response to patient/family concerns

   3. Failure to diagnose

   4. Failure to treat

   5. Improper treatment

B. Factors that contribute to patient complaints

   1. Inconsistency in communication

   2. Promises that are not kept

   3. Lack of sufficient details regarding the diagnosis and treatment plan

   4. Perceived rudeness

   5. Lack of understanding regarding known procedural/surgical complications

   6. Perception that the physician and staff are too busy to be concerned with the patient's problem

   7. Long wait times

   8. Frustration with the inability to "fix" a painful condition

C. Patient-physician communication

   1. Effective patient-physician communication will avert many patient complaints.

   2. Tools to ensure high-quality patient-physician communication

      a. Adequate time

      b. Acknowledgment of emotional distress

      c. Physician-obtained informed consent

      d. Phone calls returned in a timely fashion

D. Skills to assist with addressing complaints when first expressed

   1. Take all complaints seriously.

   2. Acknowledge the patient's concern/complaint.

   3. Provide accurate information to help clarify the situation.

   4. Be frank and honest.

   5. Avoid negative comments about other health care providers.

E. CMS requirements for complaints

   1. All complaints must be addressed with a written response to the patient in a timely manner.

   2. Situations requiring a written response to the patient

      a. When a patient specifically asks for a written report

      b. When there is a dispute about charges based on the patient's perception of quality of care

      c. Components of written response

         i. Acknowledgment of the complaint

         ii. Addressing the issue to the extent possible

         iii. Reassurance that the patient's feedback will be used to avoid a similar problem for another patient in the future

V. Standard of Disclosure

A. Varies by state

B. Two standards for assessing adequacy of disclosure

   1. Professional or reasonable physicians' standard—Based on what is customary practice in the medical community for physicians to divulge to patients (most common).

   2. Patient viewpoint standard—Based on what a reasonable person in the patient's position would want to know in similar circumstances.

   3. More information generally is revealed with patient viewpoint standard than in jurisdictions that adhere to the professional or reasonable physicians' standard.

C. Elements of informed consent

   1. Stated diagnosis

   2. Nature of the condition or illness requiring medical or surgical intervention

   3. Nature and purpose of the treatment or procedure recommended

   4. Risks and potential complications associated with the recommended treatment or procedure

   5. All feasible alternative treatments or procedures noted, including the option of taking no action

   6. Relative probability of success for treatment or procedure in terms the patient will understand

Top 10 Medicolegal Terms

1. *Abandonment:* Termination of the physician-patient relationship by the physician without reasonable notice to the patient at a time when the patient requires medical attention and without the opportunity to make arrangements for appropriate continuation and follow-up care.

2. *Burden of proof:* Typically, a plaintiff's responsibility to affirmatively prove a fact or facts in dispute on an issue raised between parties in a case.

3. *Causation:* The causal connection between the act or omission of the defendant and the injury suffered by the plaintiff. The plaintiff must show causation of an injury by the defendant to prove negligence.

4. *Damages:* Money receivable through judicial order by a plaintiff sustaining harm, impairment, or loss to his or her person or property as the result of the accidental, intentional, or negligent act of another. Damages can be grouped into two primary types: compensatory and punitive.

   • Compensatory damages are to compensate the injured party for the injury sustained and nothing more. Compensatory damages can be divided into economic, noneconomic, and special damages.

   • Economic damages include an estimate of lost wages, both past and future, of the plaintiff and affected family members, and all costs associated with residual disability of the patient.

   • Noneconomic damages include intangible damage resulting from the negligent act such as pain and suffering, disfigurement, and interference with the ordinary enjoyment of life.

   • Special damages are the actual out-of-pocket losses incurred by the plaintiff, such as medical expenses, rehabilitation expenses, and earnings lost during treatment and recovery.

   • Punitive damages are awarded to punish a defendant who has acted maliciously or in reckless disregard of the plaintiff's rights.

5. *Duty* is the obligation of the physician to care for the patient in a manner that is consistent with the quality of care provided by other physicians in treating a patient's particular condition.

6. *Fraud* is the intentional deception or misrepresentation that an individual knows to be false (or does not believe to be true) and he or she makes, knowing that the deception could result in some unauthorized benefit to himself or herself or some other person.

7. *Informed consent:* Consent is "fully informed" only when the patient knows and understands the information necessary to make an informed decision about the treatment or procedure. There is no informed consent when the treatment or procedure extends beyond the scope of consent. For example, if the risk associated with the changed treatment or procedure is substantially different from that contemplated by the patient, the courts may find the original informed consent was not sufficient. There are certain circumstances for which special informed consent rules apply. These are medical emergencies, situations involving a minor, and those rare circumstances where authorization for treatment or procedure is obtained from a court.

8. *Malpractice:* In the case of a physician, failure to exercise the degree of care and skill that a physician or surgeon of the same specialty would use under similar circumstances (professional negligence).

9. *Negligence:* In medical malpractice cases, a legal cause of action involving the failure of a defendant physician to exercise that degree of diligence and care that an average qualified physician practicing in the same specialty as that of the defendant physician would have exercised in a similar situation, and which has resulted in the breach of a legal duty owed by the physician to the patient which proximately caused an injury which the law recognizes as deserving of compensation (damages).

10. *Res ipsa loquitur* ("The thing speaks for itself"): A doctrine that may be invoked in a negligence action when the plaintiff has no direct evidence of negligence, but the injury itself leads to the inference that it would not have occurred in the absence of a negligent act. It raises an inference of the defendant's negligence, thereby altering the burden of proof so that the defendant must produce evidence that he or she did not commit a negligent act.

Bibliography

AAOS Government Relations website: www.aaos.org/govern/govern.asp.

AAOS Risk Management CME website: www5.aaos.org/OKO/RiskManagement.cfm.

Agency for Healthcare Quality and Research website: www.ahrq.gov.

Institute of Medicine website: www.iom.edu.

Joint Commission on Accreditation of Healthcare Organizations website: www.jointcommission.org.

National Patient Safety Foundation website: www.npsf.org.

2: General Knowledge

Chapter 14

Medical Ethics

Mohammad Diab, MD

I. Professionalism

A. Professionalism is a neglected curriculum area in orthopaedic education. It is currently taught by role models, review processes, rewards, and regulations.

B. Categories of unprofessional behavior

1. Criminal behavior

2. Substance abuse

3. Negligence

4. Sexual misconduct

5. Inappropriate billing

6. Inadequate medical records

7. Incomplete disclosure

8. Failure to meet the minimum standard of care

II. Informed Consent

A. Information presented to the patient

1. Clear identification of the medical condition

2. Recommended treatment(s)

3. Alternative treatment(s)

4. Risks and benefits of treatment(s) or lack thereof

B. Means of assessing comprehension of the information

1. Educating the patient—Use of discussion, written and visual aids, and referral to other health care providers or patients who have a similar condition and who have undergone the recommended treatment.

2. Answering all questions—Development of an adequately familiar and comfortable rapport that encourages a dialog between patient and physician.

3. Using simplified language—During direct discussion and in written form, both on paper and electronically.

4. Avoiding jargon—Minimize or eliminate abbreviations and technical terms on the consent form and in educational materials.

C. Voluntariness—Follows the "reasonable volunteer" standard.

1. Patient can decline recommendations or withdraw from intervention at any time.

2. Patient has adequate time for making decisions, including during the office interview and at follow-up visit(s), to allow assimilation and gathering of further information.

III. Relationships With Industry

A. Three principal interests—Patient, physician, and third party such as insurers or hospitals.

1. Patient interests must take priority when conflict arises.

2. Any alternative—and even the appearance of such—evokes suspicion of the physician's recommendations and erodes patient trust.

B. There are two principal settings for delivery of health care, each with unique financial incentives.

1. Managed care plans

a. Physicians may serve as gatekeepers and are held accountable for cost per capita.

b. Goal is to improve efficiency and reduce waste.

c. Perceived disadvantage is delay or rationing or withholding of care solely for financial reasons.

2. Fee-for-service plans

a. When reward is based on use, there is an incentive for the physician to consume greater resources, including facilities (such as laboratory work and imaging studies) and devices (as when the physician receives royalties or kickbacks for implants).

b. Financial incentives may be neutralized or elevated to acceptable ethical standards by ensuring that the patient's interests are the priority.

C. Industry sponsorship of professional and educational activities—US Food and Drug Administration (FDA) and the Accreditation Council for Continuing Medical Education (ACCME) stipulations for physicians working with industry.

1. Physicians may not accept gifts from industry valued greater than $100.

2. Industry may subsidize the costs of continuing medical education (CME) courses, but not for physician travel, lodging, recreational activities, or personal expenses.

3. Courses that do not award CME are considered commercial and subject to regulation.

IV. Stark II Regulations

A. Stark II prohibits self-referrals of Medicare patients.

B. See chapter 1, Medicolegal Issues, for details.

V. Peer Review and Medical Errors

A. Purposes of peer review

1. Quality control—To improve outcomes, reduce errors, and enhance patient safety.

2. Forms one basis of certification.

3. Grants respectability to and inspires confidence in the medical profession.

4. Facilitates consumer selection.

B. Challenges of current peer review systems

1. Current systems are largely voluntary and poor at detecting and reducing errors, with data lacking regarding true error rate and number of encounters to generate error.

2. No centralized or standardized system for reporting errors.

3. Focus on negative feedback (culpability) rather than positive feedback (learning to improve processes).

4. Threat of legal ramifications deters reporting of errors.

5. Expensive to develop, with no direct reward for participants.

C. Recommendations for peer review

1. Shift in focus

a. Focus on patient safety, not risk management.

b. Deemphasize blame because legal liability and/or professional discipline have not prevented avoidable errors. Also, avoiding blame will improve communication with colleagues and other organizations and institutions, providing the opportunity to build a knowledge base, learn from others, and devise solutions.

c. Shift from a retrospective review system to a proactive process designed to avoid errors, recognize them before they impact a patient, and identify them when they occur.

d. Shift from individual review to systems and process review.

e. Use a wide variety of tools and consult with other health care professionals when necessary, given the complex and varied nature of medical errors.

f. Include noninstitutional care in peer review.

i. Institutional care, especially in hospital, has been the traditional focus.

ii. Noninstitutional care settings such as the office setting lack the advantages of scale and resources but may provide greater reward on investment, despite the perception that they are less complicated systems with patients who are less ill.

2. Change reporting requirements.

a. Require strict confidentiality in reporting to encourage/increase voluntary reporting.

b. Report "near misses," which are more readily discussed and equally informative.

3. Encourage legal reform.

a. Work for tort reform to end open-ended legal damage awards.

i. Set limits, or caps, for legal damage awards.

ii. Develop a sliding scale proportionate to loss.

b. Shift the burden of liability from the individual to the organization (exclusive enterprise liability).

i. Removing personal liability may eliminate one significant barrier to error reporting.

ii. Shift does not eliminate sanctions from professional partners or organizations.

4. Facilitate patient selection.

a. Make information on outcomes readily available to the consumer.

b. Make patients partners in the process so that they can help improve safety through their health care dollar. This would represent part of a change from penalties for poor outcomes to support for improved outcomes.

VI. End-of-Life Issues

A. Do Not Resuscitate (DNR) orders

1. Cardiopulmonary resuscitation (CPR) is initiated in a patient who experiences a cardiopulmonary arrest unless a DNR order is on record.

2. A DNR order is appropriate if the patient or surrogate requests one or if CPR would be futile.

3. DNR orders and the reasons for them must be documented in the medical record.

4. "Slow" or "show" codes that merely appear to provide CPR in the absence of DNR orders are deceptive and therefore unacceptable.

5. A DNR order signifies that only CPR will be withheld, but the reasons that justify the DNR order may lead to a reconsideration of other plans for care.

B. Advance directives

1. Advance directives are statements by competent patients to direct care if they lose decision-making capacity. They may specify which interventions are acceptable to the patient and who serves as surrogate on behalf of the patient.

2. Types of advance directives

   a. Oral conversations—These are the most common format but can be disputed due to lack of clarity and completeness.

   b. Living wills—These direct physicians to forgo or provide life-sustaining interventions if the patient develops a terminal condition or persistent vegetative state.

   c. Health care proxy (In some states, this process is called executing a durable power of attorney for health care.)

      i. Makes decisions if the patient loses such capacity

      ii. Most flexible and comprehensive

      iii. More comprehensive than the living will, applying whenever the patient is unable to make decisions

3. Patients generally may refuse only interventions that "merely prolong the process of dying."

4. Federal Patient Self-Determination Act requires hospitals and Health Maintenance Organizations (HMOs) to inform patients of their right to make health care decisions and to provide advance directives.

5. Substituted judgment

   a. In the absence of clear advance directives, surrogates and physicians substitute their judgment for that of the patient when making decisions that respect what the patient would wish and the patient's best interests.

   b. In the event of disagreement, several resources may be accessed:

      i. Another physician, who may provide a "second opinion" that is unprejudiced.

      ii. The hospital ethics committee, which has experience in resolving such disputes.

      iii. A court of law, which should be viewed as the last resort.

VII. Confidentiality

A. The importance of confidentiality is widely accepted by the medical profession. Aspects of patient confidentiality are codified in Health Insurance Portability and Accountability (HIPAA) regulations (see chapter 1, Medicolegal Issues).

B. Breaches of confidentiality are justified in circumstances where society regards the benefits to others as outweighing the benefits to the patient:

1. When a patient is at risk (eg, when evidence arises that a treatment has unexpected or unacceptable risk).

2. When a third party is at risk (eg, in communicable disease).

3. When there is a legal obligation to do so (eg, in cases of abuse).

VIII. Institutional Review Boards

A. The modern history of the protection of human subjects began with the Nuremberg Code of Medical Ethics, which was developed by the Nuremberg Military Tribunal after the investigation of Nazi physicians (1946-1947).

1. The code was quickly adopted by the World Medical Association (1948).

2. The Department of Health, Education and Welfare (DHEW) instituted regulations protecting human subjects on May 30, 1974.

3. This was followed in July of the same year by establishment of the National Commission for the Protection of Human Subjects of Biomedical and Behavioral Research, which issued the Belmont Report (Belmont Conference Center at the Smithsonian Institute) defining the basic ethical principles that should underlie the conduct of biomedical and behavioral research involving human subjects.

2: General Knowledge

B. The Belmont Report—Elements of this 1978 report form the basis for human research in the United States.

1. Respect for individuals—Emphasizes dignity and autonomy, and encompasses informed consent (*quid vide*).

2. Beneficence—Emphasizes the need to maximize benefit and minimize risk, including for both the individual and society.

   a. Risk should be minimized, with an initial goal of avoiding the use of using human subjects if at all possible.

   b. Risk and benefit are determined by assessing information provided by the investigator and all other relevant information available in the literature.

3. Justice—Requires fair selection of subjects and distribution of the benefits and burdens of research. The subject must be considered not only as an individual but also as a member of a social, racial, sexual, or cultural group in an effort to avoid bias.

C. Specific protections were added for vulnerable populations.

1. Fetuses and pregnant women (1978)

2. Prisoners (1978)

3. Children (1991)—Specified need to obtain assent of child and consent of parent.

IX. Care of the Uninsured

A. Obligation to provide care

1. No national public policy in the United States establishes a patient's right to medical care.

2. The physician has an ethical obligation, however, to provide care consistent with the fundamental principles of the medical profession to provide care to a patient in need, regardless of ability to pay and in the absence of a legal or governmental mandate to do so. The physician must advocate for the patient in such circumstances, but not "by any means necessary," that is, not by lying, misrepresentation, or withholding necessary information, because this behavior undermines the very ethical principles that the physician wishes to uphold.

B. Allocation of health care resources

1. Directed allocation, or rationing, is unavoidable because resources are limited.

2. Ideally, allocation decisions should be a matter of public policy with physician input, and not made in the clinical setting.

3. In the clinical setting, the physician should act as a patient advocate within constraints set by society, reasonable insurance coverage, and evidence-based practice.

4. Ad hoc rationing in the clinical setting is ethically problematic because physicians may be inconsistent, unqualified, unfair, and/or ineffective.

X. Culturally Competent Care

A. Factors to be considered when tailoring health care to individual patient needs:

1. Age

2. Gender

3. Cultural competence

B. Culturally competent care

1. Enhanced by an awareness of and willingness to challenge the following features of North American medical culture:

   a. Dominance of time

   b. Individual needs over the group or society

   c. The shrinking family

   d. Undisputed belief in science

   e. Primacy of Western medicine

   f. Competition

   g. Action/goal/work/future orientation

   h. Openness

   i. Materialism

   j. Change

   k. Equality

   l. Informality

   m. Practicality and efficiency

   n. Secularism over religion

2. Components of culturally competent care

   a. Values—Perceptions of "quality" of treatment and what is regarded as "acceptable" benefit and risk.

   b. Customs

   c. Communication

   d. Nonverbal interactions and behaviors

   e. Institutions, including religious

3. Benefits of culturally competent care

   a. Improved accuracy of care—In its simplest form, this includes language.

b. Improved consistency in the delivery of care—The informed patient who can negotiate efficiently the medical system and is able to comply with proposed treatment(s).

c. Wider access to care—Surmounting barriers that may shut cultural minorities out of certain parts of the health care system.

d. Reduced cost of care—Elimination of misunderstanding and adoption of preventive measures.

e. Improved outcomes

f. Higher patient satisfaction

4. Misconceptions about culturally competent care include that it is a euphemism for segregated care, that it relies on racial quotas, that it is guided by racial stereotypes, and that it is fulfilled simply by provision of an interpreter.

Top Testing Facts

1. Breaches of medical professionalism include inappropriate billing, failure to maintain adequate medical records, and incomplete disclosure.

2. The three elements essential to informed consent are information, comprehension, and voluntariness.

3. Physicians may not accept gifts from industry valued greater than $100.

4. Physicians attending continuing medical education courses may not accept subsidies for travel, lodging, recreational activities, or personal expenses.

5. Stark II regulations prohibit a physician from referring a Medicare patient for certain designated health services to an entity with which the physician or immediate family member has a direct or indirect financial relationship.

6. Essential components to improvement of peer review and the rate or reporting of medical errors include

emphasis on the patient over the practitioner; systems over the individual; proaction over retrospection; and maintenance of confidentiality.

7. Advance directives may be established through oral conversations, living wills, or the appointment of a health care proxy.

8. Patient confidentiality may be breached justifiably when a patient is at risk, when a third party is at risk, or when there is a legal obligation to do so.

9. The three essential components of the Belmont Report are respect for persons, beneficence in maximizing benefit and minimizing risk, and justice of distribution of benefits of human research.

10. Cultural competence will improve accuracy of, delivery of, and access to health care, thereby improving patient outcomes and satisfaction.

Bibliography

Beauchamp TL, Childress JF: *Principles of Biomedical Ethics*, ed 5. New York, NY, Oxford University Press, 2001.

Berg JW, Lidz CW, Appelbaum PS: *Informed Consent: Legal Theory and Clinical Practice*, ed 2. New York, NY, Oxford University Press, 2001.

Lo B: *Resolving Ethical Dilemmas: A Guide for Clinicians*, ed 3. Baltimore, MD, Williams & Wilkens, 2005.

Meisel A: *The Right to Die*, ed 2. New York, NY, John Wiley & Sons, 1995.

Papadakis MA, Tehrani A, Banach MA, et al: Disciplinary action by medical boards and prior behavior in medical school. *N Engl J Med* 2005;353:2673-2682.

Salimbene S: *What Language Does Your Patient Hurt In? A Practical Guide to Culturally Competent Patient Care*. Amherst, MA, Diversity Resources, 2000.

Seiber JE: *Planning Ethically Responsible Research: A Guide for Students and Internal Review Boards*. Newbury Park, CA, Sage, 1992.

Snyder L, Leffler C: Ethics and Human Rights Committee of the American College of Physicians: Ethics manual, 5th ed. *Ann Intern Med* 2005;142:560-582.

2: General Knowledge

Chapter 15

Occupational Health/Work-Related Injury and Illness

Peter J. Mandell, MD

I. Workers' Compensation

A. Burden of proof

1. The injured worker does not have to prove the employer was at fault.

2. The injured worker must prove that work at least partially caused the injury/illness.

3. Causation must be proved to attribute work-related factor(s) to a particular condition.

   a. Results of the history and physical examination should identify the diagnosis and determine causation.

   b. A thorough review of the injured worker's records is also needed to support conclusions.

   c. A detailed history of the injury may reveal important facts to support an opinion on causation.

B. Assessment of the injured worker

1. The patient history should accomplish the following:

   a. Specific information regarding the how, when, where, and why of an accident or injurious exposure should be elicited.

   b. The areas of the body that were involved should be identified.

   c. The extent and onset of symptoms following the accident or injurious exposure should be identified.

   d. The treatment history should be reviewed in detail, specifically methods and effectiveness. Failure to respond at all to multiple, usually reliable treatments of common diagnoses suggests a nonorganic component.

   e. The worker's perception of events compared with those depicted in the medical records should be analyzed to assess credibility.

2. Current symptoms should be discussed to document answers to the following questions:

   a. What hurts now?

   b. What can the patient do? What can't the patient do?

   c. How does the injury impact the patient's ability to work, perform activities of daily living, and play?

3. The past medical history and review of systems should focus on other possible causes or contributors:

   a. Prior injuries to the same or related body regions

   b. Prior surgeries

   c. Prior industrial accidents of any type

   d. A family history of similar problems

   e. Diseases and habits that impact the neuromusculoskeletal system

      i. Diabetes mellitus

      ii. Rheumatoid arthritis

      iii. Obesity

      iv. Smoking

      v. Alcohol abuse

      vi. High-impact hobbies/sports activities

4. A detailed work history is essential. Knowledge of the patient's work activities and environment can determine possible causative factors and the feasibility of modified work activities. The work history should include:

   a. How long the patient has worked at the job

   b. Prior work experience

   c. Concurrent employment at a second or third job

   d. Job satisfaction

      i. Recent job changes such as increased workload resulting from layoffs

Table 1

Waddell Nonorganic Physical Signs in Low Back Pain

1. Tenderness	Tenderness related to physical disease should be specific and localized to specific anatomic structures. Superficial—tenderness to pinch or light touch over a wide area of lumbar skin Nonanatomic—deep tenderness over a wide area, not localized to a specific structure
2. Simulation tests	These tests should not be uncomfortable. Axial loading—reproduction of low back pain with vertical pressure on the skull Rotation—reproduction of back pain when shoulders and pelvis are passively rotated in the same plane
3. Distraction tests	Findings that are present during physical examination and disappear at other times, particularly while the patient is distracted
4. Regional disturbances	Findings inconsistent with neuroanatomy Motor—nonanatomic voluntary release or unexplained giving way of muscle groups Sensory—nondermatomal sensory abnormalities
5. Overreaction	Disproportionate verbal or physical reactions

Reproduced from Moy OJ, Ablove RH: Work-related illnesses, cumulative trauma and compensation, in Vaccaro AR (ed): Orthopaedic Knowledge Update 8. Rosemont, IL, American Academy of Orthopaedic Surgeons, 2005, pp 143-148.

 ii. Conflicts with a supervisor or associates

 iii. A high demand–low control (stressful) work environment

5. Musculoskeletal examination of the injured area

   a. Examine the injured body part(s).

   b. Investigate other, less obvious explanations.

     i. Cervical disk disease as a cause of shoulder pain

     ii. Hip arthritis as a cause of back or knee pain

   c. Remember that the physical findings may form a major portion of the basis for administrative and financial decisions that will significantly impact the patient.

   d. Comments on the reliability of the patient's physical findings and on whether the findings support the injured employee's degree of subjective complaints should be included.

 i. For patients with low back pain, assess Waddell signs (**Table 1**)

 ii. Three of five signs must be present to be considered a nonorganic source of pain.

II. Workplace Safety and OSHA

A. Ergonomics

1. Science that studies ways to make the workplace more congenial to human capabilities

2. Considers the realities of human anatomy and the physiology of human muscle strength and fatigue

3. Involves machine and workstation design to improve workplace safety

B. US Department of Labor's Occupational Safety and Health Administration (OSHA)

1. Developed guidelines and programs to improve worker health and safety

2. Workplace safety measures have resulted in a sharp decrease in the incidence of distinct workplace injuries in the late 20th century.

3. The decline of these specific injuries revealed a host of other conditions that may develop in the workplace and can increase in severity over time.

   a. Controversy exists about what to call these conditions and if they are indeed work related. Many call them cumulative trauma disorders (CTDs). This term is frequently cited in both the medical and legal literature.

     i. The term is problematic because some argue that CTD implies a specific etiology that generally has not been clearly and scientifically substantiated; the cause is multifactorial.

     ii. Not all CTDs become chronic problems; in fact, many disappear as workers become conditioned to specific work activities. But if rest is not provided or if activities exceed physiologic limits, then no amount of conditioning will prevent tissue damage.

   b. OSHA calls these musculoskeletal disorders (MSDs).

     i. An MSD is an injury of the musculoskeletal and/or nervous system that may be associated with or caused by repetitive tasks, forceful exertions, vibrations, mechanical compression (pressing against hard surfaces), or sustained or awkward positions.

     ii. Examples include low back pain, sciatica, bursitis, epicondylitis, and carpal tunnel syndrome.

c. Conditions such as MSDs caused by more extended exposure to employment are termed occupational *illnesses*, whereas an occupational *injury* is one arising from a distinct event.

d. The American Academy of Orthopaedic Surgeons adopted a position statement in 2004 regarding the use of these terms. It is available at www.aaos.org/about/papers/position/1165.asp.

III. Legal Issues in Occupational Orthopaedics

A. Advantages of workers' compensation

1. For injured workers—it obligates employers to

   a. Compensate the injured worker for high-quality, timely treatment needed to cure or relieve the worker of the effects of the work injury(ies).

   b. Repay lost wages, to a maximum that varies from state to state.

   c. Pay a final disability settlement (analogous to the "damages" awarded in civil cases).

2. For employers

   a. The employer is shielded from being sued for negligence, except in particularly egregious circumstances.

   b. Workers' compensation is usually the "exclusive remedy," precluding claims against employers for pain and suffering, emotional distress, punitive damages, and bad faith.

   c. The system is no-fault.

   d. The employer is required to pay benefits only when work is the cause—at least partially—of the worker's problem(s).

B. Components of the claim

1. Determining causation

2. The need for treatment and, if needed, type and duration

3. The extent of present disability

4. The ultimate disability settlement

C. Allocating or apportioning causation

1. Some causes may be work related, and some may be preexisting.

2. Legal apportionment varies by state.

   a. Many states require employers to "take their workers as they find them," which makes apportioning to preexisting (but asymptomatic) conditions such as gout, diabetes mellitus, and obesity difficult or illegal.

b. Other states seemingly allow apportionment to factors beyond the employer's control such as those listed above. Factors such as sex, race, smoking, and obesity may not survive constitutional challenge.

IV. Assignment of Impairment and Disability

A. Importance of terms and definitions of terms in workers' compensation

1. Different jurisdictions assign somewhat different meanings to the same words.

2. The same word or terms can mean different things in different contexts.

3. Check the meaning of important terms in your state.

4. Commonly accepted words and definitions (not universal)

   a. *Impairment*—A deviation or loss of body structure or of physiologic or psychologic function.

   b. *Disease*—A pathologic condition of a body part.

   c. *Illness*—Total effect of an injury or disease on the entire person.

   d. *Disability*—Any restriction or lack of ability to perform an activity in the manner or within the range considered normal for an individual.

5. Impairment and disease are purely biologic issues that usually have an objectively measurable effect on the anatomy and/or physiology of the injured organ. An injury leads to an impairment that leads to a disease that may lead to a disability and an illness.

6. Illness and disability are the final complete functional manifestations of impairment and disease, including the social, physiologic, and economic (work) consequences of the employee's injury.

B. Assessment of level of impairment

1. Only physicians can evaluate for and assign level of impairment.

2. The assessment must be based on medical probability, also known as medical certainty, which implies that a statement or opinion is correct with >50% certainty.

3. In most states, providing a medically probable opinion about an injured worker's impairment generally requires use of the American Medical Association's *Guides to the Evaluation of Permanent Impairment*.

   a. This reference provides tables and other stan-

2: General Knowledge

dardized methods (depending on the body part or parts involved) for determining impairment.

    b. It also supplies rules for combining the regional impairments into a "whole person" impairment.

4. Impairments are translated into disability ratings by state workers' compensation boards and other jurisdictions.

V. Malingering, Somatization, and Depression

A. Special considerations—Unlike most medical problems, with workers' compensation, the patient often thinks she or he knows what is wrong; there is reason to be skeptical when insurance issues are on the line.

B. Malingering

    1. Malingering is an act, not a disease. Calling someone a malingerer is an accusation, not a diagnosis.

    2. Malingering is at the far edge of a spectrum of explanations about a problem with many names, including

        a. Nonorganic findings

        b. Symptom magnification

        c. Exaggeration

        d. Submaximal, insincere, or low effort

        e. Selling oneself short

        f. Inappropriate pain or illness behavior

C. Somatization (formerly called hysteria or Briquet's syndrome)

    1. Somatization is an extreme form of body language.

    2. Patients who cannot (or whose cultures will not allow them to) express psychological problems may communicate such problems through sometimes powerful physical manifestations.

    3. Somatization may be an attempt by patients to strive for psychological homeostasis.

D. Nonorganic findings

    1. Most patients with nonorganic findings may look like malingerers but really have somatization.

    2. Patients with nonorganic findings may be adult survivors of childhood physical and/or sexual abuse.

E. Factitious disorder

    1. Another form of somatization that resembles malingering

2. A psychological disorder in which patients have an unconscious need to assume an ill role by producing their disease (eg, people who fear heights but don't know why); the most well known factitious disorder is Munchausen's syndrome.

F. Depression

    1. May affect assignment of disability because depressed patients often have a heightened perception of disability.

    2. Depression can be a vicious cycle, arising from a protracted injury and then creating at least the perception of more physical illness.

VI. Issues Relating to Return to Work

A. Statistics

    1. About 10% of injured employees who are off work have significant problems returning to their jobs within usual timeframes.

    2. Some studies cite the percentage of workers who return to full duty at only 50% after having been out of work for 6 months.

    3. Other studies report the same percentage but after only 3 months on disability.

B. Early return to work

    1. Disability itself can be pathogenic and even fatal; early return to duty usually is the best approach for all concerned in the workers' compensation system, especially the injured employee. Early return

        a. Minimizes the sense of illness

        b. Lessens the loss of camaraderie and teamwork with associates

        c. Improves self-respect and positive feedback that comes from knowing one is valued by society

        d. Lessens the effect of deconditioning

    2. Exceptions to early return to work include lack of appropriate light duty and posttraumatic stress after severe injuries such as amputations and burns.

    3. Job satisfaction and early return to work

        a. Leading factor in early return to work

        b. Workers with high levels of discretion are twice as likely to be working than those with less autonomy.

        c. An unpleasant, stressful work environment greatly reduces the chances that an injured employee will return to work.

    4. Employer factors and early return to work

a. The employer should show support for injured workers.

b. Employer hostility intensifies worker stress.

c. Some employers use disability as a way to dismiss workers.

C. Worker factors and return to work

1. Some use time off and benefits to resolve home and family problems.

2. Workers on disability tend to recover more slowly and have poorer outcomes than those with the same injuries covered by group health and other forms of insurance.

D. Other factors and return to work

1. Union rules sometimes do not allow injured workers to be assigned to lighter jobs because other workers have more seniority.

2. Work hardening can be helpful as an intermediate step in transitioning patients from physical therapy to full duty.

Top Testing Facts

1. A workers' compensation claim is valid when a patient's diagnosis is related to work exposure.

2. It is crucial that the history, review of medical records, and physical examination findings support the diagnosis and its causation analysis.

3. Workplace safety programs and OSHA activities have greatly reduced major industrial accidents.

4. Cumulative trauma/musculoskeletal disorders have become more obvious with the decline of major work injuries.

5. It is important to know the precise meanings of the terms often used in workers' compensation matters, including *impairment*, *disease*, *illness*, and *disability*.

6. Key factors in a workers' compensation case include medical decisions about causation, treatment, light work status, and residual impairments.

7. Calling someone a malingerer is an accusation, not a diagnosis.

8. Somatization is far more common than malingering.

9. Depressed patients often have a heightened sense of impairment.

10. Early return to work is an important key to obtaining a successful outcome after a work injury.

Bibliography

Amadio PC: Work-related illness, cumulative trauma, and compensation, in Koval KJ (ed): *Orthopaedic Knowledge Update 7*. Rosemont, IL, American Academy of Orthopaedic Surgeons, 2002, pp 121-126.

American Academy of Orthopaedic Surgeons: Defining musculoskeletal disorders in the workplace. Position statement 2004. www.aaos.org/about/papers/position/1165.asp.

Brady W, Bass J, Royce M, Anstadt G, Loeppke R, Leopold R: Defining total corporate health and safety costs: Significance and impact. *J Occup Environ Med* 1997;39:224-231.

Brinker MR, O'Connor DP, Woods GW, Pierce P, Peck B: The effect of payer type on orthopaedic practice expenses. *J Bone Joint Surg Am* 2002;84:1816-1822.

Gerdtham UG, Johannesson M: A note on the effect of unemployment on mortality. *J Health Econ* 2003;22:505-518.

Harris I, Multford J, Solomon M, van Gelder J, Young J: Association between compensation status and outcome after surgery. *JAMA* 2005;293:1644-1652.

Jin RL, Shah CP, Svoboda TJ: The impact of unemployment on health: A review of the evidence. *CMAJ* 1995;153: 529-540.

Lea RD: Independent medical evaluation: An organization and analysis system, in Grace TG (ed): *Independent Medical Evaluations*. Rosemont, IL American Academy of Orthopaedic Surgeons, 2001, pp 35-57.

Moy OJ, Ablove RH: Work-related illness, cumulative trauma, and compensation, in Vaccaro AR (ed): *Orthopaedic Knowledge Update 8*. Rosemont, IL, American Academy of Orthopaedic Surgeons, 2005, pp 143-148.

Stone DA: *The Disabled State*. Philadelphia, PA, Temple University Press, 1984.

Waddell G, McCulloch JA, Kummel E, Venner RM: Nonorganic physical signs in low back pain. *Spine* 1980;5:117-125.

Zeppieri JP: The physician, the illness, and the workers' compensation system, in Beaty JH (ed): *Orthopaedic Knowledge Update 6*. Rosemont, IL, American Academy of Orthopaedic Surgeons, 1999, pp 131-137.

2: General Knowledge

Chapter 16

Musculoskeletal Imaging

C. Benjamin Ma, MD   Lynne Steinbach, MD

I. Radiography

A. Principles of radiography

1. Radiographic images are obtained by projecting x-ray beams through an object onto an image detector.

2. The image produced is a projectional map of the amount of radiation absorbed by the object along the course of the x-ray beam.

3. The amount of whiteness of the image is a function of the radiodensity and thickness of the object.

4. The denser the object, the more radiation is being absorbed, and hence a lighter or whiter image is produced. Metal objects and bone are very radiodense and appear white on radiographs.

5. Digital radiography

    a. Commonly used now

    b. Image processing and distribution are achieved through a picture archiving and communication system.

    c. The process allows the images to be portable and transferable via computers or compact discs.

B. Digital radiography versus conventional film screen radiography

1. Film screen radiography has higher spatial resolution.

2. Improved contrast resolution for digital radiography means the technique is comparable in terms of diagnostic efficiency.

C. Radiation dose measurements

1. The scientific unit of measurement of radiation dose, commonly referred to as "effective dose," is the millisievert (mSv).

2. Other radiation dose measurement units include the rad, rem, roentgen, and sievert.

D. Radiation exposure

1. Continual from natural sources

2. The average person in the United States receives an effective dose of 3 mSv/year from naturally occurring radioactive materials and cosmic radiation.

3. The average radiation dose from a standard chest radiograph is 0.1 mSv.

E. Advantages of radiography

1. Most commonly used medical imaging modality

2. Relatively inexpensive

3. Real-time radiographic imaging, or fluoroscopy, allows instantaneous feedback on stress radiographs, angiography, and orthopaedic interventions.

F. Disadvantages of radiography

1. Radiation is transmitted to the patient.

2. It is not effective for soft-tissue imaging because of poor contrast resolution.

3. The images obtained are always magnified. Measurement "standards" can be placed with the object to allow determination of magnification.

4. Although most medical x-ray beams do not pose a risk to a fetus, there is a small likelihood that serious illness and developmental problems can occur. The actual risk depends on the type of imaging study and the trimester of pregnancy.

II. Computed Tomography

A. Principles of CT

1. Uses x-ray beams to produce tomographic images, or slices of an object.

2. Multiple images are obtained and reassembled to generate a three-dimensional image.

3. X-ray densities are measured in Hounsfield units (HUs) or CT numbers.

C. Benjamin Ma, MD, or the department with which he is affiliated has received research or institutional support from OREF and NIH.

2: General Knowledge

a. Water is assigned a value of 0 HU; air, a value of −1,000 HU.

b. Images are displayed as grayscale; denser objects are lighter.

c. Good for soft-tissue imaging; grayscale can be modified ("windowed") to show data that fall within a fixed range of densities, such as bone windows or lung windows.

B. Advantages of CT

1. Tomographic nature of the images

2. Higher contrast resolution

3. The latest generation of CT scanners uses multiple detector row arrays, which leads to improved resolution and shorter acquisition times.

4. Images are processed digitally; images in a plane other than the one in which the original images were obtained can be reconstructed to give a different perspective of the object/tissue of interest.

5. Magnification artifacts that occur in plain radiography do not occur with CT; direct measurements can be performed on the scans.

6. CT can be combined with arthrography or myelography to evaluate specific joint or spinal abnormalities.

7. CT is useful for injections, biopsies, and aspirations of fluid collections.

8. CT provides better detail of cortical and trabecular bone structures than MRI.

E. Disadvantages of CT

1. Most CT slices require about 1 second, which is longer than the time required for a radiographic image; thus, scans are subject to motion artifacts.

2. CT is subject to artifacts due to metal objects.

a. Metal has high x-ray density, which prevents sufficient x-ray beams from being transmitted through the body part.

b. These result in an artifact called "beam hardening." Beam hardening appears as streaks of white or black that can obscure the anatomy adjacent to the metal object.

3. CT can be impractical for obese patients.

a. Most scanners have a weight limit.

b. Above the limit, the table that carries the patient through the scanner may not move or may break.

4. CT produces higher radiation exposure than plain radiography.

5. It is generally contraindicated for pregnant patients, except in life-threatening circumstances.

III. MRI and MR Arthrography

A. General principles of MRI

1. MRI is similar to CT scanning in that images are produced by reconstruction of a data set.

2. MRI does not use radiation or have the tissue-damaging properties of radiation-based imaging modalities. It uses a strong magnet that generates a magnetic field and multiple coils that send and/or receive radio frequency (RF) signals.

3. All clinical MRI scans image the protons in hydrogen atoms. In a strong magnetic field, the protons line up like countless compasses.

4. A brief RF pulse is applied to the tissue that deflects the protons. When the pulse is terminated, the protons realign, or relax, along the strong magnetic field. The protons relax at different rates depending on their atomic environment.

5. The weak signal that the proton emits during relaxation allows the detector to detect the properties within the tissue.

6. Contrast on MRIs can be manipulated by changing the pulse sequence parameters. Two important parameters are the repetition time (TR) and the echo time (TE). The most common pulse sequences are T1-weighted and T2-weighted sequences. The T1-weighted sequence uses a short TR and short TE; the T2-weighted sequence uses a long TR and long TE. Different structures are identified more easily on each sequence (**Figure 1 and Table 1**).

7. Signals from fat also play an important role in providing contrast. Fat-suppression techniques add a useful dimension to the manipulation of image contrast. Fat-suppressed images are helpful in delineating various structural abnormalities.

8. The strength of the magnet is expressed in tesla (T) units. The stronger the magnet, the higher the intrinsic signal-to-noise ratio, which can improve imaging speed and resolution.

B. Types of MRI scanners

1. Conventional

a. Requires a large room and a small bore

b. Has weight limit for patients

c. Takes longer than CT scanning

d. Patients with claustrophobia may not tolerate the scan well.

2. Open scanners or extremity scanners

a. Usually are lower field-strength machines

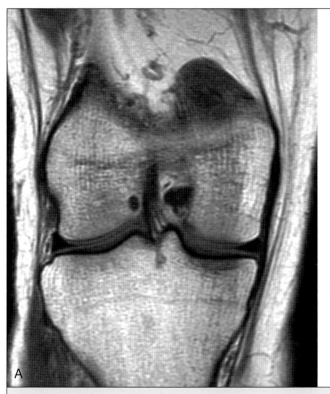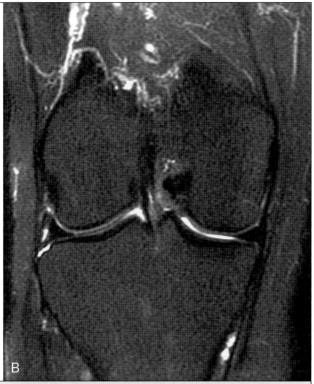

Figure 1   The appearance of different anatomic structures on T1- and T2-weighted coronal MRIs of the knee. **A,** On the T1-weighted image, fat and bone marrow are bright, whereas the menisci and tendon are dark. **B,** On the T2-weighted image, joint fluid and blood vessels are bright in contrast to other structures.

Table 1

Relative Signal Intensities of Selected Structures in MRI

Structure	T1-Weighted Image	T2-Weighted Image
Fat	Bright	Intermediate
Fluid	Dark	Bright
Bone	Dark	Dark
Ligament	Dark	Dark
Muscle	Intermediate	Dark
Bone marrow edema	Dark	Bright
Fibrocartilage	Dark	Dark
Osteomyelitis	Dark	Bright

b. Can image the extremity well

c. Can accommodate claustrophobic patients

d. Images can be of adequate quality despite the lower field strength but generally provide less resolution than conventional closed MRI scanners.

D. MR arthrography

1. Commonly used to augment MRI to diagnose soft-tissue problems.

   a. In direct MR arthrography, a dilute gadolinium-containing solution is percutaneously injected into the joint.

   b. In indirect MR arthrography, gadolinium is administered intravenously and allowed to travel through the vascular system to the region of interest.

2. MR arthrography is commonly used for diagnosis of labral tears in the shoulder and hip joints and postoperative evaluation of meniscus repairs.

E. Advantages of MRI

1. Superior images of soft tissues, such as ligaments, muscle, and fat

2. Can give tomographic images of the object of interest

3. Can be more effective than CT at detecting changes in intensity within the bone marrow to diagnose osteomyelitis, malignancy, and stress fractures

4. MRI contrast (gadolinium) is safer than iodine-based media.

F. Disadvantages of MRI

1. Prone to large and more severe types of artifacts from metal and motion

   a. Metal screws or pellets can produce significant artifact, obscuring anatomic structures.

   b. Metal suppression sequences can be used, but with loss of resolution.

2. Usually takes longer than CT

3. Patients need to remain still throughout the scanning process.

4. Sedation often is needed for pediatric patients.

G. Dangers associated with MRI

1. Because of the strong magnet in the scanner, extreme caution is needed when a patient, physician, nurse, or technician enters the room. Electrical appliances such as pacemakers and mechanical pumps can malfunction.

2. Metal objects brought into the scanner can turn into dangerous projectiles.

3. Metal foreign bodies within the eye or brain can migrate and cause blindness and brain damage.

4. Patients with metal implants in their joints or body can have a MRI scan if the implants are secured in bone or stable. Discussion with the physician and technician before the scan is important to avoid potentially disastrous outcomes.

H. Considerations in pregnant women

1. Although MRI does not use radiation, the effect of RF and magnetic field on the fetus is unknown.

2. It is usually recommended that a pregnant woman not have an MRI scan.

I. Use of gadolinium as contrast

1. Gadolinium behaves like iodinated contrast media, accumulating in highly vascular and metabolically active tissues.

2. It should not be administered to patients with a creatinine < 33 mg/dL because it can lead to nephrogenic fibrosing dermopathy.

3. The echo waves are then analyzed by the time traveled and amplitude, and the information is converted into an image.

4. Image resolution and beam attenuation depend on the wavelength and frequency.

5. A lower frequency ultrasound beam has a longer wavelength and less resolution but deeper penetration.

6. A higher frequency ultrasound beam can give higher resolution for superficial structures such as tendons and ligaments.

7. Doppler ultrasonography can be used to image blood vessels for flow velocity and direction. Color maps can be generated for color Doppler ultrasound.

B. Advantages of ultrasonography

1. Noninvasive at the frequencies used for diagnostic imaging

2. Commonly used for imaging in children and pregnant women

3. Shows nonossified structures such as the femoral head to diagnose hip dysplasia and dislocation

4. The equipment is portable and inexpensive compared with MRI and CT equipment.

5. Highly echogenic structures, such as a foreign body that may not be visible on radiographs, can be easily detected using ultrasonography.

6. Can be used for targeted therapy, such as injections and ablations

7. Useful for injections and aspirations of fluid collections

C. Disadvantages of ultrasonography

1. Image quality and interpretation depend on the experience of the ultrasonographer and radiologists.

2. Cannot image inside bone because bone cortex reflects almost all sound waves

3. Internal joint structures are not well visualized.

IV. Ultrasonography (Ultrasound)

A. Principles of ultrasonography

1. Uses high-frequency sound waves to produce images, analogous to using sonar waves to obtain images of the ocean.

2. A transducer produces sound waves that travel through the patient; echo waves are deflected back by the tissue to the same transducer.

V. Nuclear Medicine

A. Principles of nuclear medicine

1. Uses radioisotope-labeled, biologically active drugs.

2. The radioactive tracer is administered to the patient to serve as markers of biologic activity.

3. The images produced by scintigraphy are a collection of the radiation emissions from the isotopes.

B. Bone scintigraphy (bone scan)

1. Generally performed using diphosphonates labeled with radioactive technetium Tc 99m.

2. Phases

a. The initial (transient) phase is characterized by tracer delivery to the tissue, which represents the perfusion images.

b. The second (blood pool) phase follows the initial phase.

c. The final (delayed) phase shows tracer accumulation in tissues with active turnover of phosphates, mostly in bone undergoing growth and turnover.

C. Positron emission tomography (PET)

1. PET using the metabolic tracer FDG is widely used in clinical oncology.

2. FDG accumulation reflects the rate of glucose utilization in tissue.

a. FDG is transported into tissue by the same mechanisms of glucose transport and is trapped in the tissue as FDG-6-phosphate.

b. Use of FDG in evaluation of the musculoskeletal system is based on an increased glycolytic rate in pathologic tissues.

c. High-grade malignancies tend to have higher rates of glycolysis than low-grade malignancies and have greater uptake of FDG than do low-grade or benign lesions.

D. Advantages of nuclear medicine imaging

1. Scintigraphy has high sensitivity for bone pathology.

2. Scintigraphy allows imaging of metabolic activity. Most metabolic processes involving bone have slow metabolic activity compared with that of soft tissue, such as kidney and liver. Fortunately, most radioisotopes are relatively long lived.

3. White cell scintigraphy can be used to diagnose osteomyelitis.

4. Scintigraphy can be used to diagnose metastasis, stress fracture, or occult fractures.

E. Disadvantages of nuclear medicine imaging

1. Lack of detail and spatial resolution

2. Has limited early sensitivity to detect acute fractures in patients with slow bone metabolism; it may take several days for the bone scan to be positive to diagnose occult femoral neck fracture.

3. Low sensitivity can occur with lytic diseases such as multiple myeloma.

4. Scintigraphy has low specificity for bone pathology.

VI. Radiation Safety

A. Children and fetuses are especially susceptible to ionizing radiation.

B. Radiography, CT, and bone scintigraphy produce ions that can deposit energy to organs and tissues. The energy can damage DNA.

C. Radiation for radioactive-labeled tracers in scintigraphy primarily affects the patient. Some tracers (eg, iodine-131) have half lives of several days and can concentrate in excreted body fluid and breast milk.

D. Rapidly dividing tissues are the most susceptible to radiation-induced neoplasia (**Table 2**).

1. Bone marrow

2. Breast tissue

3. Gastrointestinal mucosa

4. Gonads

5. Lymphatic tissue

E. Risk of cancer is approximately 4% per sievert (100 rem).

F. Risk of fetal malformation

1. Greatest in the first trimester and with doses > 0.1 Gy (10 rad)

2. Late in pregnancy (≥ 150 days postconception), the greatest risk is an increase in childhood malignancies such as leukemia.

Table 2		
Threshold Acute Exposure Doses for Effects in Humans		
Organ Exposed	**Dose (in Gy)**	**Effect**
Ocular lens	2	Cataracts
Bone marrow	2-7	Marrow failure with infection, death
Skin	3	Temporary hair loss
Skin	5	Erythema
Testes	5-6	Permanent decrease in sperm count
Skin	7	Permanent hair loss
Intestines	7-50	Gastrointestinal failure, death
Brain	50-100	Cerebral edema, death

Adapted from Radiation safety, in Johnson TR, Steinbach LS (eds): Essentials of Musculoskeletal Imaging. Rosemont, IL, American Academy of Orthopaedic Surgeons, 2004, p 28.

2: General Knowledge

3. A 10-mGy (1-rad) dose increases childhood leukemia risk as much as 40%.

4. It is important to ensure that the patient is not pregnant when obtaining any imaging examinations other than ultrasonography. Performance of other types of imaging examinations can be discussed in consultation with the radiologist and physician.

G. Protection

1. Sensitive organs such as gonads should be shielded.

2. It is best to follow the principle of ALARA ("as low as reasonably achievable") dosing for pregnant women and children.

3. Exposure to radiation decreases as an inverse square of the distance from the source.

4. Medical personnel should wear lead aprons and be monitored using devices such as film badges.

5. CT delivers the highest amount of radiation dose among all medical imaging procedures (5-15 mSv versus 0.1-2.0 mSv for plain radiography).

Top Testing Facts

1. All clinical MRI scans image the protons in hydrogen atoms.

2. It is extremely important to screen patients with metallic objects before entering the MRI machine. Ferromagnetic objects in or on the body can be pulled toward the magnet and cause serious injuries.

3. Patients with advanced kidney failure should not receive gadolinium-containing contrast agents because exposure to the agent can cause development of nephrogenic fibrosing dermopathy.

4. A lower frequency ultrasound beam has a longer wavelength and less resolution but deeper penetration.

5. A higher frequency ultrasound beam can give higher resolution for superficial structures such as tendons and ligaments.

6. Caution is advised when ordering nuclear medicine tests for women who are breast-feeding; some of the pharmaceuticals can pass into the mother's milk and subsequently into the child.

7. Exposure to radiation decreases as an inverse square of the distance from the source.

8. CT delivers the highest radiation dosage of all imaging modalities.

9. The risk of cancer is approximately 4% per sievert (100 rem).

10. It is important to ensure that the patient is not pregnant when obtaining any imaging examinations other than ultrasonography. Performance of other types of imaging examinations can be discussed in consultation with the radiologist and physician.

Bibliography

Board on Radiation Effects Research, Commission on Life Sciences, National Research Council, Beir V: Committee on Biological Effects of Ionizing Radiation, in *Health Effects of Exposure to Low Levels of Ionizing Radiation*. Washington, DC, National Academy Press, 1990.

Brent RL, Gorson RO: Radiation exposure in pregnancy, in *Current Problems in Radiology: Technic of Pneumoencephalography*. Chicago, IL, Year Book Medical, 1972.

Johnson TR, Steinbach LS (eds): Imaging modalities, in *Essentials of Musculoskeletal Imaging*. Rosemont, IL, American Academy of Orthopaedic Surgeons, 2003, pp 3-30.

Vaccaro AR (ed): Musculoskeletal imaging, in *Orthopaedic Knowledge Update 8 Home Study Syllabus*. Rosemont, IL, American Academy of Orthopaedic Surgeons, 2005, pp 119-136.

2: General Knowledge

Chapter 17

Perioperative Medical Management

Andrew Auerbach, MD, MPH

I. Assessment

A. Goals of preoperative medical assessment

1. Assess the risk of potential perioperative mortality and morbidity.

2. Determine whether a patient's medical condition can be optimized before elective surgery.

B. Patient's "readiness" for surgery

1. Determined by the patient's anesthesiologist on the day of surgery.

2. Includes risk assessment for intraoperative and acute postoperative outcomes.

3. Includes evaluation of preexisting conditions, both related and unrelated to the planned surgical procedure.

II. Preoperative Evaluation

A. A thorough history and physical examination is necessary and can be conducted by a primary care physician, internist, hospitalist, or other physician.

B. Systems-based approach includes all body systems.

C. Goals of the history and physical examination are to identify an undiagnosed, poorly managed, or other condition. Such conditions can place the patient at a higher perioperative risk for morbidity and mortality.

III. Preoperative Testing

A. Blanket testing is not cost effective in planning care of a general population of patients.

B. Patients with specific comorbidities should be screened using tests relevant to their disease.

C. A directed bleeding history (**Table 1**) is more effec-

tive for assessing the risk of abnormal surgical bleeding than routine screening with platelet counts, International Normalized Ratio (INR), or bleeding time tests.

IV. Assessment of Cardiac Risk

A. Key preoperative steps include:

1. Identifying patients with new or unstable cardiopulmonary symptoms for additional preoperative testing (eg, noninvasive stress tests, catheterization).

2. Beginning preventive therapies, if needed, even though preoperative revascularization does not improve outcomes after orthopaedic surgery except in patients who already require angioplasty or bypass surgery.

3. Planning for postoperative monitoring in high-risk patients.

4. Ordering a preoperative electrocardiogram (ECG) for all patients with a history of coronary artery disease, vascular disease, or cerebrovascular disease.

B. Risk factors for coronary artery disease

1. Age >50 years

Table 1
Elements of a Directed Bleeding History
1. Do you have frequent unprovoked nose or gum bleeding?
2. Have you had iron deficiency from heavy periods?
3. Have you had unprovoked large bruises on your back, chest, or abdomen?
4. Have you had bleeding into a joint with mild trauma?
5. Have you previously had excessive blood loss with surgery?
6. Do you have a family history of bleeding problems?
7. Do you have kidney or liver disease?

Table 2

Revised Cardiac Risk Index (RCRI)

1. **Type of surgery** (1 pt) Abdominal aortic aneurysm repair

2. **History of coronary artery disease** (1 pt) History of angina, Q-waves on ECG, history of coronary bypass surgery or percutaneous coronary artery intervention, abnormal stress test, use of nitrates

3. **History of congestive heart failure** (1 pt) History of ejection fraction < 30%, cardiogenic pulmonary edema, paroxysmal nocturnal dyspnea, rales or clinical findings consistent with CHF on exam, chest radiograph consistent with CHF

4. **History of cerebrovascular accident/TIA** (1 pt)

5. **History of creatinine > 2.0 mg/dL** (1 pt)

6. **History of insulin-dependent diabetes** (1 pt)

TIA = transient ischemic attack

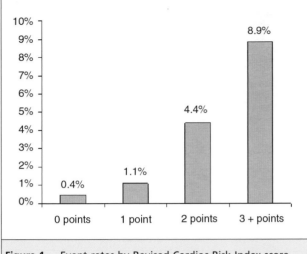

Figure 1 Event rates by Revised Cardiac Risk Index score.

2. Family history

3. Diabetes

4. Hypertension

5. Smoking

C. Use of β-blockers

1. β-blockers should be administered perioperatively only in patients at high risk (eg, Revised Cardiac Risk Index [RCRI] of 2 or more; **Table 2** and **Figure 1**), with documented coronary disease, or who are currently taking β-blockers.

2. β-blockers should be administered preoperatively (optimally 1 week or more before surgery), titrated to a therapeutic heart rate (55 to 70 beats/min) throughout hospitalization, and continued for 7 days after surgery (or indefinitely, if patients are already on β-blockers).

V. Assessment of Pulmonary Risk

A. Pulmonary complications such as pneumonia and respiratory failure are probably more common than cardiac complications.

B. Diagnostic testing

1. Chest radiographs are indicated if patients have signs or symptoms of pulmonary disease (baseline oxygen requirement, crackles, rhonchi, wheezing).

2. Arterial blood gas measurements and pulmonary function testing are indicated in the following situations:

a. With severe or unexplained symptoms.

b. If the etiology of the underlying diagnosis—eg, chronic obstructive pulmonary disease (COPD), congestive heart failure (CHF)—is unclear.

c. If the information is needed to plan for postoperative airway management (eg, extubation in the operating room, postanesthesia care unit, or requirement for intensive care unit).

C. Physical examination, particularly assessment of functional status (ability to climb one flight of stairs), is probably more predictive of pulmonary risk than preoperative tests.

D. Ways to reduce the risk for postoperative pulmonary complications

1. Treating exacerbations of COPD or asthma adequately preoperatively

2. Early mobilization of patients, including early ambulation, sitting up in bed, or sitting in a chair

3. Use of incentive spirometry every hour while awake in all patients

4. Targeted use of nebulizers

5. Use of noninvasive ventilation (eg, bilevel positive airway pressure [BiPAP] or postanesthesia care unit) or intensive care unit in selected patients whose respiratory status is tentative

VI. Special Considerations

A. Renal/hepatic insufficiency

1. Risk for complications is higher than in unaffected patients.

2. Consult or referral to the appropriate medical specialist is needed.

3. Patients on dialysis should undergo hemodialysis

Table 3

Marcantonio Delirium Risk Index

1. **Type of surgery.** Aortic aneurysm surgery (2 pts), noncardiac thoracic surgery (1 pt)

2. **Age > 70** (1 pt)

3. **Alcohol abuse** (1 pt)

4. **Severe physical impairment** (1 pt) Unable to make bed, walk 1 block, or dress without stopping

5. **Baseline dementia/confusion** ([MMSE] < 24) (1 pt)

6. **Abnormal sodium, potassium, or glucose** (1 pt) Sodium < 130 or > 150, potassium < 3 or > 6, glucose < 60 or > 300

MMSE = mini-mental state examination

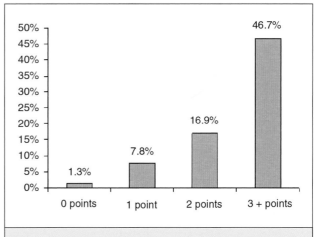

Figure 2 Event rates by Marcantonio Delirium Risk Index.

the evening before or morning of surgery, with close attention to electrolytes and fluid status afterward.

4. Close attention to bleeding risk, fluid status, and risk of oversedation and impaired hepatic clearance of opioids and benzodiazepines is needed in patients with liver disease.

5. Drug dosing in patients with cirrhosis and renal failure must be modified according to the severity of their renal or liver disease.

VII. Diabetes

A. Blood glucose levels in orthopaedic surgical patients should be maintained between 110 and 150 mg/dL throughout the perioperative period to reduce the risk of complications (eg, surgical site infections).

B. Preoperative insulin dosing

1. Patients with type II diabetes should hold or take a reduced amount of their usual oral medications the morning of surgery.

2. Patients with type I diabetes should take a smaller than usual morning dose of insulin while NPO and awaiting surgery.

3. Regardless of the type of diabetes, the management plan depends on the time of day the procedure takes place, the patient's medication regimen, and the how well blood glucose levels are controlled at baseline.

C. Other types of insulin dosing

1. Insulin infusions are optimal therapy for patients in intensive care, on enteral or parenteral feedings, and who have persistent hyperglycemia.

2. Split-dose sliding scales, which combine longer-acting insulin at regular intervals with short-acting (aspart or regular) insulin for correction, are recommended.

3. Regular insulin sliding scales (eg, sliding scales that use a single type of short-acting insulin to control blood glucose) should be avoided because they are ineffective at maintaining tight glucose control.

D. Oral agents should be resumed as soon as the patient can tolerate taking oral medications.

VIII. Postoperative Delirium

A. Incidence and risk factors

1. Postoperative delirium is a very common complication of orthopaedic surgery, particularly in patients with hip fracture.

2. Many risk factors for delirium mirror risks for postoperative cardiac complications. Risk indices for postoperative delirium also exist, and they accurately identify patients in whom delirium is likely (**Table 3** and **Figure 2**).

3. All patients should be asked if they have experienced postoperative confusion. A positive answer is highly specific, and prompt preventive measures are needed.

4. Patients with no history of postoperative delirium

a. Preoperative evaluation should include assessments for dementia or other cognitive disorders (eg, sundowning, or late-day confusion). Both the patient and the family should be questioned.

b. Risk factors for postoperative delirium in this group include a history of alcohol abuse, stroke, and marked metabolic abnormalities (eg, elevated blood urea nitrogen [BUN], elevated glucose).

B. Management

1. The overall goal is to reduce the duration and severity of symptoms so that postoperative care (eg, early mobilization, physical therapy, compliance with incentive spirometry) can continue.

2. Assess the severity of pain. The delirious patient who reports pain should be treated with the most effective therapy possible (even including opioid analgesics).

3. Assess and treat for other complications such as infection, hypoxemia, hyperglycemia, or hypovolemia.

4. Minimize iatrogenic factors, particularly the use of urinary catheters and anticholinergic medications.

5. Encourage family and friends to accompany the patient as much as possible to help reorient and reassure the patient in the immediate postoperative period.

6. Medications

a. Haloperidol (0.5 to 1.0 mg intramuscular) can be used hourly until symptoms are controlled. Monitor ECG and QT interval during its use.

b. Benzodiazepines such as lorazepam should be used in patients who are agitated and whose symptoms are not controlled by haloperidol.

7. Restraints are an option of last resort.

IX. Rheumatologic Considerations

A. Cervical instability should be suspected in any patient with rheumatoid arthritis.

B. Screen for cervical instability specifically using CT or plain radiographs of the neck.

X. Medication Management

A. Steroids

1. Despite few data to direct whether patients undergoing surgery who have been on long-standing steroid treatment require "stress dose" steroids, this practice is common.

2. If stress dose (eg, hydrocortisone 100 mg every 8 hours) steroid supplementation is used, it should be of very short duration (36 hours), after which time the outpatient steroid regimen should resume.

B. Aspirin

1. The practice of holding aspirin before surgery, while prudent in concept, is fairly unsupported by evidence.

2. Although it is reasonable to discontinue aspirin in most patients, continuing aspirin should be considered in patients with any implanted coronary device (eg, coronary stent) because of the high risk of acute coronary occlusion.

C. Warfarin

1. The plan for managing warfarin perioperatively in orthopaedic patients depends on the indication for long-term anticoagulation.

a. Low-risk groups (atrial fibrillation without prior stroke; cardiomyopathy without atrial fibrillation)

i. These patients have an annual thrombotic risk (without anticoagulation) of less than 4%.

ii. They can be managed by withholding anticoagulant medication for the 4- to 6-day perioperative period.

iii. Stop warfarin in these patients 5 days before surgery and check INR 1 day before surgery to confirm that it is below 1.5.

iv. Restart warfarin as soon as possible after surgery.

b. Moderate-risk patients (mechanical aortic valve, risk of stroke off warfarin between 4% and 7%)

i. These patients require "bridging" anticoagulation.

ii. Low-molecular-weight heparin (LMWH) is preferred for bridging therapy because it can be initiated while the patient is at home (as opposed to unfractionated heparin, which requires admission).

c. High-risk patients (mechanical mitral valve; atrial fibrillation with prior stroke)

i. These patients have an annual risk > 7%.

ii. They require "bridging" anticoagulation.

ii. LMWH is preferred for bridging therapy because it can be initiated while the patient is at home (as opposed to unfractionated heparin, which requires admission).

2. Bridging therapy

a. Discontinue warfarin 5 days before surgery and 36 hours after the last dose of warfarin.

b. Check the INR 1 day before surgery to confirm it has decreased to below 1.5.

c. Discontinue 12 to 24 hours before surgery.

d. Resume once hemostasis has been achieved; restart warfarin at the patient's usual outpa-

tient dose at the same time.

e. Unfractionated heparin or LMWH is discontinued once the INR is greater than 2.0.

Top Testing Facts

1. Choose preoperative tests that assess for stability of current comorbidities or diagnose unclear symptoms or signs. Blanket testing policies are not cost effective and can be misleading.

2. A directed bleeding history can help to identify patients for whom preoperative bleeding tests are most useful.

3. The RCRI is a simple and highly predictive way to identify patients who should be referred to cardiology or should have surgery delayed.

4. Risk for cardiac events can be substantially lowered if β-blockers are used appropriately in high-risk patients, specifically those with two or more RCRI criteria.

5. Pulmonary complications such as pneumonia and respiratory failure are probably more common than cardiac complications.

6. Risk for pulmonary complications can be managed through treating an exacerbation of asthma or COPD before surgery, as well as early mobilization, use of incentive spirometers, nebulizers, and noninvasive ventilation (such as BiPAP).

7. In general, maintaining blood glucose levels below 150 mg/dL in postoperative patients is optimal. Achieving this goal requires use of insulin infusions (ICU patients) or sliding scales, which include both short- and long-acting insulin.

8. Postoperative delirium is common, and can be managed effectively by minimizing noxious stimuli (eg, pain, indwelling urinary catheters, restraints), and by reorienting patients as often as possible.

9. Careful consideration of continuing aspirin in patients with coronary artery stents is required; these patients are at high risk for stent restenosis and death if antiplatelet agents are discontinued.

10. Management of warfarin around the time of surgery is predicated on the underlying reason for warfarin use—in general, shorter duration of time off warfarin (or bridging therapy with heparin) is required for patients at higher risk for thrombotic complications when not anticoagulated.

Bibliography

Auerbach A, Goldman L: Assessing and reducing the cardiac risk of noncardiac surgery. *Circulation* 2006;113:1361-1376.

Baker R: Pre-operative hemostatic assessment and management. *Transfus Apher Sci* 2002;27:45-53.

Douketis JD: Perioperative anticoagulation management in patients who are receiving oral anticoagulation therapy: A practical guide for clinicians. *Thromb Res* 2002;108:3-13.

Hoogwerf BJ: Perioperative management of diabetes mellitus: How should we act on the limited evidence? *Cleve Clin J Med* 2006;73(suppl 1):S95-S99.

Marcantonio ER, Flacker JM, Wright RJ, Resnick NM: Reducing delirium after hip fracture: A randomized trial. *J Am Geriatr Soc* 2001;49:516-522.

Smetana GW: Preoperative pulmonary evaluation: Identifying and reducing risks for pulmonary complications. *Cleve Clin J Med* 2006;73(suppl 1):S36-S41.

2: General Knowledge

Chapter 18

Coagulation and Thromboembolism

Craig J. Della Valle, MD

I. Coagulopathies

A. Coagulation cascade

1. The coagulation cascade is a series of enzymatic reactions that lead to the eventual formation of fibrin.

2. Fibrin forms a lattice that traps platelets to form a clot and stem bleeding (**Figure 1**).

3. Each step in the cascade involves the activation of a clotting factor that, in turn, activates the next step in the cascade.

4. There are two pathways for the initiation of clot formation, the intrinsic and extrinsic pathways.

    a. Intrinsic pathway

        i. Activated by the exposure of collagen from the subendothelium of damaged blood vessels to factor XII

        ii. Measured using partial thromboplastin time (PTT)

    b. Extrinsic pathway

        i. Activated by the release of thromboplastin (via cell damage) into the circulatory system

        ii. Measured by prothrombin time (PT)

    c. Platelet dysfunction can be identified by prolongation of the bleeding time.

B. Fibrinolytic system

1. The fibrinolytic system acts to stem clot formation and maintain vascular patency.

2. The key step is the formation of active plasmin from plasminogen.

3. Plasminogen dissolves fibrin.

C. Hemophilia

1. Hereditary factor deficiency that leads to abnormal bleeding (**Table 1**)

2. Recurrent hemarthrosis and resultant synovitis of the large joints can lead to joint destruction (the knee is most commonly affected).

3. Treatment options

    a. Initial treatment consists of factor replacement, aspiration, initial splinting, and physical therapy.

    b. If bleeding continues despite prophylactic factor infusion, radioisotope or arthroscopic synovectomy is indicated if the cartilaginous surfaces are relatively preserved.

    c. Total knee arthroplasty (TKA) in these patients can be complex secondary to severe preoperative stiffness and contracture.

4. These patients are at high risk for infection.

5. Use of factor replacement

    a. If surgical intervention is planned, intravenous factor replacement is required to maintain factor levels of 100% immediately preoperatively and for 3 to 5 days postoperatively for soft-tissue procedures and for 3 to 4 weeks postoperatively for bony procedures such as total hip arthroplasty (THA) and TKA.

    b. Although plasma derivatives were commonly used for factor replacement in the past (associated with a high risk of infection with blood-borne pathogens such as hepatitis and HIV), recombinant derived factor currently is used.

6. Inhibitors—Circulating antibodies that neutralize factor VIII or IX.

    a. These antibodies are suspected when a patient fails to respond to increasing doses of factor replacement.

    b. Diagnosis is confirmed via an in vitro assay,

Craig J. Della Valle, MD, or the department with which he is affiliated has received research or institutional support from Zimmer, miscellaneous nonincome support, commercially-derived honoraria, or other nonresearch-related funding from Zimmer and Ortho Biotech, and is a consultant for or employee of Zimmer and Ortho Biotech.

2: General Knowledge

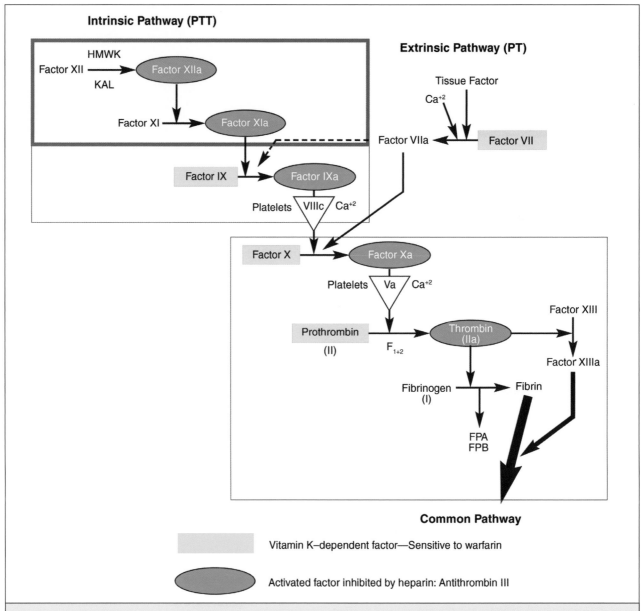

Intrinsic Pathway (PTT)

HMWK

Factor XII → Factor XIIa

KAL

Factor XI → Factor XIa

Factor IX → Factor IXa

Platelets / VIIIc / Ca⁺²

Extrinsic Pathway (PT)

Tissue Factor

Ca⁺²

Factor VIIa ← Factor VII

Factor X → Factor Xa

Platelets / Va / Ca⁺²

Prothrombin (II)

F_{1+2}

Thrombin (IIa)

Factor XIII

Factor XIIIa

Fibrinogen (I) → Fibrin

FPA
FPB

Common Pathway

Vitamin K–dependent factor—Sensitive to warfarin

Activated factor inhibited by heparin: Antithrombin III

Figure 1 The coagulation pathways. PT measures the function of the extrinsic and common pathways, whereas PTT measures the function of the intrinsic and common pathways. HMWK = high-molecular-weight kininogen; KAL = kallikrein; FPA = fibrinopeptide A; FPB = fibrinopeptide B. *(Adapted with permission from Stead RB: Regulation of hemostasis, in Goldhaber SZ (ed):* Pulmonary Embolism and Deep Venous Thrombosis. *Philadelphia, PA, WB Saunders, 1985, p 32.)*

whereby the addition of normal plasma or factor concentrate fails to correct a prolonged PTT.

   c. Although they previously were considered a contraindication to elective surgery, presently they can be overwhelmed to counteract the effect of the inhibitor.

D. von Willebrand disease

   1. von Willibrand disease is a collection of genetic coagulopathies secondary to a deficiency of von Willebrand factor (vWF).

2. Role of vWF

   a. Integral to normal platelet adhesion and the functioning of factor VIII

   b. Normally found in platelets and in the vascular endothelium

3. Types of deficiencies

   a. Type 1 (quantitative; decreased vWF levels)—A milder form that presents as heavy menstrual bleeding or excessive bleeding from the gums, easy bruising, or excessive surgical bleeding.

Table 1

Factor Deficiencies Causing Bleeding Disorders

Factor	Disease	Frequency	Inheritance
VIII	Hemophilia A	1:5,000 males	X-linked recessive
IX	Hemophilia B (Christmas disease)	1:30,000 males	X-linked recessive
XI	Hemophilia C	1:100,000	Autosomal dominant
I	Fibrinogen deficiency	1-2:1,000,000	Autosomal recessive
II	Prothrombin deficiency	1:2,000,000	Autosomal recessive
V	Parahemophilia	1:1,000,000	Autosomal recessive
VII	Alexander disease	1:500,000	Autosomal recessive
X	Factor X deficiency	1:500,000	Autosomal recessive
XII	Hageman factor deficiency	1:1,000,000	Autosomal recessive
XIII	Fibrin stabilizing factor deficiency	1:5,000,000	Autosomal recessive

   b. Type 2 (qualitative; abnormal vWF)

   c. Type 3 (quantitative; no vWF produced)—The most severe form of the disease, which is very rare (1 in 500,000).

4. Diagnosis is made via measuring the bleeding time, factor VIII activity, and both quantitative and qualitative tests for vWF.

5. Treatment

   a. Desmopressin, usually administered via a nasal spray, works via increased endogenous release of vWF from the vascular endothelium.

   b. Factor VIII concentrates combined with vWF may be required in patients with more severe deficiencies (types 2 and 3).

E. Coagulopathies

1. Coagulopathies are caused by high blood loss secondary to major trauma or extended surgical procedures.

2. Fluid volume and packed red blood cells must be replaced.

3. The need for platelet and fresh frozen plasma transfusion must be assessed by monitoring platelet counts and coagulation parameters.

II. Venous Thromboembolic Disease

A. Pathophysiology—Deep venous thrombosis (DVT) is the end result of a complex interaction of events including activation of the clotting cascade and platelet aggregation.

B. Virchow triad (predisposing factors)

1. Venous stasis

   a. Impaired mobility

   b. Intraoperative vascular congestion

2. Endothelial damage secondary to injury or surgical trauma

3. Hypercoagulability

   a. Release of tissue factors and procoagulants (such as collagen fragments, fibrinogen, and tissue thromboplastin)

   b. Large release of thrombogenic factors during preparation of the femur during THA, particularly if a cemented femoral component is used

C. Epidemiology and risk factors

1. Without prophylaxis, patients with a proximal femur fracture have a reported prevalence of fatal pulmonary embolism (PE) as high as 7%.

2. Patients undergoing elective THA and TKA have been described as having rates of symptomatic PE without prophylaxis of up to 20% and 8%, respectively.

3. Patients undergoing TKA seem to be at higher risk for venographically identified DVT but at lower risk for symptomatic PE than THA patients.

4. Risk factors for thromboembolism (Table 2)

   a. May have a cumulative effect; a combination of risk factors present in a given patient may greatly increase the risk.

   b. Patients with a prior history of a thromboembolic event deserve special attention, given the numerous inherited hypercoagulable states

Table 2

Risk Factors for Thromboembolic Disease

History of prior thromboembolic event

Advanced age

Obesity

Malignant disease

Genetic hypercoagulable state

Oral contraceptive use

Pregnancy

Extended immobilization

Major orthopaedic surgery

History of myocardial infarction/stroke/CHF

Table 3

Pharmacologic Agents for Thromboembolic Prophylaxis

Agent	Site of Action	Metabolism
UFH	Antithrombin III, IIa, Xa	Hepatic
LMWH	Antithrombin III, Xa > IIa	Renal
Fondaparinux	Xa	Renal
Warfarin	II, VII, IX, X	Hepatic
Aspirin	Platelets	Hepatic

UFH = unfractionated heparin, LMWH = low-molecular-weight heparin

(such as factor V Leiden) that have recently been identified. Preoperative consultation with a hematologist may be appropriate.

III. Prophylaxis

A. Given the high risk of thromboembolism in patients undergoing major orthopaedic surgery, the difficulty in diagnosing these events, and their potential for morbidity and mortality (approximately two thirds of patients who sustain a fatal PE die within 60 minutes of the development of symptoms), some form of prophylaxis is often necessary. Prophylaxis is required for all THA and TKA patients and for hip fracture patients.

B. The optimal duration of prophylaxis is unclear; however, patients may be at risk for thromboembolism for several weeks postoperatively.

C. Mechanical approaches

1. Sequential compression devices

a. Act via increasing peak venous flow to decrease venous stasis

b. Stimulate the fibrinolytic system

c. Present no risk of bleeding

d. Poor patient compliance and/or inappropriate application is common.

e. Good efficacy has been shown in patients who undergo TKA.

2. Plantar compression devices

a. Compression of the venous plexus of the foot produces pulsatile flow in the deep venous system of the leg (simulates walking).

b. Inadequate data are available to recommend these devices alone.

3. Graduated compression stockings

a. These stockings produce a pressure differential between the distal and proximal portions of the lower extremity, decreasing venous stasis.

b. These stocking should be used as an adjunct only and not as the sole means of prophylaxis.

4. Prophylactic inferior vena cava (IVC) filters

a. JVC filters are retrievable devices that are typically placed before surgery and then electively removed 10 to 14 days later.

b. Indications

i. Patients who require surgery in the context of a recent thromboembolic event

ii. Critically ill multiple-trauma patients (relative indication)

iii. May be considered in patients at high risk for a thromboembolism (eg, those with a hereditary hypercoagulable state). Consultation with a hematologist is useful in these cases.

D. Pharmacologic approaches (**Table 3**)

1. Unfractionated heparin (UFH)

a. Binds to antithrombin III, potentiating its inhibitory effect on thrombin (factor IIa) and factor Xa

b. Higher risk of bleeding and lower efficacy than low-molecular-weight heparin (LMWH)

c. Increased risk of heparin-induced thrombocytopenia, which is secondary to heparin-dependent antibodies that activate platelets

d. Fixed low-dose heparin (5,000 U administered subcutaneously twice daily) generally is not effective in orthopaedic patients.

e. Reversed using protamine sulfate

2. Low-molecular-weight heparin

a. LMWH is derived from the fractionation of UFH into smaller, more homogeneous molecules.

b. LMWH is unable to bind both antithrombin III and thrombin simultaneously and thus has a greater inhibitory effect on factor Xa than factor IIa (thrombin).

c. Provides superior protection against DVT and does not inhibit hemostasis as vigorously at surgical sites as to UFH

d. Less inhibition of platelet function and less vascular permeability than UFH

e. Improved bioavailability (90% versus 35% for UFH)

f. Longer half-life (less frequent dosing)

g. Laboratory monitoring is not required.

h. First full dose 12 to 24 hours postoperatively or until hemostasis obtained at the surgical site

i. Should not be used in conjunction with an indwelling epidural catheter or in patients who have had a traumatic neuraxial anesthetic placed (secondary to a risk of epidural bleeding). Neuraxial anesthesia can be performed 12 hours after administration of LMWH.

j. Compared with warfarin, LMWH is associated with a decreased risk of venographically identified DVT but a higher risk of bleeding complications.

k. Excretion is primarily renal and thus dosing needs to be adjusted in patients with chronic renal failure.

l. Several agents are presently available, and pharmacokinetics, dosing, and outcomes differ among agents.

3. Fondaparinux

a. Synthetic pentasaccharide and an indirect factor Xa inhibitor

b. Dosing is 2.5 mg/day subcutaneously; first dose is given 6 to 12 hours postoperatively.

c. Decreased incidence of venographically identified DVT compared with enoxaparin in hip fracture and TKA patients

d. Trend toward an increased risk of bleeding complications

e. Not recommended for patients who weigh less than 50 kg or those with renal insufficiency; has not been used in conjunction with indwelling epidural catheters.

Table 4
Common Drug Interactions With Warfarin
Trimethoprim-sulfamethoxazole (Bactrim or Septra)
Rifampin
Macrolide antibiotics (such as erythromycin)
Quinolone antibiotics (such as ciprofloxacin)
Metronidazole (Flagyl)
Certain cephalosporins (such as cefamandole)
Thyroid hormones (such as levothyroxine)
Phenytoin (Dilantin)
Cimetidine (Tagamet)
Antiarrhythmics such as amiodarone
Herbal medications such as garlic

4. Warfarin

a. Antagonizes vitamin K, which prevents the γ-carboxylation of glutamic acid required for the synthesis of factors II, VII, IX, and X and proteins C and S.

b. Typical dosing regimens start on the night of surgery, as soon as the patient can tolerate oral pain medication.

c. The anticoagulant effect is delayed for 24 to 36 hours after the initiation of therapy, and the target International Normalized Ratio (INR) is often not achieved until 3 days postoperatively.

d. The target level of anticoagulation has been controversial; however, a target INR of 2.0 is appropriate for orthopaedic patients.

e. Advantages—Low cost, oral administration, and efficacy in reducing symptomatic thromboembolic events.

f. Disadvantages—Difficulty in dosing and need for frequent blood monitoring. Patients with impaired hepatic function may be sensitive to the drug and thus must be dosed and monitored carefully.

g. Warfarin interacts with many other medications that can augment its effect (**Table 4**).

h. Not recommended for use in conjunction with NSAIDs secondary to a higher risk of bleeding at surgical and nonsurgical sites (particularly gastrointestinal bleeding)

i. Patients who ingest large amounts of vitamin K–rich foods (eg, green, leafy vegetables) may require increased doses to achieve the target INR.

k. Reversible with vitamin K administration; complete reversal can take several days. Fresh frozen plasma is given if immediate reversal is required.

5. Aspirin

a. Aspirin irreversibly binds to and inactivates cyclooxygenase (COX) in both developing and circulating platelets, which blocks the production of thromboxane A2, the necessary prostaglandin for platelet aggregation.

b. Advantages—Low cost, ease of administration, and low risk of bleeding-related complications.

c. The role of aspirin when used alone as a prophylactic agent is controversial given lower efficacy compared with other agents when venographic evidence of DVT is used as an end point. Randomized trials assessing the efficacy of aspirin are necessary.

6. When combined with neuraxial anesthetics and particularly hypotensive epidural techniques, aspirin seems to be associated with a lower risk of postoperative thromboembolic events secondary to enhanced blood flow in the lower extremities.

7. The Seventh American College of Chest Physicians Conference on Antithrombotic and Thrombolytic Therapy's highest recommendations for patients undergoing THA and TKA include warfarin (goal INR 2.0 to 3.0), LMWH, or fondaparinux for a minimum of 10 days. Routine screening with a duplex ultrasound at the time of hospital discharge is not recommended.

8. Data exist to support prolonged prophylaxis (up to 35 days) in THA patients, but prolonged prophylaxis has not been shown to have an effect in TKA patients.

IV. Diagnosis of Thromboembolic Events

A. Approach to diagnosing thromboembolism

1. No clinical signs are specific for diagnosis of DVT or PE.

2. Calf pain, swelling, and pain on forced dorsiflexion of the foot (Homans' sign) are common in the perioperative period secondary to postoperative pain, swelling, and abnormal gait patterns leading to muscular strain.

B. Initial patient evaluation

1. Chest radiograph—To rule out alternative causes of hypoxia such as pneumonia, congestive heart failure, and atelectasis.

2. Electrocardiogram (ECG)—To rule out cardiac

pathology; tachycardia is the most common ECG finding in PE, although a right ventricular strain pattern can be seen.

3. Arterial blood gas measurements on room air

4. Assessing oxygenation

a. Most patients are hypoxic (P_{AO_2} < 80 mm Hg), hypocapnic (P_{ACO_2} < 35 mm Hg), and have a high A-a gradient (> 20 mm Hg).

b. The A-a gradient (indicative of poor gas exchange between the alveolus and arterial blood supply) can be calculated as

$$(150 - 1.25 [P_{ACO_2}]) - P_{AO_2}.$$

c. Pulse oximetry is not an adequate alternative to arterial blood gas measurements on room air; patients can hyperventilate to maintain adequate oxygenation.

5. Ventilation/perfusion (V/Q) scanning

a. V/Q scanning has been the standard of care for diagnosing PE for many years.

b. Scans are compared to identify "mismatch defects": areas that are ventilated without associated perfusion.

c. Graded as normal, low, intermediate, or high probability based on criteria determined from prior studies that compared V/Q scans and pulmonary angiograms

i. Patients with normal or low-probability scans should be evaluated for alternative sources of hypoxemia (particularly if a search for lower extremity DVT is negative).

ii. Patients with high-probability scans require treatment.

iii. If the scan is intermediate and clinical suspicion is high, the lower extremities should be assessed for DVT; if negative, a high-resolution chest CT or pulmonary angiogram is indicated to rule out PE.

6. High-resolution (helical or spiral) chest CT angiography

a. Widely adopted as the first-line study for diagnosing PE, given the high rate of indeterminate V/Q scans and the accuracy of this technique compared with other imaging modalities

b. Advantage—Ability to identify alternative diagnosis if PE is not identified.

c. Requires contrast

d. Radiation dose can be a concern in certain patient populations (eg, pregnant women).

e. Sensitivity may be such that high rates of smaller, peripheral emboli are identified that are not clinically relevant, leading to overtreatment.

7. Pulmonary angiography

   a. Pulmonary angiography is considered the gold standard for diagnosing PE

   b. It is both expensive and invasive and therefore is rarely used in clinical practice.

8. Duplex ultrasonography

   a. Noninvasive, simple, and inexpensive

   b. Accuracy has been shown to be operator dependent.

   c. Accurate in diagnosis of symptomatic proximal clots. Ability to visualize veins in the calf and pelvis is limited.

   d. Routine screening for DVT before hospital discharge has not been shown to be cost effective.

9. Lower extremity contrast venography

   a. Still considered the gold standard for diagnosing lower extremity DVT

   b. Expensive and invasive; therefore, rarely used in clinical practice

10. D-dimer testing

    a. D-dimer testing can be used as an adjunct to diagnosing thromboembolic events.

    b. Elevated D-dimer levels indicate a high level of fibrin degradation products (which also can be seen following a recent surgery).

    c. A low D-dimer level indicates a low risk for DVT (high negative predictive value).

C. Approach to diagnosing PE

1. PE is difficult to diagnose based on classic symptoms of dyspnea and pleuritic chest pain because these are rarely seen.

2. Vague symptoms such as cough, palpitations, and apprehension or confusion are common.

3. The most common sign seen in diagnosed PE is tachypnea followed by tachycardia and fever; therefore, even vague signs and symptoms require a thorough evaluation.

4. If chest radiograph and ECG do not point to an alternative diagnosis, a D-dimer level can be obtained; if negative, the likelihood of PE is low.

5. Depending on availability, chest CT or V/Q scan is obtained.

6. If the V/Q scan is low or intermediate probability and clinical suspicion is high, duplex ultrasonography of the lower extremities can be used.

7. If the ultrasound is negative and suspicion is still high, pulmonary angiography can be used to determine the presence or absence of PE.

D. Treatment of a thromboembolic event

1. Continuous intravenous heparin for at least 5 days, followed by oral warfarin. LMWH is now commonly used because it is simple and the patient may not need to be admitted to the hospital.

   a. It prevents clot propagation while allowing the fibrinolytic system to dissolve clots that have already formed.

   b. It decreases mortality in these patients compared with those who are not anticoagulated.

   c. Risk of bleeding at the surgical site has been related to supratherapeutic levels of anticoagulation and initiation of therapy within 48 hours after surgery.

   d. Intravenous heparin is adjusted to maintain a goal PTT of 1.5 to 2.5 times the control value for 5 days.

   e. Avoiding the use of a bolus dose of intravenous heparin in the early postoperative period can reduce bleeding.

   f. Warfarin is initiated with a target of INR of 2.0 to 3.0 maintained for a minimum of 3 months.

2. In patients who have sustained a PE, elective surgery should not be considered for at least 3 months after the event, and a thorough evaluation is needed to ensure that the clot has resorbed and that there are no residual effects (such as pulmonary hypertension).

3. LMWH is an alternative to intravenous UFH therapy (dosed at 1 mg/kg administered subcutaneously twice daily).

   a. LMWH has more predictable onset, but it is associated with the potential for a higher risk of bleeding at the surgical site.

   b. Although commonly used to treat orthopaedic patients, no studies to date have specifically examined the use of LMWH for the treatment of diagnosed thromboembolic events in patients who have had orthopaedic surgery.

4. IVC filters

   a. Indications

      i. When anticoagulation is contraindicated (eg, recent spinal surgery or head injury)

      ii. Bleeding complication secondary to anticoagulant therapy

      iii. Patients who have sustained a thromboembolic event despite adequate prophylactic anticoagulation

      iv. Patients with poor cardiopulmonary reserve and at high risk for further morbidity and mortality if clot extension or recurrence occurs

b. Emboli can recur as either small emboli that pass through the filter, as collateral circulation develops, or as propagation of a large thrombus above the filter.

c. Complications include insertional problems, distal migration or tilting, vena cavae occlusion (which can lead to severe lower extremity swelling and rarely complete venous outflow obstruction) and vena cavae or aortic perforation.

d. In current practice, the IVC filter is often retrieved within 3 weeks, but certain designs allow for retrieval up to 1 year postinsertion.

5. DVT isolated to the calf is rarely associated with PE; proximal extension can occur in 10% to 20% of patients. In isolated calf vein thrombosis, serial ultrasonography can be performed and anticoagulant treatment withheld unless proximal extension is identified.

Top Testing Facts

1. LMWH inhibits factor Xa activity.

2. Fondaparinux is a synthetic pentasaccharide and an indirect inhibitor of factor X activity.

3. Both LMWH and fondaparinux are metabolized in the kidneys; warfarin is metabolized primarily in the liver.

4. Patients undergoing major elective orthopaedic surgery such as hip and knee arthroplasty and those who have sustained multiple trauma and proximal femoral fractures are at high risk for thromboembolic events.

5. The selection of a prophylactic agent requires balancing efficacy and safety.

6. The diagnosis of thromboembolic events can be difficult to make postoperatively; clinical signs and symptoms are unreliable for diagnosis.

7. Initial evaluation of the patient suspected of PE includes an arterial blood gas (ABG) on room air, a chest radiograph, and an ECG to rule out an alternative diagnosis.

8. Pulse oximetry is not an adequate alternative to an ABG as patient hyperventilation can maintain adequate oxygenation.

9. Treatment of thromboembolic events with intravenous heparin or LMWH followed by oral warfarin is effective at reducing morbidity and mortality.

10. IVC filters are indicated for patients diagnosed with a pulmonary embolus in whom anticoagulation is contraindicated or a bleeding complication has occurred, or if cardiopulmonary reserve is poor.

Bibliography

Colwell CW, Hardwick ME: Venous thromboembolic disease and prophylaxis in total joint arthroplasty, in Barrack RL, Booth RE, Lonner JH, McCarthy JC, Mont MA, Rubash HE (eds): *Orthopaedic Knowledge Update: Hip & Knee Reconstruction 3*. Rosemont, IL, American Academy of Orthopaedic Surgeons, 2006, pp 233-240.

Conduah AH, Lieberman JR: Thromboembolism and pulmonary distress in the setting of orthopaedic surgery, in Einhorn TA, O'Keefe RJ, Buckwalter JA (eds): *Orthopaedic Basic Science: Foundations of Clinical Practice*, ed 3. Rosemont, IL, American Academy of Orthopaedic Surgeons, 2007, pp 105-113.

Della Valle CJ, Mirzabeigi E, Zuckerman JD, Koval KJ: Thromboembolic prophylaxis for patients with a fracture of the proximal femur. *Am J Orthop* 2002;31:16-24.

Geerts WH, Pineo GF, Heit JA, et al: Prevention of venous thromboembolism: The seventh ACCP conference on antithrombotic and thrombolytic therapy. *Chest* 2004;126: 338S-400S.

Luck JV, Silva M, Rodriguea-Mercan EC, Ghalambor N, Zabiri CA, Finn RS: Hemophilic arthropathy. *J Am Acad Orthop Surg* 2004;12:234-245.

Morris CD, Creevy WS, Einhorn TA: Pulmonary distress and thromboembolic conditions affecting orthopaedic practice, in Buckwalter JA, Einhorn TA, Simon SR (eds): *Orthopaedic Basic Science: Biology and Biomechanics of the Musculoskeletal System*, ed 2. Rosemont, IL, American Academy of Orthopaedic Surgeons, 2000, pp 307-316.

Shen FH, Samartzis D, De Wald CJ: Coagulation and thromboembolism in orthopaedic surgery, in Vaccaro AR (ed): *Orthopaedic Knowledge Update 8*. Rosemont, IL, American Academy of Orthopaedic Surgeons, 2005, pp 169-176.

Turpie AGG, Eriksson BI, Bauer KA, Lassen MR: Fondaparinux: Advances in therapeutics and diagnostics. *J Am Acad Orthop Surg* 2004;12:271-375.

Whang PG, Lieberman JR: Low-molecular-weight-heparins: Advances in therapeutics and diagnostics. *J Am Acad Orthop Surg* 2002;10:299-302.

Zimlich RH, Fulbright BM, Frieman RJ: Current status of anticoagulation therapy after total hip and knee arthroplasty. *J Am Acad Orthop Surg* 1996;4:54-62.

Chapter 19

Blood Management

*Timothy J. Hannon, MD, MBA   *Jeffery L. Pierson, MD

I. Blood Management Programs

A. Definition of blood management—Proactive processes, techniques, drugs, or medical devices that reduce the need for allogeneic blood when used in an efficient, effective and timely manner.

B. Principles

   1. Use of evidence-based transfusion guidelines to reduce variability in transfusion practice

   2. Use of multidisciplinary teams to study, implement, and monitor local blood management strategies

C. Goals

   1. Ensure that each blood product that is transfused is appropriate.

   2. Ensure that blood-related resources are used efficiently and effectively.

D. Hospital responsibilities—By developing and implementing comprehensive blood management programs, hospitals can promote safe, efficient, and clinically effective blood utilization practices for the benefit of the health system, its patients, and the local community.

II. Issues in Blood Banking

A. Availability and use

   1. More than 29 million units of blood components were administered in the United States in 2004.

   2. As the donor pool continues to decrease, there are real concerns that in the near future, demand will outstrip supply.

   3. Blood use is suboptimal in many hospitals be-
cause of poor training and inadequate oversight, review, and monitoring of transfusion practices.

   4. Blood substitutes currently are not US Food and Drug Administration (FDA) approved given the lack of safety and efficacy data.

B. The decision to transfuse

   1. Often clouded by myths, misconceptions, and emotions, and not supported by good medical science

   2. Generalized lack of compliance with appropriate transfusion guidelines

   3. Transfusion practices vary widely among institutions and among individual physicians within the same institution.

C. Risks and benefits

   1. Although the blood supply is the safest it has ever been, transfusion of blood components remains a high-risk procedure that results in some degree of harm to all patients.

   2. The benefits of transfusion, especially the use of red cells, are not well elucidated. Few, if any, well-controlled studies demonstrate improved outcomes with red cells.

      a. In the landmark 1999 Transfusion Requirements in Critical Care (TRICC) trial, a restrictive strategy of red cell transfusions (Hgb 7.0) was at least as effective and possibly superior to a more liberal strategy (Hgb 9.0-10.0) with the possible exception of patients with acute coronary syndromes.

      b. A 2004 study by cardiologists at Duke University questioned the benefit of transfusions in high-risk cardiac populations.

   3. Bacterial contamination of platelets is one of the leading causes of transfusion-related morbidity and mortality, with a frequency of 1:2,000 to 3,000 transfusions.

   4. Transfusion of blood products to the wrong patient is also a leading risk, with the alarming frequency of 1:12,000 to 1:19,000 units transfused.

   5. Death occurs in 1:600,000 to 1:800,000 transfusions.

Timothy J. Hannon, MD, MBA, or the department with which he is affiliated has received miscellaneous nonincome support, commercially-derived honoraria, or other nonresearch-related funding from Bayer, Medtronic, and Ortho Biotech. Jeffrey L. Pierson, MD, is a consultant for or an employee of Zimmer.

2: General Knowledge

6. Prolonged storage of blood products (allogeneic and autologous) leads to a progressive decline in product quality and linear increases in debris and inflammatory mediators.

D. Costs

1. Blood product prices more than doubled between 2001 and 2007.

2. Within hospitals, the procurement, storage, processing, and transfusion of blood products involves an array of expensive resources that include laboratory supplies, pharmaceuticals, and medical devices, as well as significant technician and nursing time (**Figure 1**).

3. Resource utilization in the administration of blood products to patients results in a three- to fourfold increase in the total cost of blood beyond the base cost of their acquisition.

4. Accounting for adverse events such as increased length of stay and infection rates may make the total cost of allogeneic transfusion as high as $2,000 per unit.

5. Cost of blood products and processing must be considered when comparing allogeneic transfusions with transfusion alternatives.

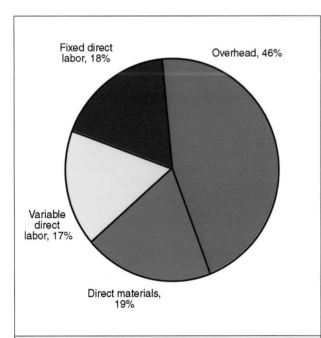

Figure 1 Transfusion costs by resource category. Direct material costs (19%) reflect the costs of acquiring blood products and supplies as a percentage of total cost. Total cost of an outpatient transfusion accounting for all resource categories was $677 to $752 in 2004 dollars. (*Adapted with permission from Cremieux PY, Barrett B, Anderson K, et al: Cost of outpatient blood transfusion in cancer patients. J Clin Oncol 2000;18:2755-2761.*)

III. General Blood Management Strategies

A. General strategies and principles are outlined in **Tables 1 and 2**.

B. Preoperative preparation and planning (**Table 1**)

1. Preoperative planning is essential to the safe and optimal management of surgical patients.

2. Early identification of high-risk patients amenable to strategies to modify those risks can improve patient outcomes and improve overall resource utilization by reducing adverse events.

3. Universal predictors for transfusion requirements

   a. Type and complexity of surgery

   b. Preoperative anemia

   c. Preexisting coagulopathy

Table 1

Orthopaedic Blood Management Strategies

Preoperative
Early identification of patients at high risk of transfusion
Blood management algorithms
Selective use of erythropoietic agents and iron therapy
Discontinuation of drugs and herbal medicines that increase bleeding
Autologous predonation (not recommended)

Intraoperative
Minimization of surgical time
Regional anesthesia
Temperature maintenance
Patient positioning
Controlled "normotension"
Cautery
Topical hemostatic agents
Intraoperative autotransfusion
Antifibrinolytics (TA, EACA) and serine protease inhibitors (aprotinin)
Point of care testing
Evidence-based transfusion decisions

Postoperative
Evidence-based transfusion decisions
Postoperative autotransfusion (washed)
Minimize iatrogenic blood loss

TA = tranexamic acid; EACA = epsilon aminocaproic acid

Table 2

Blood Management Principles

Early identification and intervention for patients at high risk for transfusions
Use of current scientific evidence and the promotion of clinical best practices
Alignment and coordination of all members of the health care team
Patient advocacy and patient safety
Stewardship of scarce and expensive hospital resources

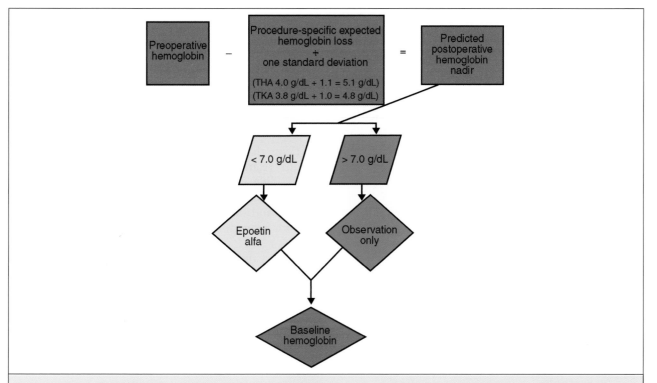

Figure 2   Blood management algorithm for primary unilateral total hip and knee arthroplasty illustrating patient-specific recommendations. The preoperative hemoglobin is the hemoglobin before the patient enters the algorithm. The baseline hemoglobin is the hemoglobin at the time of surgery. THA = total hip arthroplasty; TKA = total knee arthroplasty. (*Adapted with permission from Pierson JL, Hannon TJ, Earles DR: A blood-conservation algorithm to reduce blood transfusions after total hip and knee arthroplasty.* J Bone Joint Surg Am *2004;86:1512-1518.*)

4. Improving preoperative hemoglobin levels is the single best strategy for patients at risk of needing an allogeneic blood transfusion after orthopaedic surgery.

   a. **Figure 2** is an algorithm for the use of erythropoietin in selected patients.

   b. Established protocols should be used for discontinuation of drugs such as aspirin, coumadin, and clopidogrel, as well as certain herbal supplements that increase bleeding.

5. Anemia management protocols are essential to blood management programs because they increase red cell mass in anemic patients, reducing or eliminating the need for allogeneic blood during high blood loss surgeries.

6. Formal protocols for preoperative testing of hemoglobin for major blood loss surgeries and coagulation status testing in certain patient populations should be in place.

D. Predonated autologous blood

   1. Causes iatrogenic anemia that is treated with a return of the predonated blood, without a net benefit to the patient.

   2. Storage of autologous blood leads to a progressive decline in the quality of the red cells and increase in inflammatory mediators.

IV. Perioperative Blood Management Strategies

A. Laboratory-related considerations

   1. Measured laboratory values are needed to make evidence-based transfusion decisions.

   2. Absence of timely information often leads to excessive or improper selection of blood products, unnecessarily exposing patients to harm.

   3. Hemoglobin or hematocrit testing should be readily available perioperatively.

   4. Coagulation and platelet function testing are useful in complex cases.

B. Technique-related considerations

   1. After adequate patient preparation, the next most important orthopaedic blood management strategy is meticulous yet efficient surgical technique.

   2. Longer surgical times are strongly correlated with complications and blood loss in major orthopaedic and spine surgery.

   3. Use of regional anesthesia can lower blood loss, probably through the combined benefits of a slightly lowered blood pressure and good postoperative pain control.

4. Use of controlled hypotension is controversial and has fallen into disfavor because of marginal blood-sparing benefits and a greatly increased medicolegal risk if perioperative adverse events occur.

5. Acute normovolemic hemodilution is not widely practiced and not recommended.

   a. The theoretical benefit comes from patients bleeding "thinner" blood through the early withdrawal then late return of autologous blood in the operating room.

   b. With good patient selection and proper technique, other blood-sparing effects are available for patients who have large amounts of blood withdrawn and subsequently lose large amounts of blood intraoperatively.

C. Other patient-related considerations

   1. Proper patient positioning to reduce venous bleeding

   2. Monitoring and maintenance of patient temperature because even mild hypothermia (35°C) greatly increases bleeding time and blood loss because of the relationship between temperature and the clotting cascade.

D. Use of perioperative autotransfusion ("cell saver")

   1. This technique is safe and cost-effective when performed by properly trained and proficient personnel using properly maintained and certified devices.

   2. It should be used only when the collection and return of one unit or more of red blood cells is likely.

E. Limiting early postoperative blood loss

   1. Early postoperative blood loss often is the result of fibrinolysis, followed by a hypercoagulable state within 8 to 16 hours.

   2. Perioperative use of antifibrinolytics such as tranexamic acid, epsilon aminocaproic acid, and aprotinin have demonstrated dramatic reductions in postoperative blood loss (< 50%) without an apparent increase in thromboembolic events.

   3. Aprotinin is used extensively in cardiac surgery and has additional anti-inflammatory properties, but its orthopaedic use may be limited by costs (~ $800 per patient) and the risk of adverse events such as hypersensitivity reactions and renal dysfunction in certain patients.

V. Postoperative Blood Management Strategies

A. The key to blood management is the maintenance of endogenous red cell mass.

B. Postoperative transfusion decisions should be based on measured laboratory values using evidence-based protocols.

C. Major orthopaedic surgery is associated with large amounts of blood loss, with a 46% reported rate of allogeneic and autologous transfusions after primary hip and knee arthroplasty.

D. Most postoperative symptoms in orthopaedic patients that are attributed to anemia are more causally related to volume deficits from postoperative bleeding. Aggressive but well-monitored volume replacement generally is sufficient to allow rehabilitation and timely discharge of postoperative patients with hemoglobin levels in the 7 to 8 g/dL range.

E. Wound drainage reinfusion systems often are used for postoperative blood conservation.

   1. These devices work by drawing shed blood from the wound under low vacuum into a sterile collection reservoir and returning the blood within the first 4 to 6 hours after surgery after it is passed through a filter.

   2. It is our expert opinion that the return of unwashed shed blood is not a sound practice, and washed cell reinfusion devices are strongly recommended.

      a. Blood collected from surgical wounds typically has a low hematocrit and is usually of poor quality from surgical debris and harmful inflammatory mediators.

      b. Common complications associated with re-transfusion of shed blood include systemic inflammatory response syndrome (SIRS), transfusion-related acute lung injury (TRALI), and increased postoperative bleeding as a result of fibrin degradation-induced disseminated intravascular coagulation (DIC).

      c. Simple filtration systems are insufficient to remove cytokines and fibrin degeneration products; therefore, no "safe" amount of this blood can be returned.

      d. If shed blood is of sufficient quantity to be retransfused, it should be washed on a certified autotransfusion device that is operated by qualified personnel.

D. As with intraoperative transfusion decisions, postoperative transfusions should be based on measured laboratory values and evidence-based protocols.

Top Testing Facts

1. Optimal blood management constitutes proactive processes, techniques, drugs, or medical devices that reduce the need for allogeneic blood when employed in an efficient, effective, and timely manner.

2. Blood use is suboptimal in many hospitals because of poor training and inadequate oversight, review, and monitoring of transfusion practices.

3. Although the blood supply is the safest it has ever been, transfusion of blood components remains a high-risk procedure that results in some degree of harm to all patients.

4. Storage of blood (allogeneic and autologous) results in a progressive decline in the quality of the red cells and an increase in inflammatory mediators.

5. Formal protocols for preoperative testing of hemoglobin for major blood loss surgeries and coagulation status testing in certain patient populations are important for early identification and intervention.

6. A core element of perioperative blood management is the use of measured laboratory values to make evidence based transfusion decisions. Absence of timely information often leads to excessive or improper selection of blood products, unnecessarily exposing patients to harm. There should be ready availability of hemoglobin or hematocrit testing in the perioperative period. Coagulation and platelet function testing also are useful in complex patients.

7. After adequate patient preparation, the next most important orthopaedic blood management strategy is meticulous yet efficient surgical technique.

8. Postoperative transfusion decisions also should be based on measured laboratory values using evidence-based protocols.

9. Major orthopaedic surgery is associated with large amounts of blood loss, with a 46% reported rate of allogeneic and autologous transfusions after primary hip and knee arthroplasty.

10. Many symptoms in postoperative orthopaedic patients attributed to anemia are more causally related to volume deficits from postoperative bleeding. Aggressive but well-monitored volume replacement is generally sufficient to allow rehabilitation and timely discharge in postoperative patients with hemoglobin levels in the 7 to 8 g/dL range.

Bibliography

Bierbaum BE, Callaghan JJ, Galante JO, et al: An analysis of blood management in patients having a total hip or knee arthroplasty. *J Bone Joint Surg Am* 1999;81:2-10.

Billote DB, Glisson SN, Green D, et al: A prospective, randomized study of preoperative autologous donation for hip replacement surgery. *J Bone Joint Surg Am* 2002;84-A:1299-1304.

Buehler PW, Alayash AI: Toxicities of hemoglobin solutions: In search of in-vitro and in-vivo model systems. *Transfusion* 2004;44:1516-1530.

Carson JL, Altman DG, Duff A, et al: Risk of bacterial infection associated with allogeneic blood transfusion among patients undergoing hip fracture repair. *Transfusion* 1999;39:694-700.

Cremieux PY, Barrett B, Anderson K, et al: Cost of outpatient blood transfusion in cancer patients. *J Clin Oncol* 2000;18:2755-2761.

Hansen E, Hansen MP: Reasons against the retransfusion of unwashed wound blood. *Transfusion* 2004;44:45S-53S.

Hebert PC, Wells G, Blajchman MA, et al: A multicenter, randomized, controlled clinical trial of transfusion requirements in critical care: Transfusion requirements in critical care investigators. Canadian critical care trials group. *N Engl J Med* 1999;340:409-417.

Keating EM, Meding JB: Perioperative blood management practices in elective orthopaedic surgery. *J Am Acad Orthop Surg* 2002;10:393-400.

Parker MJ, Roberts CP, Hay D: Closed suction drainage for hip and knee arthroplasty: A meta-analysis. *J Bone Joint Surg Am* 2004;86-A:1146-1152.

Pierson JL, Hannon TJ, Earles DR: A blood-conservation algorithm to reduce blood transfusions after total hip and knee arthroplasty. *J Bone Joint Surg Am* 2004;86-A:1512-1518.

Poses RM, Berlin JA, Noveck H, et al: How you look determines what you find: Severity of illness and variation in blood transfusion for hip fracture. *Am J Med* 1998;105:198-206.

Rao SV, Jollis JG, Harrington RA, et al: Relationship of blood transfusion and clinical outcomes in patients with acute coronary syndromes. *JAMA* 2004;292:1555-1562.

Spahn DR, Casutt M: Eliminating blood transfusions: New aspects and perspectives. *Anesthesiology* 2000;93:242-255.

Spiess BD: Risks of transfusion: Outcome focus. *Transfusion* 2004;44:4S-14S.

Toy P, Popovsky MA, Abraham E, et al: Transfusion-related acute lung injury: Definition and review. *Crit Care Med* 2005;33:721-726.

2: General Knowledge

Chapter 20
Normal and Pathologic Gait

Mary Ann Keenan, MD

I. Normal Gait

A. Walking is the process by which the body moves forward while maintaining stance stability. During the gait cycle, agonist and antagonist muscle groups work in concert to advance the limb.

1. Most muscle groups undergo eccentric (lengthening with contraction) contractions.

2. The quadriceps undergoes concentric contraction (muscle shortening) during midstance.

3. Alternatively, some muscle groups undergo isocentric contracture (muscle length stays constant). An example of this is the hip abductors during midstance.

B. The gait cycle, or stride (**Figure 1**)

1. The gait cycle is the complete sequence of all of the functions of a single limb during walking, from initial contact to initial contact. The sections of the gait cycle are often expressed as a percentage, beginning with initial contact (0%) and ending with the most terminal portion of swing (100%).

2. The gait cycle comprises two periods: stance and swing.

   a. Stance—Period while the foot is in contact with the ground. At normal walking speed, stance constitutes approximately 60% of the gait cycle.

   b. Swing—Period when the foot is off the ground and the leg is moving forward. Swing constitutes 40% of the gait cycle.

   c. The percentage relationship between stance and swing periods is velocity dependent.

3. The gait cycle also can be described in terms of step and stride.

   a. Stride is the distance between consecutive initial contacts of the same foot with the ground.

   b. Step is the distance between the initial contacts of alternating feet.

4. Three tasks are required during gait: During stance, the leg must (a) accept body weight and (b) provide single-limb support; (c) during swing, the limb must be advanced.

5. Eight phases of the gait cycle

   a. Weight acceptance (stance): initial contact, limb-loading response

   b. Single-limb support (stance): midstance, terminal stance, preswing

   c. Limb advancement (swing): initial swing, midswing, terminal swing

6. Characteristic joint positions and muscle activity during each phase of gait

   a. Initial contact: begins as the foot contacts the ground.

      i. In normal gait, the heel is the first part of the foot to touch the ground.

      ii. The hip is flexed, the knee is extended, and the ankle is dorsiflexed to neutral.

      iii. The hip extensor muscles contract to stabilize the hip because the body's mass is behind the hip joint.

   b. Loading response

      i. Loading response marks the beginning of the initial double-limb stance period.

      ii. It begins when the foot contacts the floor and continues until the opposite foot is lifted for swing.

      iii. Body weight is transferred onto the supporting leg.

      iv. During the loading response, the knee flexes to 15°, and the ankle plantar flexes to absorb the downward force.

      v. The ankle dorsiflexor muscles are active with an eccentric contraction (lengthening contraction) to control the plantar flexion moment.

      vi. As the knee flexes and the stance leg accepts the weight of the body, the quadriceps muscle becomes active to counteract the flexion moment and stabilize the knee.

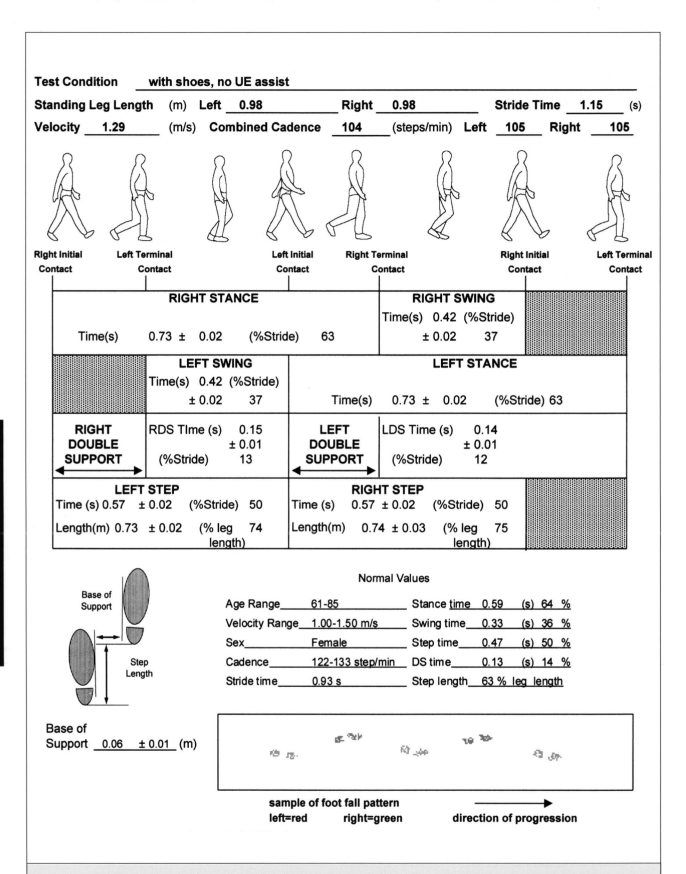

Test Condition   with shoes, no UE assist

Standing Leg Length (m) **Left** 0.98   **Right** 0.98   **Stride Time** 1.15 (s)

Velocity 1.29 (m/s) **Combined Cadence** 104 (steps/min) **Left** 105 **Right** 105

Right Initial Contact   Left Terminal Contact   Left Initial Contact   Right Terminal Contact   Right Initial Contact   Left Terminal Contact

RIGHT STANCE	RIGHT SWING
Time(s) 0.73 ± 0.02 (%Stride) 63	Time(s) 0.42 (%Stride) ± 0.02 37

LEFT SWING	LEFT STANCE
Time(s) 0.42 (%Stride) ± 0.02 37	Time(s) 0.73 ± 0.02 (%Stride) 63

RIGHT DOUBLE SUPPORT		LEFT DOUBLE SUPPORT	
	RDS Time (s) 0.15 ± 0.01 (%Stride) 13		LDS Time (s) 0.14 ± 0.01 (%Stride) 12

LEFT STEP	RIGHT STEP
Time (s) 0.57 ± 0.02 (%Stride) 50	Time (s) 0.57 ± 0.02 (%Stride) 50
Length(m) 0.73 ± 0.02 (% leg length 74	Length(m) 0.74 ± 0.03 (% leg length 75

Base of Support

Step Length

Base of Support   0.06 ± 0.01 (m)

Normal Values

Age Range	61-85	Stance time 0.59 (s) 64 %
Velocity Range	1.00-1.50 m/s	Swing time 0.33 (s) 36 %
Sex	Female	Step time 0.47 (s) 50 %
Cadence	122-133 step/min	DS time 0.13 (s) 14 %
Stride time	0.93 s	Step length 63 % leg length

sample of foot fall pattern

left=red   **right=green**   **direction of progression**

Figure 1   The gait cycle. An example of gait temporal-spatial data depicting the measurement of symmetry and timing. *(Reprinted from Esquenazi A, Biomechanics of gait, in Vaccaro AR (ed):* Orthopaedic Knowledge Update 8, *Rosemont, IL, American Academy of Orthopaedic Surgeons, 2005, p. 380.)*

c. Midstance

i. Midstance is the initial period of single-limb support.

ii. Midstance begins with the lifting of the opposite foot and continues until body weight is aligned over the supporting foot.

iii. The supporting leg advances over the supporting foot by ankle dorsiflexion while the hip and knee extend.

iv. The hip extensors and quadriceps undergo concentric contraction (muscle shortening) during midstance.

v. As the body's mass moves ahead of the ankle joint, the calf muscles become active to stabilize the tibia and ankle to allow the heel to rise from the floor.

d. Terminal stance

i. Terminal stance begins when the supporting heel rises from the ground and continues until the heel of the opposite foot contacts the ground.

ii. Body weight progresses beyond the supporting foot as increased hip extension puts the leg in a more trailing position.

iii. The heel leaves the floor, and the knee begins to flex as momentum carries the body forward.

iv. In the final portion of terminal stance, as the body rolls forward over the forefoot, the toes dorsiflex at the metatarsophalangeal joints.

v. The toe flexor muscles are most active at this time.

e. Preswing

i. Preswing marks the second double-limb stance interval in the gait cycle.

ii. This phase begins with the initial contact of the previous swing limb and ends with toe-off of the previously supporting leg.

iii. Ground contact by the opposite leg, making initial contact, causes the knee of the trailing limb to flex to 35° and the ankle to plantar flex to 20°.

iv. Body weight is transferred to the opposite limb.

v. The quadriceps should be inactive at this time to allow the knee to flex.

vi. The hip flexor muscles provide the power for advancing the limb and are active during the initial two thirds of the swing phase.

vii. Forward movement of the leg provides the inertial force for knee flexion.

f. Initial swing

i. Initial swing marks the period of single-limb support for the opposite limb.

ii. This phase begins when the foot is lifted from the floor and ends when the swinging foot is opposite the stance foot.

iii. The swing leg is advanced by concentric contraction of the hip flexor muscles.

iv. The knee flexes in response to forward inertia provided by the hip flexors.

v. The ankle partially dorsiflexes to ensure ground clearance.

g. Midswing

i. Midswing begins when the swinging foot is opposite the stance foot and continues until the swinging limb is in front of the body and the tibia is vertical.

ii. Advancement of the swing leg is accomplished by further hip flexion.

iii. The knee extends with the momentum provided by hip flexion while the ankle continues dorsiflexion to neutral.

iv. The ankle dorsiflexors become active during the latter two thirds of the phase to ensure foot clearance as the knee begins to extend.

h. Terminal swing

i. This phase begins when the tibia is vertical and ends when the foot contacts the floor.

ii. Limb advancement is completed by knee extension.

iii. The hamstring muscles decelerate the forward motion of the thigh during the terminal period of the swing phase.

iv. The hip maintains its flexed position.

v. The ankle dorsiflexors maintain their activity to ensure that the ankle remains dorsiflexed to neutral.

C. Center of mass (COM)

1. The COM is located anterior to the second sacral vertebra, midway between both hip joints (**Figure 2**).

2. The body requires the least amount of energy to move along a straight line.

3. During gait, the COM deviates from the straight line in vertical and lateral sinusoidal displacements.

a. The COM displaces vertically in a rhythmic fashion as it moves forward.

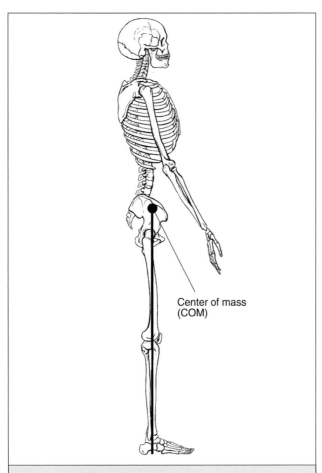

Figure 2 Illustration from a sagittal view of the COM and weight-bearing line in the standing position.

b. The highest point occurs at midstance, and the lowest point occurs at the time of double-limb support.

c. The mean vertical displacement is 5 cm, and the mean lateral displacement is approximately 5 cm.

d. The speed of movement of the COM decreases at midstance, and the peak of vertical displacement is achieved.

e. The speed of movement of the COM increases as the stance limb is unloaded.

f. The COM displaces laterally with forward movement.

g. As weight is transferred from one leg to the other, the pelvis shifts to the weight-bearing side.

h. The limits of lateral displacement are reached at midstance.

D. Gait analysis—A clinically useful way to assess lower limb function either by visual observation or with quantitative measurements.

1. Visual analysis

   a. Visual analysis begins with a general assessment, noting symmetry and smoothness of movements of the various body parts.

   b. The cadence (steps per minute), base width, stride length, arm swing, movement of the trunk, and rise of the body should be noted.

   c. Because of the speed and the complexity of walking, visual analysis does not supply the observer with enough quantitative information to enable precise diagnosis.

   d. Videotaping is useful for supplementing clinical observation.

2. Laboratory gait analysis

   a. Kinematics is the analysis of the motion produced during the gait cycle (**Figure 3**).

   b. Kinetics is the analysis of forces that produce motion (**Figure 4**).

   c. Dynamic polyelectromyography assesses the activity of multiple muscles during gait (**Figure 5**).

3. Stride can be assessed with gait pressure mats or other timing devices. Characteristics include velocity, cadence (steps per minute), stance and swing times, and single- and double-limb support times.

4. Kinematic analysis

   a. Videotaping in two planes is useful for recording motion.

   b. Electrogoniometers or tensiometers are used to record individual joint movement.

   c. Motion analysis uses multiple cameras that detect sensors on a patient. The data from the cameras can be used to recreate a three-dimensional model of the patient's gait pattern.

5. Kinetic analysis

   a. Force plate studies measure ground reactive forces and changes in the center of pressure as a patient walks.

   b. Pedobaric measurements can be used to determine the magnitude and distribution of forces under the foot.

   c. Joint moments and powers can be calculated using movement and force data.

6. Dynamic polyelectromyography measures and records the electrical activity in the multiple muscle groups that work during functional activity.

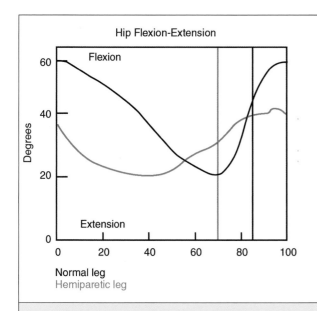
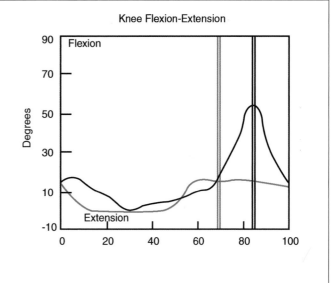

Normal leg
Hemiparetic leg

Figure 3 Three-dimensional sagittal kinematic data of the normal and hemiparetic limbs in the same patient. Data was obtained with CODA mpx motion tracking system (Charnwood Dynamics, Leicestershire, England). Normalized gait cycle expressed as percent of the gait cycle (x-axis); 0 = initial contact, vertical line indicates the beginning of swing phase, 100 = the next initial contact.

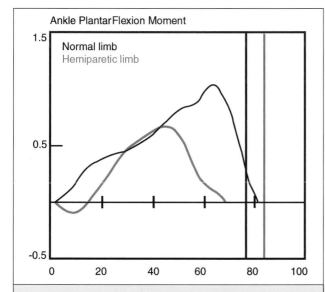

Figure 4 Kinetic data. Ankle plantar flexion moments of a normal and hemiparetic limb in the same patient.

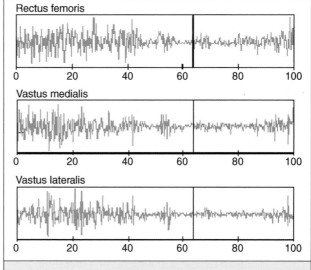

Figure 5 Dynamic polyelectromyography of the quadriceps muscles obtained from the hemiparetic limb of a patient with a stiff knee gait.

II. Pathologic Gait

A. Antalgic gait—Any gait abnormality resulting from pain. It is a nonspecific term. Different pathologies can result in similar compensations during gait.

1. Hip osteoarthritis

   a. Leaning of the trunk laterally over the painful leg during stance brings the COM over the joint.

   b. Compressive forces decrease across the joint as the need for contraction of the hip abductor muscles decreases.

2. Knee pain

   a. The knee is maintained in slight flexion throughout the gait cycle, especially if there is an effusion.

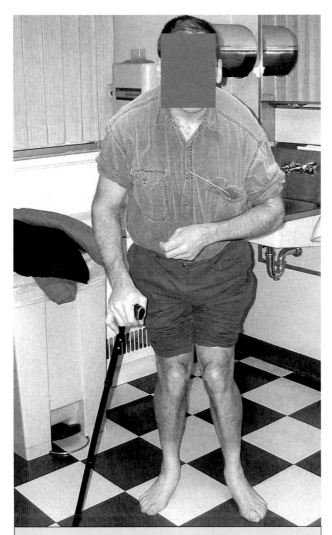

Figure 6 A knee flexion contracture is often associated with a concurrent hip flexion contracture. A crouched posture results in high energy demands because the hip, knee, and ankle extensors must be continuously active to maintain an upright posture. This limits the time and distance a person is able to walk.

    b. Moderate flexion reduces tension on the knee joint capsule.

    c. Compensation for knee flexion involves toe walking on the affected side.

    d. The time of weight bearing on the painful leg is also reduced.

  3. Foot and ankle pain

    a. Patients attempt to limit weight bearing through the affected area.

    b. The stride length is shortened.

    c. Normal heel-to-toe motion is absent.

  4. Forefoot pain

    a. Patients have a characteristic flatfoot gait.

    b. Patients avoid weight bearing on the metatarsal heads.

  5. Ankle or hindfoot pain

    a. Patients avoid heel strike at initial contact.

    b. Patients ambulate on the toes of the affected side.

B. Joint contractures

  1. Flexion contracture of the hip

    a. The contracture is compensated for by increased lumbar lordosis.

    b. Compensatory knee flexion is required to maintain the COM over the feet for stability.

    c. The characteristic crouched posture is energy inefficient and results in shorter overall walking distances.

  2. Flexion contracture of the knee

    a. Flexion contracture of the knee causes a relative limb-length discrepancy.

    b. Contractures of less than 30° become more pronounced with faster walking speeds, whereas those of greater than 30° are apparent at normal walking speeds.

    c. Gait is characterized by toe walking on the affected side.

    d. Increased hip and knee flexion (steppage gait) of the opposite limb may be required to clear the foot because the affected limb is relatively too long (**Figure 6**).

  3. Plantar flexion contracture of the ankle

    a. Results in a knee extension moment (knee extension thrust) at initial contact of the forefoot with the floor.

    b. During swing phase, hip and knee flexion of the affected limb (steppage gait) must be increased to clear the foot because the limb is relatively too long.

C. Joint instability

  1. Knee instability can result in variable gait presentations depending on the ligament involved.

  2. Knee recurvatum

    a. Knee recurvatum results from weakness of the ankle plantar flexors and quadriceps.

    b. During stance, the patient compensates by leaning the trunk forward to place the COM anterior to the knee.

    c. This leads to degenerative changes of the knee joint over time (**Figure 7**).

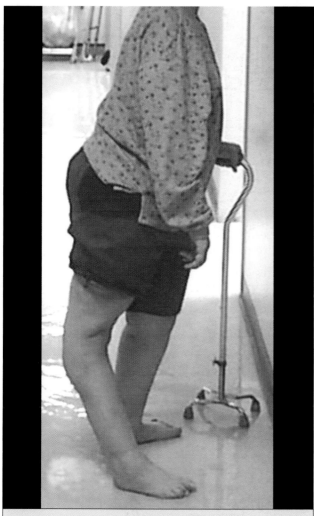

Figure 7   Weakness of the ankle plantar flexors and quadriceps muscles causes a patient to position the COM anterior to the flexion axis of the knee to prevent the knee from buckling. Over time, this compensation leads to a recurvatum deformity of the knee.

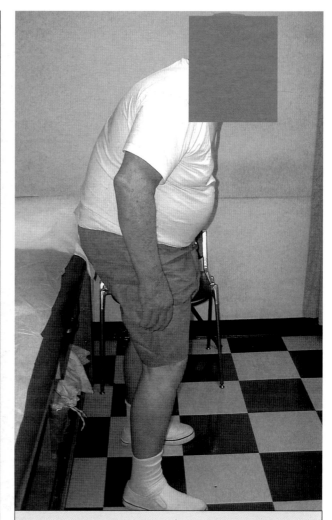

Figure 8   Assuming a posture of hip flexion places the hip extensor muscles in a position of greater mechanical advantage. This helps to compensate for moderate weakness of the hip extensor muscles (grade 4) during walking.

3. Injuries of the posterolateral corner of the knee (posterior cruciate ligament, lateral collateral ligament, posterior joint capsule, and the popliteus tendon) result in a varus thrust gait pattern during stance.

4. Quadriceps avoidance gait

   a. This type of gait occurs in patients with an anterior cruciate ligament (ACL)–deficient knee

   b. With an ACL-deficient knee, the tibia is prone to anterior subluxation because the contraction of the quadriceps provides an anterior force to the tibia.

   c. Attempts to decrease the load response phase on the affected limb are made by decreasing stride length and avoiding knee flexion during the midportion of stance.

5. Ankle instability

   a. Ankle instability results in difficulty with supporting body weight during initial contact.

   b. An unstable ankle often buckles, resulting in an antalgic gait that limits the load response phase on the affected side.

D. Muscle weakness

   1. Weakness of the hip flexor

      a. Limits limb advancement during swing

      b. Results in a shortened step length

   2. Moderate weakness of the hip extensors

      a. Compensated by forward trunk flexion

      b. This posture places the hip extensors on stretch and in a position of increased mechanical advantage (**Figure 8**).

2: General Knowledge

3. Severe weakness of the hip extensors results in the need for upper limb assistive devices to maintain an erect posture.

4. Quadriceps weakness

   a. Makes the patient susceptible to falls at initial contact

   b. The patient compensates by leaning the trunk forward to keep the COM anterior to the knee joint.

   c. The gastrocnemius muscle contracts more vigorously to maintain the knee in extension.

   d. At times, patients use the hand to push the knee into extension with initial weight bearing.

5. Ankle plantar flexor weakness

   a. Causes instability of the tibia and knee as the COM moves anterior to the knee

   b. Quadriceps activity increases to keep the knee extended.

   c. This compensation limits step length, which predisposes the patient to painful overuse syndromes of the patella and quadriceps.

6. Combined quadriceps and ankle plantar flexor weakness

   a. Causes the patient to hyperextend the knee for stability at initial contact

   b. Over time, this compensation results in a genu recurvatum deformity.

Top Testing Facts

1. A gait cycle, also known as a stride, is the complete sequence of all the functions of a single limb during walking, from initial contact to initial contact. The sections of the gait cycle are often expressed as a percentage, beginning with the initial contact of the foot with the floor (0%) and ending with the most terminal portion of swing (100%).

2. The sections of the gait cycle—initial contact, single-limb support, etc.—describe the events that occur. The three tasks required during gait are of more conceptual importance, however. During stance, the leg must (a) accept body weight and (b) provide single-limb support; (c) during swing, the limb must be advanced.

3. The normal gait cycle has two periods (stance and swing), and eight phases (initial contact, limb-loading response, midstance, terminal stance, preswing, initial swing, midswing, terminal swing).

4. The COM is located anterior to the second sacral vertebra, midway between the hip joints.

5. Antalgic gait is a nonspecific term that describes any gait abnormality resulting from pain.

6. Flexion contracture of the hip requires compensatory knee flexion to maintain the COM over the feet for stability, resulting in the characteristic crouched posture.

7. A plantar flexion contracture of the ankle results in a knee extension moment (knee extension thrust) at initial contact of the forefoot with the floor.

8. Weakness of the hip flexor limits limb advancement during swing and results in a shortened step length.

9. With quadriceps weakness, the patient compensates by leaning the trunk forward to keep the COM anterior to the knee joint.

10. Ankle plantar flexor weakness causes increased quadriceps activity, limiting step length and predisposing the patient to painful overuse syndromes of the patella and quadriceps.

Bibliography

Crosbie J, Green T, Refshauge K: Effects of reduced ankle dorsiflexion following lateral ligament sprain on temporal and spatial gait parameters. *Gait Posture* 1999;9:167-172.

Esquenazi A: Biomechanics of gait, in Vaccaro AR (ed): *Orthopaedic Knowledge Update 8*. Rosemont, IL, American Academy of Orthopaedic Surgeons, 2005.

Gage JR (ed): *The Treatment of Gait Problems in Cerebral Palsy Series: Clinics in Developmental Medicine*. Mac Keith Press, No. 164.

Keenan MA, Esquenazi A, Mayer N: The use of laboratory gait analysis for surgical decision making in persons with up-per motor neuron syndromes. *Phys Med & Rehabil State of the Art Revs* 2002;16:249-261.

Lim MR, Huang RC, Wu A, Girardi FP, Cammisa FP Jr: Evaluation of the elderly patient with an abnormal gait. *J Am Acad Orthop Surg* 2007;15:107-117.

Neumann DA: Biomechanical analysis of selected principles of hip joint protection. *Arthritis Care Res* 1989;2:146-155.

Perry J: *Gait Analysis: Normal and Pathological Function*. Slack Publishers, 1992.

Chapter 21
Orthoses, Amputations, and Prostheses

Mary Ann Keenan, MD   Douglas G. Smith, MD

I. Lower Limb Orthoses

A. Terminology

1. Orthosis (or orthotic device) is the medical term for a brace or splint. Orthoses generally are named according to body region.

2. The basic types are static and dynamic devices.

   a. Static—Rigid devices used to support the weakened or paralyzed body parts in a particular position.

   b. Dynamic—Used to facilitate body motion to allow optimal function.

3. Standard abbreviations include FO (foot orthosis), AFO (ankle-foot orthosis), KAFO (knee-ankle-foot orthosis), HKAFO (hip-knee-ankle-foot orthosis), and THKAFO (trunk-hip-knee-ankle-foot orthosis).

B. Principles

1. Orthoses are used for management of a specific disorder, including a painful joint, muscle weakness, or joint instability or contracture.

2. Orthotic joints should be aligned at the approximate anatomic joints.

3. Orthoses should be simple, lightweight, strong, durable, and cosmetically acceptable.

4. Considerations for orthotic prescription

   a. Three-point pressure control system

   b. Static or dynamic stabilization

   c. Tissue tolerance to compression and shear force

5. Construction materials include metal, plastic (most commonly polypropylene), leather, synthetic fabric, or any combination thereof.

C. Foot orthoses

1. Shoes are a type of FO and can be modified to accommodate deformities or to provide support to the limb during walking.

   a. A cushioned or negative heel is often used with a rigid ankle to reduce the knee flexion moment.

   b. Medial and lateral wedges can be added to the heel or sole of a shoe to accommodate fixed varus or valgus foot deformities. These wedges also influence the varus and valgus forces on the knee.

   c. Medial and lateral flares can be added to the heel or sole of a shoe to widen the base of support for the foot.

   d. Rocker soles help to transfer the body weight forward while walking, but they may destabilize the knee by transferring body weight forward too rapidly.

   e. An extra deep shoe allows additional room for deformities and inserts.

2. An FO placed inside the shoe can provide support, control motion, stabilize gait, reduce pain, correct flexible deformities, and prevent progression of fixed deformities.

   a. Heel cup

      i. A heel cup is a rigid plastic insert.

      ii. It covers the plantar surface of the heel and extends posteriorly, medially, and laterally up the side of the heel.

      iii. Heel cups are used to prevent lateral calcaneal shift in the flexible flatfoot.

   b. University of California Biomechanics Laboratory (UCBL) FO (**Figure 1**).

      i. The UCBL FO is constructed of plastic and is fabricated over a cast of the foot held in maximal manual correction.

      ii. It encompasses the heel and midfoot with rigid medial, lateral, and posterior walls.

   c. Arizona brace

      i. The Arizona brace combines the UCBL orthosis with a laced ankle support.

      ii. It provides more rigid hindfoot support.

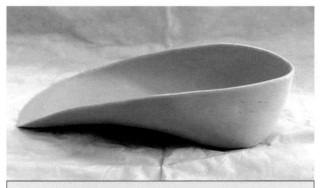

Figure 1 The UCBL foot orthosis encompasses the heel and midfoot. It has medial, lateral, and posterior walls.

D. Ankle-foot orthoses (**Table 1** and **Figure 2**)

1. AFOs are prescribed for weakness or muscle over-activity of ankle dorsiflexion, plantar flexion, inversion, and eversion.

2. AFOs are used to prevent or correct deformities.

3. The ankle position indirectly affects knee stability, with ankle plantar flexion providing a knee extension force and ankle dorsiflexion providing a knee flexion force.

4. All AFOs consist of a footplate with stirrups, uprights, and a calf band, regardless of the materials used for construction.

5. Nonarticulated AFOs

   a. Nonarticulated AFOs are more cosmetically acceptable.

   b. They place a flexion force on the knee during weight acceptance.

   c. The trim lines of plastic AFOs determine the degree of flexibility during late stance and are described as having maximal, moderate, or minimal resistance to ankle dorsiflexion.

   d. Nonarticulated AFOs may be constructed of plastic, composite materials, or leather and metal.

   e. Thermoplastic AFOs must be used with care in patients with fluctuating edema and lack of sensation.

   f. Nonarticulated AFOs are described according to the amount of rigidity of the brace, which depends on the thickness and composition of the plastic, as well as the trim lines and shape.

      i. Posterior leaf spring

      ii. Minimal resistance to ankle dorsiflexion

      iii. Moderate resistance to dorsiflexion

      iv. Maximal resistance to dorsiflexion

Table 1

Types of Ankle Motion allowed by Orthotic Ankle Joints and the Effect on Gait

Ankle Joint Motion	Effect on Gait
Unrestricted plantar flexion and dorsiflexion	Provides medial-lateral ankle stability
Unrestricted plantar flexion	Allows normal weight acceptance in early stance
Unrestricted dorsiflexion	Unrestricted dorsiflexion allows calf strengthening and stretching of the plantar flexors (Achilles tendon).
Plantar flexion stop	Limits a dynamic equinus deformity and provides a knee flexion moment during weight acceptance
Dorsiflexion assistance	Corrects a flexible foot drop during swing
Limited dorsiflexion (dorsiflexion stop)	Provides a knee extension moment in the later part of stance. Useful to stabilize the knee in the presence of quadriceps or plantar flexion weakness
Locked ankle	Limits motion for multiplanar instability or ankle pain

6. Articulated AFOs

   a. Articulated AFOs allow a more natural gait pattern and adjustment of plantar and dorsiflexion.

   b. They can be designed to provide dorsiflexion assistance to clear the toes during swing.

   c. Adjustable ankle joints can be set to the desired range of ankle dorsiflexion or plantar flexion.

   d. Mechanical ankle joints

      i. These joints can control or assist ankle dorsiflexion or plantar flexion by means of stops (pins) or assists (springs).

      ii. They also control medial-lateral stability of the ankle joint.

      iii. Limits on ankle motion affect knee stability: Unrestricted plantar flexion allows normal weight acceptance in early stance; plantar flexion stop causes a knee flexion moment during weight acceptance; dorsiflexion stop provides a knee extension moment during the later part of stance.

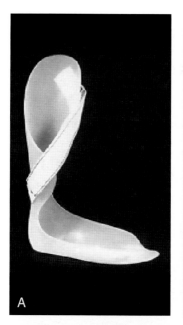
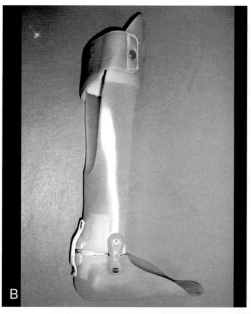
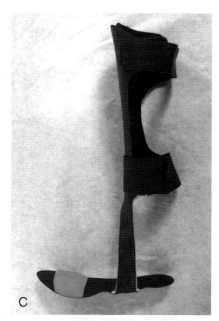
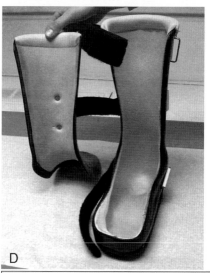
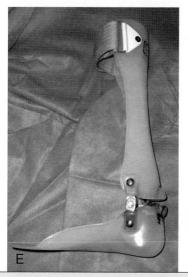
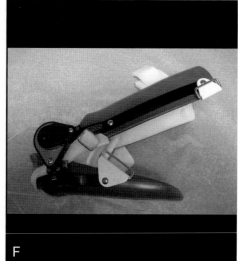

Figure 2 Examples of ankle-foot orthoses (AFOs). **A,** Posterior leaf-spring AFO. **B,** Floor reaction AFO. **C,** Carbon fiber composite AFO. **D,** Clamshell AFO for neuropathic arthropathy. **E,** Articulated AFO with simple joint. **F,** Dynamic dorsiflexion AFO.

7. Types of AFO designs

   a. Free motion ankle joints—Allow unrestricted ankle dorsiflexion and plantar flexion motion, provide only medial-lateral stability, and are useful for ligamentous instability.

   b. Unrestricted (free) plantar flexion—Allows normal weight acceptance in early stance.

   c. Unrestricted (free) dorsiflexion—Allows calf muscle strengthening and stretching of the plantar flexors (Achilles tendon).

   d. Limited motion ankle joints—Can be adjusted for use in ankle weakness affecting all muscle groups.

   e. Plantar flexion stop ankle joint

      i. These joints are used in patients with weakness of dorsiflexion during swing phase.

      ii. The plantar flexion stop limits a dynamic (flexible) equinus deformity.

      iii. These joints provide a knee flexion moment during weight acceptance. They should not be used in patients with quadriceps weakness.

   f. Dorsiflexion stop ankle joint

      i. In the setting of mild equinus, this joint can be used to promote a knee extension mo-

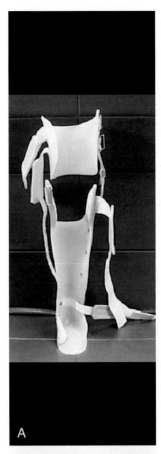
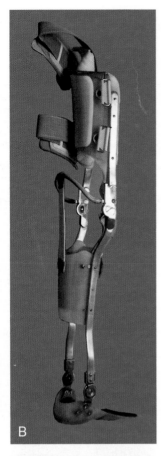
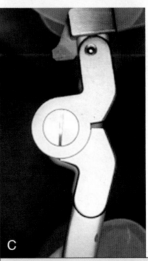
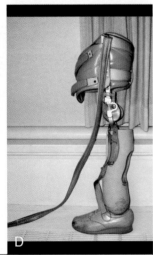

Figure 3 Examples of knee-ankle-foot orthoses (KAFOs). **A,** KAFO. **B,** KAFO with bail knee lock joint. **C,** Posterior knee joint and drop lock for a KAFO. **D,** Combined prosthesis for ankle disarticulation and KAFO for quadriceps weakness.

iii. These joints are useful for stabilizing the knee during the later part of stance in the presence of quadriceps or ankle plantar flexion weakness.

g. Locked ankle joint—Limits motion for multiplanar instability or ankle pain.

h. Dorsiflexion assist spring joint—Provides dynamic ankle dorsiflexion during swing phase and corrects a flexible foot drop during swing.

8. Varus or valgus correction straps (T-straps)

a. When used for valgus correction, this type of device contacts the skin medially and circles the ankle until buckled on the outside of the lateral upright.

b. When used for varus correction, this type of device contacts the skin laterally and is buckled around the medial upright.

E. Knee-ankle-foot orthoses

1. Construction

a. KAFOs consist of an AFO with metal uprights, a mechanical knee joint, and two thigh bands (**Figure 3**).

b. They can be made of metal-leather and metal-plastic or plastic and plastic-metal.

2. Principles of operation

a. KAFOs can be used in quadriceps paralysis or weakness to maintain knee stability and control flexible genu valgum or varum.

b. They are used to limit the weight bearing of the thigh, leg, and foot with quadrilateral or ischial containment brim.

c. A KAFO is more difficult to don and doff than an AFO.

d. KAFOs are not recommended for patients who have moderate to severe cognitive dysfunction.

3. Types of KAFO designs

a. Double upright metal KAFO (most common)

i. This type of KAFO comprises an AFO with two metal uprights extending proximally to the thigh to control knee motion and alignment.

ii. It consists of a mechanical knee joint and two thigh bands between two uprights.

b. Scott-Craig orthosis

i. The Scott-Craig orthosis includes a cushioned heel with a T-shaped foot plate for mediolateral stability, an ankle joint with anterior and posterior adjustable stops, double uprights, a pretibial band, a posterior thigh

ment during the loading response to prevent buckling of the knee.

ii. Limited ankle dorsiflexion provides a knee extension moment in the later part of stance.

Table 2

Designs of Orthotic Knee Joints and Their Uses

Knee Joint	Design	Use
Single-axis joint	The axis of rotation of the joint is aligned with the rotational axis of the anatomic knee joint.	Provides medial-lateral knee stability May allow full knee movement or be locked
Posterior offset joint	The axis of rotation of the joint is aligned posterior to the rotational axis of the anatomic knee joint.	Provides additional stability to the extended knee Limits knee recurvatum
Polycentric joint	Allows limited multiplanar motion during flexion and extension	Decreases joint contact forces in a painful arthritic knee
Dynamic extension joint	A spring or coil provides active knee extension force.	Provides active knee extension for quadriceps

band, and a knee joint with pawl locks and bail control.

  ii. Hip hyperextension allows the center of gravity to fall behind the hip joint and in front of the locked knee and ankle joint.

  iii. With 10° of ankle dorsiflexion alignment, a swing-to or swing-through gait with crutches is possible.

  iv. The Scott-Craig orthosis is used for standing and ambulation in patients with paraplegia as a result of a spinal cord injury.

c. Supracondylar plastic orthosis

  i. The ankle is immobilized in slight plantar flexion to produce a knee extension moment in stance to help eliminate the need for a mechanical knee lock.

  ii. This orthosis resists genu recurvatum and provides medial-lateral knee stability.

d. Plastic shell and metal upright orthosis—Posterior leaf spring AFO with double metal uprights that extend up to a plastic shell in the thigh with an intervening knee joint.

4. Knee joints (**Table 2**)

a. Single-axis knee joints—The axis of rotation of the joint is aligned with the rotational axis of the anatomic knee joint.

  i. The single-axis knee joint is useful for knee stabilization.

  ii. The arc of knee motion can be full or limited.

  iii. A free motion knee joint allows unrestricted knee flexion and extension with a stop to prevent hyperextension; it is used for patients with recurvatum but good strength of the quadriceps to control knee motion.

b. Posterior offset knee joint—The axis of rota-

tion of the orthotic joint is aligned posterior to the rotational axis of the anatomic knee joint.

  i. The posterior offset knee shifts the weight-bearing axis provided by the center of mass (COM) more anterior to the anatomic knee joint.

  ii. At initial contact and during weight acceptance, the ground reaction force is anterior to the flexion axis of the anatomic knee. This extends the knee and results in great stability during early stance.

  iii. It provides a knee extension moment during stance.

  iv. The knee can flex freely during swing phase.

c. Polycentric joint

  i. This joint allows limited multiplanar motion during flexion and extension.

  ii. It is useful for patients with knee arthritis.

d. Dynamic knee extension joint

  i. This type of joint provides active knee extension, usually by means of a coiled spring within the joint.

  ii. It is helpful for patients with quadriceps weakness but full knee extension.

5. Types of knee joint locking mechanisms—Orthotic knee joints can be modified to allow locking of the joint for stability during stance.

a. Drop ring lock knee joint

  i. This is the most commonly used knee lock to prevent knee flexion while walking.

  ii. Rings drop over the joint to lock the knee joint while the knee is in extension.

  iii. The knee is stable, but gait is stiff without knee motion.

  iv. This type of lock is appropriate for patients

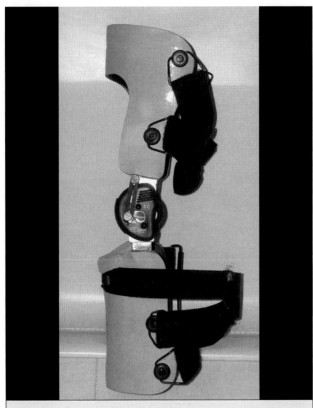

Figure 4   Dynamic knee extension orthosis.

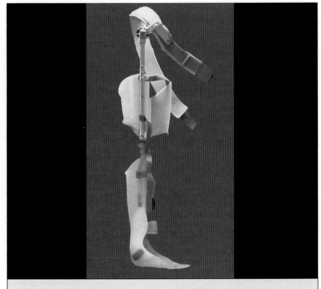

Figure 5   Hip-knee-ankle-foot orthosis (HKAFO).

with severe quadriceps weakness or gross ligamentous instability.

    v. Extensions may be added to the rings to allow the patient to unlock the joint for sitting without the need to bend forward.

  b. Pawl lock with bail release knee joint

    i. A semicircular bail attaches to the knee joint posteriorly, and the patient can unlock both joints easily by pulling up the bail or backing up to sit down in a chair.

    ii. A major drawback is that the knee can accidentally unlock, such as while the patient is pulling up his or her pants or if bumped on a chair.

  c. Adjustable knee lock joint (dial lock)

    i. This serrated adjustable knee joint allows knee locking at different degrees of flexion.

    ii. This type of lock is used for patients with knee flexion contractures that are improving gradually with stretching.

6. Additional potential modifications of a KAFO

  a. Anterior knee pad—Can be placed over the patella to prevent knee flexion.

  b. Medial strap or pad—Controls a valgus knee deformity.

  c. Lateral strap or pad—Controls a varus knee deformity.

  d. Ischial weight bearing—Upper thigh band cuff is brought up above the ischium to provide a weight bearing surface.

F. Knee orthoses—KOs provide support or control to the knee only, not the foot and ankle (**Figure 4**).

1. KOs for patellofemoral disorders—These types of KOs supply medial-lateral knee stability, control patellar tracking during knee flexion and extension, and generally include an infrapatellar strap.

2. KOs for knee control in the sagittal plane—These KOs control genu recurvatum with minimal medial-lateral stability and include a Swedish knee cage and a three-way knee stabilizer.

3. KOs for knee control in the frontal plane—This type of KO consists of thigh and calf cuffs joined by sidebars with mechanical knee joints, is usually polycentric, and closely mimics the anatomic joint motion.

4. KOs for axial rotation control—These KOs can provide angular control of flexion-extension and medial-lateral planes, control axial rotation, and are used mostly in the management of sports injuries of the knee.

G. Hip-knee-ankle-foot orthoses

1. HKAFOs consist of an AFO with metal uprights, a mechanical knee joint, thigh uprights, a thigh socket, a hip joint, and waist band (**Figure 5**).

2. The hip joint can be adjusted in two planes to control flexion and extension and to control abduction and adduction.

a. Single-axis hip joint with lock

   i. This is the most common hip joint with flexion and extension.

   ii. It may include an adjustable stop to control hyperextension.

b. Two-position lock hip joint

   i. This type of hip joint can be locked at full extension and 90° of flexion.

   ii. It is used for hip spasticity control in a patient who has difficulty maintaining a seated position.

c. Double-axis hip joint

   i. The double-axis hip joint has a flexion-extension axis to control these motions.

   ii. It also has an abduction-adduction axis to control these motions.

3. The orthotic hip joint is positioned with the patient sitting upright at 90°, whereas the orthotic knee joint is centered over the medial femoral condyle.

4. Pelvic bands

a. Pelvic bands complicate dressing after toileting unless the orthosis is worn under all clothing.

b. Pelvic bands also increase energy demands for ambulation.

H. Trunk-hip-knee-ankle-foot orthoses

1. THKAFOs consist of a spinal orthosis in addition to an HKAFO to control trunk motion and spinal alignment.

2. THKAFOs are indicated in patients with paraplegia.

3. They are very difficult to don and doff.

II. Lower Limb Amputations

A. Demographics

1. Approximately 130,000 new amputations are performed annually in the United States.

2. Causes and levels of amputations performed are listed in **Table 3**.

B. Goals of lower limb amputation

1. General goals

a. Remove diseased, injured, or nonfunctioning limb in a reconstructive procedure

b. Restore function to the level of patient need

c. Preserve length and strength

Table 3

Causes and levels of Lower Limb Amputations

	Percentage of Amputations
Causes	
Vascular disorders	80
Trauma	15
Tumor, infection, congenital	5
Levels	
Foot	50
Transtibial	25
Transfemoral	25

---

d. Balance the forces of the remaining muscles to provide a stable residual limb

2. Goals for ambulatory patients

a. Restore a maximum level of independent function

b. Ablate diseased tissue

c. Reduce morbidity and mortality

3. Goals for nonambulatory patients

a. Achieve wound healing while minimizing complications

b. Improve sitting balance

c. Facilitate position and transfers

C. Preoperative evaluation

1. The preoperative evaluation should include an assessment of skin integrity and sensation, joint mobility, and muscle strength.

2. Vascular status (to determine the viable level of amputation) should also be evaluated. Several assessment techniques are used.

a. Doppler ultrasound

   i. Ankle/brachial index >0.45 correlates with 90% healing.

   ii. Advantages—Readily available, noninvasive.

   iii. Disadvantages—Arterial wall calcification can give misleadingly elevated readings.

3. Toe systolic blood pressure

a. The minimum requirement for distal healing is 55 mm Hg.

b. Advantages—Noninvasive, readily available, and inexpensive.

2: General Knowledge

4. Transcutaneous oxygen tension

   a. Po_2 >35 is necessary for wound healing.

   b. Advantages—Noninvasive, highly accurate in assessing wound healing.

   c. Disadvantages—Results may be altered by skin disorders such as edema or cellulitis.

5. Skin blood flow measurement

   a. Xenon 133 clearance has been used in the past.

   b. Expensive and time consuming

6. Fluorescence studies have been used but provide unreliable results.

7. Arteriography

   a. Advantage—Visualize the patency of vessels.

   b. Disadvantages—Invasive and unreliable in determining successful wound healing.

D. Assessment of nutrition and immune competence

1. Total lymphocyte count of > 1,500/mL

2. Serum albumin ≥ 3 g/dL

E. Psychological preparation

1. Viewing amputation as a step in recovery, not a failure

2. Early plan for prosthetic fitting and return to function

3. Preoperative counseling for the patient and family

4. Referral to amputee support groups

F. Surgical principles

1. Blood and soft-tissue considerations

   a. Use a tourniquet to minimize blood loss if there is no significant vascular disease.

   b. Plan soft-tissue flaps for mobile and sensate skin.

   c. Balance muscle forces across the residual joints.

2. Bone considerations

   a. Bevel the bone ends to minimize skin pressure and maximize weight-bearing capacity of the residual limb.

   b. Avoid periosteal stripping to preserve bone viability and to minimize the likelihood of heterotopic bone formation.

3. Surgical procedure

   a. Myodesis is the technique in which distal muscle is sutured directly to bone or tendon, covering the distal bone end and maximizing the weight-bearing capacity of the residual limb.

   b. Divide nerves proximally and sharply to avoid painful neuromas.

   c. Close the wound with minimal tension and place a drain to decompress the underlying tissue.

4. Postoperative management

   a. Apply a compressive dressing to protect the wound and control edema.

   b. A splint or cast also may be applied to limit edema and prevent contractures.

G. Complications

1. Failure of the wound to heal properly occurs as the result of insufficient blood supply, infection, or errors in surgical technique.

2. Infection may develop postoperatively without widespread tissue necrosis or flap failure, especially if active distal infection was present at the time of the definitive amputation or if the amputation was done near the zone of a traumatic injury.

3. Postoperative edema is common, but rigid dressings help reduce this problem.

4. Phantom sensation

   a. The feeling that all or a part of the amputated limb is still present

   b. Common in nearly everyone who undergoes amputation but usually diminishes over time

5. Phantom pain

   a. A bothersome painful or burning sensation in the part of the limb that is missing

   b. Unrelenting phantom pain occurs in only a minority of patients.

6. Joint contractures

   a. Usually develop between the time of amputation and prosthetic fitting

   b. Treatment is difficult and often unsuccessful.

   c. Prevention with adequate pain control and the initial use of casts or splints is paramount.

7. Dermatologic problems

   a. The residual limb and prosthetic socket must be kept clean, rinsed well to remove all soap residue, and thoroughly dried.

   b. Shaving increases problems with ingrown hairs and folliculitis.

   c. Epidermoid cysts commonly occur at the prosthetic socket brim. The best approach is to modify the socket and relieve pressure over the cyst.

   d. Verrucous hyperplasia is a wartlike overgrowth of skin that can occur on the distal end of the residual limb. It is caused by a lack of distal contact and failure to remove normal keratin.

  e. Contact dermatitis is caused by contact with acids, bases, or caustics and frequently results from failure to rinse detergents and soaps from prosthetic socks.

  f. Candidiasis and other dermatophytoses present with scaly, itchy skin, often with vesicles at the border and clearing centrally. Dermatophytoses are diagnosed with a potassium hydroxide preparation and treated with topical antifungal agents.

III. Levels of Amputation

A. Foot

  1. Hallux amputation

    a. Save the base of proximal phalanx to preserve push-off strength.

    b. Stabilize the sesamoid bones by performing tenodesis of flexor hallucis brevis tendon.

  2. Lesser toes can be amputated through the interphalangeal joint, metatarsophalangeal joint, or the phalanx.

    a. Can use side-to-side or plantar dorsal flaps

    b. Save the base of the proximal phalanx to provide better stability and push-off strength.

  3. Ray amputations are best done on the border rays; central ray resections take longer to heal.

  4. Transmetatarsal amputations can be performed through the metatarsals or Lisfranc joints.

    a. Bevel bone cuts on plantar surface to prevent skin pressure.

    b. Create a cascade from medial to lateral side of the foot.

    c. Consider Achilles lengthening to prevent equinus.

  5. Hindfoot

    a. Chopart amputation is done through the transverse tarsal joints.

      i. Preserves the talus and calcaneus

      ii. Equinus deformity can result.

      iii. Rebalance the muscle forces by lengthening the Achilles tendon and reattaching the tibialis anterior and extensor hallucis longus tendons to the anterior talus.

    b. Boyd amputation—Combines a talectomy with calcaneotibial arthrodesis.

    c. Pirogoff amputation—The distal end of the calcaneus is excised, then rotated and fused to tibia.

    d. Both the Boyd and Pirogoff amputations prevent migration of the heel pad and provide a stable distal weight-bearing surface.

B. Ankle disarticulation (Syme)

  1. Provides superior mechanics compared with transtibial amputation

  2. Surgical procedure

    a. A long posterior flap is preferred to sagittal flaps.

    b. Preserve the length of the residual tibia.

    c. Bevel the tibia cut and perform a myodesis to protect the distal end of the limb.

    d. Distal limb is covered by heel pad and plantar skin, and the fascia is sutured.

  3. Postoperative management includes a rigid dressing or cast to control edema, protect the skin from pressure, and prevent knee flexion contracture.

C. Knee disarticulation

  1. Indicated for ambulatory patients who cannot have a transtibial amputation and nonambulatory patients

  2. Retains the length of femur for good sitting balance

  3. Prosthetic fitting is more challenging because the knee joint is distal to the opposite leg.

  4. Longer limb length provides better leverage for use of prosthesis.

D. Transfemoral amputation

  1. Usually done with equal anterior-posterior flaps

  2. Muscle stabilization is critical (**Figure 6**).

  3. Abduction and flexion forces must be balanced, even in nonambulatory patients.

  4. Without an adductor myodesis, the femur can migrate to a subcutaneous position even within a well-fitted prosthetic socket.

E. Hip disarticulation—Rarely done.

  1. Ambulation with prosthesis requires more energy than a swing-through gait with crutches.

  2. A lateral approach is preferred for several reasons:

    a. Anatomy is more familiar to orthopaedic surgeons.

    b. Dissection is simplified.

2: General Knowledge

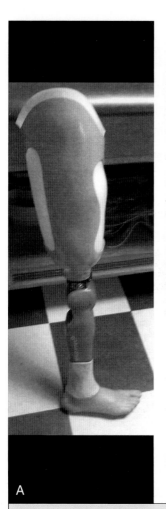
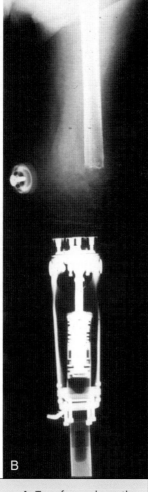

Figure 6   Transfemoral prostheses. **A,** Transfemoral prosthesis with a microprocessor knee joint. **B,** Radiograph shows abducted femur within the socket of a transfemoral prosthesis.

   c. Few perforating vessels are encountered.

   d. Results in a quick procedure with minimal blood loss.

   e. Preserves femoral and gluteal circulation.

  3. Mortality varies with the underlying disease process.

IV. Lower Limb Prostheses

A. Overview

  1. Goals

   a. Comfortable to wear

   b. Easy to don and doff

   c. Lightweight

   d. Durable

   e. Cosmetically pleasing

   f. Must function well mechanically

   g. Must have reasonably low maintenance requirements

  2. Major advances in lower limb prostheses

   a. Development of new lightweight structural materials

   b. Incorporation of elastic response ("energy-storing") designs

   c. Use of computer-assisted design and computer-assisted manufacturing technology for sockets

   d. Microprocessor control of the prosthetic knee joint

  3. Major components include the socket, suspension mechanism, knee joint, pylon, and terminal device.

B. Socket—The connection between the residual limb and the prosthesis; the socket must protect the residual limb but also must transmit the forces associated with standing and ambulation.

  1. Preparatory (temporary) socket

   a. The preparatory socket must be adjusted several times as the volume of the residual limb stabilizes.

   b. It can be created by using a plaster mold of the residual limb as a template.

  2. The most common socket used in a transtibial amputation is a patellar tendon–bearing prosthesis.

C. Suspension mechanism—Attaches the prosthesis to the residual limb using belts, wedges, straps, suction, or a combination thereof.

  1. Suction suspension—The two types are standard suction and silicon suspension.

   a. Standard suction—Form-fitting rigid or semi-rigid socket into which the residual limb is fitted (**Figure 7**).

   b. Silicon suction—Uses a silicon-based sock that slips onto the residual limb, which is then inserted into the socket. The silicon helps to form an airtight seal that stabilizes the prosthesis (**Figure 8**).

D. Knee (articulating) joint (if needed)

  1. The knee joint has three principal functions:

   a. To provide support during stance phase.

   b. To produce smooth control during swing phase.

   c. To maintain unrestricted motion for sitting and kneeling.

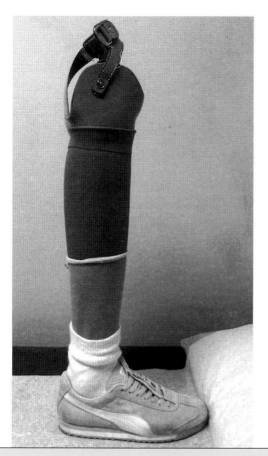

Figure 7 Transtibial prosthesis with standard socket and supracondylar suspension strap.

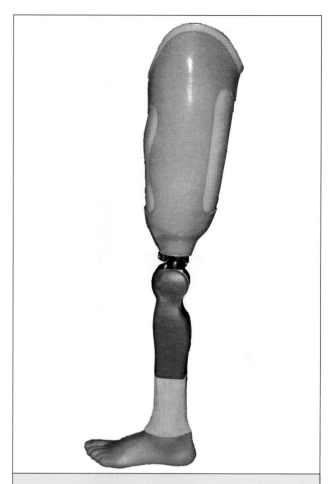

Figure 9 Transfemoral prosthesis with a microprocessor knee joint.

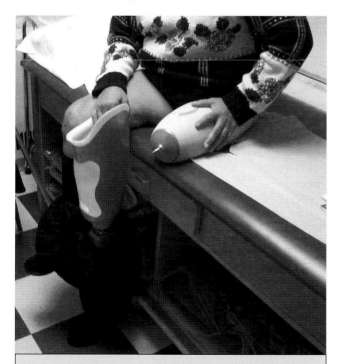

Figure 8 Transfemoral prosthesis with silicone suspension system.

2. Two types of axis

   a. A single axis with a simple hinge and a single pivot point

   b. A polycentric axis with multiple centers of rotation

3. Microprocessor control systems have been applied to the knee units for transfemoral amputees (**Figure 9**).

   a. The microprocessor alters resistance of the knee unit to flexion or extension appropriately by sensing the position and velocity of the shank relative to the thigh.

   b. Current microprocessor-controlled knee units do not provide power for active knee extension, which would assist the amputee in rising from the sitting position or going up stairs and would provide power to the amputee's gait.

   c. The new microprocessor-controlled, "intelligent" knee units do offer superior control when walking at varied speeds, descending ramps and stairs, and walking on uneven surfaces.

2: General Knowledge

E. Pylon—A simple tube or shell that attaches the socket to the terminal device.

1. This component has progressed from simple static shells to dynamic devices that allow axial rotation and absorb, store, and release energy.

2. The pylon can be an exoskeleton (soft foam contoured to match the other limb with a hard laminated shell) or an endoskeleton (internal metal frame with cosmetic soft covering).

F. Terminal device—Typically a foot, but it may take other specialized forms, as for water or other sports activities.

1. Ankle

a. Ankle function usually is incorporated into the terminal device.

b. Separate ankle joints can be beneficial in heavy-duty industrial work or in sports, but the additional weight requires more energy expenditure and more limb strength to control the additional motion.

2. Foot—The prosthetic foot has five basic functions: To provide a stable weight-bearing surface, absorb shock, replace lost muscle function, replicate the anatomic joint, and restore cosmetic appearance.

a. Non–energy-storing feet

i. Solid ankle/cushioned heel (SACH) foot—Mimics ankle plantar flexion, which allows for a smooth gait. It is a low-cost, low-maintenance foot for a sedentary patient who has had a transtibial or a transfemoral amputation.

ii. Single-axis foot—Adds passive plantar flexion and dorsiflexion, which increase stability during stance phase.

b. Energy-storing feet

i. Multiaxis foot—Adds inversion, eversion, and rotation to plantar flexion and dorsiflexion; handles uneven terrain well and is a good choice for the individual with a minimal-to-moderate activity level.

ii. Dynamic-response foot—This top-of-the-line foot is commonly used by young active individuals and athletic individuals with amputations.

G. Prosthetic prescription—Includes the type of prosthesis and its components. Considers the patient's functional level.

1. Functional level 1—Has the ability or potential to use a prosthesis for transfers or ambulation on level surfaces at a fixed cadence.

2. Functional level 2—Has the ability or potential for ambulation with the ability to traverse low-level environmental barriers such as curbs, stairs, or uneven surfaces.

3. Functional level 3—Has the ability or potential for ambulation with a variable cadence.

4. Functional level 4—Has the ability or potential for prosthetic ambulation that exceeds the basic ambulation skills, exhibiting high impact, stress, or energy levels.

H. Prosthetic training

1. Basics of prosthesis care

a. How to don and doff the prosthesis

b. How to inspect the residual limb for signs of skin breakdown; should be checked daily

c. How to perform safe transfers

2. Skills training—The end goal is for the patient to safely ambulate on all usual surfaces without adaptive equipment. Training includes:

a. Weight bearing with the prosthesis

b. Ambulation on level surfaces with a walker or other assistive device

c. Training on stairs, uneven surfaces, and ramps/inclines

I. Problems with prosthesis use

1. Choke syndrome

a. Venous outflow can be obstructed when the proximal part of the socket has too snug a fit on the residual limb. When combined with an empty space more distally in the socket, swelling can occur until that empty space is filled.

b. With acute choke syndrome, the skin is red and indurated and may have an orange-peel appearance with prominent skin pores.

c. If the constriction is not resolved, chronic skin changes with hemosiderin deposits and venous stasis ulcers can develop.

2. Dermatologic problems

a. Contact dermatitis—The usual culprits are the liner, socks, and suspension mechanism, with the socket a less likely cause. Treatment consists of removal of the offending item and symptomatic treatment with topical diphenhydramine or cortisone creams.

b. Cysts and excessive sweating—Can be signs of excessive shear forces and components that are improperly fitted.

c. Scar management—Focuses on massaging and lubricating the scar to obtain a well-healed result without dog ears or adhesions.

3. Painful residual limb

   a. Prosthesis-related pain—Possible causes:

      i. Excessive pressure over anatomic bony prominences

      ii. Excessive pressure over heterotopic ossification

      iii. Excessive friction between the skin and prosthetic socket from a poor fit

   b. Residual limb–related pain—Possible causes:

      i. Insufficient soft-tissue coverage over bony prominences

      ii. An unstable residual limb from lack of myodesis to balance muscle forces (eg, no adductor myodesis in a transfemoral amputation leads to unopposed hip abductor force)

      iii. Unstable soft-tissue pad over the distal residual limb

      iv. Neuroma formation in a superficial location

4. Prosthetic gait—The ability to walk with a prosthesis is related to the mechanical quality of the prosthesis and the physiologic quality of the residual limb. The physiologic quality of the residual limb is related to passive joint mobility and muscle strength.

   a. Transtibial amputation

      i. The demands of weight acceptance require heightened muscle control and strength.

      ii. The increased muscle demand results from insufficient knee flexion and persistent ankle dorsiflexion of the prosthesis.

      iii. A knee flexion contracture >10° is the most significant obstacle to walking with a transtibial prosthesis.

   b. Transfemoral amputation

      i. Walking is an arduous task for the transfemoral amputee, requiring significant functional contributions from the trunk and intact limb.

      ii. Residual limb function is hampered by the loss of musculature, the lack of direct contact between the thigh and the prosthetic knee joint, and limitations of the prosthetic foot, which ideally should provide increased flexibility without loss of stance stability.

J. Energy requirements of prosthetic gait (**Table 4**)

1. The increase in energy requirements can be the limiting factor in ambulation.

2. An individual who has a lower limb amputation and requires a walker or crutches to ambulate uses 65% more energy than someone with a normal gait.

Table 4

Metabolic Cost of Ambulation per Level and Nature of Amputation

Amputation Level	Metabolic Cost
Syme	Increased 15%
Traumatic transtibial	Increased 25%
Vascular transtibial	Increased 40%
Traumatic transfemoral	Increased 68%
Vascular transfemoral	Increased 100%

(Reprinted from Munin MC, Galang GF: Limb amputation and prosthetic rehabilitation, in Vaccaro AR (ed): Orthopaedic Knowledge Update 8, Rosemont, IL, American Academy of Othropaedic Surgeons, 2005, p. 652. Data from Czerniecki JM: Rehabilitation in limb deficiency: Gait and motion analysis. Arch Phys Med Rehabil 1996;77:S3-S8.)

3. Increased levels of energy consumption (percentage above normal)

   a. Below-knee unilateral amputation: 10% to 20%

   b. Below-knee bilateral amputation: 20% to 40%

   c. Above-knee unilateral amputation: 60% to 70%

   d. Above-knee bilateral amputation: >200%

4. Energy consumption is actually less with a transtibial prosthesis than ambulating with crutches. Ambulating with a transfemoral prosthesis, however, requires more energy, which makes the cardiopulmonary status of the patient more significant.

V. Upper Limb Amputations

A. Traumatic amputation

1. Overview—The initial management of traumatic amputations often occurs at centers that do not have the expertise to replant the amputated body part or appropriately treat the amputee. It is important for the physicians involved in the initial care of the patient to understand the indications for replantation as well as proper care of the patient, the residual limb, and the amputated limb segment. Knowledge of the basics of initial care and management of the residual limb and amputated body part is crucial.

B. Replantation

1. Indications—The decision whether to replant depends on patient factors (eg, age, comorbidities) and the condition of the residual limb and amputated body part.

2: General Knowledge

2. Common replantations—The most commonly replanted parts are the thumb, multiple digits in adults, and amputated digits in children.

3. Initial patient management

   a. Initial management of the trauma patient includes stabilization of the patient and evaluation for other conditions that may supersede the amputation.

   b. Life-threatening injuries always take precedence over amputation or replantation.

   c. Consultation with a hand center helps to determine whether a replantation is indicated. The goal is to expedite patient transfer to a hand center if a replantation is possibly needed.

4. Initial management of the amputated body part

   a. The amputated part should never be placed directly on ice because direct exposure of the amputated part to ice or ice water will result in tissue damage.

   b. Wrap the amputated body part in moist gauze, place inside a plastic bag, and place the bag on ice.

5. Preoperative management for replantation

   a. Patient should be placed on nothing-by-mouth (NPO) status, and tetanus prophylaxis, antibiotic therapy, and intravenous fluids should be administered.

   b. Other emergent medical conditions should be treated.

   c. Radiographs of both the residual limb and the amputated part should be obtained.

   d. Delay in treatment should be minimized because the likelihood of success of the replantation decreases with prolonged tissue ischemia.

6. Contraindications to replantation

   a. Replantation of a single digit may result in a stiff, painful, and nonfunctional finger. Ray resection may be more useful.

   b. In patients with factors that contraindicate single-digit replantation (eg, advanced age, diabetes mellitus, smoking), revision amputation is indicated.

   c. Amputations of the distal thumb or fingers can be shortened and closed primarily.

C. Surgical amputation

1. Indications for amputation—Irreparable loss of the blood supply or tissue of a diseased or injured upper limb is the only absolute indication for amputation regardless of all other circumstances.

   a. Vascular compromise or occlusion—Patients present very differently, depending on the etiology.

   b. Trauma—Most cases of involve significant avulsion and crush components.

   c. Thermal burns and frostbite—These cases rarely require amputation proximal to the hand.

   d. Neglected compartment syndromes

   e. Systemic sepsis—Amputations may be necessary to control an otherwise rampant infection.

   f. Malignant tumors

2. Incidence

   a. Published estimates of the annual incidence of upper limb amputations in the United States vary significantly, from 20,000 to 30,000 new amputations per year.

   b. Prevalence—350,000 to 1,000,000 persons with all types of amputations in the United States.

3. Goals of upper limb amputation surgery

   a. Preservation of functional length

   b. Durable skin and soft-tissue coverage

   c. Preservation of useful sensation

   d. Prevention of symptomatic neuromas

   e. Prevention of adjacent joint contractures

   f. Controlled short-term morbidity

   g. Early prosthetic fitting

   h. Early patient return to work and recreation

4. Levels of amputation

   a. Ray resection—A digital ray resection (eg, index or little finger) may be preferable to a digital replantation if the result of the replantation would be a stiff, useless, or painful digit.

   b. Transcarpal amputation

      i. Advantages—Preserves supination and pronation of the forearm and limited flexion and extension of the wrist. The long lever arm increases the ease and power with which a prosthesis can be used.

      ii. Disadvantages—Prosthetic fitting is more difficult than with a wrist disarticulation.

      iii. Surgical technique—Long full-thickness palmar and shorter dorsal flap should be created in a ratio of 2:1. The finger flexor and extensor tendons should be transected. The wrist flexors and extensors should be anchored to the remaining carpus in line with their insertions to preserve active wrist motion.

c. Wrist disarticulation

   i. Indications—Wrist disarticulation is the procedure of choice in children because it preserves the distal radial and ulnar physes. It also provides a longer lever arm for strength in both adults and children.

   ii. Advantages—Preserves the distal radioulnar joint to preserve pronation and supination.

   iii. Surgical technique—The prominent styloid processes should be rounded off. The radial styloid flare should be preserved to improve prosthetic suspension.

d. Transradial amputation

   i. Advantages—Despite resection of the distal radioulnar joint, some degree of pronation and supination is preserved.

   ii. Surgical technique—Amputation at the junction of the distal and middle third of the forearm appears to provide a good compromise between adequate functional length and adequate wound healing. If amputation at this level is not possible, a shorter residual limb is still preferable to a transhumeral amputation. Detaching the biceps tendon and reattaching it proximally to the ulna at a position approximating its resting length is advisable to facilitate prosthetic fitting. Distal reattachment may cause a flexion contracture at the elbow.

e. Transhumeral amputation

   i. Efforts should be made to retain as much of the bone length that has suitable soft-tissue coverage as possible.

   ii. Even if only the humeral head remains and no functional length is salvageable, an improved shoulder contour and cosmetic appearance results.

   iii. Myodesis helps preserve biceps and triceps strength, prosthetic control, and myoelectric signals.

f. Shoulder disarticulation

   i. Incidence and indications—Shoulder disarticulations are performed only rarely, usually in cases of cancer or severe trauma.

   ii. Disadvantages—Results in a loss of the normal shoulder contour and causes the patient difficulty because clothing does not fit well.

   iii. Surgical considerations—The humeral head should be saved if possible because this can improve the contour of a shoulder disarticulation tremendously.

D. Postoperative management of upper limb amputations

1. A soft compressive dressing is applied.

2. An elastic bandage is applied to prevent edema.

3. If a drain is used, it is removed within 24 to 48 hours.

4. If no contraindications exist, anticoagulation may be administered for deep venous thrombosis prophylaxis.

5. Immediate active range of motion of the shoulder and elbow (and wrist) is implemented to prevent joint contractures.

E. Immediate or early postoperative prosthetic fitting

1. Advantages include decreased edema, postoperative pain, and phantom pain; accelerated wound healing; improved rehabilitation; and shorter hospital stays.

2. Benefits are less pronounced at amputation levels above the elbow.

VI. Upper Limb Prostheses

A. Overview

1. Terminology

   a. Relief—A concavity within the socket designed for pressure-sensitive bony prominences.

   b. Buildup—A convexity designed for areas tolerant to high pressure.

   c. Terminal device—Most distal part of the prosthesis used to do work (eg, hand).

   d. Myodesis—Direct suturing of muscle or tendon to bone.

   e. Myoplasty—Suturing of muscle to periosteum.

   f. Prehensile—Designed for grasping.

2. Considerations for upper limb prostheses

   a. Amputation level

   b. Expected function of the prosthesis

   c. Cognitive function of the patient

   d. Vocation of the patient (desk job versus manual labor)

   e. Avocational interests of the patient

   f. Cosmetic importance of the prosthesis

   g. Financial resources of the patient

B. Types of upper limb prostheses

1. Body-powered prostheses

a. Advantages

   i. Moderate cost and weight

   ii. Most durable prostheses

   iii. Have higher sensory feedback

b. Disadvantages

   i. Less cosmetically pleasing than a myoelectric unit

   ii. Require more gross limb movement

2. Myoelectric prostheses—Function by transmitting electrical activity that the surface electrodes on the residual limb muscles detect to the electric motor.

a. Advantages

   i. Provide more proximal function

   ii. Better cosmesis

b. Disadvantages

   i. Heavy and expensive

   ii. Less sensory feedback

   iii. Require more maintenance

c. Types of myoelectric units

   i. 2-site/2-function device—Has separate electrodes for flexion and extension.

   ii. 1-site/2-function device—Has one electrode for both flexion and extension. The patient uses muscle contractions of different strengths to differentiate between flexion and extension (eg, a strong contraction opens the device, and a weak contraction closes it).

C. Prosthesis characteristics by amputation level

1. Transradial (below-elbow)

a. Voluntary opening split hook

b. Friction wrist

c. Double-walled plastic laminate socket

d. Flexible elbow hinge, a single-control cable system

e. Biceps or triceps cuff

f. Figure-of-8 harness

2. Transhumeral (above-elbow)—Similar to transradial, with several differences

a. Substitutes an internal-locking elbow for the flexible elbow hinge

b. Uses a dual-control instead of single-control cable

c. No biceps or triceps cuff

D. Components

1. Terminal devices

a. Passive terminal devices

   i. Advantages—The main advantage of a passive terminal device is its cosmetic appearance. With newer advances in materials and design, a device that is virtually indistinguishable from the native hand can be manufactured.

   ii. Disadvantages—Passive terminal devices usually are less functional and more expensive than active terminal devices.

b. Active terminal devices

   i. Active terminal devices usually are more functional than cosmetic.

   ii. Active devices can be divided into two main categories: hooks and prosthetic hands with cables, and myoelectric devices.

c. Grips—Five types

   i. Precision grip (pincer grip)

   ii. Tripod grip (palmar grip, 3-jaw chuck pinch)

   iii. Lateral pinch (key pinch)

   iv. Hook power grip (carrying a briefcase)

   v. Spherical grip (turning a doorknob)

d. Considerations for choice of terminal device (prehension device)

   i. Handlike devices—These devices are composed of a thumb and an index and long finger. The thumb and fingers are oriented to provide palmar prehension. The fingers are coupled as one unit with the thumb in a plane perpendicular to the axis of the finger joints. The device may be covered with a cosmetic silicone glove simulating the appearance of an intact hand. Often the device of choice for a person working in an office environment.

   ii. Non-hand prehension devices—Hooks or two-finger pincer designs with parallel surfaces. Good for work situations that require higher prehension force. May be fitted with quick release mechanisms to attach task-specific tools for both vocational and avocational activities. Often used in an environment requiring physical labor.

   iii. Externally powered myoelectric devices—Use force-sensing resistors. Offer freedom from a control suspension harness. Provide stronger prehension. Can be used only in a non-hostile environment, free from dirt, dust, water, grease, or solvents.

iv. Many upper extremity amputees have both a body-powered and a myoelectric prosthesis to use for specific activities.

e. Terminal device mechanisms

i. Voluntary opening mechanism—The terminal device is closed at rest. This type of mechanism is more common than a voluntary closing mechanism. The patient uses the proximal muscles to open a hook-based device against the resistive force of rubber bands or cables. Relaxation of the proximal muscles allows the terminal device to close around the desired object. In a myoelectric device, contraction of the proximal muscles activates the electric motor.

ii. Voluntary closing mechanism—The terminal device is open at rest. The patient uses the residual forearm flexors to grasp the desired object. These devices are usually heavier and less durable than a voluntary opening mechanism.

2. Wrist units

a. Quick-disconnect wrist unit—Allows easy swapping of terminal devices with specialized functions.

b. Locking wrist unit—Prevents rotation during grasping and lifting.

c. Wrist flexion unit—In a patient with bilateral upper limb amputations, a wrist flexion unit can be placed on the longer residual limb (regardless of premorbid hand dominance) to allow midline activities such as shaving or manipulating buttons.

3. Elbow units—Chosen based on the level of the amputation and the amount of residual function.

a. Rigid elbow hinge—When a patient cannot achieve adequate pronation and supination but does have adequate native elbow flexion, such as in a short transradial amputation, a rigid elbow hinge provides additional stability.

b. Flexible elbow hinge—When a patient has sufficient voluntary pronation and supination as well as elbow flexion and extension, such as in a wrist disarticulation or a long transradial amputation, a flexible elbow hinge usually works well.

4. Prostheses for amputations about the shoulder

a. When an amputation is required at the shoulder or forequarter level, function is very difficult to restore because of the weight of the prosthetic components as well as the increased energy expenditure necessary to operate the prosthesis.

b. For this reason, some individuals with this level of amputation choose a purely cosmetic prosthesis to improve body image and the fit of their clothes.

E. Problems associated with upper limb prostheses

1. Dermatologic problems

a. Contact dermatitis—The usual culprits are the liner, socks, and suspension mechanism, with the socket a less likely cause. Treatment consists of removal of the offending item and symptomatic treatment with topical diphenhydramine or cortisone creams.

b. Cysts and excessive sweating—Can be signs of excessive shear forces and components that are improperly fitted.

c. Scar management—Focuses on massaging and lubricating the scar to obtain a well-healed result without adhesions.

2. Painful residual limb

a. Prosthesis-related pain—Possible causes:

i. Excessive pressure over anatomic bony prominences

ii. Excessive pressure over heterotopic ossification

iii. Excessive friction between the skin and prosthetic socket from a poor fit

b. Residual limb–related pain—Possible causes:

i. Insufficient soft-tissue coverage over bony prominences

ii. An unstable residual limb from lack of myodesis to balance muscle forces.

iii. An unstable soft-tissue pad over the distal residual limb

iv. Neuroma formation in a superficial location

Top Testing Facts

1. Articulated AFOs allow a more natural gait pattern and allow adjustment of plantar and dorsiflexion. The joints can be designed to provide stability in terminal stance and to provide dorsiflexion assistance to clear the toes during swing.

2. A KAFO can be used in quadriceps paralysis or weakness to maintain knee stability and control flexible recurvatum, valgus, or varus.

3. A polycentric knee joint allows limited multiplanar motion during flexion and extension that decreases specific areas of joint contact forces. This is helpful for persons with osteoarthritis.

4. Lower limb amputation is a reconstructive procedure with the goals of preserving length and strength and balancing the forces of the remaining muscles to provide a stable residual limb.

5. The Syme ankle disarticulation provides superior mechanics and is the most common level of amputation in the foot.

6. The major advances in lower limb prostheses include (a) the development of new lightweight structural materials; (b) the incorporation of elastic response ("energy-storing") designs; (c) the use of computer-assisted design and computer-assisted manufacturing technology in sockets; and (d) microprocessor control of the prosthetic knee joint.

7. Increased levels of energy (percentage over normal) are associated with amputations: below-knee, 10% to 20%; bilateral below-knee, 20% to 40%; above-knee, 60% to 70%.

8. Patient management for replantation includes the following: emergent medical conditions should be treated; radiographs of both the residual limb and the amputated part should be obtained; the patient should be made NPO; and tetanus prophylaxis, antibiotic therapy, and intravenous fluids should be administered. The amputated part should be wrapped in wet gauze and placed in a plastic bag on ice.

9. Goals of upper limb amputation surgery include preservation of functional length, durable skin and soft-tissue coverage, preservation of useful sensation, prevention of symptomatic neuromas, prevention of adjacent joint contractures, controlled short-term morbidity, early prosthetic fitting, and early patient return to work and recreation.

10. A voluntary opening mechanism (the terminal device is closed at rest) is commonly used for the hand.

Bibliography

Friel K: Componentry for lower extremity prostheses. *J Am Acad Orthop Surg* 2005;13:326-335.

Garst RJ: The Krukenberg hand. *J Bone Joint Surg Br* 1991;73:385-388.

Goel A, Navato-Dehning C, Varghese G, Hassanein K: Replantation and amputation of digits: User analysis. *Am J Phys Med Rehabil* 1995;74:134-138.

Martin C, Gonzalez del Pino J: Controversies in the treatment of fingertip amputations: Conservative versus surgical reconstruction. *Clin Orthop Relat Res* 1998;353:63-73.

Potter BK, Scoville CR: Amputation is not isolated: An overview of the us army amputee patient care program and associated amputee injuries. *J Am Acad Orthop Surg* 2006;14:S188-S190.

Smith DG: Amputations, in Skinner HB (ed): *Current Diagnosis and Treatment in Orthopedics*, ed 4. New York, NY, Lange Medical Books/McGraw-Hill, 2006, pp 645-670.

Wilkinson MC, Birch R, Bonney G: Brachial plexus injury: When to amputate? *Injury* 1993;24:603-605.

Wright TW, Hagen AD, Wood MB: Prosthetic usage in major upper extremity amputations. *J Hand Surg [Am]* 1995;20:619-622.

2: General Knowledge

Chapter 22

Neuro-Orthopaedics and Rehabilitation

Mary Ann Keenan, MD

I. Spinal Cord Injuries

A. General principles

1. Approximately 400,000 people in the United States have spinal cord damage.

2. Leading causes of spinal cord injury are motor vehicle accidents, gunshot wounds, falls, and sports and water injuries.

3. Patients are generally categorized into two groups:

   a. Younger individuals who sustained the injury from significant trauma

   b. Older individuals with cervical spinal stenosis caused by congenital narrowing or spondylosis; these patients often sustained the injury from minor trauma and commonly have no vertebral fracture spinal injury.

B. Definitions

1. Tetraplegia—Loss or impairment of motor or sensory function in the cervical segments of the spinal cord with resulting impairment of function in the arms, trunk, legs, and pelvic organs.

2. Paraplegia—Loss or impairment of motor or sensory function in the thoracic, lumbar, or sacral segments of the spinal cord. Arm function is intact, but, depending on the level of the cord injured, impairment in the trunk, legs, and pelvic organs may be present.

3. Complete injury—An injury with no spared motor or sensory function in the lowest sacral segments. Patients with complete spinal cord injury who have recovered from spinal shock have a negligible chance for any useful motor return (Table 1).

4. Incomplete injury—An injury with partial preservation of sensory or motor function below the neurologic level and includes the lowest sacral segments.

C. Neurologic impairment and recovery

1. Spinal shock

   a. Diagnosis of complete spinal cord injury cannot be made until spinal shock has resolved, as evidenced by the return of the bulbocavernosus reflex. To elicit this reflex, the clinician digitally examines the patient's rectum, feeling for contraction of the anal sphincter while squeezing the glans penis or clitoris.

   b. If trauma to the spinal cord causes complete injury, reflex activity at the site of injury does not return because the reflex arc is permanently interrupted.

   c. When spinal shock disappears, reflex activity returns in the segments below the level of injury.

Table 1		
ASIA Impairment Scale		
Level	Injury	Description
A	Complete injury	No motor or sensory function is preserved in the sacral segments S4-S5.
B	Incomplete Injury	Sensory but not motor function is preserved below the neurologic level and includes the sacral segments S4-S5.
C	Incomplete injury	Motor function is preserved below the neurologic level, and more than half of key muscles below the neurologic level have a muscle grade <3.
D	Incomplete injury	Motor function is preserved below the neurologic level, and at least half of key muscles below the neurologic level have a muscle grade ≥3.
E	Normal function	Motor and sensory functions are normal.

2. Recovery

a. The *International Standards for Neurologic and Functional Classification of Spinal Cord Injury*, published by the American Spinal Injury Association (ASIA) and the International Medical Society of Paraplegia (IMSOP), represents the most reliable instrument for assessing neurologic status in the spinal cord. These standards provide a quantitative measure of sensory and motor function.

b. Assessment

i. The change in ASIA Motor Score (AMS) between successive neurologic examinations should be determined. The AMS is the sum of strength grades for each of the 10 key muscles tested bilaterally that represent neurologic segments from C5 to T1 and L2 to S1.

ii. In a neurologically intact individual, the total possible AMS is 100 points.

D. Spinal cord syndromes

1. Anterior cord syndrome

a. Anterior cord syndrome results from direct contusion to the anterior cord by bone fragments or from damage to the anterior spinal artery.

b. Depending on the extent of cord involvement, only posterior column function (proprioception and light touch) may be present.

c. The ability to respond to pain and light touch signifies that the posterior half of the cord has some intact function.

2. Central cord syndrome

a. Central cord syndrome can be understood on the basis of the spinal cord anatomy. Gray matter in the spinal cord contains nerve cell bodies and is surrounded by white matter consisting primarily of ascending and descending myelinated tracts. Central gray matter has a higher metabolic requirement and is therefore more susceptible to the effects of trauma and ischemia.

b. Central cord syndrome often results from a minor injury such as a fall in an older patient with cervical spinal canal stenosis.

c. Most patients can walk despite severe paralysis of the upper limb.

3. Brown-Séquard syndrome

a. Brown-Séquard syndrome is caused by a complete hemisection of the spinal cord.

b. This results in a greater ipsilateral proprioceptive motor loss and greater contralateral loss of pain and temperature sensation.

c. Affected patients have an excellent prognosis and usually will ambulate.

4. Mixed syndrome

a. Mixed syndrome is characterized by a diffuse involvement of the entire spinal cord.

b. Affected patients have a good prognosis for recovery.

c. As with all incomplete spinal cord injury syndromes, early motor recovery is the best prognostic indicator.

E. General management strategies

1. Prevention of contractures and maintaining range of motion should begin immediately following the injury.

2. Maintaining skin integrity is crucial to spinal injury care. Only 4 hours of continuous pressure on the sacrum is sufficient to cause full-thickness skin necrosis.

3. Intermittent catheterization has been the factor most responsible for decreasing urologic problems and for providing an increased life span of patients with spinal cord injuries.

F. Complications

1. Autonomic dysreflexia

a. Splanchnic outflow conveying sympathetic fibers to the lower body exits at the T8 region.

b. Patients with lesions above T8 are prone to autonomic dysreflexia.

c. Signs and symptoms include episodes of hypertension that may be heralded by dizziness, sweating, and headaches.

2. Heterotopic ossification (HO)

a. HO occurs between the muscles and joint capsule in 20% of patients with spinal cord injury, with a higher incidence in 20- to 30-year-olds.

b. HO is more common in cervical and thoracic-level injuries than in lumbar injuries.

c. A higher incidence of HO is seen in patients with complete lesions.

d. HO is most common at the hip, but it can occur at the knee.

e. If the functional range of motion of a joint is limited, the HO should be surgically excised.

G. Management of tetraplegia

1. C4 level function

a. The key muscles are the diaphragm and the trapezius and neck muscles.

b. Head control is present.

c. With a functioning diaphragm, long-term ventilatory support is generally not needed.

d. Tracheostomy and mechanical ventilatory assistance may be required initially.

2. C5 level function

a. Key muscles are the deltoid and biceps, which are used for shoulder abduction and elbow flexion.

b. Surgical goals are to provide active elbow and wrist extension and to restore the ability to pinch the thumb against the index finger.

c. Transferring the posterior deltoid to the triceps muscle provides active elbow extension.

d. Transferring the brachioradialis to the extensor carpi radialis brevis provides active wrist extension.

e. Attaching the flexor pollicis longus tendon to the distal radius and fusing the interphalangeal joint of the thumb provides for key pinch by tenodesis when the wrist is extended.

3. C6 level function

a. Key muscles are the wrist extensors, which enable the patient to manually propel a wheelchair, transfer from one position to another, and even live independently.

b. Surgical goals are to restore lateral pinch and active grasp.

c. Lateral pinch can be restored either by tenodesis of the thumb flexor or by transfer of the brachioradialis to the flexor pollicis longus.

d. Active grasp can be restored by transfer of the pronator teres to the flexor digitorum profundus.

4. C7 level function

a. The key muscle is the triceps.

b. All patients with intact triceps function should be able to transfer and live independently, if no other complications are present.

c. Surgical goals are active thumb flexion for pinch, active finger flexion for grasp, and hand opening by extensor tenodesis.

d. Transfer of the brachioradialis to the flexor pollicis longus provides active pinch.

e. Transfer of the pronator teres to the flexor digitorum profundus allows for active finger flexion and grasp.

f. If the finger extensors are weak, tenodesis of these tendons to the radius provides hand opening with wrist flexion.

5. C8 level function

a. Key muscles are the finger and thumb flexors, which enable a gross grasp.

b. A functioning flexor pollicis longus enables lateral pinch between the thumb and the side of the index finger.

c. Intrinsic muscle function is lacking, and clawing of the fingers usually is present.

d. Capsulodesis of the metacarpophalangeal joints corrects clawing and improves hand function.

e. Active intrinsic function can be achieved by splitting the superficial finger flexor tendon of the ring finger into four slips and transferring these tendons to the lumbrical insertions of each finger.

II. Stroke and Traumatic Brain Injury

A. Demographics

1. The annual incidence of stroke (cerebrovascular accident, or CVA) in the United States is 1 in 1,000.

a. Cerebral thrombosis causes nearly 75% of cases.

b. More than half of stroke victims survive; of those, 50% have hemiplegia.

2. In the United States, 410,000 new cases of traumatic brain injury can be expected each year.

a. Injury resulting from multiple traumatic injuries is twice as common in men as in women.

b. Most commonly, 15- to 24-year-olds are affected.

c. Half of all traumatic brain injuries result from motor vehicle accidents.

B. Management during neurologic recovery

1. Spasticity must be managed aggressively to prevent permanent deformities and joint contractures.

2. Spasmolytic drugs such as baclofen can be administered either orally or intrathecally.

3. Dantrolene is the drug of choice for treating clonus.

4. Casting and splinting have been shown to temporarily reduce muscle tone and are used to correct contractures. Dynamic splints must be monitored closely for skin effects.

5. Botulinum toxin injections into the spastic muscle provide a focal but temporary decrease in muscle tone.

C. Definitive management

1. Most motor recovery occurs within 6 months of onset in both types of patients.

2. Surgery can be considered to correct residual limb deformities at this time.

3. Surgical lengthening of musculotendinous units permanently decreases muscle tone and spasticity.

III. Lower Limb Deformities

A. Limb scissoring

1. Limb scissoring is a common problem caused by overactive hip adductor muscles.

2. It results in an extremely narrow base of support while standing and causes balance problems.

3. Surgical treatment options

a. If there is no fixed contracture of the hip adductors, transection of the anterior branches of the obturator nerve denervates the adductors, which allows the patient to stand with a broader base of support.

b. If there is a fixed hip contracture, surgical release of the adductor muscles is indicated.

B. Stiff-knee gait

1. Characteristics—Inability to flex the knee during swing phase, unrestricted passive knee motion, and a limb that appears to be functionally longer, but no difficulty sitting.

2. Inappropriate activity in the rectus femoris from preswing through terminal swing blocks knee flexion.

3. Abnormal activity is also common in the vastus intermedius, vastus medialis, and vastus lateralis muscles.

4. Circumduction of the involved limb, hiking of the pelvis, or contralateral limb vaulting may occur as compensatory maneuvers.

5. Surgical treatment options

a. Transfer of the rectus femoris to the gracilis tendon not only removes it as a deforming muscle force but also converts the rectus into a corrective flexion force.

b. When any of the vasti muscles are involved, they can be selectively lengthened at their myotendinous junction.

C. Hip and knee flexion deformity

1. Hip and knee flexion occur in concert and result in a crouched posture, which increases the physical demand on the quadriceps and hip extensor muscles, which must continually fire to hold the patient upright.

2. Surgical treatment options

a. Simultaneous surgical correction of the hip and knee flexion deformities is preferred.

b. The hip is approached through a medial incision, and the adductor longus and pectineus muscles are released.

c. The iliopsoas is recessed from the lesser trochanter.

d. Hamstring tenotomy eliminates the deformity, generally resulting in a 50% correction of the contracture at the time of surgery.

3. The residual joint contracture is then corrected by physical therapy or serial casting.

D. Equinus or equinovarus foot deformity

1. Surgical correction of an equinus deformity is achieved with Achilles tendon lengthening or a Strayer procedure.

2. Surgical correction of a claw toe deformity is achieved with release of the flexor digitorum longus and brevis tendons at the base of each toe. Transfer of the flexor digitorum longus tendon to the calcaneus offers additional support to the weakened calf muscles.

3. Surgical correction of a varus deformity

a. The tibialis anterior, tibialis posterior, and extensor hallucis longus are potentially responsible for the deformity.

b. Tendon transfers are indicated to rebalance the foot (**Figure 1**).

i. A split anterior tibial tendon transfer diverts the inverting deforming force of the tibialis anterior to a corrective force. In this procedure, half of the tendon is transferred laterally to the cuboid.

ii. When the extensor hallucis longus muscle is overactive, it can be transferred to the dorsum of the foot.

iii. Lengthening of the tibialis posterior is indicated when this muscle exhibits increased activity.

c. After healing, 70% of patients can walk without an orthosis.

IV. Upper Limb Deformities

A. Shoulder deformities

1. Shoulder adduction and internal rotation deformities

a. These deformities are caused by spasticity and

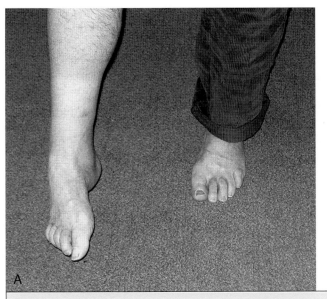 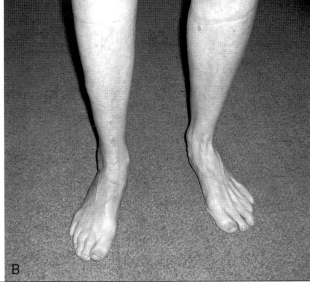

Figure 1 Equinovarus is the most common musculoskeletal deformity seen following a stroke or traumatic brain injury. **A,** Patient with an equinovarus foot deformity after a stroke. **B,** Same patient after surgery to correct the equinovarus foot deformity.

myostatic contracture of four muscles: the pectoralis major, the subscapularis, the latissimus dorsi, and the teres major.

b. Muscle contractures in a nonfunctional arm are surgically released through an anterior deltopectoral incision.

c. The subscapularis muscle can be released without violating the glenohumeral joint capsule.

2. Limited shoulder flexion

a. Antagonistic activity of the latissimus dorsi, teres major, and long head of the triceps muscles can obscure the fact that there is volitional control of the agonist muscles, the shoulder flexors.

b. Diminishing the increased muscle activity by fractional lengthening of the antagonist muscles can improve shoulder flexion.

B. Elbow flexion deformities

1. The patient has active movement.

a. Myotendinous lengthening of the spastic elbow flexors is indicated to correct the flexion deformity and improve function.

b. Surgical technique

i. The long and short biceps are lengthened proximally in the arm.

ii. The brachialis is lengthened at the elbow.

iii. The brachioradialis is lengthened in the forearm.

c. The patient can begin active motion immediately after surgery.

2. The patient has no active movement and a fixed elbow flexion contracture.

a. For fixed contracture in a nonfunctional arm, release of the contracted muscles is done through a lateral incision.

b. The brachioradialis muscle and biceps tendon are transected.

c. The brachialis muscle is released.

C. Wrist and finger flexion deformities in a functional hand

1. With active movement, myotendinous lengthening of the spastic wrist and finger flexors is indicated in the forearm.

2. The pronator teres and pronator quadratus also can be lengthened.

D. Clenched-fist deformity in a nonfunctional hand (**Figure 2**)

1. Characteristics—Palmar skin breakdown and hygiene problems, recurrent infections of the nail beds, and compression of the median nerve when combined with a wrist flexion contracture.

2. Adequate flexor tendon lengthening to correct the deformity cannot be attained by fractional or myotendinous lengthening without causing discontinuity at the musculotendinous junction.

3. Recommended surgical technique is a superficialis-to-profundus tendon transfer.

2: General Knowledge

a. This technique provides sufficient flexor tendon lengthening and preserves a passive tether to prevent a hyperextension deformity.

b. The wrist deformity is corrected by release of the wrist flexors.

c. Wrist arthrodesis maintains the hand in a neutral position and eliminates the need for a permanent splint.

d. Because intrinsic muscle spasticity occurs in conjunction with severe spasticity of the extrinsic flexors, a neurectomy of the motor branches of the ulnar nerve in the Guyon canal also is routinely performed to prevent postoperative development of intrinsic deformities.

e. A neurectomy of the recurrent median nerve is also routinely performed to prevent a thumb-in-palm deformity.

V. Heterotopic Ossification

A. Characteristics

1. HO is characterized by formation of bone in nonskeletal tissue, usually between the muscle and joint capsule (**Figure 3**).

2. HO usually develops within 2 months after a neurologic injury such as traumatic brain or spinal cord injuries.

   a. In patients with spinal cord injuries, the hip is the site most commonly involved, followed by the knee, elbow, and (least commonly) the shoulder.

   b. In patients with traumatic brain injury, the hip is most often affected, followed by the elbow, shoulder, and knee.

3. HO is generally visible on plain radiographs.

4. The etiology of HO is unknown, but a genetic predisposition is suspected.

B. Risk factors

1. Trauma greatly increases the incidence of HO in brain-injured patients.

2. Patients with massive HO usually have severe

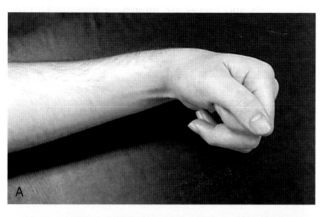
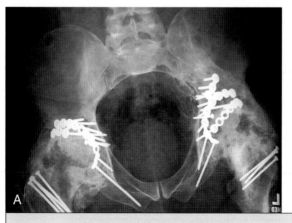

Figure 2   **A**, Patient with a clenched-fist deformity and no active function of the hand. **B**, Same patient after a superficialis-to-profundus transfer and wrist arthrodesis to correct the clenched-fist deformity.

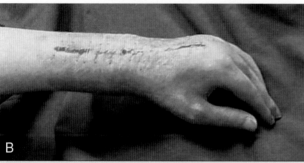
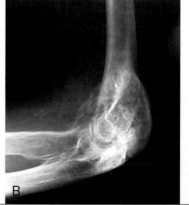
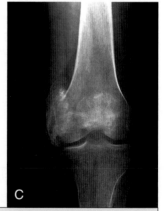

Figure 3   **A**, Radiograph of the pelvis showing HO of both hips associated with trauma in a brain-injured patient. **B**, Radiograph of an elbow with posterior HO. **C**, Radiograph demonstrating HO of the medial knee in a brain-injured patient.

spasticity and a higher recurrence rate following resection.

3. The completeness of a spinal cord lesion seems to be more predictive than the level of injury, although cervical and thoracic lesions seem to produce HO more often than lumbar lesions.

4. Soft-tissue damage, as occurs with decubitus ulcers, can be a predisposing factor.

5. Prolonged coma and young patient age (20 to 30 years) appear to increase the likelihood of HO formation.

C. Complications

1. Significant functional impairment, which can lead to a decline in a patient's ability to perform activities of daily living

2. Decreased joint range of motion, which increases the likelihood of pathologic fractures of osteoporotic bone during transfers or patient positioning and can lead to peripheral neuropathy by impinging adjacent nervous structures

3. Soft-tissue contractures of the surrounding skin, muscles, ligaments, and neurovascular bundles, which can contribute to the formation of decubitus ulcers

4. Skin maceration, often resulting in significant hygiene problems

5. Complex regional pain syndrome, which is more prevalent in patients with HO

6. Joint ankylosis, which frequently occurs as a result of HO

D. Treatment

1. Early treatment and prophylaxis

   a. Although there is no proven prophylaxis, bisphosphonates and nonsteroidal anti-inflammatory drugs (NSAIDs) are the mainstays of early treatment.

   b. Radiation is thought to inhibit HO formation by disrupting the process whereby mesenchymal cells differentiate into osteoblasts; however, no data support this.

   c. Maintaining joint motion by treating spasticity and gentle physical therapy is the goal of early treatment.

2. Surgical treatment

   a. Surgical excision is indicated when the HO interferes with function.

   b. Preoperative assessment and planning are essential.

      i. Radiographs—The maturity of HO can be assessed by the appearance of a bony cortex

on radiographs. Judet views of the pelvis are useful to assess hip HO. Limited mobility and ability to position the patient makes radiographic studies difficult.

      ii. CT is used in planning the surgical approach, with three-dimensional reconstructions particularly helpful in complex cases.

3. Surgical techniques

   a. Wide exposure and identification of major vessels and nerves are important because HO often encases neurovascular tissues and can displace and/or compress adjacent tissues, which distort the normal anatomy.

   b. Meticulous hemostasis and elimination of dead space decrease the risk of infection.

4. Complications

   a. Hematoma and infection

   b. Fractures of osteoporotic bone, either during surgery or later with physical therapy

   c. Intraoperative bleeding requiring transfusion

   d. Recurrence

   e. Late development of osteonecrosis in patients who require extensive dissection

5. Postoperative management

   a. Early gentle joint mobilization

   b. Passive limb positioning for function

   c. Prophylaxis for recurrence with bisphosphonates, NSAIDs, radiation, or a combination of these treatments. NSAIDs must be used with caution because of the risk of increased bleeding and hematoma formation.

VI. Physical Therapy and Occupational Therapy

A. Muscle weakness and physiologic deconditioning

1. Prolonged immobilization of extremities, bed rest, and inactivity lead to pronounced muscle wasting and physiologic deconditioning in a short period of time.

2. Disabled patients expend more energy than normal individuals in performing activities of daily living.

B. Aerobic metabolism

1. During sustained exercise, metabolism is mainly aerobic.

2. The principal fuels for aerobic metabolism are carbohydrates and fats.

3. In aerobic oxidation, substrates are oxidized

2: General Knowledge

through a series of enzymatic reactions that lead to the production of adenosine triphosphate (ATP) for muscular contraction.

4. A physical conditioning program can increase aerobic capacity by improving cardiac output, increasing hemoglobin levels, enhancing the capacity of cells to extract oxygen from the blood, and increasing the muscle mass by hypertrophy.

C. Areas of concern

1. Patient positioning

2. Mobility

3. Performance of activities of daily living

4. Making it possible for bedridden patients to sit can significantly improve quality of life and greatly enhance the opportunities to interact with other people.

5. For some patients, casts or orthotic devices may be required to maintain desired limb positions.

6. Aggressive joint motion exercises are necessary to prevent contractures.

D. Factors influencing a patient's ability to walk

1. Limb stability

2. Motor control

3. Good balance reactions

4. Adequate proprioception

E. Equipment and devices to aid in movement (eg, canes, walkers, wheelchairs)

1. These aids should always be of the least complex design to accomplish the goal.

2. They should be selected based on the patient's cognitive and physical levels of function.

F. Developing appropriate exercises and activities

1. Considerations include joint range of motion, muscle tone, motor control, and cognitive function of the patient.

2. Cognitive function considerations

a. Even confused and agitated patients may respond to simple, familiar functional activities such as face washing and teeth brushing.

b. Patients with higher cognitive function should be encouraged to carry out hygiene, grooming, dressing, and feeding activities.

G. Physical therapy prescription

1. Components include the diagnosis, functional deficits to be addressed, treatment goals, and any precautions or restrictions.

2. The prescription also should specify whether modalities can be used, the need for orthoses, and the weight-bearing capacity of the arm or leg.

3. The frequency and duration of the therapy also should be specified.

Top Testing Facts

1. A diagnosis of a complete spinal cord injury cannot be made until spinal shock has resolved as evidenced by return of the bulbocavernosus reflex.

2. Neurologic recovery after spinal cord injury is assessed by determining the change in AMS (the sum of strength grades for each of the 10 key muscles tested bilaterally that represent neurologic segments from C5 to T1 and L2 to S1) between successive neurologic examinations. (Review C4 through C7 levels of function.)

3. Management of the spinal cord–injured patient includes prevention of contractures and maintaining range of motion, maintaining skin integrity, and intermittent catheterization.

4. The incidence of HO is approximately 20% in patients with spinal cord injury. Surgical excision is indicated when the HO interferes with function.

5. A crouched posture increases the physical demand on the quadriceps and hip extensor muscles, which must

continually fire to hold the patient upright. Simultaneous surgical correction of the hip and knee flexion deformities is the most desirable treatment.

6. Surgical correction of claw toe deformity requires release of the flexor digitorum longus and brevis tendons at the base of each toe.

7. Surgical correction of an equinovarus deformity is achieved with tendon transfers to rebalance the foot, including a split anterior tibial tendon transfer.

8. Wrist and finger flexion deformities in a functional hand are treated with myotendinous lengthenings.

9. The recommended surgical treatment for clenched-fist deformity in a nonfunctional hand is a superficialis-to-profundus tendon transfer.

10. Factors that influence a patient's ability to walk include limb stability, motor control, balance reactions, and adequate proprioception.

Bibliography

Ditunno JF Jr, Apple DF, Burns AS, et al: A view of the future Model Spinal Cord Injury System through the prism of past achievements and current challenges. *J Spinal Cord Med* 2003;26:110-115.

Garland DE: A clinical perspective on common forms of acquired heterotopic ossification. *Clin Orthop Relat Res* 1991; 263:13-29.

Keenan MA: Orthopaedic management of upper extremity dysfunction following stroke or brain injury, in Green DP, Hotchkiss RN, Pederson WC (eds): *Operative Hand Surgery*, ed 5. New York, NY, Churchill Livingstone, 2005, pp 287-324.

Kaplan FS, Glaser DL, Hebela N, Shore EM: Heterotopic ossification. *J Am Acad Orthop Surg* 2004;12:116-125.

Kirshblum SC, Priebe MM, Ho CH, Scelza WM, Chiodo AE, Wuermser LA: Spinal cord injury medicine 3: Rehabilitation phase after acute spinal cord injury. *Arch Phys Med Rehabil* 2007;88(3, suppl 1)S62-S70.

Mehta S, Keenan MA: Rehabilitation, in Skinner HB (ed): *Current Diagnosis and Treatment in Orthopedics*, ed 4. New York, NY, Lange Medical Books/McGraw-Hill, 2006, pp 671-727.

2: General Knowledge

Chapter 23

Statistics: Practical Applications for Orthopaedics

Mohit Bhandari, MD, MSc, FRCSC

I. Presentation of Study Results

A. Terminology

1. Absolute risk increase—The difference in the absolute risk (percentage or proportion of patients with an outcome) between exposed and unexposed, or experimental and control group patients; typically used with regard to harmful exposure.

2. Absolute risk reduction—The difference in the absolute risk (percentage or proportion of patients with an outcome) between exposed (experimental event rate) and unexposed (control event rate); used only with regard to a beneficial exposure or intervention.

3. Bayesian analysis—An analysis that starts with a particular probability of an event (the prior probability) and incorporates new information to generate a revised probability (a posterior probability).

4. Blind (or blinded or masked)—Type of study/assessment in which the participant of interest is unaware of whether patients have been assigned to the experimental group or the control group. Patients, clinicians, those monitoring outcomes, judicial assessors of outcomes, data analysts, and those writing the paper all can be blinded or masked. To avoid confusion, the term *masked* is preferred in studies in which vision loss of patients is an outcome of interest.

5. Dichotomous outcome—A yes or no outcome (ie, an outcome that either happens or does not happen), such as reoperation, infection, or death.

6. Dichotomous variable—A variable that can take one of two values, such as male or female, dead or alive, infection present or not present.

7. Effect size—The difference in outcome between the intervention group and the control group divided by some measure of the variability, typically the standard deviation.

8. Hawthorne effect—Human behavior that is changed when participants are aware that their behavior is being observed. In a therapeutic study, the Hawthorne effect might affect results such that the treatment is deemed effective when it actually is ineffective. In a diagnostic study, the Hawthorne effect might be responsible if the patient does not have the target condition but the test suggests the patient does.

9. Intention-to-treat principle, or intention-to-treat analysis—Analyzing patient outcomes based on the group into which they were randomized, regardless of whether the patient actually received the planned intervention. This type of analysis preserves the power of randomization so that important unknown factors that influence outcome are likely to be distributed equally in each comparison group.

10. Meta-analysis—An overview that incorporates a quantitative strategy for combining the results of multiple studies into a single pooled or summary estimate.

11. Null hypothesis—In the hypothesis-testing framework, a null hypothesis is the starting hypothesis the statistical test is designed to consider and, possibly, reject.

12. Number needed to harm—The number of patients who would need to be treated over a specific period of time before one adverse side effect of the treatment would be expected to occur. The number needed to harm is the inverse of the absolute risk increase.

13. Number needed to treat—The number of patients who would need to be treated over a specific period of time to prevent one bad outcome. When discussing number needed to treat, it is important to specify the treatment, its duration, and the bad outcome being prevented. The number needed to treat is the inverse of the absolute risk reduction.

14. Odds—The ratio of probability of occurrence to probability of nonoccurrence of an event.

	Infection			No Infection
Treatment Group	10	A	B	90
Control Group	50	C	D	50

Treatment Event Rate (TER): A/A+B = 10/100 = 10%
  The incidence of infection in the treatment group

Control event rate (CER): C/(C+D) = 50/100 = 50%
  The CER is the incidence of infection in the
  control group.

Relative risk (RR): TER/CER = 10/50 = 0.2
  The RR is the relative risk of infection in the
  treatment group relative to the control group.

Relative risk reduction (RRR): 1 – RR = 1 – 0.2 = 0.8, or 80%
  An RRR of 80% means that treatment reduces
  the risk of infection by 80% compared to controls.

Absolute risk reduction (ARR): CER – TER = 50% – 10% = 40%
  The ARR is the actual numerical difference in infection
  rates between treatment and controls.

Number needed to treat (NNT): 1/ARR = 1/0.40 = 2.5
  An NNT of 2.5 means that for every 2.5 patients who
  receive the treatment, 1 infection can be prevented.

Odds ratio (OR): AD/BC = (10)(50)/(90)(50) = 500/4500 = 0.11
  An OR of 0.11 means that the odds of infection in
  treatment compared to controls is 0.11.

Figure 1 Presentation of study results. A hypothetical example of a study evaluating infection rates in 200 patients with a treatment and control group is presented. A 2 x 2 table is constructed, and multiple approaches to describing the results are presented. *(Reproduced with permission from Bhandari M, Devereaux PJ, Swiontkowski M, et al: Internal fixation compared with arthroplasty for displaced fractures of the femoral neck. J Bone Joint Surg Am 2003;85:1673-1681.)*

15. Odds ratio—The ratio of the odds of an event occurring in an exposed group to the odds of the same event occurring in a group that is not exposed.

16. Relative risk—The ratio of the risk of an event occurring among an exposed population to the risk of it occurring among the unexposed.

17. Relative risk reduction—An estimate of the proportion of baseline risk that is removed by the therapy; calculated by dividing the absolute risk reduction by the absolute risk in the control group.

18. Reliability—Refers to consistency or reproducibility of data.

19. Treatment effect—The results of comparative clinical studies can be expressed using various treatment effect measures. Examples are absolute risk reduction, relative risk reduction, odds ratio, number needed to treat, and effect size. The appropriate measure to use to express a treatment effect and the appropriate calculation method to use—whether probabilities, means, or medians—depends on the type of outcome variable used to measure health outcomes. For example, relative risk reduction is used for dichotomous variables, whereas effect sizes are normally used for continuous variables.

20. Continuous variable—A variable with a potentially infinite number of possible values. Examples include range of motion, blood pressure.

21. Categorical variable—A variable with possible values in several different categories. An example would be types of fractures.

B. **Figure 1** illustrates a typical presentation of study results.

C. Bias in research

1. Definition—Bias is a systematic tendency to produce an outcome that differs from the underlying truth.

   a. Channeling effect, or channeling bias—The tendency of clinicians to prescribe treatment based on a patient's prognosis. As a result of the behavior, comparisons between treated and untreated patients will yield a biased estimate of treatment effect.

   b. Data completeness bias—May occur when an information system (eg, a hospital database) is used to enter data directly for the treatment group but manual data entry is used for the control group.

   c. Detection bias, or surveillance bias—The tendency to look more carefully for an outcome in one of two or more groups being compared.

   d. Incorporation bias—When investigators study a diagnostic test that incorporates features of the target outcome.

   e. Interviewer bias—Greater probing or any subjectivity that affects how the interview is conducted by an interviewer in one of two or more groups being compared.

   f. Publication bias—When the publication of research results depends on the direction of the study results and whether they are statistically significant.

   g. Recall bias—When patients who experience an adverse outcome have a different likelihood of recalling an exposure than do the patients who do not have an adverse outcome, independent of the true extent of exposure.

   h. Surveillance bias—See detection bias, above.

i. Verification bias—When the results of a diagnostic test influence whether patients are assigned to a treatment group.

2. Limiting bias—In a clinical research study, bias can be limited by randomization, concealment of treatment allocation, and blinding.

a. Random allocation (randomization)

i. Random allocation is the allocation of individuals to groups by chance, usually by using a table of random numbers. A sample derived by selecting sampling units (eg, individual patients) such that each unit has an independent and fixed (generally equal) chance of selection.

ii. Random allocation should not be confused with systematic allocation (eg, on even and odd days of the month) or allocation at the convenience or discretion of the investigator.

b. Concealment of treatment allocation

i. Allocation is concealed when individuals cannot determine the treatment allocation of the next patient to be enrolled in a clinical trial, such as when remote telephone- or Internet-based randomization systems are used to assign treatment.

ii. Use of even/odd days or hospital chart numbers to allocate patients to a treatment group is not considered concealed allocation.

c. Blinding (see definition in I.A.4).

II. Basic Statistical Concepts

A. A statistician should be consulted when a study or analysis of a study is planned.

B. Hypothesis testing

1. Null hypothesis

a. The investigator starts with a null hypothesis that the statistical test is designed to consider and, possibly, disprove. Typically, the null hypothesis is that there is no difference between treatments being compared. Therefore, the investigator starts with the assumption that the treatments are equally effective and adheres to this position unless data make it untenable.

b. In a randomized trial in which investigators compare an experimental treatment with a placebo control, the null hypothesis can be stated as follows: "The true difference in effect on the outcome of interest between the experimental and control treatments is zero."

C. Errors in hypothesis testing—Any comparative study can have one of four possible outcomes (**Figure 2**).

Results of Study	Truth	
	Difference Exists in Actuality	No Difference Exists in Actuality
Study Shows a Difference	Correct conclusion $(1 - \beta)$	False positive (α, or type I, error)
Study Shows No Difference	False negative (β, or type II, error)	Correct conclusion $(1 - \alpha)$

Figure 2   Errors in hypothesis testing. A 2 x 2 table is used to depict the results of a study comparing two treatments (difference, no difference) and the "truth" (whether or not there is a difference in actuality). Common errors are presented, including type I and II errors. *(Reproduced with permission from Bhandari M, Devereaux PJ, Swiontkowski M, et al: Internal fixation compared with arthroplasty for displaced fractures of the femoral neck. J Bone Joint Surg Am 2003;85: 1673-1681.)*

1. A true positive result (the study correctly identifies a true difference between treatments)

2. A true negative result (the study correctly identifies no difference between treatments)

3. A false-negative result, called a type II (β) error (the study incorrectly concludes no difference between treatments when a difference really exists). By convention, the error rate is set at 0.20 (20% false-negative rate). Study power (see section D, below) is derived from the $1 - \beta$ error rate ($1 - 0.2 = 0.80$, or 80%).

4. A false-positive result, called a type I (α) error (the study incorrectly concludes a difference between treatments exists when the effects are really due to chance). By convention, most studies in orthopaedics adopt an α-error rate of 0.05. Thus, investigators can expect a false-positive error about 5% of the time.

D. Study power—The ability of a study to detect the difference between two interventions if one in fact exists. The power of a statistical test is typically a function of the magnitude of the treatment effect, the designated type I (α) and type II (β) error rates, and the sample size n.

E. *P* value—The *P* value is defined as the probability, under the assumption of no difference (null hypothesis), of obtaining a result equal to or more extreme than what was actually observed if the experiment were repeated over and over. The setting of the *P*-value threshold for significance has been set arbitrarily at 0.05 by convention. The meaning of a statistically significant result, therefore, is one that is sufficiently unlikely to be due to chance alone that the investigator is ready to reject the null hypothesis.

F. Confidence interval—Range defined by two values within which it is probable (to a specified percent-

Table 1

Common Statistical Tests

		Data Type and Distribution		
		Categorical	Ordered Categorical or Continuous and Non-normal	Continuous and Normal
Two samples	Different individuals	χ^2 test Fisher exact test	Mann-Whitney test Wilcoxon rank sum test	Unpaired *t*-test
	Related or matched samples	McNemar test	Wilcoxon signed rank test	Paired *t*-test
Three or more samples	Different individuals	χ^2 test Fisher exact test	Kruskal-Wallis test	ANOVA
	Related samples	Cochran *Q* test	Friedman test	Repeated measures ANOVA

ANOVA = analysis of variance
(Reproduced with permission from Bhandari M, Devereaux PJ, Swiontkowski M, et al: Internal fixation compared with arthroplasty for displaced fractures of the femoral neck. J Bone Joint Surg Am *2003;85:1673-1681.)*

age) that the true value lies for the whole population of patients from whom the study patients were selected. Various percentages can be used, but by convention, the 95% confidence interval is typically reported in clinical research.

III. Basic Statistical Inference

A. Normal distribution (**Table 1**)

1. Definition—A normal distribution is a distribution of continuous data that forms a bell-shaped curve; ie, one with many values near the mean and progressively fewer values toward the extremes.

2. Several statistical tests assume a normal distribution. If a sample is not normally distributed, a separate set of statistical tests should be applied. These tests are referred to as nonparametric tests because they do not rely on parameters such as the mean and standard deviation.

B. Descriptive statistics

1. Measures of central tendency

a. Mean—The sample mean is equal to the sum of the measurements divided by the number of observations.

b. Median—The median of a set of measurements is the number that falls in the middle.

c. Mode—The mode is the most frequently occurring number in a set of measurements.

d. Use of measures of central tendency

i. Continuous variables (such as blood pressure or body weight) can be summarized with a mean if the data is normally distributed.

ii. If the data are not normally distributed, the median may be a better summary statistic.

iii. Categorical variables (eg, pain grade [0,1, 2,3,4,5]) can be summarized with a median.

2. Measures of spread

a. Standard deviation—Derived from the square root of the sample variance. The variance is calculated as the average of the squares of the deviations of the measurements about their mean.

b. Range—Reflects the smallest and largest reported values.

C. Comparing means

1. Comparing two means

a. When two independent samples of normally distributed continuous data are compared, the *t*-test (often called Student, leading to the common attribution Student's *t*-test) is used.

b. When the data are non-normally distributed, a nonparametric test such as the Mann-Whitney test or Wilcoxon rank sum test can be used. When the means are paired, such as left and right knees, a paired *t*-test is most appropriate. The nonparametric correlate of this test is the Wilcoxon signed rank test.

2. Comparing three or more means—When three or more different means are compared (eg, hospital stay among patients treated for tibial fracture with plate fixation, intramedullary nail, and external fixation), the test of choice is single-factor analysis of variance.

D. Comparing proportions

1. Independent proportions—The chi-square (χ^2) test is a simple method of comparing two proportions, such as a difference in infection rates (%)

between two groups. A Yates correction factor is sometimes used to account for small sample sizes, but when measured values are very small (eg, less than 5 events in any of the treatment or control groups), the χ^2 test is unreliable and the Fisher exact test is the test of choice.

2. Paired proportions—When proportions are paired (eg, before and after study on the same patients), a McNemar test is used to examine differences between groups.

E. Regression and correlation

1. Regression analysis—Used to predict (or estimate) the association between a response variable (dependent variable) and a series of known explanatory (independent) variables.

   a. Simple regression—When a single independent variable is used.

   b. Multiple regression—When multiple independent variables are used.

   c. Logistic regression—When the response variable is dichotomous (yes or no; infection present or not).

   d. Cox proportional hazards regression—Used in survival analysis to assess the relationship between two or more variables and a single dependent variable (the time to an event).

2. Correlation—The strength of the relationship between two variables (eg, age versus hospital stay in patients with ankle fractures) can be summarized in a single number, the correlation coefficient, denoted by the letter r. The correlation coefficient can range from –1.0 to 1.0.

   a. A correlation coefficient of –1.0 represents the strongest possible negative relationship, in which the person who scores the highest on one variable scores the lowest on the other variable.

   b. A correlation coefficient of 1.0 represents the strongest possible positive relationship.

   c. A correlation coefficient of 0 denotes no relationship between the two variables.

   d. The Pearson correlation r is used to assess the relationship between two normally distributed continuous variables. If one of the variables is not normally distributed, the Spearman correlation is the better option.

F. Survival analysis

1. Time-to-event analysis involves estimating the probability that an event will occur at various time points.

2. Survival analysis estimates the probability of survival as a function of time from a discrete start point (time of injury, time of operation).

3. Survival curves, also called Kaplan-Meier curves, are often used to report the survival of one or more groups of patients over time.

IV. Determining Sample Size for a Comparative Study

A. Difference in means—The anticipated sample size for this continuous outcome measure is determined by the following equation:

$$N = 2 \left\{ \frac{(Z\alpha + Z\beta)\sigma}{\delta} \right\}^2$$

where $Z\alpha$ = type I error , $Z\beta$ = type II error, σ = standard deviation, and δ = mean difference between groups.

B. Difference in proportions—For dichotomous variables, the following sample size calculation is used:

$$N = \left\{ \frac{PA(100 - PA) + PB(100 - PB)}{(PB - PA)^2} \right\} f(\alpha,\beta)$$

where PA, PB = % successes in A and B, and $f(\alpha,\beta)$ = function of type I and II errors.

V. Reliability

A. Test-retest reliability measures the extent to which the same observer rating a subject on multiple occasions achieves similar results. Because time elapses between ratings, the characteristics being rated may also change. For example, the range of motion of a hip may change substantially over a 4-week period.

B. Intra-observer reliability is the same as test-retest reliability except that the characteristics being rated are fixed. Because time is the only factor that varies between administrations, this form of study design will typically yield a higher reliability estimate than test-retest or inter-observer reliability studies.

C. Inter-observer reliability measures the extent to which two or more observers obtain similar scores when rating the same subject. Inter-observer reliability is the broadest and—when error related to observers is highly relevant—the most clinically useful measure of reliability.

1. The κ coefficient, or κ statistic, the most commonly reported statistic in orthopaedic fracture reliability studies, can be thought of as a measure of agreement beyond chance.

2. The κ coefficient has a maximum value of 1.0 (indicating perfect agreement). κ = 0.0 indicates no agreement beyond chance; negative values indicate agreement worse than chance.

2: General Knowledge

3. The κ coefficient can be used when data are categorical (categories of answers such as definitely healed, possibly healed, or not healed) or binary (a yes or no answer such as infection or no infection).

D. Intraclass correlation coefficients (ICCs) are a set of related measures of reliability that yield a value that is closest to the formal definition of reliability. One ICC measures the proportion of total variability that is due to true between-subject variability. ICCs are used when data are continuous.

VI. Diagnostic Tests

A. Definition of terms

1. Specificity—The proportion of individuals who are truly free of a designated disorder who are so identified by the test.

2. Sensitivity—The proportion of individuals who truly have a designated disorder who are so identified by the test.

3. Positive predictive value—The proportion of individuals with a positive test who have the disease.

4. Negative predictive value—The proportion of individuals with a negative test who are free of the disease.

5. Likelihood ratios—For a screening or diagnostic test (including clinical signs or symptoms), the likelihood ratio expresses the relative likelihood that a given test result would be expected in a patient with (as opposed to one without) a disorder of interest.

6. Accuracy—For a screening or diagnostic test, its accuracy is its overall ability to identify patients

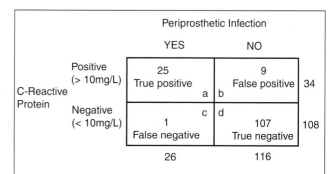

Likelihood ratio = (a/a + c)/(b/b + d) = sensitivity/(1 − specificity)
(for positive test) = (25/26)/(9/116) = 0.96/0.077 = 12.5

Likelihood ratio = (c/a + c)/(d/b + d) = (1 −t sensitivity/specificity)
(for negative test) = (1/26)/(107/116) = 0.038/0.92 = 0.041

Sensitivity: a/(a + c) = 25/26 = 96%
Specificity: d/(b + d) = 107/116 = 92%
Positive predictive value: a/(a + b) = 25/34 = 74%
Negative predictive value: d/(c + d) = 107/108 = 99%
Accuracy: a + d/(a + b + c + d) = 132/142 = 93%
Prevalence: (a + c)/(a + b + c +d) = 26/142 = 18%

Figure 3 Diagnostic tests. A 2 x 2 table depicts C-reactive protein thresholds for diagnosing infection. Several test characteristics are presented, including sensitivity, specificity, and likelihood ratios. (*Reproduced with permission from Bhandari M, Devereaux PJ, Swiontkowski M, et al: Internal fixation compared with arthroplasty for displaced fractures of the femoral neck. J Bone Joint Surg Am 2003;85:1673-1681.*)

with disease (true positives) and without disease (true negatives) in the study population.

B. **Figure 3** illustrates the application of these concepts to C-reactive protein thresholds.

Top Testing Facts

1. Bias in clinical research is best defined as a systematic deviation from the truth.

2. Randomization, concealment of allocation, and blinding are key methodologic principles to limit bias in clinical research.

3. Type II (β) error occurs when a study concludes there is no difference between treatments when in fact a difference really exists.

4. The power of a study is its ability to find a difference between treatments when a true difference exists.

5. The P value is defined as the probability, under the assumption of no difference (null hypothesis), of obtaining a result equal to or more extreme than what was actually observed.

6. A 95% confidence interval is the interval within which the true estimate of effect lies 95% of the time.

7. Two means can be compared with a Student's *t*-test.

8. Two proportions can be compared statistically with a chi-square (χ^2) test.

9. The specificity of a test is the proportion of individuals who are free of the disorder who are so identified by the test.

10. The sensitivity of a test is the proportion of individuals who have a designated disorder who are so identified by the test.

Bibliography

Bhandari M, Guyatt GH, Montori V, Swiontkowski MF: User's Guide to the Orthopaedic Literature IV: How to use an article about a diagnostic test. *J Bone Joint Surg Am* 2003;85: 1133-1140.

Bhandari M, Guyatt GH, Swiontkowski MF: User's guide to the orthopaedic literature I: How to use an article about a surgical therapy. *J Bone Joint Surg Am* 2001;83:916-927.

Dorrey F, Swiontkowski MF: Statistical tests: What they tell us and what they don't. *Ad Orthop Surg* 1997;21:81-85.

Griffin D, Audige L: Common statistical methods in orthopaedic clinical studies. *Clin Orthop Relat Res* 2003;413:70-79.

Guyatt GH, Jaeschke R, Heddle N, Cook DJ, Shannon H, Walter SD: Basic statistics for clinicians: Hypothesis testing. *Can Med Assoc J* 1995;152:27-32.

Guyatt GH, Jaeschke R, Heddle N, Cook DJ, Shannon H, Walter SD: Basic statistics for clinicians: Interpreting study results and confidence intervals. *Can Med Assoc J* 1995;152: 169-173.

Guyatt GH, Rennie D (eds): *User's Guides to the Medical Literature: A Manual for Evidence-Based Clinical Practice.* Chicago, IL, American Medical Association Press, 2001.

Moher D, Dulberg CS, Wells GA: Statistical power, sample size, and their reporting in randomized controlled trials. *JAMA* 1994;272:122-124.

Chapter 24

Evidence-Based Medicine

Khaled J. Saleh, MD, MSc(Epid), FRCSC   Wendy M. Novicoff, PhD

I. Basics of Evidence-Based Medicine

A. Definition—Evidence-based medicine is the practice of integrating individual clinical expertise with the best available clinical evidence from systematic research to maximize the quality and quantity of life for individual patients.

B. Goal—To achieve the best possible patient management and patient outcomes through the combination of empirical evidence, clinical expertise, and patient values.

C. Steps in evidence-based medicine

1. Formulate an answerable question

2. Track down the best evidence of outcomes available

3. Appraise the evidence

4. Apply the evidence (integrate with clinical expertise)

5. Evaluate the effectiveness and efficiency of the process

D. Assessing evidence

1. Not restricted to randomized trials and meta-analyses

2. Cluster evidence of similar validity and provide indications of similarity across the different sorts of questions (prognosis, diagnosis, etc)

3. Grade is matched directly to the level of evidence and quality of study

II. Types of Studies

A. Therapeutic studies—Investigate the results of treatment.

Khaled J. Saleh, MD, or the department with which he is affiliated has received research or institutional support from Stryker and Smith & Nephew, has received royalties from Smith & Nephew, and is a consultant for or an employee of Stryker and Smith & Nephew.

1. Level I

a. High-quality randomized controlled trial with statistically significant difference or no statistically significant difference but narrow confidence interval (CI)

b. Systematic review of level I randomized controlled trials (in which study results are homogeneous)

2. Level II

a. Lesser-quality randomized controlled trial (eg, <80% follow-up, no blinding, or improper randomization)

b. Prospective comparative study

c. Systematic review of level II studies or level I studies with inconsistent results

3. Level III

a. Case-control study

b. Retrospective comparative study

c. Systematic review of level III studies

4. Level IV—Case series or poor-quality cohort and case-control studies.

5. Level V—Expert opinion.

B. Prognostic studies—Investigate the effect of a patient characteristic on the outcome of disease.

1. Level I

a. High-quality prospective study (eg, all patients enrolled at the same point in their disease with ≥80% follow-up)

b. Systematic review of level I studies

2. Level II

a. Retrospective study

b. Untreated controls from a randomized controlled trial

c. Lesser quality prospective study (eg, patients enrolled at different points in their disease or < 80% follow-up)

d. Systematic review of level II studies

3. Level III—Case-control study.

4. Level IV—Case series.

5. Level V—Expert opinion.

C. Diagnostic studies—investigating a diagnostic test

1. Level I

a. Testing of previously developed diagnostic criteria in series of consecutive patients (with universally applied reference gold standard)

b. Systematic review of level I studies

2. Level II

a. Development of diagnostic criteria on basis of consecutive patients (with universally applied reference gold standard)

b. Systematic review of level II studies

3. Level III

a. Study of nonconsecutive patients (without consistently applied reference "gold" standard)

b. Systematic review of level III studies

4. Level IV

a. Case-control study

b. Poor reference standard

5. Level V—Expert opinion.

D. Economic and decision analyses—Developing an economic or decision model.

1. Level I

a. Sensible costs and alternatives; values obtained from many studies; multi-way sensitivity analyses

b. Systematic review of level I studies

2. Level II

a. Sensible costs and alternatives; values obtained from limited studies; audits and chart reviews

b. Systematic review of level II studies

3. Level III

a. Analyses based on limited alternatives and costs; poor estimates

b. Systematic review of level III studies

4. Level IV—No sensitivity analyses.

5. Level V—Expert opinion.

Examples of Study Types in Orthopaedic Surgery

Therapeutic study, evidence level I

Moseley JB, O'Malley K, Peterson NJ, et al: A controlled trial of arthroscopic surgery for osteoarthritis of the knee. *N Engl J Med* 2002;347:81-88.

Therapeutic study, evidence level II

Jaeger M, Maier D, Kern WV, Sudkamp NP: Antibiotics in trauma and orthopedic surgery—A primer of evidence-based recommendations. *Injury* 2006;37 (Suppl 1):S74-S80.

Prognostic study, evidence level II

Leadbetter WB, Ragland PS, Mont MA: The appropriate use of patellofemoral arthroplasty: An analysis of reported indications, contraindications, and failures. *Clin Orthop Relat Res* 2005;436:91-99.

Shervin N, Rubash HE, Katz JN: Orthopaedic procedure volume and patient outcomes: A systematic literature review. *Clin Orthop Relat Res* 2007;457:35-41.

Diagnostic study, evidence level II

Harris MB, Sethi RK: The initial assessment and management of the multiple-trauma patient with an associated spine injury. *Spine* 2006;31 (Suppl 11):S9-S15.

Diagnostic study, evidence level III

Vaccaro AR, Kreidel KO, Pan W, et al: Usefulness of MRI in isolated upper cervical spine fractures in adults. *J Spinal Disord* 1998;11:289-294.

Economic and decision analysis study, evidence level II

Brauer CA, Neumann PJ, Rosen AB: Trends in cost effectiveness analysis in orthopaedic surgery. *Clin Orthop Relat Res* 2007;457:42-48.

Economic and decision analysis study, evidence level IV

Hurwitz SR, Tornetta P III, Wright JG: An AOA critical issue: How to read the literature to change your practice: An evidence-based medicine approach. *J Bone Joint Surg Am* 2006;88:1873-1879.

Glossary of Evidence-Based Medicine Terms

Absolute risk reduction (ARR)—Difference in the event rate between control group (control event rate, CER) and treated group (experimental event rate, EER): ARR = CER − EER.

Blinded—Study in which any or all of the clinicians, patients, participants, outcome assessors, or statisticians are unaware of who received which study intervention. A double-blind study usually means the patient and clinician are blinded but is ambiguous, so it is better to state who is blinded.

Case-control study—Identifying patients who have the outcome of interest (cases) and control patients without the same outcome, and looking back to see if they had the exposure of interest.

Case series—Report on a series of patients with an outcome of interest. No control group is involved.

Clinical practice guideline—Systematically developed statement designed to assist practitioner and patient make decisions about appropriate health care for specific clinical circumstances.

Cohort study—Identification of two groups (cohorts) of patients, one that received the exposure of interest and one that did not, and following these cohorts forward for the outcome of interest.

Confidence interval (CI)—Quantification of the uncertainty in measurement; usually reported as 95% CI, which is the range of values within which we can be 95% sure that the true value for the whole population lies.

Control event rate (CER)—*see* Event rate.

Cost–benefit analysis—Converts effects into the same monetary terms as the costs and compares them.

Cost-effectiveness analysis—Converts effects into health terms and describes the costs for some additional health gain (eg, cost per additional event prevented).

Cost–utility analysis—Converts effects into personal preferences (or utilities) and describes how much it costs for some additional quality gain (eg, cost per additional quality-adjusted life-year [QALY]).

Crossover study design—Administration of two or more experimental therapies one after the other in a specified or random order to the same group of patients.

Cross-sectional study—Observation of a defined population at a single point in time or time interval. Exposure and outcome are determined simultaneously.

Decision analysis—Application of explicit, quantitative methods to analyze decisions under conditions of uncertainty.

Ecological survey—Based on aggregated data for some population as it exists at some point or points in time; to investigate the relationship of an exposure to a known or presumed risk factor for a specified outcome.

Experimental event rate (EER)—*see* Event rate.

Event rate—Proportion of patients in a group in whom the event is observed. Thus, if out of 100 patients, the event is observed in 27, the event rate is 0.27. Control event rate (CER) and experimental event rate (EER) are used to refer to this in control and experimental groups of patients, respectively.

Evidence-based health care—Extends the application of the principles of evidence-based medicine to all professions associated with health care, including purchasing and management.

Evidence-based medicine—The conscientious, explicit, and judicious use of current best evidence in making decisions about the care of individual patients. The practice of evidence-based medicine means integrating individual clinical expertise with the best available external clinical evidence from systematic research.

Likelihood ratio—Likelihood of a given test result in a patient with the target disorder compared with the likelihood of the same result in a patient without that disorder.

Meta-analysis—Systematic review or overview that uses quantitative methods to summarize the results.

N-of-1 trials—Patient undergoes pairs of treatment periods organized so that one period involves the use of the experimental treatment and one period involves the use of an alternate or placebo therapy. The patients and physician are blinded, if possible, and outcomes are monitored. Treatment periods are replicated until the clinician and patient are convinced that the treatments are definitely different or definitely not different.

Negative predictive value (−PV)—Proportion of people with a negative test who are free of disease.

Number needed to treat (NNT)—Number of patients who need to be treated to prevent one bad outcome; the inverse of the absolute risk reduction.

Odds—Ratio of events to nonevents. If the event rate for a disease is 0.2 (20%), its nonevent rate is 0.8 (80%), then its odds are 0.2/0.8 = 0.25. *See also* Odds ratio.

Odds ratio—Odds of an experimental patient suffering an event relative to the odds of a control patient.

Overview—Systematic review and summary of the medical literature.

P value—Probability of obtaining the same or more extreme data assuming the null hypothesis of no effect; *P* values are generally (but arbitrarily) considered significant if $P < 0.05$.

Positive predictive value (+PV)—Proportion of people with a positive test who have disease. Also called the posttest probability of disease after a positive test.

Posttest probability—Proportion of patients with that particular test result who have the target disorder (posttest odds/[1 + posttest odds]).

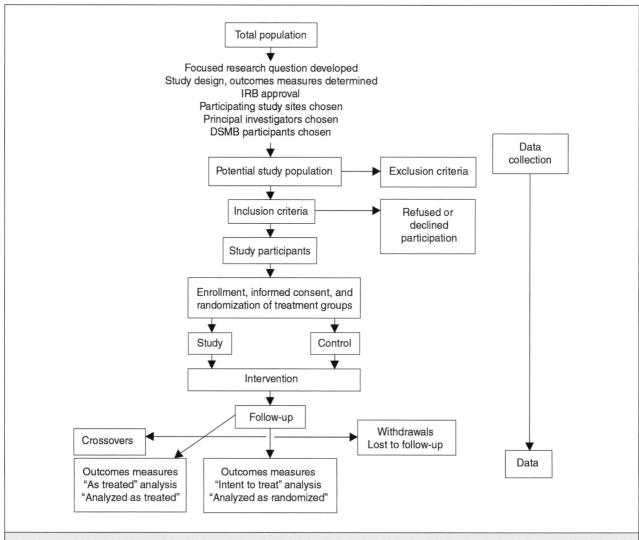

Figure 1 Basic design of a randomized clinical trial. IRB = Institutional Review Board; DSMB = Data and Safety Monitoring Board. *(Adapted from Abdu, WA: Outcomes Assessment and Evidence-Based Practice Guidelines in Orthopaedic Surgery, in Vaccaro, AR:* Orthopaedic Knowledge Update 8, *2005, pp 99-107.)*

Power—Probability that the sample mean will be sufficiently different from the mean under null hypothesis to allow rejection of the null hypothesis.

Randomized controlled clinical trial—Group of patients is randomized into an experimental group and a control group. These groups are followed up for the variables/outcomes of interest (**Figure 1**).

Relative risk reduction (RRR)—Percent reduction in events in the treated group event rate (EER) compared to the control group event rate (CER).

Sample size—Calculations performed before the inception of a study to determine the number of subjects needed to participate to avert a type I error or type II error. See **Table 1**.

Type I error—Probability of rejecting the null hypothesis when it is really true. The probability of making a type I error is denoted by the Greek letter α.

Type II error—Probability of failing to reject a null hypothesis that is really false. The probability of making a type II error is denoted by the Greek letter β.

Table 1

Common Formulas for the Determination of Sample Size

Study Design and Type of Error	Sample Size Formula
Studies using paired t test (before and after studies) with α (type I) error only	$N = \dfrac{(z_a)^2 \cdot (s)^2}{(\bar{d})^2}$ = total number of subjects
Studies using t test (randomized controlled trials with one experimental and one control group, considering α error only)	$N = \dfrac{(z_a)^2 \cdot 2 \cdot (s)^2}{(\bar{d})^2}$ = number of subjects/group
Studies using t test considering α and β errors	$N = \dfrac{(z_a + z_b)^2 \cdot 2 \cdot (s)^2}{(\bar{d})^2}$ = number of subjects/group
Tests of difference in proportions considering α and β errors	$N = \dfrac{(z_a + z_b)^2 \cdot 2 \cdot \bar{p}(1-\bar{p})}{(\bar{d})^2}$ = number of subjects/groups

N = sample size, za = value for α error (equals 1.96 for $P = 0.05$ in two-tailed test), zb = value for β error (equals 0.84 for 20% β error = 80% power in one-tailed test), $(s)^2$ = variance, p = mean proportion of success, d = smallest clinically important difference to be detected. (*Reproduced from Abdu WA: Outcomes assessment and evidence-based practice guidelines in orthopaedic Surgery, in vaccaro AR: Orthopaedic Knowledge Update 8. Rosemont, IL, American Academy of Orthopaedic Surgeons, 2005, pp 99-107.*)

Top Testing Facts

1. Evidence-based medicine is the practice of integrating individual clinical expertise with the best available clinical evidence from systematic research.

2. Evidence-based practice guidelines serve to assist the practicing orthopaedic surgeon in his or her quest to improve patient care by consolidating the relevant evidence and indicating the strength of the recommendation for treatment options.

3. Grades I through V of studies are matched directly to the level of evidence.

4. Therapeutic studies investigate the results of treatment.

5. A study's power is the probability that the sample mean will be sufficiently different from the mean under null hypothesis to allow one to reject the null hypothesis. Sample size plays a critical role in power analysis. When trying to detect small differences between groups, larger sample sizes are necessary.

6. A type II error is the probability of determining that there is no difference between treatment groups when there actually is a difference. Type II errors often occur when the sample size of the treatment group is too small and leads to a false-negative result.

7. A type I error is a false-positive conclusion that occurs when one rejects a null hypothesis that is actually true.

8. The P value is the probability of obtaining the same or more extreme data, assuming the null hypothesis is of no effect ($P < 0.05$).

9. The confidence interval (CI) is a quantification of the uncertainty of measurement. Typically, a 95% CI reports the range of values within which one can be 95% certain that the true value for the whole population lies.

Bibliography

Centre for Evidence-Based Medicine (www.cebm.net).

The Cochrane Collaboration (www.cochrane.org).

Online EBM: www.ebm.bmj.com.

Evidence-Based Medicine Working Group: Evidence-based medicine: a new approach to teaching the practice of medicine. JAMA 1992;268:2420-2425.

Evidence-Based Medicine Working Group. Users' guides to the medical literature I-XXV. *JAMA* 1993-2000.

Davidoff F, Haynes B, Sackett D, Smith R: Evidence-based medicine: A new journal to help doctors identify the information they need. *BMJ* 1995;310:1085-1086.

Greenhalgh T: *How to Read a Paper: The Basics of Evidence-Based Medicine*, ed 3. Malden, MA, Blackwell Publishing, 2006.

Sackett DL, Richardson WS, Rosenberg WS, Haynes RB (eds): *Evidence-Based Medicine*. London, England, Churchill-Livingstone, 1996.

2: General Knowledge

Sackett DL, Rosenberg WM, Gray JA, Haynes RB, Richardson WS: Evidence based medicine: What it is and what it isn't. *BMJ* 1996;312:71-72.

Thoma A, Farrokhyar F, Bhandari M, Tandan V: Users' guide to the surgical literature: How to assess a randomized controlled trial in surgery. *Can J Surg* 2004;47:200-208.

Section 3

Pediatrics

Section Editors

David L. Skaggs, MD
Robert M. Kay, MD

Chapter 25

Pediatric Multiple Trauma and Upper Extremity Fractures

Robert M. Kay, MD

I. General Considerations

A. Skeletal differences between children and adults

1. Pediatric bone is more elastic, leading to unique fracture patterns, including torus (buckle) fractures and greenstick fractures.

2. The thicker periosteum generally remains intact on the side of the bone toward which the distal fragment is displaced.

   a. This periosteal hinge serves to facilitate reduction.

   b. Overly aggressive reduction attempts can disrupt the hinge and increase the difficulty of obtaining and maintaining a satisfactory reduction.

3. Open physes (growth plates) can allow remodeling and straightening of a malunited fracture; however, in the case of growth disturbance, ongoing growth can result in angular deformity, limb-length discrepancy, or both.

   a. Remodeling occurs more rapidly and fully in the plane of joint motion (eg, sagittal malalignment at the wrist will remodel more successfully than will a coronal plane deformity).

   b. In the upper extremity, the fastest growth is at the upper and lower ends of the extremity (ie, at the proximal humerus and distal radius and ulna), whereas in the lower extremity, most growth is in the middle (ie, at the distal femur and proximal tibia and fibula).

B. Growth plate (physeal) fractures—The most commonly used classification for growth plate fractures is the Salter-Harris classification (Figure 1).

1. Advantages—Ease of use and prognostic value.

2. One disadvantage of this classification is that Salter-Harris V fractures (which occur rarely) cannot be distinguished from Salter-Harris I fractures at initial presentation; the differentiation often is not made until a growth arrest has occurred.

II. Multiple Trauma

A. Epidemiology

1. Trauma is the most common cause of death in children older than 1 year.

2. The most common causes are falls and motor vehicle accidents (MVAs).

   a. Many injuries and deaths could be avoided by appropriate use of child seats and restraints.

   b. Cervical spine injuries following an MVA are more common in children younger than 8 years because restraints often do not fit young children optimally.

B. Initial evaluation, resuscitation, and transport

1. Initial attention and care is directed to the life-threatening injuries.

   a. Airway, breathing, and circulation (the ABCs) are addressed immediately.

   b. Care from a trauma team is requisite to maximize the child's chance of survival.

   c. Fluid resuscitation is essential; if venous access is difficult, an intraosseous infusion with a large-bore needle may be necessary.

   d. Children often remain hemodynamically stable for significant periods of time following significant blood loss.

      i. Hypovolemic shock eventually ensues if fluid resuscitation is inadequate.

      ii. The "triad of death" (acidosis, hypothermia, and coagulopathy) may occur if hypovolemia persists.

2. Because of large head size in young children, a special transport board with an occipital cutout is necessary when transporting children younger than 6 years to the hospital, to prevent cervical spine flexion and potential iatrogenic cervical spinal cord injury.

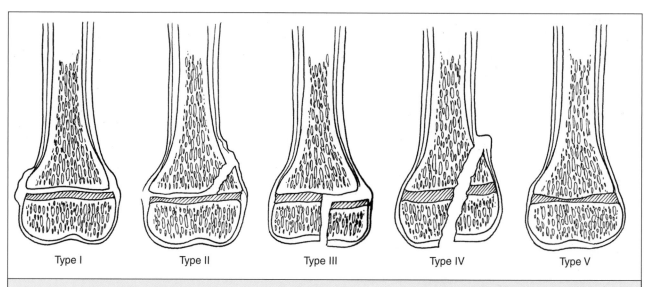

Figure 1 Salter-Harris classification of physeal fractures. Type I is characterized by a physeal separation; type II by a fracture that traverses the physis and exits through the metaphysis; type III by a fracture that traverses the physis before exiting through the epiphysis; type IV by a fracture that passes through the epiphysis, physis, and metaphysis; and type V by a crush injury to the physis. *(Reproduced from Kay RM, Matthys GA: Pediatric ankle fractures: Evaluation and treatment.* J Am Acad Orthop Surg *2001;9:268-278.)*

C. Secondary evaluation

1. Trauma rating systems

    a. Although no single system is optimal for determining prognosis, several trauma rating scores frequently are used, including the Injury Severity Score, the Modified Injury Severity Score (MISS), and the Pediatric Trauma Score.

    b. The Glasgow Coma Scale (GCS; see **Table 1**), scored on a scale of 3 to 15 points, is the tool most commonly used for evaluating head injury.

        i. GCS <8 at presentation in verbal children indicates a higher risk of mortality.

        ii. GCS motor score 72 hours postinjury is predictive of permanent disability following traumatic brain injury.

2. Abdominal bruising often heralds abdominal visceral injuries and spine fractures.

3. Up to 10% of injuries are initially missed by the treating team because of head injury and/or severe pain in other locations.

D. Imaging studies

1. Plain radiographs suffice for most extremity fractures.

2. CT scans

    a. Only about half of pelvic fractures identified on CT scan appear to be effected by AP pelvic radiographs.

    b. CT also helps to delineate fracture patterns in spinal, calcaneal, or other intra-articular fractures.

3. Intravenous pyelography is used to assess for bladder or urethral injuries, which may occur with anterior pelvic fractures (especially straddle fractures).

E. Head and neck injuries

1. The two most important prognostic indicators of long-term neurologic recovery and function are oxygen saturation at the time of presentation and the GCS score 72 hours after injury.

2. Children can make remarkable recoveries following severe traumatic brain injury and must be treated as though such a recovery will occur.

3. Intracranial pressure (ICP) must be controlled in these patients to minimize ongoing brain damage. ICP can be controlled by elevating the head of the bed, hyperventilation (which lowers pCO2), limiting intravenous fluids, administration of diuretics, and appropriate pain control (including appropriate fracture immobilization before definitive treatment).

4. Musculoskeletal manifestations of head injuries

    a. Spasticity begins within days to weeks; splinting helps prevent contractures.

        i. Part-time positioning of the hip and knee in flexion can decrease the plantar flexor tone to help prevent equinus contracture.

Table 1			

Pediatric Glasgow Coma Scale

Score	Older Than Age 5 Years	Age 1 to 5 Years	Younger Than Age 1 Year
Best Motor Response			
6	Obeys commands	Obeys commands	
5	Localizes pain	Localizes pain	Localizes pain
4	Withdrawal	Withdrawal	Abnormal withdrawal
3	Flexion to pain	Abnormal flexion	Abnormal flexion
2	Extensor rigidity	Extensor rigidity	Abnormal extension
1	None	None	None
Best Verbal Response			
5	Oriented	Approriate words	Smiles/cries appropriately
4	Confused	Inappropriate words	Cries
3	Inappropriate words	Cries/screams	Cries inappropriately
2	Incomprehensible	Grunts	Grunts
1	None	None	None
Eye Opening			
4	Spontaneous	Spontaneous	Spontaneous
3	To speech	To speech	To shout
2	To pain	To pain	To pain
1	None	None	None

(Reproduced from Sponseller PD, Paidas C: Management of the pediatric trauma patient, in Sponseller PD (ed): Orthopaedic Knowledge Update: Pediatrics 2. Rosemont, IL, American Academy of Orthopaedic Surgeons, 2002, pp 73-79.)

    ii. Pharmacologic intervention with botulinum toxin A may be helpful acutely to control spasticity and facilitate rehabilitation.

  b. Heterotopic ossification (HO), especially around the elbow, is more common following traumatic brain injury.

    i. An increase in serum alkaline phosphatase may herald the onset of HO.

    ii. Treatment is generally with observation, although early administration of salicylates or nonsteroidal anti-inflammatory drugs decreases the likelihood of severe HO.

  c. Fractures heal rapidly following traumatic brain injury, but the mechanism is not yet understood.

F. Abdominal visceral injuries

  1. Abdominal bruising, swelling, and/or tenderness are worrisome clinical signs.

  2. CT scans are the most reliable screening examinations for abdominal injuries.

G. Genitourinary injuries

  1. Rare in most multiple-trauma patients but common in those with pelvic fractures

  2. The risks are greatest with anterior pelvic fractures (especially straddle fractures).

H. Peripheral nerve injuries

  1. Most commonly occur in association with closed fractures. Observation in such cases is warranted; electrodiagnostic studies should be obtained if there is no return of nerve function by 2 to 3 months.

  2. If nerve function was intact preoperatively and absent postoperatively, nerve exploration is warranted.

  3. In the case of an open fracture associated with nerve injury, surgical exploration is generally warranted.

I. Treatment of the patient with multiple injuries

  1. Surgical fracture treatment is much more common in multiple-trauma patients.

  2. Surgical fixation of fractures facilitates patient care and mobilization and decreases the risk of pressure sores from immobilization.

  3. Open fractures are discussed below, in section III.

J. Complications in the patient with multiple injuries

  1. Mortality rates can be as high as 20% following pediatric multiple trauma.

  2. Long-term morbidity is present in one third to one half of children following multiple trauma.

    a. Most of this long-term morbidity is due to head injuries and orthopaedic injuries.

    b. The orthopaedic surgeon can minimize such late orthopaedic morbidity by assuming that the injured child will make a full recovery from the nonorthopaedic injuries.

3: Pediatrics

3. Fat embolism syndrome is a rare but life-threatening complication.

   a. The syndrome is heralded by an acute change in mental status, tachypnea, tachycardia, and hypoxemia.

   b. Treatment is via intubation, mechanical ventilation, and intravenous hydration.

K. Rehabilitation

   1. Pediatric patients often improve for 1 year or more following injury, with many making dramatic neurologic and functional gains.

   2. Splinting and bracing are needed to prevent contractures and to enhance function.

III. Open Fractures

A. Epidemiology

   1. Open fractures are often high-energy injuries, and associated injuries are common.

   2. Lawnmower injuries are another common cause of open fractures. These are often devastating injuries, with high rates of amputation and associated injuries of the head, neck, and upper extremities.

B. Initial evaluation and management

   1. For high-energy injuries, initial evaluation and management is as discussed in section II, Multiple Trauma.

   2. Thorough evaluation for other injuries is essential, because many children with open fractures have injuries to the head, abdomen, chest, or multiple extremities.

   3. Tetanus status should be confirmed and updated; children with an unknown vaccination history or who have not had a booster within 5 years should receive a dose of tetanus toxoid.

   4. Prompt administration of intravenous antibiotics is essential to minimize the risk of infection (Table 2).

C. Classification—As in adults, the Gustilo-Anderson classification is used to grade open fractures (Table 3).

D. Treatment

   1. Prompt administration of intravenous antibiotics appears to be the most important factor in preventing infection following open fractures.

   2. Irrigation and débridement (I & D) must be performed in all open fractures.

Table 2

Antibiotics Used in the Treatment of Pediatric Open Fractures

Antibiotic	Dose	Interval	Maximum Dose	Indications
Cefazolin	100 mg/kg/d	Q8 h	6 g/d	All open fractures
Gentamicin	5-7.5 mg/kg/d	Q8 h	None specified	Severe grade II and III injuries
Penicillin	150,000 units/kg/d	Q6 h	24 million units/d	Farm-type or vascular injuries
Clindamycin	15-40 units/kg/d	Q6-8 h	2.7 g/d	Patients with allergies to cefazolin or penicillin

Table 3

Gustilo-Anderson Classification of Open Fractures

Grade	Contamination	Wound Length	Defining Feature
I	Clean	<1 cm	
II	Moderate	1-10 cm	
III	Severe	>10 cm	
IIIA	Severe	>10 cm	Adequate soft-tissue coverage
IIIB	Severe	>10 cm	Bone exposure without adequate soft-tissue coverage; soft-tissue coverage often required
IIIC	Severe	Any length	Major vascular injury in injured segment

a. Type I fractures generally need only a single I & D, whereas grade II and III injuries are generally treated with serial I & D every 48 to 72 hours until all remaining tissue appears clean and viable.

b. Recent studies have demonstrated that the risk of infection following open fractures is no higher if I & D is performed 8 to 24 hours postinjury than if it is performed within 8 hours of injury.

c. Because of better soft-tissue envelope and vascularity in children, tissue of apparently marginal viability may be left in the child at the time of initial débridement. Tissue viability will often declare itself by the time of re-exploration, 2 to 3 days later.

d. Because of enhanced periosteal new bone formation in children, some bone defects may fill in spontaneously, particularly in young children.

3. Wound cultures

a. Wound cultures are contraindicated in the absence of clinical signs of infection.

b. The correlation of both pre- and postdébridement cultures with the development of infection is low, and such cultures should not be performed routinely.

4. Fracture fixation (internal or external) is almost universally indicated to stabilize the soft tissues, allow wound access, and maintain alignment.

E. Complications

1. Complications associated with specific fractures are discussed in section IV, with the discussion of the particular fracture type.

2. Compartment syndrome is a significant risk, particularly in children with a head injury or other distracting injuries.

3. Infection risk is minimized with the prompt administration of intravenous antibiotics and appropriate I & D.

4. Chronic pain and psychological sequelae are common manifestations following severe trauma.

IV. Fractures of the Shoulder and Humeral Shaft

A. Clavicle fractures

1. General information—Clavicle fractures account for 90% of obstetric fractures. There is a high incidence of concomitant clavicle fracture and obstetric brachial plexus palsy.

2. Fracture location

a. Medial clavicle fractures

i. The medial clavicular physis is the last physis in the body to close, at 23 to 25 years of age.

ii. Most medial clavicle fractures are physeal fractures; sternoclavicular joint dislocations are rare.

iii. Posteriorly displaced fractures may impinge on the mediastinum (including the great vessels and trachea).

b. Clavicle shaft fractures—Displaced fractures rarely cause problems, although compression of the subclavian vessels and brachial plexus can occur.

c. Lateral clavicle fractures—A lateral clavicle fracture may be confused with an acromioclavicular joint dislocation, which is very rare in children.

3. Treatment

a. Medial clavicle fractures

i. Nonsurgical treatment, with a sling for 3 to 4 weeks as needed, is sufficient.

ii. Percutaneous reduction with a towel clip may be indicated for posteriorly displaced fractures impinging on the mediastinum. Some authors recommend that a vascular surgeon be present because of potential vascular complications.

iii. Open reduction may be needed for open fractures or if percutaneous reduction fails. Suture fixation generally suffices in such cases.

b. Clavicle shaft fractures

i. Nonsurgical treatment (with a figure-of-8 harness or sling for 4 to 6 weeks) is appropriate for most of these fractures. A swathe may be used in infants.

ii. Open reduction and internal fixation (ORIF) may be indicated in the instance of floating shoulder injuries or potentially with multiple trauma. Fixation with pins should be avoided because of the risk of pin migration.

c. Lateral clavicle fractures

i. Most of these fractures are treated symptomatically with a sling.

ii. For markedly displaced fractures, the consideration of surgical treatment is controversial.

4. Complications

a. Medial fractures—Compression of the mediastinal structures may occur with posteriorly displaced fractures.

b. Shaft fractures

   i. Complications are rare with closed treatment, although prominence at the fracture site is expected.

   ii. Compression of the subclavian vessels and brachial plexus is rare.

   iii. Surgical treatment increases the risks of infection, delayed union, and malunion. Fixation with pins may result in pin migration.

c. Lateral fractures—Complications are rare with closed treatment.

B. Proximal humerus fractures

1. General—Because 90% of humeral growth is proximal, these are very forgiving fractures.

2. Evaluation

a. Plain radiographs are almost universally sufficient for evaluation of fracture configuration and to rule out associated shoulder dislocation.

b. Because of its proximity, the brachial plexus may be injured with these fractures. Most associated brachial plexus palsies are neurapraxias, which resolve rapidly.

3. Classification—The Neer and Horwitz classification is used to define the amount of fracture displacement. Grade I fractures are displaced ≤5 mm, grade II fractures ≤1/3 of the humeral diameter, grade III fractures ≤2/3 of the humeral diameter, and grade IV fractures >2/3 of the humeral diameter.

4. Nonsurgical treatment

a. Most of these fractures can be treated nonsurgically.

b. Reduction may be performed for Neer and Horwitz III and IV fractures.

   i. Reduction is generally obtained by shoulder abduction to 90° and external rotation to 90°.

   ii. Impediments to reduction may include the long head of the biceps, the periosteum, or the glenohumeral joint capsule.

c. Nonsurgical treatment options include sling and swathe, shoulder immobilizer, or coaptation splint.

d. Gentle shoulder range-of-motion (ROM) exercises should be started 1 to 2 weeks after injury.

5. Surgical treatment

a. Surgical treatment is indicated only for adolescents with Neer and Horwitz grade III and IV injuries and for children of any age with open fractures.

b. Closed reduction and percutaneous pinning is used in most surgical cases. The pins are removed 2 to 3 weeks postinjury.

c. Open reduction and pinning is necessary if interposed structures (biceps tendon, periosteum, and/or joint capsule) prevent closed reduction in adolescents with grade III or IV injuries.

6. Complications

a. Malunion, growth arrest, and other complications are rare.

b. Brachial plexus injuries are almost always stretch injuries, which resolve spontaneously.

C. Humeral shaft fractures

1. Evaluation—Radial nerve palsy occurs in <5% of humeral shaft fractures and is almost always a neurapraxia following middle or distal third fractures.

2. Nonsurgical treatment

a. Nonsurgical therapy is the mainstay of treatment.

b. Significant displacement and angulation (up to 30°) are acceptable because range of shoulder motion is generally excellent.

c. Typical immobilization is via sling and swathe, sugar-tong splint, or fracture brace; ROM exercises are started by 2 to 3 weeks postinjury.

3. Surgical treatment

a. Indications for surgical treatment include open fractures, multiple trauma, and floating elbow or shoulder injuries.

b. Procedures

   i. Intramedullary rod fixation (flexible titanium nails) is the preferred surgical treatment of most shaft fractures requiring fixation.

   ii. Plate fixation results in increased scarring and puts the radial nerve at risk during the procedure.

4. Complications

a. Malunion rarely has functional consequences because normal shoulder ROM is excellent.

b. Primary radial nerve palsies (present at the time of injury) are almost always due to neurapraxia and resolve spontaneously. Primary nerve palsies should be observed. If they do not resolve spontaneously by 3 to 4 months, then electrophysiologic studies are indicated and surgical exploration may be needed.

c. Secondary nerve palsies (present after intervention) are often more complete injuries and require exploration acutely.

d. Stiffness is rare; early ROM minimizes this risk.

e. Limb-length discrepancy is common but is generally mild and of no functional consequence.

V. Supracondylar Humerus Fractures

A. Epidemiology

1. Supracondylar humerus (SCH) fractures account for more than half of pediatric elbow fractures.

2. 95% to 98% are extension-type injuries.

B. Relevant anatomy

1. Distal humeral anatomy is shown in **Figure 2**.

2. The Baumann angle may be measured on AP radiographs of the distal humerus to assess the coronal plane fracture alignment, but it is used less commonly now because of difficulty and variability in its measurement.

C. Associated injuries

1. Vascular injuries occur in ~1% of SCH fractures. Because of the rich collateral flow at the elbow, distal perfusion may remain good despite a vascular injury (**Table 4**).

2. Nerve injuries—see **Table 5**.

D. Classification—The modified Gartland classification is widely used to classify SCH fractures (**Figure 3**).

E. Nonsurgical treatment

1. Type I fractures are treated closed with a long-arm cast in ~90° of elbow flexion.

2. A minority of type II fractures may be treated closed in a cast.

3. Closed treatment is considered for type II fractures only if the following criteria are met:

a. No significant swelling is present.

b. The anterior humeral line intersects the capitellum.

c. There is no medial cortical impaction of the distal humerus.

4. In essentially all cases, the casts are removed after fracture healing at 3 weeks.

F. Surgical treatment

1. Indications—Most type II and all type III (and IV) fractures are treated with reduction and pinning.

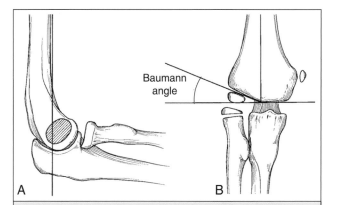

Figure 2 Typical anatomic relationships in the elbow. **A**, The anterior humeral line, shown as would be drawn on a lateral radiograph, should bisect the capitellum. In extension-type supracondylar fractures, the capitellum moves posterior to the anterior humeral line. **B**, The Baumann angle (shown as would be measured on an AP view) is the angle subtended by a line perpendicular to the long axis of the humerus and a line along the lateral condylar physis. The Baumann angle may be used to assess the adequacy of the reduction in the coronal plane and may be compared to the contralateral elbow. (*Reproduced from Skaggs DL: Elbow fractures in children: Diagnosis and management. J Am Acad Orthop Surg 1997;5:303-312.*)

Table 4

Treatment for Vascular Injuries With Supracondylar Humerus Fractures

Vascular Status	Treatment
Pulse lost after reduction and pinning	Explore brachial artery and treat.
Pulseless, well-perfused hand	Observe for 24-72 h.
Pulseless, cool hand	Explore brachial artery and treat.

Table 5

Nerve Injuries With Supracondylar Humerus Fractures

Nerve Injury	Association
Anterior interosseous nerve	Most common nerve injury with supracondylar humerus fracture
Median nerve	Associated with posterolateral fracture displacement
Radial nerve	Seen with posteromedial fracture displacement
Ulnar nerve	Rare traumatic injury. Cause is almost always iatrogenic (due to medial pin).

3: Pediatrics

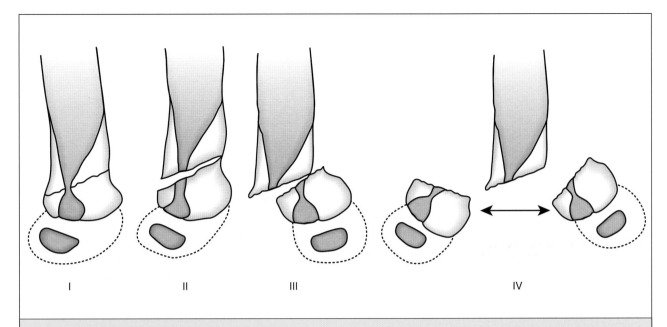

Figure 3 Gartland classification of supracondylar fractures. Type I injuries are nondisplaced. Type II injuries are displaced but have an intact hinge of bone (located posteriorly in extension-type fractures). Type III fractures are completely displaced and there is no intact hinge. Type IV fractures are completely displaced fractures that are unstable in both flexion and extension.

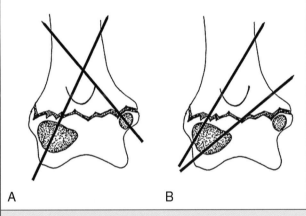

Figure 4 Typical pin configurations for crossed pinning (**A**) and lateral-entry pinning (**B**) for SCH fractures. Regardless of pin configuration, both the medial and lateral columns should be engaged proximal to the fracture site. *(Reproduced from Flynn JM, Cornwall R: Elbow: Pediatrics, in Vaccaro AR (ed): Orthopaedic Knowledge Update 8. Rosemont, IL, American Academy of Orthopaedic Surgeons, 2005, pp 705-713.)*

Table 6

Comparison of Crossed Pins and Lateral-Entry Pins for Supracondylar Humerus Fractures

	Laboratory Testing	Clinical Stability	Iatrogenic Ulnar Nerve Injury
Crossed pins	More stable	Comparable	3%-8%
Lateral-entry pins	Less stable	Comparable	0%

2. Pin configuration (**Figure 4** and **Table 6**)

  a. Crossed pins

    i. Crossed pins have been found to be more stable biomechanically in laboratory studies than are lateral-entry pins.

    ii. Use of a medial pin results in a significant risk (3% to 8%) of iatrogenic ulnar nerve in-jury. The risk is highest if the medial pin is inserted with the elbow in hyperflexion.

  b. Lateral-entry pins

    i. Lateral-entry pins should be separated sufficiently to engage both the medial and lateral columns of the distal humerus at the level of the fracture.

    ii. When inserted with appropriate technique, lateral-entry pins have comparable success in maintaining reduction of SCH fractures.

    iii. Iatrogenic ulnar nerve injury does not occur with lateral-entry pins.

G. Complications

  1. Volkmann ischemic contracture is the most disastrous result and is more commonly due to compression of the brachial artery with casting in >90° of flexion than to arterial injury.

2. Cubitus varus (gunstock deformity) is generally a cosmetic deformity with few functional sequelae. The rates of cubitus varus are much lower with reduction and pinning than with closed reduction and casting.

3. Recurvatum is common following cast treatment of type II and III fractures and remodels poorly because of the limited growth of the distal humerus.

4. Stiffness is rare following casting or reduction and pinning, particularly with cast removal at 3 weeks.

VI. Other Elbow Fractures

A. Relevant anatomy

1. Ossification centers of the elbow (**Table 7**)

2. Distal humerus—The alignment (including anterior humeral line and Baumann angle) as noted in SCH fractures is essential to remember.

3. Proximal radius

a. There is normally a 12° valgus angle of the proximal radius.

b. The proximal radius should be directed toward the capitellum on all radiographs.

c. The relationships between the proximal radius and the capitellum and the ulna and the humerus often facilitate fracture identification (**Figure 5**).

B. Lateral condyle fractures

1. Classification

a. The most widely used classification of lateral condyle fractures is based on the amount of fracture displacement (**Figure 6**). The oblique view is most sensitive for detecting maximal displacement and must be obtained if closed treatment is contemplated.

Table 7		
Order of Appearance of Ossification Centers of the Elbow on Radiographs*		
	Age of Appearance in Girls (years)	**Age of Appearance in Boys (years)**
Capitellum	1	1
Radius (proximal)	4-5	5-6
Medial epicondyle	5-6	7-8
Trochlea	8-9	10-11
Olecranon	9	11
Lateral epicondyle	10	11-12

*A rough guide is that the capitellum appears at age 1 year, and in girls, 2 years should be added for each additional ossification center (except the proximal radius, which appears in girls at 4 to 5 years). There is a 2-year delay for boys for all centers except the capitellum.

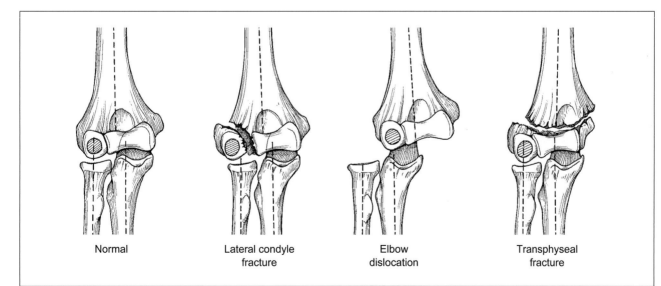

Normal   Lateral condyle   Elbow   Transphyseal
                    fracture   dislocation   fracture

Figure 5   Osseous relationships about the elbow as seen on AP radiographs of the elbow. In transphyseal fractures the radius is directed toward the capitellum; in elbow dislocations, the proximal radius is not directed toward the capitellum. *(Reproduced from Skaggs DL: Elbow fractures in children: Diagnosis and management. J Am Acad Orthop Surg 1997;5:303-312.)*

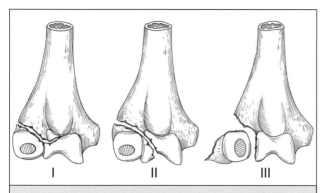

Figure 6 Illustration of types of lateral condyle fractures as typically classified. Type I fractures are displaced <2 mm and generally have an intact intra-articular surface. Type II fractures are displaced 2 to 4 mm and have a displaced joint surface. Type III injuries are displaced >4 mm and often are completely displaced and rotated. *(Reproduced from Sullivan JA: Fractures of the lateral condyle of the humerus. J Am Acad Orthop Surg 2006;14:58-62.)*

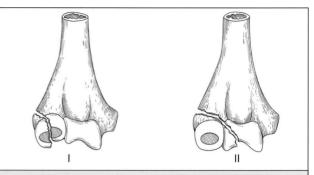

Figure 7 Milch classification of lateral condyle fractures. In Milch I fractures, the fracture traverses the ossific nucleus of the capitellum, and in type II fractures, the fracture line is medial to the ossific nucleus. *(Reproduced from Sullivan JA: Fractures of the lateral condyle of the humerus. J Am Acad Orthop Surg 2006;14:58-62.)*

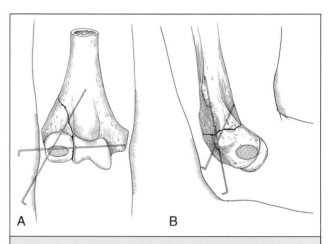

Figure 8 Typical pin configuration for lateral condyle fractures. The pins must be divergent, and the distal pin should engage metaphyseal bone (rather than simply unossified cartilage). *(Reproduced from Sullivan JA: Fractures of the lateral condyle of the humerus. J Am Acad Orthop Surg 2006;14:58-62.)*

b. The Milch classification (**Figure 7**) is rarely used because it is irrelevant to patient care. Milch I fractures are considered Salter-Harris IV fractures and are very rare. Milch II fractures are considered Salter-Harris II fractures.

2. Treatment algorithm

   a. Type I fractures are treated with casting for 3 to 6 weeks, although 2% to 10% of these fractures displace sufficiently in a cast to require reduction and pinning.

   b. Type II fractures are treated surgically with closed versus open reduction and percutaneous fixation (generally with smooth pins).

      i. Closed reduction and pinning is appropriate if there is no intra-articular incongruity following pinning (as assessed on an intraoperative arthrogram).

      ii. Open reduction is required if joint congruity cannot be obtained with closed treatment.

   c. Type III fractures—ORIF (with percutaneous pins or screws) is requisite.

3. Surgical technique

   a. Pin configuration (**Figure 8**)—The pins must be divergent to minimize the risk of fracture displacement, and the distal pin must engage at least a portion of the ossified distal humeral metaphysis.

   b. Open reduction

      i. The posterior soft tissues should never be dissected off the lateral condyle because the blood supply enters posteriorly and posterior dissection can result in osteonecrosis.

      ii. The entire length of the fracture, including the joint line, must be visualized to ensure an anatomic reduction.

4. Complications

   a. Stiffness is minimized by mobilizing the elbow once fracture healing is complete, generally by 4 weeks.

   b. Osteonecrosis can be minimized by avoiding posterior soft-tissue dissection.

   c. Nonunion is rare if the above protocol is followed.

      i. If nonunion is evident within the first 6 to 12 months after injury, the nonunion may be treated with bone grafting and screw fixation.

ii. Cubitus valgus is frequent in the case of non-union.

d. Tardy ulnar nerve palsy may occur following nonunion and cubitus valgus, but it generally does not occur for decades after the injury, if ever. Treatment is ulnar nerve transposition.

C. Medial condyle fractures

1. Classification—Classification is based on the amount of displacement and is comparable to that noted above for lateral condyle fractures.

2. Treatment—Treatment is as described for lateral condyle fractures; however, type I medial condyle injuries are rare.

3. Complications—The most common complication is failure to recognize this fracture, though a metaphyseal fragment can generally be seen on plain radiographs in cases of medial condyle fracture. Elbow MRI or arthrogram may be indicated to accurately assess whether surgery is necessary.

D. Medial epicondyle fractures

1. Overview

a. The mechanism of injury is generally avulsion of the medial epicondyle apophysis.

b. Half of medial epicondyle fractures are associated with elbow dislocations.

2. Classification—The classification is based on the amount of displacement and whether the medial epicondyle is entrapped in the elbow joint.

3. Nonsurgical treatment

a. Nonsurgical care is the mainstay of treatment. (Exceptions are listed under Surgical treatment, below.)

b. Closed attempts to extricate an entrapped medial condyle may be undertaken by supinating the forearm, placing a valgus stress on the elbow, and extending the wrist and fingers.

c. Early motion (within 3 to 5 days) minimizes the risk of elbow stiffness.

4. Surgical treatment

a. Indications

i. Absolute—Intra-articular entrapment of the medial epicondyle.

ii. Relative—Dominant arm in a throwing athlete, weight-bearing extremity in an athlete (eg, gymnast), ulnar nerve dysfunction.

b. Technique—Open reduction with screw fixation is preferred to allow early motion. (Kirschner wires may be used in young children.) It is important to remember that the medial epicondyle is relatively posterior on the humerus.

5. Complications

a. Stiffness is almost universal, although rarely of functional consequence.

b. Ulnar neuropathy is generally a neurapraxia, which spontaneously resolves.

c. Chronic instability is rare.

d. Failure to diagnose an incarcerated medial epicondyle may lead to elbow stiffness and degenerative changes.

E. Lateral epicondyle fractures

1. Nonsurgical treatment is indicated for most of these fractures.

2. Surgery is indicated when the epicondyle has displaced into the elbow joint.

F. Distal humeral physeal fractures

1. Epidemiology—These fractures are most common in children younger than 3 years of age, but they may occur up to 6 years of age.

2. Evaluation

a. These fractures almost always displace posteromedially (**Figure 9**) and are frequently misdiagnosed as elbow dislocations.

b. Elbow dislocations are very rare in young children, so a physeal fracture should be assumed in young children with displacement of the proximal radius and ulna relative to the distal humerus.

c. Elbow arthrography or MRI may be used to clarify the diagnosis.

3. Classification—The Salter-Harris classification is used, with all fractures being type I or II.

4. Treatment

a. Closed reduction and percutaneous pinning is the mainstay of treatment.

b. Pin configuration is similar to that used for supracondylar fractures.

c. Closed reduction should not be performed if the injury is diagnosed late (after 5 to 7 days postinjury), to minimize the risk of iatrogenic physeal injury.

5. Complications are rare following prompt diagnosis and treatment, and misdiagnosis is the most common complication.

G. Proximal radius fractures

1. General—Most fractures are radial neck and/or physeal fractures and are typically associated with valgus loading of the elbow or elbow dislocation.

2. Classification—These fractures are most commonly classified based on the location of the frac-

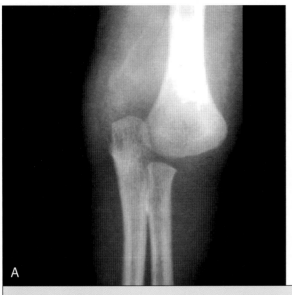 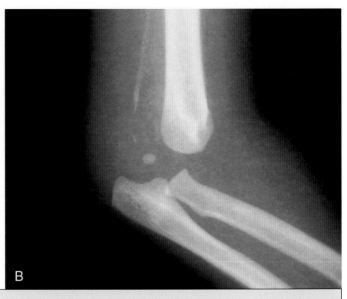

Figure 9 AP (**A**) and lateral (**B**) radiographs of the elbow of an 18-month-old infant with a physeal fracture of the distal humerus demonstrate typical alignment of the elbow following these injuries. Although the appearance resembles an elbow dislocation, the age of the child is younger and the radius can be noted to be directed at the capitellum in these radiographs. The vast majority of these injuries are displaced posteromedially. Periosteal new bone is evident in this 2-week-old fracture. *(Reproduced from Sponseller PD: Injuries of the arm and elbow, in Sponseller PD (ed): Orthopaedic Knowledge Update: Pediatrics 2. Rosemont, IL, American Academy of Orthopaedic Surgeons, 2002, pp 93-107.)*

ture (neck or head) and the angulation and/or displacement.

3. Nonsurgical treatment

   a. Most of these fractures are treated closed.

   b. Manipulative techniques

      i. Patterson maneuver—Hold the elbow in flexion and varus while applying direct pressure to the radial head.

      ii. Israeli technique—Direct pressure is held over the radial head with the elbow flexed 90° while the forearm is pronated and supinated.

      iii. Elastic bandage—Spontaneous reduction may occur with tight application of an elastic bandage around the forearm and elbow.

   c. Early mobilization (within 3 to 7 days) is indicated to minimize stiffness.

4. Surgical treatment

   a. Indications following reduction:

      i. >30° of residual angulation

      ii. >3 to 4 mm of translation

      iii. <45° of pronation and supination

   b. Procedures

      i. Percutaneous manipulation is usually attempted using a Kirschner wire, awl, elevator, or other metallic device.

   ii. The Metaizeau technique involves retrograde insertion of a flexible pin or nail. The pin is passed across the fracture site, and the fracture is reduced by rotating the pin.

   iii. Open reduction via a lateral approach is rarely necessary, but it may be required for severely displaced fractures.

   iv. Internal fixation is used only for fractures that are unstable following reduction.

5. Complications

   a. Elbow stiffness is extremely common, even after nondisplaced fractures.

   b. Overgrowth of the radial head is common.

H. Olecranon fractures

1. Evaluation—Palpation over the radial head is necessary to rule out a Monteggia fracture. Tenderness over a reduced radial head is indicative of a Monteggia fracture with spontaneous reduction of the radial head.

2. Classification—It is important to distinguish apophyseal fractures from metaphyseal olecranon fractures because the former may be the first indication of osteogenesis imperfecta.

3. Nonsurgical treatment—Most olecranon fractures are treated nonsurgically, with casting in relative extension (usually 10° to 45° of flexion) for 3 weeks.

4. Surgical treatment—Indicated for fractures that are displaced more than 2 to 3 mm using tension band fixation. (In children, an absorbable suture rather than a wire is often used as the tension band.)

5. Complications are rare and rarely of clinical significance, though failure to diagnose associated injuries (such as radial head dislocation) may be a cause of significant morbidity.

I. Nursemaid's elbow

1. Epidemiology—Nursemaid's elbow occurs with longitudinal traction on the outstretched arm of a young child (generally younger than 5 years of age) as the orbicular ligament subluxates over the radial head.

2. Evaluation

a. The history and physical examination are classic, with the child holding the elbow extended and the forearm pronated.

b. Radiographs are not needed unless the classic history and arm positioning are absent. If radiographs are obtained, they are normal in nursemaid's elbow.

3. Treatment—With one thumb held over the affected radial head (to feel for a "snap" as the orbicular ligament reduces), the forearm is supinated and the elbow is flexed past 90°.

4. Complications—Recurrent nursemaid's elbow is relatively common, although recurrences are rare after age 5 years.

VII. Fractures of the Forearm, Wrist, and Hand

A. Diaphyseal forearm fractures

1. Evaluation—Open wounds are often punctate and are commonly missed when the injury is not evaluated by an orthopaedic surgeon.

2. Classification

a. Greenstick fractures are incomplete fractures and are common in children. These should be described as apex volar or apex dorsal to facilitate reduction.

b. Complete fractures are categorized the same as in adults, by fracture location, fracture pattern, angulation, and displacement.

3. Nonsurgical treatment

a. Most pediatric forearm fractures can be treated without surgery.

b. Greenstick fractures are generally rotational injuries. Apex volar fractures (supination injuries) may be treated by forearm pronation, and

apex dorsal injuries (pronation injuries) by forearm supination.

c. Casting for 6 weeks is typical.

4. Surgical treatment

a. Indications

i. Unacceptable alignment following closed reduction may necessitate open reduction. Unacceptable alignment includes angulation >15° in children younger than 10 years and >10° in children 10 years of age or older, and bayonet apposition in children older than 10 years.

ii. Significantly displaced fractures in adolescents are at high risk for redisplacement and are a relative indication for surgery.

iii. Open fractures are commonly treated surgically.

b. Technique

i. Advantages of intramedullary fixation are a smaller dissection, use of a load-sharing device, and fewer stress risers.

ii. Unlike in adults, intramedullary fixation in children results in rapid healing, and nonunion is rare.

iii. Fixation of one bone is often sufficient to stabilize an unstable forearm (especially in children younger than 10 years).

5. Complications

a. Refracture occurs in 5% to 10% of children following forearm fractures.

b. Malunion is unusual if serial radiographs are obtained during healing (usually weekly for the first 2 to 3 weeks after complete fractures).

c. Compartment syndrome may occur, particularly in high-energy injuries. The rate after intramedullary fixation is high, likely due to selection bias and multiple attempts at reduction and rod passage.

d. Loss of pronation and supination is common, though generally mild.

B. Monteggia fractures

1. Evaluation

a. Palpation over the radial head must be performed for all children with ulnar fractures because spontaneous relocation of the radial head is relatively common in pediatric Monteggia injuries.

b. Isolated radial head dislocations almost never occur in children. Such presumed "isolated" injuries are almost universally due to plastic

Table 8		
Bado Classification of Monteggia Fractures		
Bado Type	Apex of Ulnar Fracture	Radial Head Pathology
I	Anterior	Anterior dislocation
II	Posterior	Posterior dislocation
III	Lateral	Lateral dislocation
IV	Any direction (typically anterior)	Proximal radius dislocation and fracture

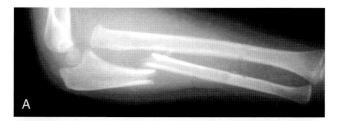

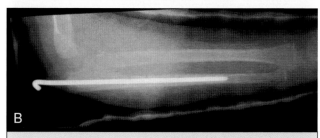

Figure 10   Bado I Monteggia fracture-dislocation. **A,** Preoperative radiograph. **B,** Postoperative radiograph shows that the fracture was treated by closed reduction and intramedullary nail fixation. (*Reproduced from Waters PM, Injuries of the shoulder, elbow, and forearm, in Abel MF (ed): Orthopaedic Knowledge Update: Pediatrics 3. Rosemont, IL, American Academy of Orthopaedic Surgeons, 2006, pp 303-314.*)

deformation of the ulna with concomitant radial head dislocation.

2. Classification

    a. The Bado classification (**Table 8**) is most commonly used to describe these fractures.

    b. Fractures may be classified as acute or chronic (>2 to 3 weeks since injury).

3. Nonsurgical treatment

    a. Nonsurgical treatment is much more common (and successful) in children with Monteggia fractures than in adults.

    b. Reestablishment of ulnar length is of primary importance to maintain reduction of the radial head.

    c. For type I and III fractures, the forearm should be supinated in the cast.

4. Surgical treatment

    a. Acute fractures should be operated on if they are open and/or unstable. For closed fractures, reduction is frequently successful, and an intramedullary nail is often used to maintain ulnar length (**Figure 10**). For comminuted fractures, plate fixation may be needed. Annular ligament reconstruction is almost never needed for acute fractures.

    b. Chronic Monteggia fractures should be reduced surgically (preferably within 6 to 12 months postinjury). They require an ulnar osteotomy and annular ligament reconstruction.

5. Complications

    a. Posterior interosseous nerve palsy occurs in up to 10% of acute injuries but almost always resolves spontaneously.

    b. Delayed or missed diagnosis is common when the child is not seen by an orthopaedic surgeon.

    c. Complication rates and severity are much greater if the diagnosis is delayed more than 2 to 3 weeks.

C. Distal forearm fractures

1. Classification

    a. Physeal fractures are categorized by the Salter-Harris classification.

    b. For metaphyseal fractures, distinction is made between buckle fractures and complete fractures.

2. Nonsurgical treatment

    a. Most of these fractures are treated by closed means.

    b. Physeal fractures heal in 3 to 4 weeks and metaphyseal fractures in 4 to 6 weeks. Buckle fractures heal in 3 weeks.

3. Surgical treatment

    a. Indications

      i. The most common indications for surgical intervention are ipsilateral elbow fractures, open fractures, or unacceptable alignment following reduction. Unacceptable alignment for complete metaphyseal fractures is >15° to 20° of angulation in any age child and bayonet apposition in children older than 10 years. For physeal fractures, residual displacement >50% is unacceptable.

      ii. For children with ipsilateral elbow fractures, percutaneous pinning of the distal radius results in much lower rates of loss of reduction and malunion.

iii. For physeal fractures, no more than one or two reduction attempts should be attempted in the emergency department. Physeal fractures should not be manipulated more than 5 to 7 days postinjury.

b. Procedures

i. Closed reduction is successful in reducing most of these fractures.

ii. Percutaneous pinning (avoiding the superficial radial nerve) is generally sufficient to maintain reduction.

4. Complications

a. Malunion generally results in cosmetic deformity rather than functional deficits and often remodels spontaneously.

b. Growth arrest occurs in <1% to 2% of distal radius physeal fractures and <1% of metaphyseal fractures.

D. Carpal injuries

1. Nonsurgical treatment

a. Scaphoid fractures are most commonly treated with a thumb spica cast. There is no consensus regarding short- or long-arm thumb spica use.

i. Distal pole fractures routinely heal with closed treatment.

ii. Waist fractures (especially in adolescents) have worse results and may result in osteonecrosis and/or nonunion.

b. Triangular fibrocartilage complex (TFCC) tears may be seen with distal radial and/or ulnar styloid fractures and are generally treated closed.

2. Surgical treatment

a. Scaphoid fractures may be treated with ORIF for displaced waist fractures or with ORIF and bone grafting for established nonunions.

b. If there is ongoing wrist pain following closed treatment of a wrist fracture, TFCC tears may be repaired arthroscopically.

3. Complications

a. Scaphoid waist fractures can result in osteonecrosis and nonunion.

b. TFCC tears may result in chronic wrist pain.

E. Metacarpal fractures

1. Classification

a. For growth plate injuries, the Salter-Harris classification is used.

b. For nonphyseal fractures, classification is based on fracture location, configuration, angulation, and displacement, as in adults.

c. Some of these fractures are "open" injuries ("fight bites" or "clenched-fist" injuries), and lacerations over the knuckles should be sought to rule out such an injury.

2. Nonsurgical treatment

a. Most of these fractures are treated closed.

i. Rotational alignment must be good for closed treatment to be acceptable.

ii. Acceptable sagittal angulation increases from radial to ulnar as in adults, with the following general guidelines: second metacarpal, 10° to 20°; third metacarpal, 20° to 30°; fourth metacarpal, 30° to 40°; and fifth metacarpal, 40° to 50°.

b. Closed treatment is generally successful for diaphyseal and metaphyseal fractures of the thumb metacarpal.

3. Surgical treatment

a. Surgical indications are unacceptable rotational, sagittal, and/or coronal alignment.

b. Physeal fractures of the base of the thumb metacarpal often require surgery because of instability and/or intra-articular step-off.

4. Complications—The most common complication is malalignment (including rotational deformity with overlapping fingers) requiring late osteotomy.

F. Phalangeal fractures

1. Classification

a. Physeal fractures are assessed via the Salter-Harris classification.

b. Shaft and neck fractures are categorized by fracture type and displacement.

2. Nonsurgical treatment suffices for most fractures, with healing in ~3 weeks.

3. Surgical treatment

a. Indications—Surgical treatment is needed for most intra-articular phalangeal fractures.

b. Procedures

i. Closed reduction and pinning is indicated for most minimally displaced intra-articular fractures.

ii. Open reduction and pinning is often needed for more displaced unicondylar and bicondylar fractures.

4. Complications—Stiffness, fixation loss, growth disturbance, and malunion are relatively uncommon given the frequency of these injuries in children.

3: Pediatrics

Top Testing Facts

Multiple Trauma

1. Children can remain hemodynamically stable following significant blood loss, but then can rapidly decline into hypvolemic shock and the "triad of death" (acidosis, hypothermia, and coagulopathy).

2. The orthopaedic surgeon should assume that complete recovery from other injuries (including head injuries) will occur, as many children make excellent recoveries from such injuries.

3. In a child without a head injury, the acute onset of mental status changes, tachypnea, tachycardia, and hypoxemia are classic for fat embolism syndrome.

Open Fractures

1. Prompt administration of intravenous antibiotics is the most important factor in decreasing the rate of infection following open fractures.

2. Routine wound cultures are misleading and should not be performed in the absence of clinical signs of infection.

Fractures of the Shoulder and Humeral Shaft

1. Obstetric clavicle fractures are frequently associated with brachial plexus palsies.

2. The medial clavicular physis is the last physis in the body to close, at age 23 to 25 years.

3. Posteriorly displaced medial clavicle fractures can impinge on the mediastinal structures, including the great vessels and trachea.

4. Proximal humerus fractures have tremendous remodeling potential, so surgery is rarely needed.

5. With fractures of the humeral shaft, primary radial nerve palsies should be observed; however, secondary radial nerve palsies require urgent exploration.

Fractures of the Elbow and Nursemaid's Elbow

1. A pulseless, well-perfused hand may be observed following SCH fracture because of the excellent collateral circulation around the elbow.

2. Injury to the anterior interosseous nerve is the most common nerve injury associated with SCH fractures.

3. Ulnar nerve injury with SCH fractures is almost always iatrogenic and is due to medial pin insertion. The risk is greatest if the medial pin is inserted with the elbow in a hyperflexed position.

4. Cubitus varus (gunstock deformity) after treatment of SCH is generally a cosmetic deformity with few functional consequences. Tardy ulnar nerve palsy is rare.

5. The oblique radiograph is the most sensitive for detecting maximal displacement of lateral condyle fractures and must be obtained when contemplating closed treatment.

6. During open reduction of lateral condyle fractures, posterior soft-tissue dissection must be avoided to avoid osteonecrosis.

7. The only absolute indication for surgical treatment of medial epicondyle fractures is entrapment of the medial condyle within the joint.

8. Elbow dislocations in young children are exceedingly rare, so transphyseal fractures should be suspected in patients with displacement of the proximal radius and ulna relative to the humerus. Elbow arthrography or MRI may be performed to confirm the diagnosis if the diagnosis is unclear.

9. To diagnose nursemaid's elbow, the classic position of elbow extension and forearm pronation should be sought. If the classic history and positioning are absent, then radiographs should be obtained before manipulation.

Fractures of the Forearm, Wrist, and Hand

1. With forearm fractures, bayonet apposition is acceptable in children younger than 10 years of age.

2. Isolated radial head dislocations almost never occur in children. These presumed "isolated" injuries are almost always the result of plastic deformation of the ulna with concomitant radial head dislocation (Monteggia fracture).

3. Closed treatment is often successful in pediatric Monteggia fractures (unlike in adults).

4. Late treatment of Monteggia fractures has far worse results than does acute treatment, so a delayed or missed diagnosis must be avoided.

5. Reduction loss and malunion are much higher for distal radius fractures with a concomitant elbow fracture. These rates can be minimized with internal fixation of the distal radius fracture.

6. With distal forearm physeal fractures, to minimize the risk of iatrogenic physeal injury, no more than one or two reduction attempts should be performed in the emergency department, and rereduction should not be performed more than 5 to 7 days after injury.

7. Distal pole fractures of the scaphoid are common in children and uniformly do well, though scaphoid waist fractures, particularly in adolescents, have poorer outcomes and may result in osteonecrosis and/or nonunion.

8. With metacarpal fractures, check for lacerations over the knuckles ("fight bites" or "clenched-fist injuries"), which are indicative of open injuries.

9. Intra-articular physeal fractures of the phalanges generally require surgery.

Bibliography

Kay RM, Skaggs DL: Pediatric polytrauma management. *J Pediatr Orthop* 2006;26:268-277.

Noonan KJ, Price CT: Forearm and distal radius fractures in children. *J Am Acad Orthop Surg* 1998;6:146-156.

Ring D, Jupiter JB, Waters PM: Monteggia fractures in children and adults. *J Am Acad Orthop Surg* 1998;6:215-224.

Skaggs DL: Elbow fractures in children: Diagnosis and management. *J Am Acad Orthop Surg* 1997;5:303-312.

Sponseller PD: Injuries of the arm and elbow, in Sponseller PD (ed): *OKU Pediatrics 2*. Rosemont, IL, American Academy of Orthopaedic Surgeons, 2002, pp 93-107.

Sponseller PD, Paidas C: Management of the pediatric trauma patient, in Sponseller PD (ed): *Orthopaedic Knowledge Update: Pediatrics 2*. Rosemont, IL, American Academy of Orthopaedic Surgeons, 2002, pp 73-79.

Stewart DG, Kay RM, Skaggs DL: Open fractures in children: Principles of evaluation and management. *J Bone Joint Surg Am* 2005;87:2784-2798.

Sullivan JA: Fractures of the lateral condyle of the humerus. *J Am Acad Orthop Surg* 2006;14:58-62.

3: Pediatrics

Chapter 26

Pediatric Pelvic and Lower Extremity Fractures and Child Abuse

Robert M. Kay, MD

I. Pelvic Fractures

A. Evaluation—Approximately half of all pelvic fractures identified on CT scan are not identified on plain AP pelvis radiographs.

B. Classification

1. The most common classification systems used for pelvic fractures are the Tile classification system and the Torode and Zieg classification system.

   a. Tile classification

      i. Type A—stable

      ii. Type B—rotationally unstable but vertically stable

      iii. Type C—rotationally and vertically unstable

   b. Torode and Zieg classification

      i. Type I—avulsions

      ii. Type II—iliac wing fractures

      iii. Type III—simple ring fractures without segmental instability

      iv. Type IV—ring disruptions with segmental instability

2. Regardless of the classification system used, it is essential to determine whether the pelvic fracture is stable.

C. Treatment

1. Nonsurgical—Good results can be expected from nonsurgical treatment of almost all pediatric pelvic fractures with bed rest and bed-to-chair transfers for 3 to 4 weeks, followed by progressive weight bearing.

2. Surgical indications

   a. Rapid application of an external fixator is occasionally indicated to close down the volume of the pelvis in open book injuries.

   b. Surgery is most commonly indicated in adolescents with vertically unstable injuries or significantly displaced acetabular fractures.

D. Complications—Malunion and nonunion are extremely rare, though limb-length discrepancy may occur in vertically unstable fractures.

II. Avulsion Fractures of the Pelvis

A. Epidemiology—These fractures typically occur in adolescent athletes involved in explosive-type activities (such as sprinting, jumping, and/or kicking). The most common avulsion sites (and the causative muscles) are the ischium (because of the hamstring/adductor muscles), the anterior superior iliac spine (sartorius), the anterior inferior iliac spine (rectus femoris), the iliac crest (abdominals), and the lesser trochanter (iliopsoas).

B. Treatment

1. Nonsurgical—Treatment is with local measures, including rest, ice, and anti-inflammatory medication for 2 to 3 weeks. Activities are then resumed gradually.

2. Surgical—Surgery is almost never indicated for these injuries, although it may be considered for symptomatic nonunions.

C. Complications—There are few, if any, long-term sequelae of these injuries.

III. Hip Fractures

A. Classification—The Delbet classification is used most commonly for these fractures (**Figure 1**).

1. Type I—transphyseal

2. Type II—transcervical

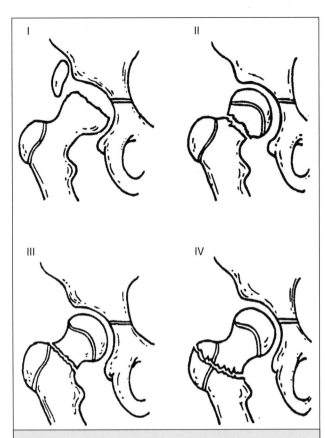

Figure 1 The Delbet classification of pediatric hip fractures. Type I fractures are physeal fractures; type II, transcervical; type III, cervicotrochanteric; and type IV, intertrochanteric. *(Reproduced with permission from Hughes LO, Beaty JH: Fractures of the head and neck of the femur in children. J Bone Joint Surg Am 1994;76:283-292.)*

3. Type III—cervicotrochanteric

4. Type IV—intertrochanteric

B. Treatment

1. Nonsurgical—Nonsurgical treatment is rarely indicated because of the increased risks of coxa vara and nonunion with closed treatment.

2. Surgical procedures

 a. When feasible, closed treatment and internal fixation is preferred.

 b. Decompression of the intracapsular hematoma by aspiration or arthrotomy has been advocated by some to decrease the risk of osteonecrosis (ON); however, the supporting data are equivocal.

 c. Fixation

  i. When possible, fixation should not cross the physis.

  ii. Fixation is with Kirschner wires (K-wires) or cannulated screws for Delbet type I frac-

tures, cannulated screws for type II and III fractures, and a pediatric hip screw or dynamic hip screw for type IV fractures.

C. Complications

1. Osteonecrosis is the most common, and most devastating, complication and is directly related to fracture level. The risk of ON is 90% to 100% for type I fractures, 50% for type II fractures, 25% for type III fractures, and 10% for type IV fractures.

2. Coxa vara and nonunion are much more common after nonsurgically treated fractures, particularly for Delbet II and III fractures.

3. Limb-length discrepancy is common after hip fractures in young children because the proximal femoral physis accounts for approximately 15% of total leg length.

IV. Femoral Shaft Fractures

A. Epidemiology

1. Child abuse is the cause of the vast majority of femur fractures before walking age.

2. Although abuse must be considered in children up to 5 years of age, it is a less common cause of femur fractures after walking age.

B. Treatment

1. Nonsurgical

 a. Spica casting is routinely performed in children younger than 6 years. This may be either immediate spica casting or traction followed by delayed spica casting.

 b. When skeletal traction is used, it should be inserted into the distal femur rather than into the proximal tibia. (Proximal tibial traction pins risk damage to the tibial tubercle apophysis with resultant genu recurvatum.)

 c. Shortening exceeding 2.5 to 3.0 cm is a relative contraindication and multiple trauma is an absolute contraindication to immediate spica casting.

2. Surgical treatment

 a. Indications—Most children older than 6 years are treated surgically, as are many younger multiple trauma patients.

 b. Procedures

  i. Flexible intramedullary (IM) rodding is the treatment of choice for the vast majority of pediatric femoral shaft fractures. Comminuted or very distal or proximal fractures are harder to control with IM rods. Complication rates are higher in children > 10 years of age.

ii. External fixation has become less popular over the past 10 years. External fixation may be used for comminuted or segmental fractures. It has higher rates of delayed union and refracture than other forms of fixation.

iii. Open plating of femoral shaft fractures is rarely used in most centers because of the increased dissection required, the increased blood loss, the desire to avoid load-bearing implants, and the presence of multiple stress risers following hardware removal.

iv. Submuscular bridge plating is becoming increasingly popular, especially for comminuted femoral shaft fractures. Insufficient data are currently available to assess outcomes accurately. Drawbacks for these devices are that they are load-bearing, there are many stress risers in the femoral shaft following hardware removal, and there is a significant learning curve.

v. Antegrade, rigid femoral nails are indicated in children with closed proximal femoral physes. In children with open physes, the risk of ON is up to 1% to 2%.

vi. Trochanteric entry nails are gaining in popularity for larger children (most commonly those older than 10 years and those with extensive comminution). These nails appear to cause abnormalities of proximal femoral growth (resulting in a narrow femoral neck), and the risk of ON is unknown.

C. Complications

1. Limb-length discrepancy

a. Typically 7 to 10 mm of ipsilateral overgrowth occurs in children who sustain a femur fracture between the ages of 2 and 10 years.

b. Limb-length discrepancy may occur as a result of either excessive overgrowth or excessive shortening at the time of fracture healing following cast treatment.

2. Malunion

a. Angular malunion is typically due to varus and/or procurvatum deformity, is unusual following surgical treatment, and can be minimized following spica treatment by careful technique.

b. Torsional malunion is common but rarely of clinical consequence.

3. Refracture is most common following external fixation and typically occurs following fixator removal. Refracture is most common following transverse or short oblique fractures.

4. Delayed union and nonunion are typically seen only after surgical treatment and are much more common when load-bearing devices (external fixators or plates) are used.

5. ON of the femoral head has been reported following rigid antegrade nailing of femoral fractures in skeletally immature individuals with both piriformis fossa and trochanteric nail entry points.

V. Distal Femur Fractures

A. Distal femoral metaphyseal fractures

1. Nonsurgical treatment—Casting suffices for the vast majority of low-energy insufficiency fractures in children with neuromuscular disease.

2. Surgical treatment—For displaced fractures, surgical treatment (with closed reduction and pinning) is almost always indicated. The physis should be avoided, if possible.

3. Complications—Malunion is the most common complication following displaced fractures because accurate assessment of coronal plane alignment is difficult following casting.

B. Distal femoral physeal fractures

1. Classification—The Salter-Harris classification is used to describe these fractures.

2. Nonsurgical treatment is indicated for nondisplaced Salter-Harris I and II fractures.

3. Surgical treatment

a. Indications—Surgical care is indicated for displaced fractures of the distal femoral physis.

b. Procedures

i. Closed reduction and internal fixation is appropriate for most of these fractures, although open reduction and internal fixation (ORIF) may be needed for irreducible fractures.

ii. Fixation avoids the physis when possible. When fixation must cross the physis, smooth K-wires are used and should be removed by 3 to 4 weeks after surgery.

4. Complications

a. Popliteal artery injury and compartment syndrome are rare but are more likely when the epiphysis displaces anteriorly.

b. Growth arrest occurs in ~30% to 50% of distal femoral physeal injuries.

3: Pediatrics

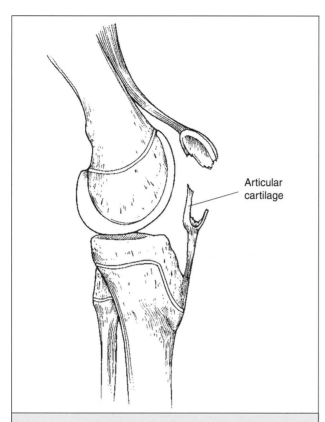

Articular
cartilage

Figure 2 Lateral view of a patellar sleeve fracture. The only sign on plain radiographs may be patella alta. *(Adapted with permission from Tolo VT: Fractures and dislocations around the knee, in Green NE, Swiontkowski MF (eds): Skeletal Trauma in Children. Philadelphia, PA, WB Saunders, 1994, vol 3, pp 369-395.)*

  i. Sequelae of distal femoral physeal fractures include limb-length discrepancy and angular deformity.

  ii. These sequelae are often severe because of the rapid growth of the distal femur.

VI. Patellar Fractures

A. Evaluation—Bipartite patella is a normal variant that occurs in up to 5% of knees. It differs from a patellar fracture in two ways.

  1. Typically a bipartite patella has rounded borders.

  2. It is located superolaterally.

B. Classification

  1. Fractures are generally categorized based on location, fracture configuration, and the amount of displacement (if any).

  2. Patellar sleeve fractures are a relatively common type of pediatric patellar fracture in which a

chondral "sleeve" of the patella separates from the main portion of the patella and ossific nucleus. The only finding on plain radiographs may be apparent patella alta for distal fractures (**Figure 2**) or patella baja for proximal fractures, so these fractures are often missed on initial presentation.

C. Treatment

  1. Nonsurgical—Nonsurgical treatment is indicated for nondisplaced and minimally displaced fractures in children without a knee extensor lag.

  2. Surgical

    a. Indications

      i. Surgical fixation is generally performed for fractures displaced >2 mm at the articular surface. The indication for surgery is confirmed by an extensor lag or the inability to actively extend the knee.

      ii. Patellar sleeve fractures require surgery.

    b. Procedures

      i. For osseous fractures, fixation (as in adults) with tension banding is indicated. A cerclage wire may be needed for extensively comminuted fractures.

      ii. For patellar sleeve fractures, repair of the torn medial and lateral retinaculum along with the use of sutures through the cartilaginous and osseous portions of the patella generally suffice.

VII. Tibia and Fibula Fractures

A. Tibial spine fractures

  1. Evaluation—Children with fractures of the tibial spine present with a mechanism consistent with an anterior cruciate ligament (ACL) tear and an acutely unstable knee. Although it is the result of avulsion of the ACL insertion (rather than a tear in the ACL itself), the presentation and physical examination are comparable to those following a ligamentous ACL tear.

  2. Classification—The Meyers and McKeever classification (**Figure 3**) is used to categorize these fractures: type I, minimally displaced; type II, hinged with displacement of the anterior portion; and type III, completely displaced.

  3. Nonsurgical treatment—Closed reduction and casting suffices for type I and some type II fractures. For type II fractures, the reduction must be within a few millimeters of anatomic to accept closed treatment. The optimal amount of knee flexion for reduction is controversial, though gen-

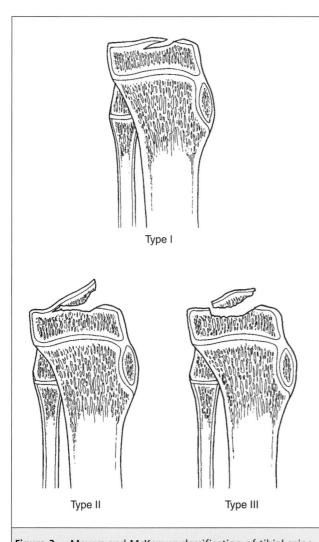

Figure 3   Meyers and McKeever classification of tibial spine fractures. *(Adapted with permission from Tolo VT: Fractures and dislocations around the knee, in Green NE, Swiontkowski MF (eds): Skeletal Trauma in Children. Philadelphia, PA, WB Saunders, 1994, pp 369-395.)*

erally recommended to be 0° to 20°. Arthrocentesis may be needed before casting if there is a large hemarthrosis.

   4. Surgical treatment

      a. Indications—Type II fractures that do not reduce with casting and type III fractures are treated surgically.

      b. Procedures—ORIF and arthroscopic reduction and internal fixation are both effective, and fixation with sutures and/or screws should avoid the physis. The meniscus is often entrapped and must be moved to allow for reduction.

   5. Complications

      a. ACL laxity is common, but it is generally not clinically significant.

      b. Malunion with persistent elevation of the fracture fragment may result in impingement in the notch.

B. Proximal tibial physeal fractures

   1. Classification—The Salter-Harris classification is used to categorize these fractures (**Figure 4**).

   2. Nonsurgical treatment

      a. Nondisplaced fractures account for 30% to 50% of Salter-Harris I and II fractures.

      b. Nondisplaced fractures may be treated with cast immobilization.

   3. Surgical treatment

      a. Indications—Closed (or open) reduction and internal fixation should be performed for displaced fractures.

      b. Procedures

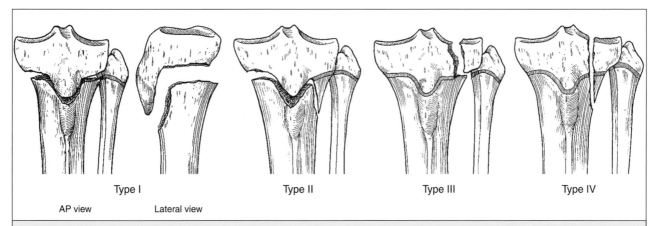

Figure 4   Salter-Harris fractures of the proximal tibial physis. *(Adapted with permission from Hensinger RN (ed): Operative Management of Lower Extremity Fractures in Children. Park Ridge, IL, American Academy of Orthopaedic Surgeons, 1992, p 49.)*

3: Pediatrics

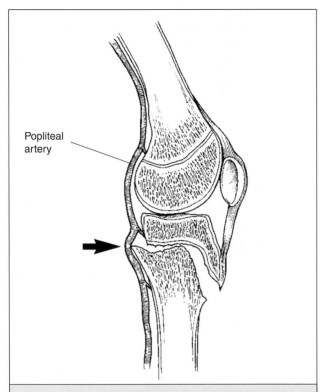

Figure 5 Lateral view of the knee depicting the potential for popliteal artery injury due to proximal tibial physeal fracture. *(Adapted with permission from Tolo VT: Fractures and dislocations around the knee, in Green NE, Swiontkowski MF (eds): Skeletal Trauma in Children. Philadelphia, PA, WB Saunders, 1994, pp 369-395.)*

Popliteal artery

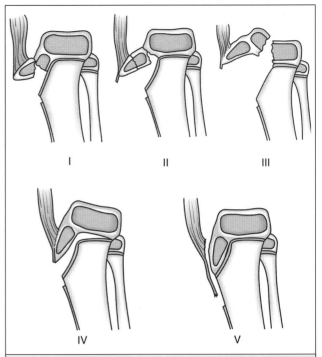

Figure 6 Classification of tibial tubercle injuries. Types I through IV are true fractures, while type V is actually a soft-tissue injury with detachment of the periosteal sleeve.

    i. For most Salter-Harris I and II fractures, fixation is with crossed smooth K-wires, which are removed by 3 to 4 weeks after surgery.

    ii. For Salter-Harris III and IV fractures (and Salter-Harris II fractures with large metaphyseal fragments), cannulated screws parallel to the physis are indicated.

4. Complications

    a. Popliteal artery injuries (~5%), compartment syndrome (~3% to 4%), and peroneal nerve injury (5%) are relatively common. Vascular complications are particularly common with hyperextension injuries (**Figure 5**).

    b. Redisplacement of the fracture is common for displaced fractures treated without internal fixation.

    c. Growth arrest occurs in 25% of patients and can result in limb-length discrepancy and/or angular deformity.

C. Proximal tibial metaphyseal fractures

1. Classification—No specific classification is used for these fractures.

2. Nonsurgical treatment—Nonsurgical treatment (with a long-leg cast) is the mainstay of treatment of low-energy injuries in children younger than 10 years.

3. Surgical treatment—Surgery is generally necessary for high-energy proximal tibia fractures in older children because these fractures are often significantly displaced and unstable.

4. Complications

    a. For low-energy injuries (so-called Cozen fractures), the most common complication is genu valgum in the first 6 to 12 months after fracture that is due to medial proximal tibial overgrowth. No treatment is needed for this acutely because most of these deformities improve spontaneously.

    b. For high-energy fractures in older children, neurovascular damage, compartment syndrome, and malunion may occur.

D. Tibial tubercle fractures

1. Classification—The classification has evolved since Watson-Jones first described three types of fractures. The current classification is shown in **Figure 6**.

2. Nonsurgical treatment is rarely indicated, but it may be used in children with minimally displaced fractures (<2 mm) and no extensor lag.

3. Surgical treatment

a. Indications—Most children with these fractures require surgery. The only exceptions are those with minimally displaced fractures and no extensor lag.

b. Procedures—Surgery is via ORIF with screws for fracture types I through IV. For type III fractures, the joint must be visualized to accurately reduce the joint surface and to assess for meniscal injury. For type V fractures, the periosteal sleeve is reattached with suture, and this may be supplemented with small screws.

4. Complications—Compartment syndrome and genu recurvatum are both rare.

E. Tibial shaft fractures

1. Nonsurgical treatment

a. Most tibia fractures in children can be treated with reduction and casting.

b. Healing takes 3 to 4 weeks for toddler fractures and 6 to 8 weeks for other tibial fractures.

2. Surgical treatment

a. Indications include open fractures, marked soft-tissue injury, unstable fractures, multiple trauma, >1 cm of shortening, and unacceptable closed reduction (>10° of angulation).

b. Fixation options include external fixation, intramedullary rod fixation, percutaneous pins or plates.

3. Complications

a. When closed reduction is lost, it is typically due to a drift into varus for isolated tibial fractures and into valgus for combined tibia and fibula fractures.

b. Delayed union and nonunion are almost never seen in closed fractures but are more common following external fixation.

c. Compartment syndrome, although relatively uncommon, can occur with open or closed fractures.

VIII. Ankle Fractures

A. Classification

1. An anatomic classification system is most typically used for ankle fractures. The Salter-Harris classification is commonly used for physeal fractures.

2. A mechanistic classification system (typically, the Dias-Tachdjian classification) may be used. The Dias-Tachdjian classification is patterned after the Lauge-Hansen categorization of adult fractures and describes four main mechanisms: supination-inversion, supination–plantar flexion, supination–external rotation, and pronation/eversion–external rotation.

B. Distal tibial physeal fractures

1. Salter-Harris I and II fractures

a. Closed treatment suffices for most of these fractures. To minimize the risk of iatrogenic physeal injury, no more than one or two attempts at reduction should be made in the emergency department. Acceptable reduction is to within 2 to 3 mm of anatomic alignment and <10° of angulation.

b. Open treatment may be needed for irreducible fractures (usually the result of interposed periosteum, tendons, or neurovascular structures). Hardware is rarely needed following open reduction.

c. Complications—Physeal injury with growth arrest and angular deformity and/or limb-length discrepancy is rare in these fractures.

2. Salter-Harris III fractures

a. Overview—Medial malleolus and Tillaux fractures are the most common Salter-Harris III ankle fractures.

b. Pathoanatomy

i. Tillaux fractures (**Figure 7**) are Salter-Harris III fractures of the anterolateral tibial epiphysis that occur with supination–external rotation injuries.

ii. Tillaux fractures (as well as triplane fractures) occur in this location because the distal tibial physis closes centrally, then medially, and then laterally.

c. Closed treatment suffices for most minimally displaced fractures. A postreduction CT is used to confirm that there is less than 2 mm of joint step-off and fracture diastasis.

d. Open treatment is indicated when there is >2 mm of displacement based on postreduction CT. Percutaneous manipulation with a K-wire may aid in reduction. Fixation is with one or two cannulated screws. Ideally, the screws are inserted parallel to the physis.

e. Complications

i. Joint incongruity is a risk, as with any Salter-Harris III physeal fracture.

ii. The risk of physeal arrest is less when reduction within 2 mm of anatomic alignment is obtained.

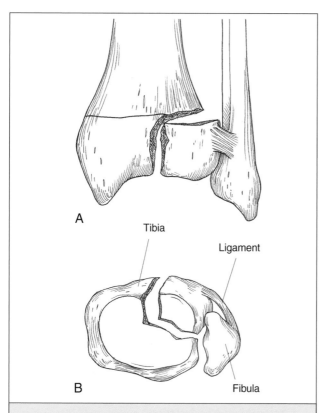

Figure 7   Tillaux fracture as seen from anterior (**A**) and inferior (**B**). The anterolateral fragment is avulsed by the anterior inferior tibiofibular ligament. *(Part A adapted with permission from Weber BG, Sussenbach F: Malleolar fractures, in Weber BG, Brunner C, Freuler F (eds): Treatment of Fractures in Children and Adolescents. New York, NY, Springer-Verlag, 1980.)*

3. Salter-Harris IV fractures

   a. Medial malleolus shear fractures

      i. Closed treatment—Closed reduction and casting suffices for minimally displaced fractures.

      ii. Open treatment—Open treatment is indicated for fractures displaced >2 mm following reduction. ORIF (with 2 epiphyseal screws) is required for the vast majority of these fractures to optimize joint and physeal alignment (and minimize the risk of growth arrest).

      iii. Complications—Medial malleolar Salter-Harris IV fractures have the highest rate of growth disturbance of any ankle fracture.

   b. Triplane fractures

      i. Pathoanatomy—Triplane fractures (**Figure 8**) are Salter-Harris IV fractures that include an anterolateral fragment of the distal tibial epiphysis (as in a Tillaux fracture) in conjunction with a metaphyseal fracture. These may be 2- or 3-part fractures.

      ii. Closed treatment—Closed reduction and casting suffices for minimally displaced fractures. Postreduction CT is used to confirm <2 mm of joint step-off and fracture diastasis.

      iii. Open treatment—Open treatment is indicated for fractures with >2 mm of displacement based on postreduction CT. Fixation is

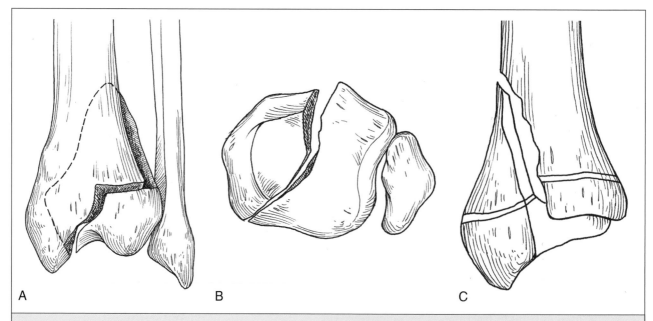

Figure 8   A two-part lateral triplane fracture as seen from anterior (**A**) and inferior (**B**). *(Adapted with permission from Jarvis JG: Tibial triplane fractures, in Letts RM (ed): Management of Pediatric Fractures. Philadelphia, PA: Churchill Livingstone, 1994, p 739.)* **C,** A two-part medial triplane fracture. *(Adapted with permission from Rockwood CA Jr, Wilkins KE, King RE: Fractures in Children. Philadelphia, PA, JB Lippincott, 1984, p 933.)*

with one or two cannulated screws (ideally, parallel to the physis); the screws may cross the physis (if necessary) once distal tibial physeal closure has begun. Comminuted and/or high fibula fractures may require concomitant fixation in children with high-energy injuries.

iv. Complications—Joint incongruity is a risk, as with any Salter-Harris IV physeal fracture. Ankle pain and degenerative changes are both relatively common, especially in those fractures not reduced within 2 mm of anatomic alignment.

4. Salter-Harris V fractures appear to be Salter-Harris I fractures on initial presentation and are noted to be type V fractures only retrospectively, when the child presents with a growth arrest and limb-length discrepancy.

C. Distal fibula fractures

1. Isolated distal fibula fractures

   a. Epidemiology

      i. Isolated distal fibula fractures are very common after inversion ankle injuries and are almost exclusively Salter-Harris I and II fractures.

      ii. These fractures are much more common than ankle sprains following an ankle inversion injury in a child.

   b. Treatment—Closed treatment with a short-leg walking cast for 3 weeks is typical for Salter-Harris I and II fractures, but for the very rare Salter-Harris III and IV fractures, surgical fixation may be necessary.

   c. Complications are rare for distal fibula physeal fractures, and growth disturbance occurs in <1%. Complex regional pain syndrome should be considered if the pain does not resolve promptly with appropriate treatment.

2. Distal fibula fractures associated with tibia fractures

   a. These fractures are reduced in conjunction with the tibia fracture.

   b. ORIF may be needed in cases of high fibula fracture and/or severe comminution in a child approaching skeletal maturity.

IX. Foot Fractures

A. Pathoanatomy—Accessory ossicles in the foot (Figure 9) are common and must be differentiated from acute injuries.

B. Talar fractures and dislocations

1. Overview

   a. Most talar fractures are avulsion fractures.

   b. Talar neck and body fractures are generally high-energy injuries, with falls from a height and motor vehicle accidents accounting for 70% to 90%.

2. Classification

   a. Talar fractures are categorized as avulsion fractures, talar neck fractures, or talar body fractures. Osteochondral lesions are considered fractures by some authors.

   b. Talar neck fractures are classified by the Hawkins classification (as are adult fractures) (Table 1).

3. Nonsurgical treatment is indicated for nondisplaced talar neck and body fractures, and closed reduction should be attempted for displaced fractures. Because talar neck fractures are dorsiflexion injuries, these fractures are generally most stable in plantar flexion.

4. Surgical treatment—Although surgical indications are not well defined, surgery should be considered for displaced intra-articular talar fractures.

5. Complications—Chronic pain and ON are common following talar neck and body fractures. ON risk is highest for Hawkins III and IV injuries and lowest for type I injuries.

C. Calcaneus fractures

1. Classification—Although a variety of classification schema have been described, the most important distinctions are whether the fracture is intra- or extra-articular and whether the fracture is displaced.

2. Nonsurgical treatment is the mainstay of treatment of pediatric calcaneal fractures because of relatively favorable results and potential calcaneal remodeling.

3. Surgical treatment is often indicated in adolescent children with displaced intra-articular calcaneal fractures.

D. Other tarsal fractures

1. Avulsion fractures of the navicular, cuneiforms, and cuboid are the most common type of fracture and are generally low-energy injuries. Treatment is with a walking cast for 2 to 3 weeks; the results are excellent.

2. Displaced fractures of the navicular, cuneiforms, and cuboid are generally high-energy injuries, with high rates of associated injuries and compartment syndrome. ORIF is generally required.

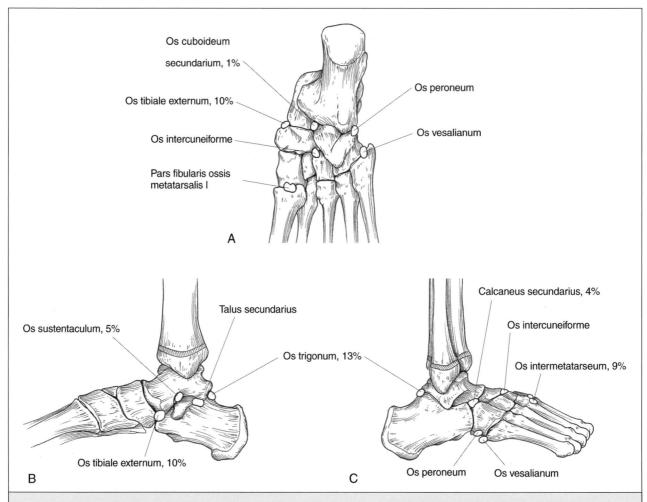

Figure 9 Accessory ossicles of the foot and their frequency of occurrence (when data are available) as viewed from the plantar **(A)**, medial **(B)**, and lateral **(C)** aspects of the foot. *(Adapted with permission from Tachdijian MO (ed): Pediatric Orthopedics, ed 2. Philadelphia, PA, WB Saunders, 1990, p 471.)*

Table 1

Hawkins Classification of Talar Neck Fractures

Hawkins Type	Talar Fracture	Subluxated or Dislocated Joint(s)
I	Nondisplaced	None
II	Displaced	Subtalar
III	Displaced	Subtalar and tibiotalar
IV	Displaced	Talonavicular and subtalar and/or tibiotalar

E. Lisfranc injuries

  1. Treatment

    a. Closed treatment is indicated for nondisplaced fractures and is attempted for displaced fractures (often with the aid of finger traps).

    b. Fixation in adolescents is with cannulated screws and in younger children with smooth K-wires.

  2. Complications—Compartment syndrome and chronic pain are both common and often result in poor outcomes.

F. Metatarsal fractures

  1. Classification—There is no specific classification system for most metatarsal fractures.

  2. Treatment

    a. Nonsurgical treatment suffices for most metatarsal fractures. Weight bearing is allowed for almost all such fractures; one exception is a fifth metatarsal base fracture at or distal to the metaphyseal-diaphyseal junction.

    b. Surgical—The rare indications for surgical intervention include:

      i. Marked displacement of the metatarsal head in the sagittal plane

ii. Fractures of the fifth metatarsal distal to the metaphyseal-diaphyseal junction that fail closed treatment

3. Complications—Complications are rare, though delayed union or nonunion are relatively common for fifth metatarsal base fractures distal to the metaphyseal-diaphyseal junction.

G. Phalangeal fractures

1. Treatment

a. Nonsurgical treatment suffices for almost all phalangeal fractures.

b. Surgical—The few indications for surgical intervention include:

i. Open fractures

ii. Significantly displaced intra-articular fractures

2. Complications—Complications are rare, although growth arrest may occasionally occur following a physeal fracture of the great toe.

H. Occult foot fractures

1. General

a. Occult foot fractures are a common cause of limp in preschool-age children.

b. If a child crawls without difficulty but limps or refuses to weightbear when standing, the pathology is distal to the knee.

2. Evaluation

a. Radiographs are typically negative.

b. Bone scans (although rarely necessary) will show increased uptake in the affected tarsal bones.

3. Treatment is with a short-leg walking cast for 2 to 3 weeks. If the child does not feel better within days of cast application, another source of pain should be sought.

X. Child Abuse

A. Evaluation

1. Child abuse should be suspected in the following circumstances:

a. Any fracture before walking age

b. Multiple injuries in a child without a witnessed and reasonable explanation

c. Multiple injuries in a child <2 years

d. A child with long-bone injury(ies) and a head injury

2. Corner fractures (seen at the junction of the metaphysis and physis) and posterior rib fractures are essentially pathognomonic for nonaccidental trauma, but isolated, transverse long-bone fractures are actually more common.

3. A skeletal survey must be obtained in all children suspected of child abuse to rule out other fractures of differing ages (including examination for skull and rib fractures).

4. Thorough examination of the child by nonorthopaedists is necessary to rule out other evidence of abuse, including skin bruising (especially bruises of different ages) or scarring, retinal hemorrhages, intracranial bleeds, or evidence of sexual abuse.

B. Treatment

1. Reporting of suspected child abuse is mandatory.

a. The orthopaedic surgeon is protected from litigation when reporting cases of suspected abuse.

b. Failure to report suspected abuse puts the abused child at a 50% risk of repeat abuse and up to a 10% risk of being killed.

2. Many fractures are sufficiently healed at the time of presentation to the orthopaedic surgeon that they do not require treatment.

Bibliography

Flynn JM, Schwend RM: Management of pediatric femoral shaft fractures. *J Am Acad Orthop Surg* 2004;12:347-359.

Flynn JM, Skaggs DL, Sponseller PD, Ganley TJ, Kay RM, Leitch KK: The surgical management of pediatric fractures of the lower extremity. *Instr Course Lect* 2003;52:647-659.

Gray DW: Trauma to the hip and femur in children, in Sponseller PD (ed): *OKU Pediatrics 2*. Rosemont, IL, American Academy of Orthopaedic Surgeons, 2002, pp 81-91.

Kay RM, Matthys GA: Pediatric ankle fractures: Evaluation and treatment. *J Am Acad Orthop Surg* 2001;9:268-278.

Kay RM, Tang CW: Pediatric foot fractures: Evaluation and treatment. *J Am Acad Orthop Surg* 2001;9:308-319.

Kocher MS, Kasser JR: Orthopaedic aspects of child abuse. *J Am Acad Orthop Surg* 2000;8:10-20.

Zionts LE: Fractures around the knee in children. *J Am Acad Orthop Surg* 2002;10:345-355.

3: Pediatrics

Top Testing Facts

Fractures of the Pelvis, Hip, and Femur

1. Plain AP pelvis radiographs fail to identify about half of all pediatric pelvic fractures found on CT scan.

2. Most pediatric pelvic fractures can be treated nonsurgically with good results.

3. The rate of ON of the hip is inversely related to the Delbet fracture category (90% to 100% for type I fractures, 50% for type II, 25% for type III, and 10% for type IV).

4. Surgical fixation of hip fractures (particularly Delbet II and III fractures) significantly decreases the risks of coxa vara and nonunion.

5. Child abuse is by far the most common reason for a femoral shaft fracture in a child younger than 1 year. Child abuse can also be causative in children up to 5 years of age.

6. Spica casting for femoral shaft fractures is appropriate for most children younger than 6 years.

7. Surgical treatment of femoral shaft fractures is indicated for most children older than 6 years.

8. Femoral overgrowth of 7 to 10 mm is typical in children who sustain a femoral shaft fracture between the ages of 2 and 10 years.

9. Most displaced distal femoral metaphyseal fractures are treated surgically to prevent malunion.

10. Distal femoral physeal fractures have a worse prognosis than other physeal fractures because of the high rate of growth arrest (up to 50%) and the rapid growth of the distal femur.

11. Fixation should be used for all displaced fractures of the distal femoral physis to minimize the risk of redisplacement.

Fractures of the Knee

1. Bipartite patella is seen in up to 5% of knees. Classically, these appear different from patellar fractures because they have rounded borders and are located superolaterally.

2. Patella sleeve fractures are common in children. Radiographs may only only patella alta or baja.

3. Because of the fact that ligaments in children are generally stronger than bone, tibial spine fractures, rather than ACL injuries, often occur in children.

4. An entrapped meniscus often prevents type II tibial spine fractures from reducing closed.

5. Vascular injury and/or compartment syndrome occurs in nearly 10% of patients with fractures of the proximal tibial physis; the risk is highest with hyperextension injury.

6. Proximal tibial metaphyseal fractures in children younger than 10 years typically grow into valgus in the first 6 to 12 months after injury. Observation is indicated in these cases because the genu valgum usually resolves spontaneously.

7. Tibial tubercle fractures may be treated closed only if there is minimal displacement and no extensor lag.

Fractures of the Lower Leg and Foot

1. Isolated tibia fractures tend to drift into varus; combined tibia and fibula fractures tend toward valgus.

2. Medial malleolar Salter-Harris IV fractures have the highest rate of growth arrest of any ankle fracture and often result in varus ankle deformity and limb-length discrepancy.

3. Tillaux fractures and triplane fractures both occur in the anterolateral distal tibial physis because of the order of distal tibial physeal closure (the central portion closes first, then the medial, and finally the lateral).

4. When a child sustains an inversion injury to the ankle, a distal fibula physeal fracture is much more likely than an ankle sprain.

5. Osteonecrosis is common following talar neck and body fractures. The risk is highest for Hawkins IV fractures and lowest in type I injuries.

6. Calcaneal fractures can remodel in children and generally have favorable long-term outcomes, though ORIF may be indicated in adolescents with significantly displaced intra-articular calcaneal fractures.

7. Even in children, long-term outcomes following Lisfranc injuries appear poor.

8. If a child crawls without difficulty but limps or refuses to bear weight when standing, the pathology is below the knee.

9. If a child who is treated for an occult foot fracture does not feel better almost immediately in the cast, another source of pain should be sought.

Child Abuse

1. Reporting of suspected child abuse is mandatory.

2. Many of the findings of child abuse are nonorthopaedic, so involvement of a child abuse team or specialists is requisite.

Chapter 27
Pediatric Spine Conditions

*Scott J. Luhmann, MD   *David L. Skaggs, MD

I. Idiopathic Scoliosis (Infantile/Juvenile/Adolescent)

A. Overview (epidemiology)

1. Definition of idiopathic scoliosis (IS)—A coronal plane deformity of >10° (by Cobb method) with no known cause.

2. Normal thoracic kyphosis is 20° to 45°; normal lumbar lordosis is 30° to 60°.

3. Genetics—Autosomal dominant with variable penetrance.

B. Pathoanatomy

1. Scoliometer measurement >5°

   a. 2% to 5% false-negative rate for curve >20°

   b. 50% false-positive rate for curve <20°

2. Infantile IS can dramatically impair alveolar growth and thoracic cage development, causing significant cardiopulmonary impairment with restrictive lung disease and possibly cor pulmonale.

   a. Growth velocity of the T1-L5 segment is fastest in the first 5 years of life, with the height of the thoracic spine doubling between birth and skeletal maturity.

   b. Male to female ratio is 1:1.

   c. The most common curve location is the thoracic spine; 75% of curves are left convex.

   d. Risk of progression overall is 10%. Curves with apical rib-vertebra angle difference (RVAD), or Mehta angle, >20° (**Figure 1**) and phase 2 apical rib-vertebrae relationship (overlap of the rib head with the apical vertebral body)

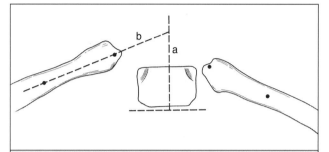

Figure 1   To measure the rib-vertebra angle difference (RVAD), a line is drawn perpendicular to the end plate of the apical vertebrae (a). Next, a line is drawn from the midpoint of the neck of the rib through the midpoint of the head of the rib to the perpendicular on the convex side (b). The resultant angle is calculated. The angle on the concave side is calculated in a similar manner. Concave – convex = RVAD. (*Adapted with permission from Mehta MH: The rib-vertebra angle in the early diagnosis between resolving and progressive infantile scoliosis.* J Bone Joint Surg Br *1972;54:230-243.*)

(**Figure 2**) are at the greatest risk of progression.

   e. 22% of patients with curves ≥20° have neural axis abnormality; approximately 80% of these patients will require neurosurgical care.

3. Juvenile IS

   a. Incidence is higher in females than in males.

   b. Right thoracic curves are most common.

   c. Spontaneous resolution is uncommon.

   d. Curves with RVAD >20° and phase 2 rib-vertebrae relationship are at increased risk of progression.

   e. 95% of curves will progress.

   f. Incidence of neural axis abnormalities is 20% to 25%; hence MRI is necessary.

4. Adolescent IS

   a. Polygenetic interaction is suspected.

   b. Female to male ratio is 1:1 for small curves but increases to 10:1 for curves >30°.

   c. Risk of progression is related to curve size and

Scott J. Luhmann, MD, is a consultant or employee of Stryker and Medtronic. David L. Skaggs, MD, or the department with which he is affiliated has received research or institutional support and miscellaneous nonincome support, commercially derived honoraria, or other non–research-related funding from Medtronic and Stryker Spine, and is a consultant or employee for Medtronic and Stryker Spine.

3: Pediatrics

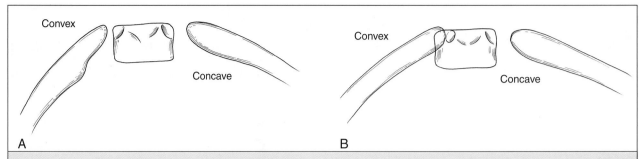

Figure 2   Rib-vertebra relationships. **A,** Phase 1 rib-vertebra relationship demonstrating no overlap of the rib head and vertebral body. **B,** Phase 2 rib-vertebrae relationship. The overlap of the rib head on the vertebral body is indicative of curve progression. (*Adapted with permission from Mehta MH: The rib-vertebra angle in the early diagnosis between resolving and progressive infantile scoliosis. J Bone Joint Surg Br 1972;54:230-243.*)

remaining skeletal growth, which is assessed by Tanner stage, Risser grade, age of menarche, and presence of open triradiate cartilages.

   i. Girls at greatest risk for progression are premenarchal, Risser grade 0, Tanner stage <3, and have open triradiate cartilage.

   ii. Peak height velocity (fastest growth) generally occurs before Risser grade 1.

   iii. Peak height velocity in adolescence is approximately 10 cm/year and occurs just before the onset of menses in girls.

   iv. If the curve is >30° at peak height velocity, the curve is likely to require surgery.

5. Long-term implications of scoliosis are dependent on the size of the curve at skeletal maturity.

   a. Thoracic curves >50° and lumbar curves >40° have been shown to progress up to a mean of 1°/year after skeletal maturity.

   b. Curves >60° can have a negative impact on pulmonary function tests, but symptomatic cardiopulmonary impact traditionally is seen with curves >90°.

   c. With significant curves, a mild increase in the incidence of back pain is likely in adulthood.

C. Evaluation

1. Physical examination

   a. The physical examination should include a detailed neurologic examination of the lower extremities (sensory examination, motor examination, and reflexes).

   b. Skin evaluation should include inspection for café-au-lait spots (neurofibromatosis).

   c. Lower extremity evaluation should rule out cavovarus feet (associated with neural axis abnormalities) and document normal strength, gait, and coordination.

   d. Hairy patches, dimples, nevi, or tumors over the spine may be indicative of spinal dysraphism.

   e. Dimples outside the gluteal fold are generally benign.

   f. Asymmetric abdominal reflexes are associated with a syrinx and are an indication for MRI of the spine.

2. Radiographic evaluation

   a. PA and lateral upright (weight-bearing) views (36-inch cassette) should be obtained.

   b. Bending or traction films are useful for surgical planning.

3. MRI of spine

   a. MRI is used to rule out intraspinal anomalies (tethered cord, syringomyelia, dysraphism, and spinal cord tumor).

   b. Indications

      i. Atypical curve patterns (eg, left thoracic curve, short angular curves, absence of apical thoracic lordosis, absence of rotation and congenital scoliosis)

      ii. Patients <10 years of age with a curve >20°

      iii. Abnormal neurologic finding on examination, abnormal pain, rapid progression of curve (>1°/mo)

   c. Intraspinal anomalies are referred to a neurosurgeon for evaluation.

   d. A syrinx (**Figure 3**) is commonly associated with scoliosis without rotation and an asymmetric umbilicus reflex.

D. Classification

1. Age

   a. Infantile (<3 years of age) represents 4% of IS cases.

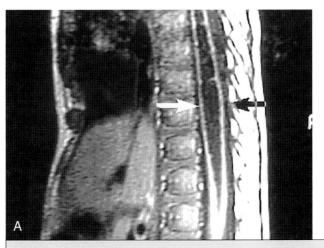 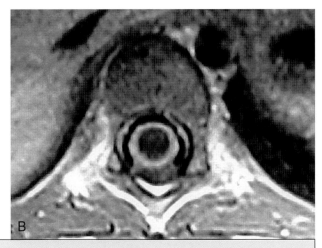

Figure 3 Large syrinx involving the entire spine of a 2-year-old boy. **A,** Sagittal T1-weighted MRI scan shows the syrinx to be largest at the level of the lower thoracic spine (arrows). **B,** Axial T1-weighted image confirms that the syrinx is located within the center of the spinal cord. (*Reproduced from Khanna AJ, Wasserman BA, Sponseller PD: Magnetic resonance imaging of the pediatric spine.* J Am Acad Orthop Surg *2003;11:248-259.*)

Table 1

Lenke Classification of Idiopathic Scoliosis*

Type	Proximal Curve	Main Thoracic	Thoracolumbar/Lumbar	Curve Type
1	Nonstructural	Structural†	Nonstructural	Main Thoracic
2	Structural	Structural†	Nonstructural	Double Thoracic
3	Nonstructural	Structural†	Structural	Double Major
4	Structural	Structural†	Structural	Triple Major
5	Nonstructural	Nonstructural	Structural†	Thoracolumbar/Lumbar
6	Nonstructural	Structural†	Structural†	Thoracolumbar/Lumbar-Main Thoracic

*The Lenke classification system also includes modifiers to describe the associated thoracic sagittal profile and deviation of the apical lumbar vertebra (see Figure 4)
†Major; largest Cobb measurement, always structural
(*Reproduced with permission from Lenke LG, Betz RR, Haher TR, et al: Multisurgeon assessment of surgical decision making in adolescent idiopathic scoliosis: Curve classification, operative approach, and fusion levels.* Spine *2001;26(21):2347-2353.*)

b. Juvenile (3 to 10 years of age) represents 15% of IS cases.

c. Adolescent (>10 years of age) represents 80% of IS cases. Prevalence: 2% to 3% for curves 10° to 20°, 0.3% for curves >30°.

2. Curve location

    a. Cervical (C2 through C6)

    b. Cervicothoracic (C7-T1)

    c. Thoracic (T2-T11/12 disk)

    d. Thoracolumbar (T12-L1)

    e. Lumbar (L1-2 disk through L4)

3. Surgical classification of adolescent idiopathic scoliosis

    a. King-Moe

    b. Lenke classification (**Table 1**) describes six major curve types with modifiers for the lumbar curve and amount of thoracic kyphosis (T5 through T12).

E. Treatment—Recommendations are based on the natural history of scoliosis.

1. Nonsurgical

    a. Infantile: Patients with RVAD >20°, phase 2 rib-vertebrae relationship, and Cobb angle >30° are at high risk of progression (**Figures 1 and 2**). Bracing may be considered when the Cobb angle is >20°, but many curves of this size improve spontaneously, so it is reasonable not to brace until a curve reaches 30°.

    b. Bracing

        i. Bracing is usually started for juveniles with curves >20° and adolescents >25°; smaller curves are treated with observation.

3: Pediatrics

ii. Bracing is used for skeletally immature patients (Risser 0, 1, or 2). Recommended for 16 to 23 h/day and continued until completion of skeletal growth or curve progression to >45° (at which point bracing is no longer considered effective).

iii. The aim of bracing is to halt progression of curve during growth, not to correct scoliosis.

iv. Thoracic hypokyphosis is relative contraindication for bracing.

v. An underarm brace, or thoracolumbosacral orthosis (TLSO), is most effective when the curve apex is at T7 or below.

vi. The efficacy of brace treatment is controversial.

2. Surgical

a. Indications

i. Infantile/juvenile—Cobb >50° to 60°.

ii. Adolescent—Thoracic curves >45° to 50°. Lumbar curves >45° or marked trunk imbalance with curve >40° (relative).

b. Contraindications

i. Patients with active infections

ii. Poor skin at surgical site

iii. Inability to adhere to postoperative activity limitation

iv. Significant concomitant medical comorbidities

c. Procedures

i. Infantile/juvenile—Dual growing rod constructs can permit growth of affected spine up to 5.0 cm over the instrumented levels.

ii. Adolescent—Both anterior and posterior fusions have been reported to be effective in correcting and maintaining correction during the postoperative period. Anterior release has been performed in addition to posterior fusion for large (>70° to 80°), stiff (<50% flexibility index) curves but may not be necessary with newer generation spinal implants. For large, rigid curves, Smith-Petersen osteotomies (Ponte), pedicle subtraction osteotomies, and vertebral column resections can help improve correction and spinal balance. In Risser 0 patients with open triradiate cartilage and Risser 0, anterior diskectomy and fusion has been recommended to avoid the crankshaft phenomenon, although the use of thoracic pedicle screws in this population may obviate the need for anterior fusion.

F. Complications

1. Crankshaft phenomenon

a. Progression of spine deformity after a solid posterior fusion due to continued anterior spinal growth

b. Can be avoided by concomitant anterior spine fusion at the time of posterior fusion

2. Short-term postoperative complications include ileus, syndrome of inappropriate antidiuretic hormone release, atelectasis, pneumonia, and superior mesentertic artery syndrome.

3. Infections occur in up to 5% of patients.

a. Early infection (<6 months after surgery) is treated with irrigation and débridement and antibiotics without removal of implants because fusion is assumed to not have occurred.

b. Chronic deep infections of spinal implants are treated with implant removal and intravenous antibiotics, although progression of deformity over time may occur.

4. Implant failure and pseudarthrosis occur in up to 3% of patients, but this is uncommon in the skeletally immature.

5. Neurologic injury occurs in up to 0.7% of patients as a result of compressive, tensile, or vascular phenomenon. Current recommendations are for intra-operative spinal cord monitoring of somatosensory-evoked potentials (SSEPs) and neurogenic motor-evoked potentials (MEPs).

6. Decreased pulmonary function has been reported following anterior fusion and posterior thoracoplasty.

a. Thoracoscopic approaches to the thoracic spine have less negative impact on pulmonary function than open thoracotomy.

b. Similarly, open anterior thoracolumbar fusion has less impact than open thoracic fusion.

G. Spinal cord monitoring

1. The current standard of care is spinal cord monitoring using both SSEPs, which will detect many but not all neurologic difficulties, and MEPs, which can detect neurologic injury earlier than SSEPs.

2. Monitoring of the upper extremities with SSEPs can identify positional injury to the upper extremity, which is the most common intraoperative neurologic injury that is reversible.

3. When spinal cord monitoring suggests neurologic injury, either technical problems or real neurologic problems may be responsible.

a. Technical problems

   i. Loose electrodes

   ii. Use of inhalational agents makes MEPS monitoring difficult.

b. Real neurologic problems

   i. If changes occurred following deformity correction, reverse or lessen the correction.

   ii. Raise blood pressure

   iii. If hematocrit is low, give a blood transfusion.

   iv. Give intravenous steroids (eg, solumedrol 30 mg/kg bolus, and 6.5mg/kg × 23 hours).

   v. Administer the wake-up test.

   vi. If all else fails and if the spine is stable, remove instrumentation.

H. Rehabilitation

1. Participating in activities of daily living (ADL) should be encouraged in the early postoperative phase.

2. Besides encouraging ambulation and ADLs, little active physical therapy is indicated.

3. Return to sports is surgeon-dependent.

II. Congenital Scoliosis

A. Overview (epidemiology)

1. Genetics—No specific inheritance pattern; isolated occurrences.

2. Estimated prevalence in general population is 1% to 4%.

B. Pathoanatomy

1. Three categories—failure of formation, failure of segmentation, and mixed (**Figure 4 and Table 2**).

a. Failure of formation—The mildest form is wedge vertebra, followed by a hemivertebra.

   i. Three types of hemivertebrae are fully segmented (disk space present above and below hemivertebra), semisegmented (hemivertebra fused to adjacent vertebra on one side with disk on the other), and unsegmented (hemivertebra fused to vertebra on each side).

   ii. Hemimetameric shift is the presence of contralateral hemivertebrae separated by one normal vertebra.

b. Failure of segmentation—Implies bony bars between vertebrae.

   i. Block vertebrae have bilateral bony bars.

   ii. Unilateral bars cause scoliosis by tethering growth on one side and are thus present at the concavity of the curve.

   iii. A unilateral unsegmented bar associated with a contralateral hemivertebra has the worst prognosis for development of scoliosis.

   iv. The best prognosis is for the block vertebra (bilateral failure of segmentation).

c. The presence of a congenital vertebral anomaly in the thoracolumbar region with fused ribs has a high risk of progression.

d. Incarcerated hemivertebrae do not cause scoliosis because deficiencies above and below the hemivertebrae compensate.

2. Thoracic insufficiency syndrome (TIS)

a. TIS is defined as the inability of the thorax to support normal respiration or lung growth.

b. It is usually associated with significant scoliosis (idiopathic or congenital), a shortened thorax, rib fusions or rib aplasia, or poor rib growth (Jeunes syndrome).

c. Jarcho-Levin syndrome, extensive congenital fusions of the thoracic spine, is a common cause of TIS, with two important subtypes:

   i. Spondylothoracic dysplasia (primarily vertebral involvement)

   ii. Spondylocostal dysplasia (fused or missing ribs)

d. Left untreated, TIS can cause significant cardiopulmonary insufficiency or an early demise.

3. Progression of deformity correlates with growth, which is rapid the first 3 years of life.

C. Evaluation

1. Associated systemic abnormalities are present in up to 61% of patients with vertebral anomalies.

a. Congenital heart defects (26%)

b. Congenital urogenital defects (21%)

c. Limb abnormalities (hip dysplasia, limb hypoplasia, Sprengel deformity)

d. Anal atresia

e. Hearing deficits

f. Facial asymmetry

2. Approximately 38% to 55% of patients with vertebral anomalies present with a constellation of defects that constitute a syndrome, such as VACTERL (*v*ertebral, *a*nal, *c*ardiac, *t*racheal, *e*sophageal, *r*enal, and *l*imb defects) and Goldenhar syndrome (dysplastic or aplastic ears, eye

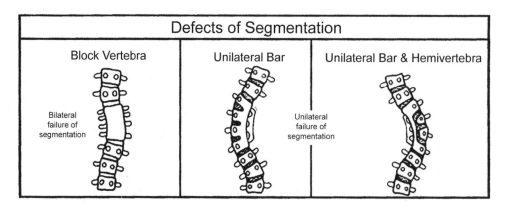

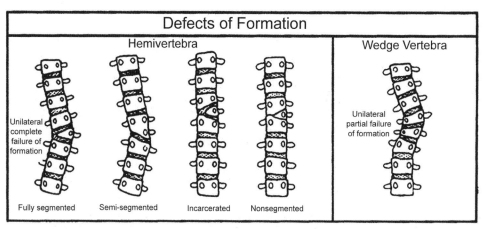

Figure 4 Classification of congenital vertebral anomalies resulting in scoliosis. Defects of segmentation include block vertebra, unilateral bar, and unilateral bar with contralateral hemivertebra. *(Reproduced with permission from McMaster MJ: Congenital scoliosis, in Weinstein SL (ed): The Pediatric Spine: Principles and Practices. New York, NY, Raven Press, 1994, pp 227-244.)*

Table 2	
Rates of Progression for Specific Anomalies*	
Type of Anomaly	**Progression (per year)**
Block vertebra	<2°
Wedge vertebra	<2°
Hemivertebra	2° to 5°
Unilateral bar	5° to 6°
Unilateral bar with contralateral hemivertebra	5° to 10°

*Data taken from McMaster MJ, Ohtsuka K: The natural history of congenital scoliosis: A study of two hundred and fifty-one patients. *J Bone Joint Surg Am* 1982;64:1128-1147.
(Reproduced from Hedequist D, Emans J: Congenital scoliosis. J Am Acad Orthop Surg *2004;12:266-275.)*

growths or absent eye, asymmetric mouth/chin, usually affecting one side of face).

3. Workup of patients with congenital scoliosis includes renal (MRI or ultrasound) and cardiologic evaluation.

4. Pulmonary function should also be evaluated, with attention to TIS.

5. MRI is indicated for all patients with congenital spinal deformity because 20% to 40% will have a neural axis abnormality (Chiari type 1 malformation, diastematomyelia, tethered spinal cord, syringomyelia, low conus, intradural lipoma).

6. MRI in young children who would require general anesthesia may be delayed if the curve is not progressive or requiring surgery.

7. The presence of chest dysplasia (fused or absent ribs) impacts treatment options.

D. Treatment

1. Nonsurgical—Bracing has no effect on congenital scoliosis.

2. Surgical

   a. Indications

      i. Significant progression of scoliosis

      ii. Known high risk of progression, such as a unilateral bar opposite a hemivertebra

      iii. Declining pulmonary function

      iv. Neurologic deficit

   b. Contraindications

      i. Poor skin at surgical site

      ii. Minimal soft-tissue coverage over spine

      iii. Significant medical comorbidities

   c. Procedures

      i. Unilateral unsegmented bars with minimal deformity are best treated with early in situ arthrodesis, either anterior and posterior or posterior alone.

      ii. Progressive fully segmented hemivertebrae in children <5 years of age with <40° curve without notable spinal imbalance have traditionally been treated with an in situ anterior and/or posterior contralateral hemiepiphysiodesis with hemiarthrodesis.

      iii. Hemivertebra excision is recommended for patients with progressive curve with marked trunk imbalance caused by a hemivertebra. This technique has the best results for patients <6 years of age with flexible curves <40°.

      iv. Anterior and/or posterior osteotomy/vertebrectomy approaches are recommended for more severe, rigid deformities, fixed pelvic obliquity, or decompensated deformities that present late.

      v. Growing rod constructs may attach to the spine and/or ribs and attempt to control deformity and encourage spinal growth. Better results are reported with lengthening the construct about every 6 months.

      vi. TIS—A shortened hemithorax with fused ribs may benefit from an opening wedge thoracostomy, expansion of the hemithorax, and growing implant(s) across the hemithorax.

   d. Rehabilitation is usually not needed.

E. Complications

1. Iatrogenic shortening of spinal column due to fusion

   a. Younger age at surgery and more fused levels have a greater impact on growth.

   b. The goal of growth constructs is to optimize spinal growth.

2. Neurologic injury—Can occur secondary to over-distraction or overcorrection, harvesting of segmental vessels, or spinal implant intrusion into the canal.

3. Soft-tissue problems over the spinal implants

   a. Children with congenital scoliosis, especially those with pulmonary compromise, often have insufficient subcutaneous tissue volume to safely pad the implants.

   b. Maximation of preoperative nutrition is vital.

3. The importance of nutrition in this population cannot be overemphasized.

III. Kyphosis

A. Overview (epidemiology)

1. The most common types are postural, Scheuermann (**Figure 5**), and congenital (**Figures 6 and 7**) kyphosis.

2. Less commonly, kyphosis is secondary to trauma, infection, or spinal instrumentation.

3. The incidence of Scheuermann kyphosis is 1% to 8%, with a male to female ratio between 2:1 and 7:1.

4. Scheuermann kyphosis is defined as thoracic hyperkyphosis caused by three consecutive vertebrae with >5° of anterior wedging (Sorensen's criteria). Increased kyphosis with gibbus on clinical examination may be considered diagnostic.

B. Pathoanatomy

1. Scheuermann kyphosis

   a. Believed to be a developmental error in collagen aggregation leading to disturbance of enchondral ossification of the vertebral end plates; this leads to wedge-shaped vertebra and increased kyphosis.

   b. It is most common in the thoracic spine; less common in the lumbar spine.

   c. The natural history of Scheuermann kyphosis in adults with mild forms of the disease (mean 71°) is back pain that only rarely interferes with daily activities or professional careers.

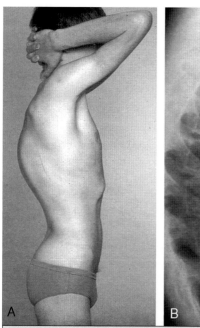
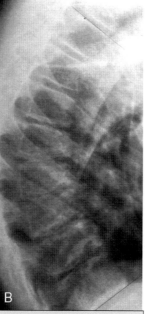

Figure 5 Patient with Scheuermann kyphosis. **A,** Clinical photograph showing sharp angulation typical of Scheuermann kyphosis. **B,** Lateral radiograph showing wedging of vertebrae and irregularity of end plates. (*Reproduced from Arlet V, Schlenzka D: Scheuermann kyphosis: Surgical management. Eur Spine J 2005;14(9):817-827.*)

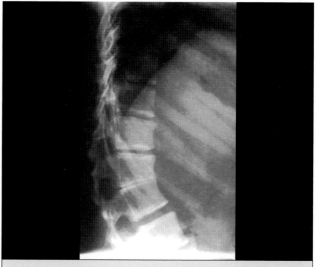

Figure 6 Lateral radiograph demonstrating congenital kyphosis with failure of segmentation.

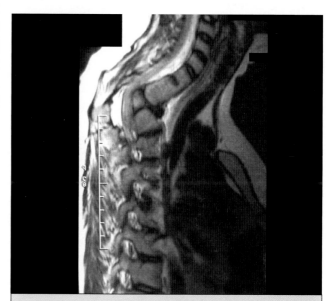

Figure 7 Sagittal MRI demonstrating congenital kyphosis primarily from posterior hemivertebra, with block vertebra immediately cephalad.

    d. More severe deformities (>75°) are more likely to cause severe thoracic pain.

    e. Pulmonary compromise is not generally a concern unless kyphosis exceeds 100°.

2. Congenital kyphosis—Divided into four types, with type I and type III associated with the greatest risk of neurologic injury.

    a. Type I—Failure of formation. Rate of progression for this type is 7° to 9°/year.

    b. Type II—Failure of segmentation. Rate of progression is 5° to 7°/year.

    c. Type III (mixed)—Has worst prognosis for sagittal plane deformity.

    d. Type IV—Rotatory/congenital dislocation of spine.

C. Evaluation

1. Normal thoracic kyphosis is 20° to 45° with no kyphosis at the thoracolumbar junction.

2. The patient usually presents because of cosmetic concerns or pain, which can be at the thoracic region or in the hyperlordotic lumbar spine.

    a. Thoracolumbar kyphosis is typically painful, whereas thoracic kyphosis is typically not painful.

    b. Patients with congenital and Scheuermann kyphosis will clinically demonstrate an acute gibbus at the site of pathology.

3. Postural kyphosis presents a more gentle, rounded contour (without gibbus) of the back with up to 60° of kyphosis.

4. Classic plain radiographic findings in Scheuermann kyphosis are vertebral end plate abnormalities, loss of disk height, Schmorl nodule, and wedge vertebra. The lumbar spine needs to be evaluated to rule out concomitant spondylolisthesis.

5. Magnetic resonance imaging

  a. MRI is indicated for all patients with congenital kyphosis, which has a 56% incidence of intraspinal anomalies.

  b. It may be indicated preoperatively in Scheuermann kyphosis to rule out potential thoracic disk herniation, epidural cyst, or spinal stenosis, which may cause neurologic symptoms at the time of deformity correction.

D. Treatment

  1. Nonsurgical

    a. Congenital kyphosis—Bracing is ineffective.

    b. Scheuermann kyphosis

      i. Bracing can be effective if >1 year of growth remains and kyphosis is between 50° and 70° with the apex at or below T7.

      ii. Bracing is continued for a minimum of 18 months.

      iii. Pain can respond to physical therapy and NSAIDs.

      iv. Patient noncompliance with bracing is common.

  2. Surgical

    a. Indications—Congenital kyphosis.

      i. Surgery is indicated for most patients with type II (failure of segmentation) or type III (mixed) kyphosis, especially those with neurologic deficits.

      ii. For those with type I (failure of formation), an indication for surgery is progressive local kyphosis >40° or neurologic symptoms.

    b. Scheuermann kyphosis—Relative indications for surgery:

      i. Kyphosis >75°

      ii. Deformity progression

      iii. Cosmesis

      iv. Neurologic deficits

      v. Significant pain unresponsive to nonsurgical management

    b. Contraindications—Asymptomatic Scheuermann kyphosis in a child without cosmetic concerns.

    c. Procedures

      i. Congenital kyphosis—For children with failure of segmentation who are <5 years of age with <55° kyphosis, posterior fusion is recommended to stabilize the kyphosis and permit some correction. Anterior decompres-

sion (which may be performed through a posterior approach) is performed for compromised neural structures.

      ii. Scheuermann kyphosis surgery—Posterior spinal fusion with instrumentation. Anterior release has been recommended for deformities that do not correct to >50° on hyperextension lateral radiograph over an apical bolster. Newer thoracic pedicle screw constructs with multiple posterior osteotomies may obviate the need for anterior releases. Traditional recommendations are to limit correction to <50% of deformity to prevent proximal or distal junctional kyphosis or implant pull-out.

  d. Rehabilitation—Generally not needed.

E. Complications

  1. Neurologic injury (paralysis, nerve root deficit) can occur due to mechanical impingement or stretch of cord, by spine implants or bony/soft-tissue structure, or vascular.

  2. Anterior approaches to the thoracic spine can injure the artery of Adamkiewicz, the main blood supply to the T4-T9 spinal cord, generally arising variably from T8-L2 on the left.

  3. Junctional kyphosis occurs in 20% to 30% of patients, although this is usually not clinically significant.

IV. Spondylolysis/Spondylolisthesis

A. Overview (epidemiology)

  1. Incidence of spondylolysis is 5% (males > females). Incidence is 53% in Eskimos.

  2. 25% of patients with spondylolysis have associated spondylolisthesis.

  3. Of patients with isthmic spondylolisthesis, males are affected more commonly than females, but females are four times more likely to develop high-grade slip.

  4. Primarily affects L5 (in 87% to 95% of patients); less frequently, L4 (in up to 10%) and L3 (in up to 3%).

B. Pathoanatomy

  1. Spondylolysis is an acquired condition presumed to be a stress fracture through the pars interarticularis.

  2. Spondylolisthesis is anterior slippage of one vertebra relative to another and is most common in the lumbar spine.

  3. Progression is associated with the adolescent growth spurt, lumbosacral kyphosis (slip angle

3: Pediatrics

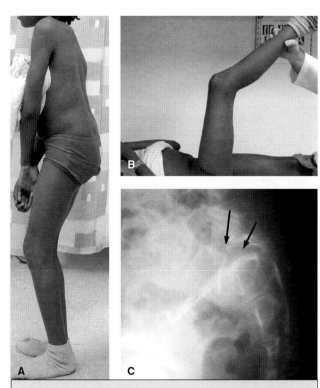

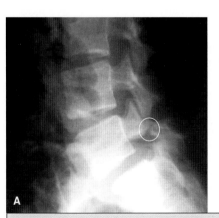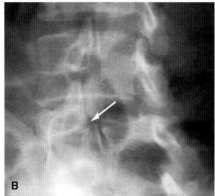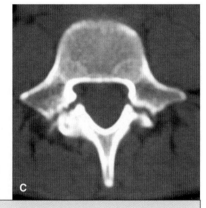

Figure 8 Grade IV dysplastic (Wiltse type I) spondylolisthesis of L5-S1 in a 9-year-old girl. **A,** Clinical photograph. Note the position of flexion of her hips and knees. **B,** Popliteal angle measurement of 55° secondary to contracture of hamstring muscles. **C,** Lateral weight-bearing radiograph of the lumbosacral spine of the same patient, illustrating high-grade dysplastic spondylolisthesis with severe lumbosacral kyphosis (*arrows*). (*Reproduced from Cavalier R, Herman MJ, Cheung EV, Pizzutillo PD: Spondylolysis and spondylolisthesis in children and adolescents: I. Diagnosis, natural history, and nonsurgical management. J Am Acad Orthop Surg 2006;14:417-424.*)

>40°), higher Meyerding grade (>II or >50% translation), younger age, female sex, dysplastic posterior elements, and dome-shaped sacrum.

4. Dysplastic spondylolistheses have an intact posterior arch, increasing the risk of neurologic symptoms due to entrapment of the cauda equina and the exiting nerve roots (**Figure 8**).

C. Evaluation

1. Back pain is usually localized to the lumbosacral area but may run down the legs.

2. Pain is exacerbated by lumbar extension activities and improved with rest.

3. Physical examination findings include paraspinal muscle spasms, tight hamstrings, and limited lumbar mobility.

   a. High-grade spondylolisthesis can produce a waddling gait and hyperlordosis of the lumbar spine.

   b. The nerve root most commonly affected by a spondylolisthesis at L5-S1 is L5.

4. Imaging

   a. Oblique radiographs, in addition to AP and lateral views, may aid in identifying pars defects; this has been described as the "Scotty dog sign."

   b. In high-grade slips with significant angulation of the cephalad vertebra, a Napoleon's hat sign may be seen on the AP views.

   c. Dynamic flexion-extension lateral radiographs can be helpful in assessing translational stability.

Figure 9 Patient with spondylolytic defect of the pars interarticularis of L5. Lateral weight-bearing **(A)** and supine oblique **(B)** radiographs demonstrating the defect (circle, arrow). **C,** Axial CT image through the L5 vertebra, demonstrating the bilateral spondylolytic defects. (*Reproduced from Cavalier R, Herman MJ, Cheung EV, Pizzutillo PD: Spondylolysis and spondylolisthesis in children and adolescents: I. Diagnosis, natural history, and nonsurgical management. J Am Acad Orthop Surg 2006;14:417-424.*)

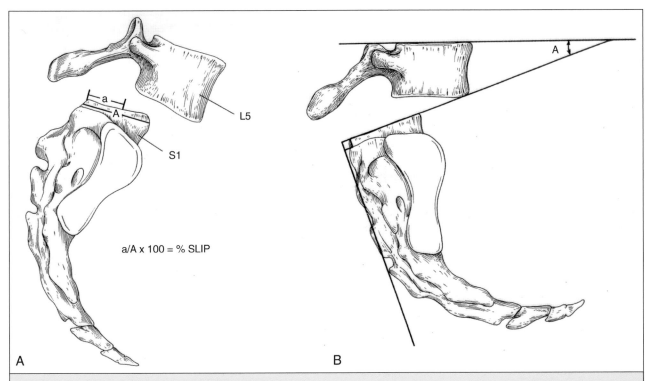

a/A x 100 = % SLIP

Figure 10   Diagrams illustrating the measurements used in the Meyerding classification. **A,** The Meyerding classification is used to quantify the degree of spondylolisthesis. Grade I is 0% to 25% slip, grade II is 26% to 50% slip, grade III is 51% to 75% slip, and grade IV is 75% to 99% slip. A = width of the superior end plate of S1, a = distance between the posterior edge of the inferior end plate of L5 and the posterior edge of the superior end plate of S1. **B,** Slip angle A quantifies the degree of lumbosacral kyphosis. A value >50° correlates with a significantly increased risk of progression of spondylolisthesis. (*Adapted with permission from Herman MJ, Pizzutillo PD, Cavalier R: Spondylolysis and spondylolisthesis in the child and adolescent athlete.* Orthop Clin North Am *2003;34:461-467.*)

d. Single photon emission CT (SPECT) is highly sensitive for pars defects (**Figure 9**).

e. MRI is suboptimal for evaluating pars defects but has a role in assessing nerve entrapment.

D. Classification

1. Wiltse system

a. Describes types based on etiology: dysplastic (congenital, type 1), isthmic (acquired, type 2), degenerative, traumatic, pathologic, iatrogenic.

b. The isthmic type (type 2), which occurs 85% to 95% of the time at L5 and 5% to 15% at L4, is most common in adolescents.

2. Meyerding classification (**Figure 10**)

a. Based on amount of forward slippage of superior vertebra on inferior vertebra and reported in quadrants.

b. Grade V is spondyloptosis, or 100% translation anteriorly of the superior vertebra.

E. Treatment

1. Nonsurgical

a. Asymptomatic patients with spondylolysis and grade I or II spondylolisthesis do not require treatment or activity restrictions.

b. Symptomatic patients (spondylolysis and grade I or II spondylolisthesis) are treated with lumbosacral orthoses for up to 4 to 6 months.

2. Surgical

a. Indications for surgery

i. Uncontrolled pain (after nonsurgical management)

ii. Neurologic symptoms (ie, radicular symptoms or cauda equina syndrome)

iii. Grade III or higher slip or progressive slip to 50% slip

b. Procedures

i. Spondylolysis can be treated with pars repair. If disk desiccation is present (dark disk), L5-S1 fusion should be performed.

ii. Posterolateral fusion (with or without instrumentation) may be performed for spondylolysis and spondylolisthesis. With uninstrumented fusions, the deformity may progress over many years. Pedicle screw constructs may increase fusion rates and decrease postoperative slip progression.

    iii. In the presence of neurologic deficit, decompression is generally recommended, although neurologic improvement has been demonstrated by in situ fusion alone.

    iv. Indications for reduction are controversial, with no universally accepted guidelines. Reduction of spondylolistheses >50% is associated with L5 nerve root stretch and neurologic injury.

F. Complications

1. Cauda equina syndrome (rare) is most likely to occur in type 1 (dysplastic/congenital) slips, with the intact posterior neural arch trapping the sacral roots against the posterosuperior corner of the sacrum. This may occur without surgery.

2. Implant failure (rare)

3. Pseudarthrosis (occurs in up to 45% of high-grade fusions without implants, up to 30% in high-grade slips with posterior instrumentation, rare in high-grade slips with circumferential fusion)

4. Postoperative slip progression

5. Pain (occurs in approximately 14% of patients at 21 years postoperatively)

V. Cervical Spine Abnormalities

A. Overview (epidemiology)

1. In Down syndrome, 61% of patients have atlanto-occipital hypermobility and 21% have atlantoaxial instability; the subaxial cervical spine is not affected.

2. Klippel-Feil syndrome is characterized by failure of segmentation in the cervical spine with a short, broad neck, torticollis, scoliosis, low hairline posteriorly, high scapula, and jaw anomalies. Sprengel deformity is seen in 33% of patients with Klippel-Feil.

3. Intervertebral disk calcification is most common in the cervical spine.

B. Pathoanatomy of os odontoideum

1. The odontoid develops from two ossification centers that coalesce at <3 months of age.

2. The tip of the dens is not ossified at birth but appears at 3 years of age and fuses to the dens by age 12 years.

3. Os odontoideum is usually due to nonunion and may result in atlantoaxial instability. The odontoid is separated from the body of the axis by a synchondrosis (appears as "cork in a bottle"), which usually fuses by age 6 to 7 years.

C. Evaluation

1. Physical examination findings in patients with basilar invagination include loss of upper/lower extremity strength, spasticity, and hyperreflexia. Patients with intervertebral disk calcification present with neck pain but have normal neurologic examination.

2. Radiographic imaging of the cervical spine includes primarily plain AP, lateral, and odontoid views.

    a. Basilar invagination is evaluated on the lateral view and is defined by protrusion of the dens above McRae's line or 5 mm above McGregor's line.

    b. Atlantoaxial instability is present when the ADI (atlanto-dens interval) is >5 mm (**Figure 11**).

    c. Instability is also evaluated with the Powers ratio (**Figure 11**), which is the ratio of the length of the line from the basion to the posterior margin of the atlas divided by the length from the opisthion to the anterior arch of the atlas. A normal Powers ratio is <1.0.

    d. Space available for spinal cord (SAC) should be ≥13 mm (**Figure 11**).

    e. At the level of the odontoid, the rule of thirds prevails, with the odontoid taking one third of the inner diameter of C1, the cerebrospinal fluid taking one third, and the spinal cord taking the final third of the distance.

D. Classification

1. Basilar invagination

    a. Commonly associated with Klippel-Feil syndrome, hypoplasia of the atlas, bifid posterior arch of the atlas, and occipitocervical synostosis.

    b. Also commonly found in systemic disorders such as achondroplasia, osteogenesis imperfecta, Morquio syndrome, and spondyloepiphyseal dysplasia.

    c. Motor and sensory disturbances occur in 85% of individuals with basilar invagination. Patients may present with headache, neck ache, and neurologic compromise.

2. In occipitocervical synostosis, clinical findings are a short neck, low posterior hairline, and limited neck range of motion. Atlantoaxial instability is present in 50%.

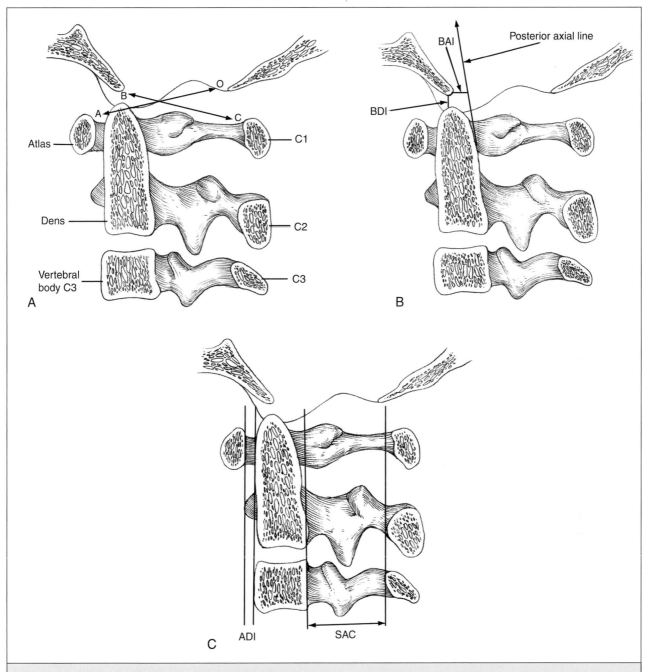

Figure 11 Upper cervical spine and occiput (C1-C3). **A,** Powers ratio = BC/AO. B = basion, C = posterior arch of the atlas, A = anterior arch of the atlas, O = opisthion. **B,** Basion-dental interval (BDI) and basion-axial interval (BAI) each should measure <12 mm. **C,** ADI and SAC. Atlantoaxial instability should be suspected with an ADI >5 mm. If the ADI is ≥10 to 12 mm, the SAC becomes negligible and cord compression occurs. (*Reproduced from Eubanks JD, Gilmore A, Bess S, Cooperman DR: Clearing the pediatric cervical spine following injury. J Am Acad Orthop Surg 2006;14:552-564.*)

3. Odontoid anomalies range from aplasia to varying degrees of hypoplasia, which secondarily causes atlantoaxial instability.

4. Congenital muscular torticollis is associated with developmental hip dysplasia (5%). Its etiology is presumed secondary to compartment syndrome.

5. The etiology of torticollis also includes oph-thalmologic, vestibular, congenital, and traumatic causes as well as tumors. If a tight sterno-cleidomastoid is not present, look for other causes.

6. Atlantoaxial rotatory displacement (AARD)

a. Ranges from mild displacement to fixed, sub-luxated C1 on C2. Most often caused by upper respiratory infection (Grisel syndrome) or trauma.

    b. CT is used to confirm the diagnosis and rule out grades III and IV AARD, which are associated with neurologic injury and sudden death.

7. Patients with Morquio syndrome commonly have atlantoaxial instability due to odontoid hypoplasia.

E. Treatment

  1. Nonsurgical

    a. Intervertebral disk calcification is treated with analgesics.

      i. Biopsy and antibiotics are not needed.

      ii. Calcifications usually resolve over 6 months.

    b. Congenital muscular torticollis—Initial treatment is passive stretching.

    c. AARD is initially managed with NSAIDs, rest, soft collar.

    d. In patients with Down syndrome who have ADI >5 mm without symptoms, restrict from stressful weight bearing on head, such as gymnastics and diving.

  2. Surgical

    a. Indications

      i. Basilar invagination

      ii. Occipitocervical synostosis with atlantoaxial instability

      iii. Odontoid anomalies: neurologic involvement, instability of >10 mm on flexion-extension radiographs, persistent neck symptoms

      iv. Congenital muscular torticollis if limitation is >30° or condition persists >1 year.

      v. Klippel-Feil—Not clearly defined.

      vi. In patients with Down syndrome, ADI >5 mm with neurologic symptoms or >10 mm without symptoms

      vii. Morquio and spondyloepiphyseal dysplasia—>5 mm of instability (regardless of symptoms)

    b. Procedures

      i. Basilar invagination is treated with decompression and fusion to C2 or C3.

      ii. Occipitoaxial synostosis requires atlantoaxial reduction with fusion of occiput-C1 complex to C2. If neural impairment exists, then consider adding decompression to fusion.

      iii. Odontoid anomalies with instability undergo C1-2 fusion.

      iv. Congenital muscular torticollis has been effectively treated with distal bipolar release of sternocleidomastoid.

      v. Atlantoaxial rotatory displacement—If persistent for >1 week and reducible, use head halter traction (at home or in hospital). If symptoms persist for >1 month, consider a halo or rigid brace. C1 to C2 fusion may be indicated if neurologic involvement or persistent deformity is present.

F. Complications

  1. Halo complications are common.

    a. Anterior pins most commonly injure the supraorbital nerve.

    b. More pins (6 to 12) with less insertional torque (≤5 inch-pounds) are used in young children.

    c. Head CT is helpful to measure calvarial thickness and optimal pin placement.

    d. The sixth cranial nerve (abducens) is the most commonly injured with halo traction, which is seen as a loss of lateral gaze. If neurologic injury is noted with halo traction, remove traction.

  2. Nonunions and up to 25% mortality rate are reported with C1-C2 fusion in patients with Down syndrome.

  3. Posterior cervical fusions have a high union rate with iliac crest bone grafting, but the union rate is reported to be much lower with allograft.

VI. Spine Trauma

A. Overview (epidemiology)

  1. Injuries to the cervical spine account for 60% of pediatric spinal injuries.

  2. Mortality from cervical injury in pediatric trauma victims is 16% to 17%.

  3. Across all pediatric age groups, the most common mechanisms of injury involve motor vehicle accidents. Toddlers and school-age children are injured most commonly in falls, and adolescents also suffer sports-related injuries.

B. Pathoanatomy

  1. Children younger than 8 years have an increased risk of cervical spine injuries due to their larger head-to-body ratio, greater ligamentous laxity, and relatively horizontal facet joints.

Table 3

Normal Radiographic Findings Unique to the Pediatric Cervical Spine

Increased atlanto-dens interval	> 5 mm abnormal
Pseudosubluxation C2 on C3	> 4 mm abnormal
Loss of cervical lordosis	
Widened retropharyngeal space	> 6 mm at C2; > 22 mm at C6
Wedging of cervical vertebral bodies	
Neurocentral synchondroses	Closure by 7 years of age

(Reproduced from Hedequist D: Pediatric spine trauma, in Abel MF (ed): OKU Pediatrics, ed 3. Rosemont, IL, American Academy of Orthopaedic Surgeons, 2006, p 324.)

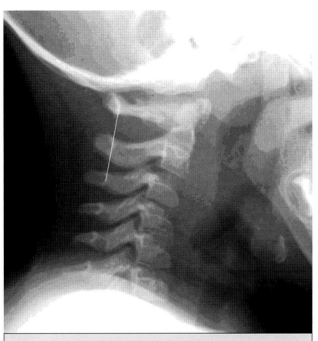

Figure 12 Radiograph demonstrating pseudosubluxation of C2-C3. The Swischuk line (white line) connects the spinolaminar junction of C1 to C3. As long as the spinolamiar junction of C2 is no more than 1 mm anterior to this line, the subluxation is physiologic.

2. In children with cervical spine injuries, 87% of those who are <8 years of age have injuries at C3 or higher. These children also have a higher mortality rate than do older children, with rates ranging from 17% at C1 to 3.7% at C4.

3. The immature spinal column can stretch up to 5 cm without rupture; the spinal cord ruptures at 5 to 6 mm of traction.

4. In children with cervical spine injuries, 33% will manifest evidence of neurologic deficit.

5. Injuries to other organ systems occur in 42% of children with spine injuries.

C. Evaluation

1. Initial management—Transport on backboard with cut-out for occiput or mattress to elevate the body, to prevent inadvertent flexion of the cervical spine due to the child's disproportionately large head.

2. Physical examination

   a. A detailed neurologic examination should be conducted, including sensation (look for sacral sparing), motor function, and reflexes (absence of anal wink indicates spinal shock).

   b. Upper cervical spine injuries should be suspected in young children with facial fractures and head trauma.

3. Imaging

   a. Initial imaging should be plain radiographs of the injured region (**Table 3 and Figure 12**).

      i. Atlantoaxial instability is evaluated using the ADI, which should be <5 mm in children. When the ADI >10 mm, all ligaments have failed, creating cord compression due to neg-

ligible space available for the spinal cord (SAC).

   ii. On a lateral radiograph, the retropharyngeal space should be <6 mm at C2 and <22 mm at C6. These spaces may be enlarged due to crying, however, and therefore this is not necessarily a sign of underlying injury in children.

   iii. Instability of the subaxial cervical spine should be suspected with intervertebral angulation of >11° or translation of >3.5 mm.

   iv. It is crucial to always visualize the C7-T1 junction on the lateral view.

   b. Three-dimensional imaging—CT and MRI help to assess injury and amount of spinal canal intrusion.

   c. Atlanto-occipital junction injuries are assessed with the Powers ratio, the C1-C2:C2-C3 ratio, and the BAI (basion-axial interval) (**Figure 11**).

      i. The Powers ratio is determined by the ratio of the line from the basion to the posterior arch of the atlas and a second line from the opisthion to the anterior arch of the atlas; a ratio >1.0 or <0.55 represents a disruption of the atlanto-occipital joint.

      ii. The C1-C2:C2-C3 ratio (interval between the posterior arches) is <2.5 in normal children.

3: Pediatrics

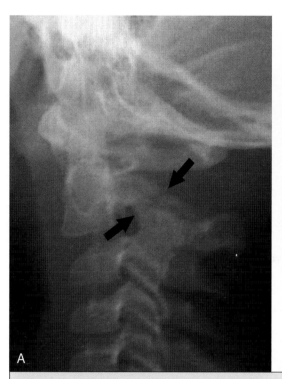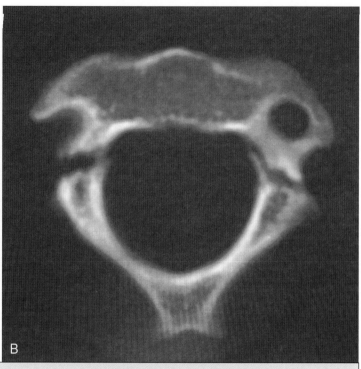

Figure 13 Lateral radiograph **(A)** and CT scan **(B)** of a 5-year-old boy who sustained a hangman's fracture (arrows) in a motor vehicle accident. *(Reproduced with permission from Children's Orthopaedic Center, Los Angeles.)*

d. The BAI is the distance from the basion to the tip of the odontoid and should be <12 mm in all children.

D. Classification

1. Cervical

    a. Atlanto-occipital junction injuries are highly unstable ligamentous injuries that are rare but commonly fatal. Common mechanisms are motor vehicle accidents and pedestrian-vehicle collisions.

    b. Atlas fractures (also known as Jefferson fractures) are uncommon injuries that are usually due to axial loading.

        i. Neurologic dysfunction is atypical.

        ii. Widening of lateral masses of >7 mm beyond the borders of the axis on the AP view indicates injury to the transverse ligament

    c. Atlantoaxial injuries are usually ligamentous injuries to the main stabilizers (transverse ligament) or secondary stabilizers (apical and alar ligaments).

    d. Odontoid fractures usually occur through synchondrosis by a flexion moment causing anterior displacement.

    e. Hangman's fractures are usually due to hyperextension causing angulation and anterior subluxation of C2 on C3 (**Figure 13**).

f. Lower (C3 through C7) cervical spine injuries are more common in adolescents.

2. Thoracolumbar

    a. Flexion injuries result in compression or burst fractures.

        i. Compression fractures rarely exceed more than 20% of vertebral body.

        ii. With >50% loss of vertical height, consider a burst fracture and obtain a CT scan.

    b. Distraction and shear injuries are highly unstable and usually associated with spinal cord injury.

    c. Chance fractures are caused by hyperflexion over automobile lap belts and are frequently associated with intra-abdominal injuries.

    d. Spinal cord injury without radiographic abnormality (SCIWORA)

        i. MRI is the study of choice.

        ii. SCIWORA is the cause of paralysis in approximately 20% to 30% of children with injuries of the spinal cord.

        iii. Approximately 20% to 50% of patients with SCIWORA have delayed onset of neurologic symptoms or late neurologic deterioration.

iv. Children <10 years of age are more likely to have permanent paralysis than older children.

E. Treatment

1. Nonsurgical

   a. Cervical

      i. Intervertebral disk calcification—Treated with rest and NSAIDs.

      ii. Atlas fractures—Treated with cervical collar or halo.

   b. Thoracolumbar

      i. Compression fractures—Bracing for 6 weeks.

      ii. Burst fractures—Bracing if stable.

      iii. Chance fractures with <20° of segmental kyphosis—Treated in a hyperextension cast.

      iv. SCIWORA—Immobilization for 6 weeks to prevent further spinal cord injury.

2. Surgical

   a. Indications

      i. Craniocervical instability

      ii. Atlantoaxial instability with ADI >5 mm

      iii. Displaced odontoid fracture

      iv. Displaced and angulated hangman's fracture

      v. Thoracolumbar burst fractures with neurologic injury and canal compromise

      vi. Distraction and shear injuries with displacement

      vii. Chance fractures that are purely ligamentous injuries and bony injuries with >20° kyphosis

   b. Procedures

      i. Craniocervical instability is treated with an occiput-to-C2 fusion with halo stabilization, preferably with internal fixation.

      ii. Atlantoaxial instability requires a C1-C2 posterior fusion with transarticular C1-C2 screw with a Brooks-type posterior fusion or lateral mass screws.

      iii. Odontoid—Reduction of displacement with extension or hyperextension with halo immobilization for 8 weeks.

      iv. Hangman's fractures with minimal angulation and translation can be treated with closed reduction in extension with immobilization in a Minerva cast or halo device for 8 weeks. Fractures with significant angulation or translation require a posterior fusion or anterior C2-C3 fusion.

      v. Halo placement—In toddlers and children <8 years of age, use more pins (8 to 12) with only finger tightness (2 to 4 inch-pounds). Anterior pins should be placed lateral enough to avoid the frontal sinus and supraorbital and supratrochlear nerves. Place pins anterior enough to avoid temporalis muscle. The posterior pins should be placed on the opposite side of the ring from the anterior pins.

      vi. Thoracolumbar burst fractures with canal compromise require canal decompression, fusion, and instrumentation. Indirect canal decompression is accomplished by surgical distraction of injured level.

      vii. Distraction and shear injuries are treated with reduction with decompression, instrumentation, and arthrodesis.

      viii. Chance injuries that are purely ligamentous injuries should be surgically stabilized with instrumentation and arthrodesis. Bony injuries with >20° kyphosis or inadequate reduction are treated with posterior compression instrumentation and arthrodesis.

F. Complications

1. Os odontoideum

   a. Caused by nonunion of an odontoid fracture that may have episodic or transient neurologic symptoms.

   b. Instability when >8 mm of motion; requires C1-2 fusion.

2. Posttraumatic kyphosis usually does not remodel and may worsen.

3. Pseudarthrosis

4. Implant failure

VII. Other Conditions

A. Diskitis

1. Pathoanatomy—Presumed infection likely begins by seeding the vascular vertebral end plate and then extending into the disk space.

2. Evaluation

   a. Symptoms

      i. Fever

      ii. Back pain

      iii. Abdominal pain

      iv. Refusal to ambulate

      v. Painful limp

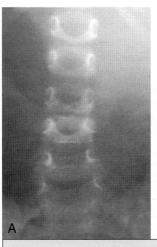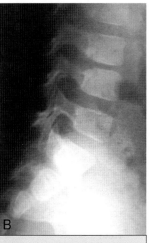

Figure 14　A 3-year-old girl with a 2-week history of irritability and refusal to walk for 2 days. PA **(A)** and lateral **(B)** radiographs demonstrate disk-space narrowing at L3-4 consistent with discitis. *(Reproduced from Early SD, Kay RM, Tolo VT: Childhood diskitis. J Am Acad Orthop Surg 2003;11:413-420.)*

vi. Lower extremity discomfort

b. 25% will be febrile.

c. Laboratory studies of ESR and CRP will be elevated.

d. Radiographs can demonstrate disk-space narrowing with vertebral end plate irregularities (**Figure 14**). Further imaging generally is not needed.

4. Classification

a. Typical organism is *Staphylococcus aureus*.

b. Must consider Langerhans cell histiocytosis (the "great imitator").

5. Treatment

a. Nonsurgical

i. Typically parenteral antibiotics (to cover *S aureus*) for 7 to 10 days; then switch to oral antibiotics for several more weeks.

ii. If the discitis fails to respond to antibiotics, biopsy should be performed for cultures and pathologic tissue evaluation.

b. Surgical

i. Indications—Paraspinal abcess in the presence of neurologic deficit; unresponsive to nonsurgical care.

ii. Contraindications—Standard discitis.

iii. Procedures—Culture, irrigation and débridement.

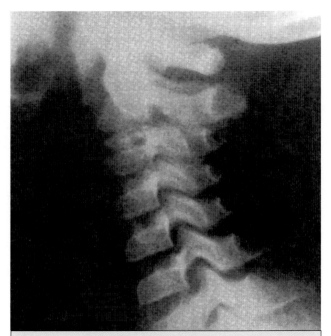

Figure 15　A 7-year-old boy was admitted with pain and a stiff neck. Lateral radiograph shows calcification of the disk space between C2 and C3. *(Reproduced with permission from Dai LY, Ye H, Qian QR: The natural history of cervical disc calcification in children. J Bone Joint Surg Am 2004;86:1467-1472.)*

6. Complications

a. Long-term disk-space narrowing

b. Intervertebral fusions

c. Back pain

7. Pearls and pitfalls—Think of salmonella in the setting of sickle cell anemia.

B. Cervical disk calcification

1. Presents with neck pain universally.

2. Radiographs show calcification of the cervical disk (**Figure 15**).

3. May have fever and elevated erythrocyte sedimentation rate (ESR) and C-reactive protein (CRP).

4. Treatment

a. Observation—Biopsy and surgery are not indicated.

b. Mean time to resolution is just over 1 month.

C. Sacroiliac joint septic arthritis

1. Epidemiology—More common in children >10 years of age.

2. Pathoanatomy

a. *S aureus* is most common.

b. Think of salmonella in association with sickle cell anemia.

3. Evaluation

a. Tenderness is usually present directly over the sacroiliac joint and the FABER test (hip flexed, abducted, externally rotated) reproduces pain.

b. MRI or bone scan confirms the diagnosis; needle biopsy is technically possible but not necessary.

VIII. Back Pain

A. Overview (epidemiology)

1. More than 50% of children will experience back pain by age 15 years. In 80% to 90%, the pain resolves within 6 weeks.

2. Differential diagnosis of back pain is shown in **Table 4**.

B. Pathoanatomy

1. In children younger than 10 years, consider serious underlying pathology, although standard mechanical back pain is still most common.

2. Older children and adolescents will commonly suffer "adult" low back pain.

3. Spinal deformities (scoliosis and kyphosis) can cause pain.

4. Consider intra-abdominal pathology such as pyelonephritis, pancreatitis, and appendicitis.

5. Studies suggest that more weight in a backpack is associated with a higher incidence of back pain.

C. Evaluation

1. History

a. Pain at night is traditionally associated with tumors.

b. Visceral pain is not relieved by rest or exacerbated by activity.

2. A detailed musculoskeletal, abdominal, and neurologic examination is necessary.

3. Imaging studies

a. Plain radiographs

b. Technetium Tc 99m bone scan is helpful to localize tumor, infection, or fracture.

c. CT is best for bone problems (spondylolysis).

d. MRI is recommended for any neurologic signs or symptoms.

Table 4
Differential Diagnosis of Back Pain in Children
Common
Muscular strain/apophysitis/overuse
Spondylolysis
Spondylolisthesis
Trauma: microfracture
Less common
Infection (diskitis/osteomyelitis)
Scheuermann disease
Trauma: fracture
Uncommon
Herniated nucleus pulposus
Ankylosing spondylitis
Juvenile rheumatoid arthritis
Bone tumor
Spinal cord tumor
Psychogenic

(Reproduced from Garg S, Dormans JP: Tumors and tumor-like conditions of the spine in children. J Am Acad Orthop Surg 2005;13:372-381.)

5. Laboratory studies such as complete blood counts, CRP, ESR, and a peripheral smear are indicated for patients with back pain and constitutional symptoms.

D. Classification

1. Possible specific causes include discitis, spinal deformity (scoliosis and kyphosis), neoplasms, spondylolysis/spondylolisthesis, disk herniations, and vertebral apophyseal end plate fracture.

2. Posteriorly, common tumors include osteoid osteoma (**Figure 16**), osteoblastoma, and aneurysmal bone cyst (**Figure 17**). Anteriorly, histiocytosis X has a predilection for the vertebral body, causing vertebrae plana (**Figure 18**).

3. The most common malignant cause of back pain is leukemia.

E. Treatment

1. Nonsurgical—Osteoid osteomas are initially treated with NSAIDs and observation.

2. Surgical

a. Indications

i. Lumbar disk herniation—If unresponsive to nonsurgical management for a minimum of 6 weeks or if neurologic symptoms are present.

3: Pediatrics

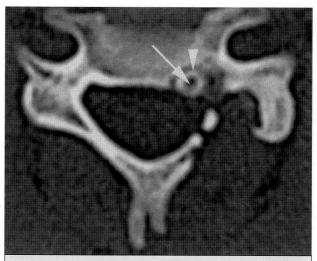

Figure 16   Axial CT scan at C5 in a 12-year-old girl with an osteoid osteoma of the left pedicle. The arrow indicates the center of the lesion (nidus). The nonlesional, reactive sclerotic bony rim around the nidus (arrowhead) is characteristic of osteoid osteoma on CT. (*Reproduced from Garg S, Dormans JP: Tumors and tumor-like conditions of the spine in children.* J Am Acad Orthop Surg *2005;13:372-381.*)

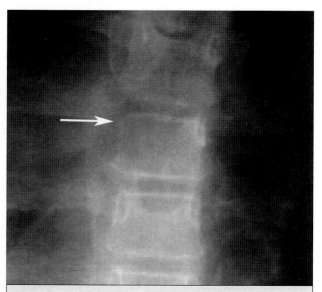

Figure 17   AP radiograph of the thoracic spine demonstrating the "winking owl" sign in an 8-year-old girl with an aneurysmal bone cyst at T5. The left pedicle of T5 is missing (arrow). (*Reproduced from Garg S, Dormans JP: Tumors and tumor-like conditions of the spine in children.* J Am Acad Orthop Surg *2005;13:372-381.*)

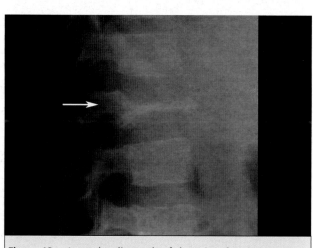

Figure 18   Lateral radiograph of the spine showing vertebra plana at L2 in a 5-year-old girl with Langerhans cell histiocytosis. The collapse of the vertebral body of L2 (arrow) without soft-tissue extension or loss of disk-space height is characteristic of Langerhans cell histiocytosis. (*Reproduced from Garg S, Dormans JP: Tumors and tumor-like conditions of the spine in children.* J Am Acad Orthop Surg *2005;13:372-381.*)

ii. Osteoid osteomas—If nonsurgical pain management fails. Radioablation is not commonly used in the spine for fear of risking neurologic injury.

iii. Osteoblastomas—Surgical treatment is always indicated because these tumors do not respond to nonsurgical interventions.

b. Procedures—Benign bone lesions can be marginally excised.

F. Red flags for pathologic back pain

1. History

a. Pain is well localized. Positive finger test: patient points to pain in one location with one finger.

b. Pain becomes progressively worse over time.

c. Pain is not associated with activities and is present at rest or nighttime.

d. Bowel or bladder incontinence

2. Physical examination

a. Tight hamstrings—Popliteal angle >50°.

b. Localized bony tenderness

c. Neurologic abnormalities

Top Testing Facts

Idiopathic Scoliosis

1. In patients with idiopathic scoliosis curves that are not standard, such as a left primary thoracic curve, an MRI is indicated because intraspinal anomalies are common in this population.

2. The general indication for surgical treatment in patients with adolescent idiopathic scoliosis is a curve >45° to 50°.

Congenital Scoliosis

1. Congenital scoliosis is associated with a significant risk of cardiac and renal anomalies; therefore, a cardiac workup and renal ultrasound are generally indicated prior to surgery.

2. Congenital scoliosis is also associated with intraspinal pathology in up to 40% of patients, so a preoperative MRI is indicated.

Kyphosis

1. Do not try to correct more than 50%.

2. The lower end of the instrumentation should include the first two lordotic vertebrae or risk junctional kyphosis.

3. When segmental pedicle screws are used in combination with multiple posterior osteotomies, anterior approaches can generally be avoided.

4. Scheuermann kyphosis is defined as thoracic hyperkyphosis caused by three consecutive vertebrae with >5° of anterior wedging.

Spondylolysis and Spondylolisthesis

1. Spondylolysis or spondylolisthesis occurs in 5% of the population, and most are asymptomatic.

2. Even though a patient has spondylolysis, continue to look for other causes of back pain if the clinical picture is not typical.

3. The end point of treatment in a slip <50% is absence of pain, not necessarily radiographic demonstration of healing.

4. Reduction of the slip >50% is associated with L5 nerve root stretch and neurologic injury, and should generally be avoided.

Spine Trauma

1. Ligamentous injuries seen in a purely soft-tissue Chance fracture do not heal and usually require surgical stabilization.

2. Bony fractures without significant angulation may be treated nonsurgically.

3. Ecchymosis in the distribution of the seatbelt should raise suspicion of a Chance fracture and/or interabdominal injuries.

4. Children younger than 8 years tend to have cervical injuries C3 and above; children older than 8 years tend to have injuries below C3.

5. On radiographs, the atlanto-dens interval should be <5 mm in children, and the retropharyngeal space should be <6 mm at C2 and <22 mm at C6.

Bibliography

Copley LA, Dormans JP: Cervical spine disorders in infants and children. *J Am Acad Orthop Surg* 1998;6:204-214.

Gillingham BL, Fan RA, Akbarnia BA: Early onset idiopathic scoliosis. *J Am Acad Orthop Surg* 2006;14:101-112.

Hedequist D, Emans J: Congenital scoliosis. *J Am Acad Orthop Surg* 2004;12:266-275.

Lenke LG, Betz RR, Harms J, et al: Adolescent idiopathic scoliosis: A new classification to determine extent of spinal arthrodesis. *J Bone Joint Surg Am* 2001;83:1169-1181.

Weinstein SL, Dolan LA, Spratt KF, Peterson KK, Spoonamore MJ, Ponseti IV: Health and function of patients with untreated idiopathic scoliosis: A 50-year natural history study. *JAMA* 2003;289:559-567.

Wenger DR, Frick SL: Scheuermann's kyphosis. *Spine* 1999; 24:2630-2639.

3: Pediatrics

Chapter 28

Osteoarticular Infection

Howard R. Epps, MD

I. Osteomyelitis

A. Overview

1. Usually occurring in the first decade of life, osteomyelitis affects 1 in 5,000 children younger than 13 years.

2. It is 2.5 times more common in boys than girls.

3. Advances in antimicrobial therapy have decreased the mortality from 50% to less than 1%.

4. The emergence of more resistant, virulent strains of bacteria has added complexity to the management of affected children.

B. Acute hematogenous osteomyelitis (AHO)

1. Overview

   a. AHO is the most common type of osteomyelitis.

   b. Risk factors for developing AHO

      i. Diabetes mellitus

      ii. Chronic renal disease

      iii. Hemoglobinopathies

      iv. Rheumatoid arthritis

      v. Concurrent varicella infection

      vi. Immune compromise

   c. Healthy children are often affected.

2. Pathophysiology

   a. Pathoanatomy

      i. Acute osteomyelitis

         (a) Most cases of acute osteomyelitis are hematogenous.

         (b) Bacteremia may result from a violation of the skin, a concurrent infection, or something as simple as brushing the teeth.

         (c) Slow blood flow in the capillaries of the metaphysis allows bacteria to exit the vessel walls.

         (d) If a sufficient number of bacteria lodge in the bone to overwhelm the local defenses, an infection occurs.

         (e) Osteoblast necrosis, activation of osteoclasts, release of inflammatory mediators, recruitment of inflammatory cells, and blood vessel thrombosis cause a purulent exudate.

         (f) A subperiosteal abscess forms when the exudate penetrates the porous metaphyseal cortex.

         (g) In bones with an intra-articular metaphysis, the exiting exudate can enter the joint and cause an associated septic arthritis.

      ii. Chronic osteomyelitis

         (a) Periosteal elevation may deprive the underlying cortical bone of its blood supply, creating a necrotic piece of bone (sequestrum).

         (b) The periosteum may form an outer layer of new bone (involucrum).

   b. Mechanism

      i. Local trauma has been associated with the development of AHO because the bone becomes more susceptible to bacterial seeding.

      ii. The combination of trauma and bacteremia seems requisite. Either one in isolation does not appear to cause AHO.

   c. Bacteriology (Table 1)

      i. In all age groups, most cases of AHO are caused by *Staphylococcus aureus*.

      ii. There has been a tremendous increase in infections caused by community-acquired, methicillin-resistant *S aureus* (CA-MRSA).

         (a) Some strains of CA-MRSA harbor genes encoding for Panton-Valentine leukocidin (PVL).

         (b) PVL-positive strains of CA-MRSA are associated with complex infections with more multifocal infections, prolonged fever, myositis, pyomyositis, intra-

3: Pediatrics

Table 1

Causative Organisms and Initial Empiric Therapy for Osteomyelitis and Septic Arthritis

Patient Type	Probable Organism	Initial Antibiotic
Neonates	Group B streptococci, *S aureus*, or gram-negative bacilli	Oxacillin plus gentamicin or oxacillin plus cefotaxime
Infants and children younger than 4 years	*S aureus*, *Streptococcus pneumoniae*, Group A streptococcus, *Haemophilus influenza* if not vaccinated	Oxacillin, nafcillin, or clindamycin
If allergic to penicillin or in areas endemic with CA-MRSA		Clindamycin or vancomycin
Children older than 4 years	*S aureus* (coagulase positive)	Nafcillin, clindamycin (CA-MRSA isolates ≥ 10%)
Septic shock requiring intensive care admission	CA-MRSA, MSSA	Vancomycin and gentamicin for synergy
Postoperative and nosocomial infections	MRSA, coagulase negative *S aureus*	Vancomycin
Shoe puncture	*Pseudomonas*, *S aureus*	Aminoglycosides (gentamicin) and cefepime, cefotaxime, ciprofloxacin (best for adolescents)
Patients with sickle cell disease	*S aureus* or *Salmonella*	Oxacillin and cefotaxime

CS-MRSA = community-acquired methicillin-resistant *S aureus*, MSSA = methicillin-susceptible *S aureus*
(Reproduced from Kocher M, Dolan M, Weinberg J: Pediatric orthopaedic infections, in Abel M (ed): Orthopaedic Knowledge Update: Pediatrics, ed 3. Rosemont, IL, American Academy of Orthopaedic Surgeons, 2006, p 60.)

osseous or subperiosteal abscesses, chronic osteomyelitis, and deep venous thrombosis.

3. Evaluation—The presentation of children with AHO can vary from an intermittent limp and low-grade fever to septic shock.

a. History

   i. The history should cover fever, pain, limp, refusal to bear weight, and recent local trauma or infections.

   ii. Immunization history must be obtained, particularly with regard to *Haemophilus influenza* vaccination.

   iii. Use of antibiotics may mask symptoms.

b. Examination

   i. The child should be examined for

   (a) General appearance

   (b) The ability to bear weight or walk

   (c) Point tenderness (including the pelvis, spine, and lower extremities)

   (d) Range of motion (ROM) of adjacent joints (including spine ROM)

   (e) Increased warmth, edema, and erythema

   ii. Temperature and vital signs should be measured to rule out hemodynamic instability.

c. Laboratory findings

   i. Initial blood work should include C-reactive protein (CRP), erythrocyte sedimentation rate (ESR), blood cultures, and white blood cell (WBC) count with differential.

   ii. The CRP is elevated in 98% percent of patients with AHO and becomes abnormal within 6 hours.

   iii. The ESR becomes elevated in 90% of patients with osteomyelitis, and peaks in 3 to 5 days.

   iv. Blood cultures may yield an organism 30% of the time.

   v. The WBC is elevated in only 25% of patients.

d. Diagnostic imaging

   i. Plain radiographs do not show bone changes for 7 days but can demonstrate deep soft-tissue swelling and loss of tissue planes.

   ii. Technetium Tc 99m bone scan can help localize the focus and will demonstrate a multifocal infection.

   (a) The overall accuracy is 92%.

(b) A "cold" bone scan is associated with more aggressive infections, possibly requiring surgical treatment.

 iii. MRI

  (a) Has sensitivity of 88% to 100%.

  (b) MRI detects marrow and soft-tissue edema seen early in infection as well as abscesses requiring surgical drainage.

  (c) MRI assists with preoperative or postoperative planning when there is a poor clinical response to antibiotic therapy or after surgical drainage.

 iv. CT demonstrates abscess formation and bony changes but is most helpful later in the disease course.

c. Differential diagnosis—The differential diagnosis for AHO includes cellulitis, septic arthritis, toxic synovitis, fracture, thrombophlebitis, rheumatic fever, bone infarction, Gaucher disease, and malignancy (including leukemia).

4. Treatment

a. Aspiration—Aspiration of the suspected area is the first step in management.

 i. Aspiration is performed before commencing antibiotics if the clinical condition of the patient allows.

 ii. Diagnostic aspiration helps guide the medical management when the organism is identified (50% of cases).

 iii. Susceptibilities and resistant strains of CA-MRSA vary by community, adding to the importance of cultures.

 iv. A large-bore needle is used to aspirate both the subperiosteal space and the intraosseous space.

 v. After aspiration, antibiotics may be started according to the guidelines in **Table 1**.

b. Nonsurgical

 i. If no purulent material is aspirated, the child can be admitted for intravenous antibiotics. Because of its frequency, CA-MRSA should be covered in most (if not all) cases.

 ii. Surgery is not indicated if the patient demonstrates clinical improvement within 48 hours.

 iii. Duration of intravenous antibiotics is usually 4 to 6 weeks.

c. Surgical

 i. Indications for surgical drainage

  (a) Aspiration of pus

  (b) Abscess formation on imaging studies

  (c) Failure to respond adequately to nonsurgical treatment

 ii. Contraindications—Hemodynamic instability is a contraindication to emergent surgery, and the child should be stabilized first.

 iii. Procedures

  (a) Surgical drainage requires evacuation of all collections of pus, débridement of devitalized tissue, and drilling the cortex to drain intraosseous collections.

  (b) Samples should be sent for culture and histology to rule out neoplasm.

  (c) The wound can be closed over drains if deemed adequately débrided, or packed and re-débrided after 2 to 3 days before closure over drains.

  (d) With chronic osteomyelitis, a more aggressive débridement may be necessary, at times including excision of the sequestrum.

5. Complications of AHO

a. Meningitis

b. Chronic osteomyelitis

c. Septic arthritis

d. Growth disturbance

e. Pathologic fracture

f. Limb-length discrepancy

g. Gait abnormality

h. Deep venous thrombosis

C. Subacute osteomyelitis

1. Overview

a. Subacute osteomyelitis is an uncommon infection characterized by bone pain and radiographic changes without systemic signs.

b. Delayed diagnosis is common.

c. Usually affects lower extremity long bones, but it can occur in other sites.

2. Pathoanatomy

a. The genesis of subacute osteomyelitis is the same as acute osteomyelitis.

b. The difference in presentation results from increased host resistance, less virulent organisms, prior antibiotic exposure, or a combination of these factors.

c. Bacteriology—*S aureus* causes most cases.

3: Pediatrics

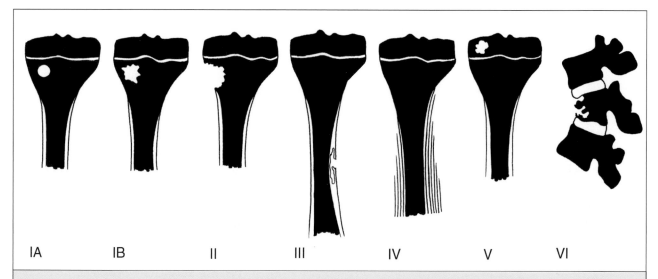

Figure 1   Radiographic classification of subacute osteomyelitis. Types IA and IB indicate lucency; type II, metaphyseal with loss of cortical bone; type III, diaphyseal; type IV, onion skinning; type V, epiphyseal; and type VI, spine. *(Reproduced from Dormans JP, Drummond DS: Pediatric hematogenous osteomyelitis: New trends in presentation, diagnosis, and treatment. J Am Acad Orthop Surg 1994;2:333-341.)*

3. Evaluation

   a. History

      i. The history is notable for the absence of fever, malaise, or anorexia.

      ii. The only symptom may be an intermittent limp or pain.

   b. Physical examination—Point tenderness over the involved bone is often the only clinical finding.

   c. Laboratory findings

      i. Blood tests are usually not helpful.

      ii. The WBC is usually normal or slightly elevated, the ESR slightly elevated, the CRP normal, and blood cultures negative.

   d. Diagnostic imaging

      i. Plain radiographs are positive for changes that range from a well-circumscribed radiolucency in the metaphysis or epiphysis to periosteal new bone formation suggestive of an aggressive malignancy.

      ii. Bone scan is usually positive.

      iii. CT and MRI help characterize the lesion, but MRI provides more information.

4. Classification

   a. The classification is based on the appearance of the lesion on plain radiographs (**Figure 1**).

   b. In all cases, the plain radiograph differential diagnosis includes neoplasm.

5. Treatment

   a. Nonsurgical

      i. Lesions without malignant features may respond to antibiotic therapy covering *S aureus*.

      ii. Surgery is most commonly needed in cases of subacute osteomyelitis.

   b. Surgical

      i. Indications

         (a) Surgical treatment is indicated in all patients with aggressive features on radiographs (types II, III, and IV).

         (b) A biopsy is required to rule out a malignancy if such radiographic features are present.

      ii. Procedures

         (a) A biopsy and culture is performed, using an approach that does not contaminate more than one muscle compartment (in case a malignancy, rather than infection, is present).

         (b) Once osteomyelitis is confirmed, the lesion can be treated with curettage and antibiotics.

6. Complications

   a. Growth disturbance (unusual)

   b. Chronic osteomyelitis

II. Septic Arthritis

A. Overview

1. Septic arthritis is a surgical emergency.

   a. Delayed treatment can cause permanent joint damage, deformity, and long-term disability.

   b. Poor outcomes follow delayed diagnosis.

2. The incidence of septic arthritis peaks in the first few years of life.

   a. 50% of cases of septic arthritis occur in children younger than 2 years.

   b. Large joints like the hip (35%) and knee (35%) are most commonly involved.

B. Pathoanatomy

1. Pathophysiology

   a. Most cases of septic arthritis result from:

      i. Bacteremia seeding the joint

      ii. Direct inoculation of the joint from trauma or surgery

      iii. Contiguous spread from adjacent osteomyelitis

   b. Release of proteolytic enzymes from inflammatory cells, synovial cells, cartilage, and bacteria may cause damage to the articular cartilage within 8 hours.

   c. Increased joint pressure in the hip may cause osteonecrosis of the femoral head if not promptly relieved.

2. Bacteriology (**Table 1**)

   a. *S aureus* causes >50% of cases.

   b. The incidence of *H influenza* septic arthritis has decreased markedly since the advent of the *H influenza* vaccine.

C. Evaluation

1. History

   a. The history of septic arthritis is similar to osteomyelitis.

   b. A history of rash or swollen lymph nodes is important for their association with other conditions in the differential diagnosis.

   c. The vaccination history must be obtained.

2. Physical examination

   a. Patients have fever and often appear toxic.

   b. There is disuse of the extremity and/or refusal to bear weight.

   c. Septic joints have an associated effusion, tenderness, and warmth; any motion causes severe pain.

   d. The extremity rests in the position that maximizes the volume of the joint; for the hip, this results in hip *f*lexion, *ab*duction, and *ex*ternal *r*otation (FABER).

3. Laboratory findings

   a. The WBC is elevated (leukocytosis) in 30% to 60% of patients, and 60% of those will have a left shift.

   b. The ESR is often elevated but may be normal early in the course.

   c. An elevated CRP is the most helpful.

   d. Blood cultures should be drawn because these are often positive, even when local cultures are negative.

4. Diagnostic imaging

   a. Plain radiographs may show joint space widening and are needed to identify any possible bone involvement.

   b. Ultrasound confirms the presence of a hip effusion and can be used to guide joint aspiration; ultrasound cannot differentiate between septic and sterile effusions.

   c. MRI detects a joint effusion and can assess for adjacent osseous involvement, but it can be difficult to obtain expeditiously.

5. Aspiration

   a. Joint aspiration is necessary for diagnosis.

   b. Fluid samples should be analyzed for cell count with differential (**Table 2**), Gram stain, and culture.

6. Differential diagnosis

   a. The differential diagnosis includes osteomyelitis, toxic synovitis, viral arthritis, inflammatory bowel disease-associated arthritis, postgastroenteritis arthritis, tuberculosis (TB), Lyme disease, poststreptococcal arthritis, juvenile arthritis, Reiter syndrome, reactive arthritis, villonodular synovitis, leukemia, sickle cell disease, hemophilia, serum sickness, and Henoch-Schönlein purpura.

      i. Children with septic arthritis appear sicker and are in more distress than those with toxic synovitis.

      ii. Children with synovitis appear comfortable and may be playful when the hip remains still.

      iii. Juvenile rheumatoid arthritis (JRA) rarely presents in the hip.

Table 2		

Synovial Fluid Analysis

Disease	Leukocytes (cells/mL)	Polymorphonucleocytes (%)
Normal	<200	<25
Traumatic effusion	<5,000, with many erythrocytes	<25
Toxic synovitis	5,000-15,000	<25
Acute rheumatic fever	10,000-15,000	50
Juvenile rheumatoid arthritis	15,000-80,000	75
Septic arthritis	>50,000	>75

(Reproduced with permission from Stans A: Osteomyelitis and septic arthritis, in Morrissy R, Weinstein S (eds): Lovell and Winter's Pediatric Orthopaedics, ed 6. Philadelphia, PA, Lippincott Williams & Wilkins, 2006, p 453.)

b. For the hip, slipped capital femoral epiphysis, Legg-Calvé-Perthes disease, fracture, and psoas abscess belong in the differential.

7. Diagnosis—Accurate diagnosis requires synthesis of the clinical findings, laboratory studies, imaging, and judgment.

　a. If all four of the following are present, the probability of septic arthritis ranges from 59% to 99.6% in various series:

　　i. Fever >38.5°C

　　ii. Inability to bear weight

　　iii. ESR >40 mm/h

　　iv. WBC >12,000/μL

　b. A CRP >2.0 mg/dL is an independent risk factor for septic arthritis.

　c. The order of importance of predictors is: fever >38.5°C, elevated CRP, elevated ESR, refusal to bear weight, and an elevated WBC.

D. Treatment

1. Initial

　a. Treatment starts with joint aspiration, preferably before starting antibiotics empirically (**Table 1**).

　b. Intravenous antibiotics are started after samples are sent for culture, and are usually administered for 3 weeks. The child's immunization status should be checked to determine whether *H influenzae* needs to be covered by the empiric antibiotics.

2. Nonsurgical—There is rarely a role for nonsurgical treatment, although some authors advocate intravenous antibiotics and serial aspirations for accessible joints.

3. Surgical

　a. Indications—Surgical drainage and irrigation is the standard of care for almost all septic joints, to clear the joint of damaging enzymes. With possible septic arthritis of the hip, it is better to err on the side of drainage. The morbidity from surgical drainage is much less than that from a neglected septic hip.

　b. Contraindications—Surgical treatment is contraindicated when the patient's clinical status prevents surgical treatment.

　c. Procedures

　　i. An arthrotomy is performed to remove all the purulent fluid and irrigate the joint.

　　ii. For the hip, an anterolateral or medial approach is performed emergently to decrease the risk of developing osteonecrosis.

　　iii. Joints like the shoulder, elbow, knee, and ankle can be drained open or with an arthroscope.

　d. Rehabilitation—Patients may start ROM exercises in the first few days after surgery.

E. Complications

1. Complications of septic arthritis are joint contracture, hip dislocation, growth disturbance, limb-length discrepancy, joint destruction, gait disturbance, and osteonecrosis.

2. The risk of meningitis is highest with *H influenza* infections.

III. "Special" Infections

A. Neonates

1. Overview

　a. Neonates younger than 8 weeks of age deserve

special consideration because their immune systems are immature.

b. Neonates are more susceptible to infection and often do not manifest the symptoms and signs that normally assist in diagnosis.

2. Patient groups

a. Neonatal intensive care unit (NICU) infants

i. NICU infants are at risk for infection because of phlebotomy sites, indwelling catheters, invasive monitoring, peripheral alimentation, and intravenous drug administration.

ii. Multiple sites of infection are present in 40% of NICU infants with musculoskeletal infection, typically due to *S aureus* or gram-negative organisms.

b. Otherwise healthy infants who develop an infection between 2 and 4 weeks of age at home

i. Group B streptococcus is usually the causative organism.

ii. Usually only one site is involved.

c. Patients with *Kingella kingae* septic joints have fewer systemic signs and less joint irritability than do those with septic joints due to other organisms.

3. Anatomy

a. Before the secondary center of ossification appears, the metaphyseal vessels also supply the epiphysis, so osteomyelitis in the metaphysis often (76% of cases) spreads to the epiphysis and the adjacent joint.

b. Growth disturbance and physeal arrest can occur.

4. Diagnosis—Diagnosis in the neonate can be difficult.

a. Fever is usually absent.

b. Early signs are pain with motion, decreased extremity use, pseudoparalysis, difficulty feeding, and temperature instability.

c. Tenderness, swelling, and erythema occur later.

5. Laboratory findings

a. The WBC is usually normal.

b. Blood cultures are positive in 40%, and the ESR may be elevated.

c. For *K kingae*, the yield of positive cultures is higher if the sample is sent in a blood culture bottle. These should be used if there is a sufficient amount of specimen.

6. Treatment

a. Neonates with documented sepsis should have aspiration and culture of all suspicious areas.

b. Positive areas should be surgically drained, with care taken to avoid additional damage to growth centers.

B. Shoe puncture—Shoe punctures can cause a simple laceration, cellulitis, septic arthritis, or osteomyelitis.

1. When an object has penetrated a sneaker, *Pseudomonas* is an organism of concern, although infection by *S aureus* is more common.

2. Tetanus status should be ascertained and coverage provided if deficient.

3. Radiographs should be taken to look for a retained foreign body.

4. Initial treatment

a. Initial treatment is soaks, elevation, rest, and antibiotic therapy that cover both *S aureus* and *Pseudomonas*.

b. A poor response to this regimen indicates a more extensive problem.

5. Bone scan or MRI can help diagnose more complex infections requiring surgical débridement.

6. Superficial infections occur in 10% to 15% of children following shoe puncture wounds, and deep infection in approximately 1%.

7. Surgery is indicated for a foreign body, abscess, septic arthritis, or failure to respond to antibiotics.

8. Late, deep infections are due to *Pseudomonas* in >90% of cases.

C. Diskitis

1. Diskitis usually occurs in children younger than 5 years.

2. The infection starts in the vertebral end plates and moves to the disk through vascular channels.

3. *S aureus* causes most cases.

4. Blood cultures should be obtained, but local cultures are not routinely needed.

5. Patients present with low-grade fever, limp, or refusal to bear weight; the child refuses to move the spine.

6. Plain radiographs are normal for the first 2 to 3 weeks, but they may show loss of the normal sagittal contour early; bone scan or MRI confirms the diagnosis earlier.

7. Antibiotics successfully treat most cases; patients who do not respond to antibiotics should have a biopsy.

D. Vertebral osteomyelitis

   1. Vertebral osteomyelitis affects older children.

   2. More constitutional symptoms are usually present with vertebral osteomyelitis than with diskitis, and there is more focal tenderness on examination.

   3. MRI or bone scan is sensitive early; plain radiographs show bone destruction later.

   4. Treatment with antistaphylococcal agents is curative.

E. Sacroiliac infections

   1. Infections of the sacroiliac joint cause fever, pain, and a limp.

   2. Patients have pain with lateral compression of the pelvis, the FABER hip test, and tenderness over the sacroiliac joint.

   3. MRI is the most sensitive test.

   4. Initial antibiotic treatment should cover *S aureus*, the most common cause.

   5. If aspiration or drainage is necessary, it can usually be done with CT guidance.

F. Sickle cell disease

   1. Children with sickle cell disease are at increased risk for both septic arthritis and osteomyelitis.

   2. The frequent bone infarcts, sluggish circulation, and decreased opsonization of bacteria all contribute to the susceptibility.

   3. *S aureus* and *Salmonella* are the most common organisms, so initial antibiotic treatment should cover both.

   4. Differentiation between sickle cell crisis and infection can be challenging.

     a. Both entities may cause fever, pain, tenderness, swelling, and warmth.

     b. The WBC, CRP, and ESR may be elevated in both.

     c. Bone scan and MRI are often not specific as well.

   5. Only approximately 2% of children with sickle cell disease admitted to a hospital with musculoskeletal pain have osteoarticular infection.

   6. A positive blood culture or a positive osteoarticular aspirate is diagnostic.

G. Notable organisms

   1. Tuberculosis

     a. The incidence of TB has been rising in developed countries over the past 30 years because of immunocompromised patients and the emergence of multidrug-resistant strains.

     b. Children are more likely to have extrapulmonary involvement, with bone and/or joint involvement occurring in 2% to 5% of children with TB.

       i. The most common sites of musculoskeletal involvement are the spine (50%), large joints (25%), and long bones (11%).

       ii. Polyostotic involvement has been reported in 12%.

     c. Presentation

       i. Patients can present with fever, night sweats, weight loss, and pain.

       ii. Patients with skeletal infections, however, may have more subtle findings, with absence of fever, only mild pain, and normal blood studies.

     d. In the spine, the anterior one third of the vertebral body is usually involved, most often in the region of the thoracolumbar junction; a paravertebral abscess may cause neurologic deficits.

     e. Long bone lesions are radiolucent, with poorly defined margins and surrounding osteopenia.

     f. The hip and knee are the joints most commonly affected. Involved joints have diffuse osteopenia and subchondral erosions.

     g. Laboratory findings—The WBC is normal, the ESR is usually elevated, and the purified protein derivative test (PPD) is usually positive.

     h. A biopsy with stains and culture for acid-fast bacilli is diagnostic.

     i. Treatment is usually medical, for at least 1 year.

       i. Surgical débridement of long-bone lesions may hasten resolution of constitutional symptoms, but incisions should be closed to avoid chronic sinus formation.

       ii. Drainage and stabilization of spine lesions is indicated for neurologic deficits, instability, progressive kyphosis, or failure of medical therapy.

   2. Lyme disease

     a. Epidemiology

       i. Lyme disease is infection caused by *Borrelia burgdorferi*, which causes erythema migrans, intermittent reactive arthritis, neuropathies, cardiac arrhythmias, and occasionally an acute arthritis.

       ii. The infection is caused by a bite from the deer tick, which is prevalent in New England and the upper Midwest.

b. History and physical examination

  i. The arthritis is generally less painful than bacterial arthritis. Patients can present with fever and a swollen, irritable joint but will still bear weight.

  ii. Erythema migrans is the rash typically seen after infection with *B burgdorferi*, although it is not always present. Classically, it is an expanding, "bulls-eye" rash.

c. Laboratory findings

  i. The WBC may be normal or elevated, but the ESR and CRP are usually elevated.

  ii. Joint aspirates have a markedly elevated WBC count.

  iii. Serologic testing is positive for *B burgdorferi*.

  iv. The rapid Lyme immunoassay should be included in the septic joint evaluation in endemic areas.

d. The factors most helpful to differentiate between bacterial arthritis and Lyme arthritis are the ability to bear weight and a normal serum WBC with the latter.

e. Lyme arthritis is treated with antibiotics, including doxycycline, amoxicillin, and cefuroxime.

4. Gonococcal arthritis

a. Gonococcal arthritis is caused by a *Neisseria gonorrhea* infection. It affects sexually active adolescents, sexually abused children, and neonates with infected mothers.

b. Because of the association with sexual abuse, children with a suspected infection should have cultures taken of all mucous membranes.

c. The knee is most commonly involved, but the infection is polyarticular in 80% of cases.

d. *N gonorrhea* is difficult to culture, so synovial aspirates should be cultured on chocolate blood agar.

e. Treatment is usually medical in confirmed cases. Typical antibiotics include ceftriaxone or cefixime because of the increased prevalence of penicillin-resistant organisms.

f. Arthrotomy is required for hip infections, but other joints can be observed or treated with serial aspiration.

4. Coccidiomycosis

a. *Coccidioides immitis* is a fungus endemic to the Southwestern United States that can cause a polyostotic osteomyelitis in affected individuals.

b. The infection starts as an upper respiratory infection but can progress to disseminated disease in a small percentage of patients. Diagnosis is usually delayed.

c. The WBC and ESR are often normal.

d. In addition to antifungal medical therapy, surgical débridement is usually required to eradicate the infection.

IV. Chronic Recurrent Multifocal Osteomyelitis

A. Overview

1. Diagnosis of chronic recurrent multifocal osteomyelitis (CRMO), an idiopathic inflammatory disease of the skeleton, is a diagnosis of exclusion.

2. CRMO is characterized by a prolonged course with periodic exacerbations.

3. When there is associated *s*ynovitis, *a*cne, *p*ustulosis, *h*yperostosis, and *o*steitis, the condition is called SAPHO syndrome.

4. The condition is characterized by periods of exacerbation, but usually goes into remission after 3 to 5 years.

5. The incidence is unknown.

6. CRMO occurs primarily in children and adolescents and is more common in girls; the peak age of onset is 10 years.

7. The metaphyses of long bones and the clavicle are most commonly involved. Clavicle involvement is common in CRMO, unlike in true infections.

B. Pathoanatomy

1. The pathophysiology is unknown.

2. Theories include an infection by an organism with fastidious growth requirements, or an autoimmune disorder.

C. Evaluation

1. History—Patients have insidious onset of episodic fever, malaise, local pain, tenderness, and swelling.

2. Physical examination

  a. Patients have swelling and point tenderness over the involved bones.

  b. They may have low-grade fever.

3. Laboratory findings

  a. The WBC is usually normal.

  b. The ESR and CRP may be elevated.

  c. Bone cultures are negative.

4. Diagnostic imaging

a. Plain radiographs show eccentric metaphyseal lesions with sclerosis, osteolysis, and new bone formation that frequently is symmetric.

b. Bone scan helps identify all the sites of involvement.

c. Because of the shared characteristics between CRMO and malignancy, MRI is helpful to judge the extent and the soft-tissue involvement of the lesion.

D. Treatment

1. Nonsurgical

a. Although many children have biopsies and local cultures at the time of initial presentation to establish the diagnosis, treatment is always nonsurgical once the diagnosis is established.

b. Scheduled nonsteroidal anti-inflammatory medications during exacerbations successfully manage the symptoms in 90% of patients.

2. Surgical—Surgery is indicated only when a biopsy is needed to establish the diagnosis.

Top Testing Facts

Acute Hematogenous Osteomyelitis

1. A child with bone pain and fever should be assumed to have osteomyelitis until proven otherwise.

2. AHO without abscess can generally be treated medically.

3. In areas with a high prevalence of CA-MRSA, surgical drainage may be necessary even in the absence of documented abscess on imaging studies.

4. If the response to antibiotics is poor, preoperative MRI aids surgical planning by delineating the extent of the infection and the location of abscesses.

5. Most cases of AHO are caused by S aureus.

6. Because of the prevalence of CA-MRSA, empiric coverage should cover CA-MRSA in most (if not all) cases.

7. Susceptibilities and resistant strains of CA-MRSA vary by community, adding importance to aspiration or biopsy for culture.

8. The metaphyseal blood supply crosses the physis to the epiphysis in children younger than 12 to 18 months, so severe sequelae are more common.

9. In neonates, the most common organism is group B streptococci.

Subacute Osteomyelitis

1. Subacute osteomyelitis may be indistinguishable from tumors on radiographic studies.

2. Surgery is most commonly required in cases of subacute osteomyelitis.

Septic Arthritis

1. Septic arthritis more commonly occurs in younger children, with 50% of cases in children ≤2 years old.

2. Septic arthritis is a surgical emergency.

3. When managing the hip, err toward drainage in equivocal cases; the morbidity of an arthrotomy is minimal compared to the sequelae of a neglected septic hip.

4. Kingella kingae infections tend to have more subtle findings—fewer systemic signs and less impressive joint irritability.

5. If there is sufficient fluid from arthrocentesis, a portion of the sample should be placed in a blood culture bottle because K kingae grows more readily in this medium.

6. Children with septic arthritis appear sicker and are in more distress than those with toxic synovitis.

7. Children with synovitis appear comfortable and may be playful if the hip remains still.

8. Check the child's immunization status to see if H influenza coverage is necessary during empiric therapy.

9. Juvenile rheumatoid arthritis rarely presents in the hip.

Special Infections

1. Of NICU babies with musculoskeletal infection, 40% have multiple site involvement.

2. Infections in infants frequently cross the physis, with resultant infection of the metaphysis and adjacent joint.

3. Following nail puncture through a shoe, soft tissue infection occurs in 10% to 15% of cases and deep infection in 1%.

4. Pseudomonas accounts for more than 90% of late deep infections following nail puncture through sneakers.

5. S aureus and Salmonella are the most common infecting organisms in children with sickle cell anemia with musculoskeletal infection.

6. In children with TB, the most common sites of musculoskeletal infection are the spine (50%), large joints (25%), and long bones (11%). Polyostotic involvement occurs in 12%.

7. Lyme disease is often heralded by the typical skin lesion, erythema migrans.

Chronic Recurrent Multifocal Osteomyelitis

1. CRMO is a diagnosis of exclusion.

2. Cultures are negative in CRMO.

3. Unlike true infections, involvement of the clavicle is common in CRMO.

Bibliography

Caird MS, Flynn JM, Leung YL, Millman JE, D'Italia JG, Dormans JP: Factors distinguishing septic arthritis from transient synovitis of the hip in children. *J Bone Joint Surg Am* 2006;88:1251-1257.

Gonzalez BE, Martinez-Aguilar G, Hulten K, et al: Severe staphylococcal sepsis in adolescents in the era of community acquired methicillin-resistant *Staphylococcus aureus*. *Pediatrics* 2005;115:642-648.

Kaplan SL: Osteomyelitis in children. *Infect Dis Clin North Am* 2005;19:787-797.

Kocher M, Dolan M, Weinberg J: Pediatric orthopaedic infections, in Abel M (ed): *Orthopaedic Knowledge Update: Pediatrics*, ed 3. Rosemont, IL, American Academy of Orthopaedic Surgeons, 2006, pp 57-73.

Kocher MS, Mandiga R, Zurakowski D, Barnewolt C, Kasser JR: Validation of a clinical prediction rule for the differentiation between septic arthritis and transient synovitis of the hip in children. *J Bone Joint Surg Am* 2004;86:1629-1635.

Levine MJ, McGuire KJ, McGowan KL, Flynn JM: Assessment of the test characteristics of C-reactive protein for septic arthritis in children. *J Pediatr Orthop* 2003;23:373-377.

Luhmann SJ, Jones A, Schootman M, Gordon JE, Schoenecker PL, Luhmann JD: Differentiation between septic arthritis and transient synovitis of the hip in children with clinical prediction algorithms. *J Bone Joint Surg Am* 2004;86:956-962.

Martinez-Aguilar G, Avalos-Mishaan A, Hulten K, Hammerman W, Mason E Jr, Kaplan S: Community-acquired, methicillin-resistant and methicillin-susceptible *Staphylococcus aureus* musculoskeletal infections in children. *Pediatr Infect Dis J* 2004;23:701-706.

Martinez-Aguilar G, Hammerman W, Mason E Jr, Kaplan S: Clindamycin treatment of invasive infection caused by community-acquired, methicillin-resistant and methicillin-susceptible *Staphylococcus aureus* in children. *Pediatr Infect Dis J* 2003;22:593-598.

McCarthy JJ, Dormans JP, Kozin SH, Pizzutillo PD: Musculoskeletal infections in children: Basic treatment principles and recent advances. *Instr Course Lect* 2005;54:515-528.

Stans A: Osteomyelitis and septic arthritis, in Morrissy R, Weinstein S (eds): *Lovell and Winter's Pediatric Orthopaedics*, ed 6. Philadelphia, PA Lippincott Williams & Wilkins, 2006, pp 439-491.

Vaz A, Pineda-Roman M, Thomas A, Carlson R: Coccidioidomycosis: An update. *Hosp Pract (Minneap)* 1998;33:105-120.

Willis AA, Widmann RF, Flynn JM, Green DW, Onel KB: Lyme arthritis presenting as acute septic arthritis in children. *J Pediatr Orthop* 2003;23:114-118.

Chapter 29
Musculoskeletal Conditions and Injuries in the Young Athlete

Jay C. Albright, MD

I. Overview

A. Child versus adult athlete

1. A child athlete is not a small adult.

2. Children have open physes growing at variable rates, making them prone to injury.

3. Children are less coordinated, with poorer mechanics, when compared with adult athletes.

4. Children have less efficient thermoregulatory mechanisms than adults, which is manifested as a poorer ability to acclimatize rapidly because of a less efficient sweating response.

B. Participation levels/preparticipation examination

1. Almost 4 million males and 3 million females participated in high school level sports in 2005-2006, compared with approximately 3.6 million males and 300,000 females participating in the early 1970s, according to the National Federation of State High School Associations.

2. Preparticipation physical examinations provide a good screening tool to identify most risk factors for injury as well as an opportunity to develop strategies and recommendations for preventing as well as treating them.

C. Sex-specific considerations

1. The "female athlete triad" of amenorrhea, disordered eating, and osteoporosis places the female athlete at higher risk of insufficiency or stress fractures, overuse injuries, and recurrent injuries.

2. Knee injuries

   a. The female knee is also at increased risk of injury from the start of puberty on.

   b. Differences in anatomy, sex hormone levels, neuromuscular control, and overall strength and coordination have been implicated in the higher incidence of knee injuries in females compared with males in the same sport.

II. Little Leaguer Shoulder

A. Overview/epidemiology

1. Little Leaguer shoulder is an epiphysiolysis, or fracture through the proximal humeral epiphysis, caused by repetitive microtrauma.

2. This injury occurs most commonly in skeletally immature overhead athletes such as pitchers and tennis players.

3. The injury is a result of repeated high loads of torque in a rapidly growing child athlete.

B. Presentation/evaluation

1. Patients present with generalized shoulder pain that is typically at its worst during the late cocking or deceleration phases, pain with resisted elevation of the shoulder and with extremes of motion in any direction, and point tenderness over the physis of the proximal humerus, which is hard to discern from subdeltoid bursal pain.

2. Radiographs show a widened proximal humeral physis compared with the opposite side (**Figure 1**).

C. Treatment

1. Treatment is the same as for a fracture, with no throwing for a minimum of 2 to 3 months.

2. When painless full range of motion is obtained, physical therapy for rotator cuff strengthening is initiated.

3. After 2 to 3 months of no throwing, a progressive throwing program is started.

   a. The athlete begins with short tosses at low velocity and gradually progresses to longer tosses; eventually the longer tosses are made with increasing velocity.

   b. After long tosses at higher velocities have been achieved, the patient can start full playing.

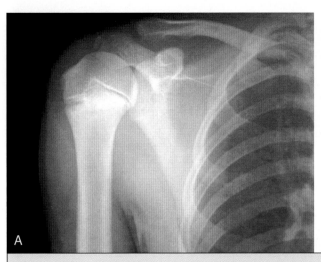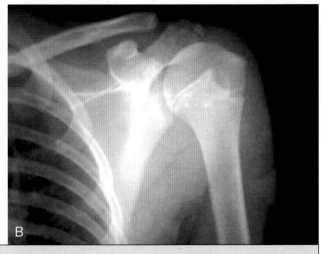

Figure 1   AP radiographs of the shoulders of a 12-year-old pitcher with right shoulder pain in the deceleration phase of throwing. Compare the physeal widening of the right shoulder (**A**) with the normal left shoulder (**B**).

Table 1		

Pitching Recommendations for the Young Baseball Player

Age	Maximum Pitches Per Game	Maximum Games per Week
8-10	52 ± 15	2 ± 0.6
11-12	68 ± 18	2 ± 0.6
13-14	76 ± 16	2 ± 0.4
15-16	91 ± 16	2 ± 0.6
17-18	106 ± 16	2 ± 0.6

(Reproduced from Pasque CB, McGinnis DW, Griffin LY: Shoulder, in Sullivan JA, Anderson ST [eds]: Care of the Young Athlete. Rosemont, IL, American Academy of Orthopaedic Surgeons, 2000, p 347.)

D. Complications

   1. A low incidence of premature growth arrest with or without angular deformity is seen.

   2. Subsequent Salter-Harris fractures can also occur.

E. Prevention—The key to prevention of this injury is avoiding overuse by adherence to guidelines set forth by multiple entities, including the American Academy of Orthopaedic Surgeons, USA Baseball, and the American Orthopaedic Society for Sports Medicine (**Table 1**).

III. Little Leaguer Elbow

A. Overview

   1. Little Leaguer elbow is a generic term covering any injury to the elbow in a child that is accom-panied by pain along the medial aspect of the proximal forearm or elbow. The term derives from the fact that these injuries are commonly related to the excessive stresses experienced by the immature skeleton during pitching.

   2. The forces are similar to those that occur in the adult elbow; ie, valgus-hyperextension overloading of the elbow during throwing.

   3. The syndrome is often associated with a habit of throwing curveballs and other "junk" pitches, or when an infielder-type bent-elbow throw that involves a whipping mechanism to gain adequate speed is used. The mechanism of all injuries in this category is similar to those seen with adult injuries, but the symptoms of each different injury in a child can be much more varied. Children often experience pain on the compressed radial side of the joint as well as the distracted ulnar side.

B. Pathoanatomy

   1. Little Leaguer elbow is a progressive problem resulting from repetitive microtrauma. Therefore, most of the early symptoms are assumed to be a result of soft-tissue strains and sprains.

   2. By the time the symptoms are severe enough to require referral to an orthopaedic surgeon, more serious ligament, cartilage, physis, and bone pathology should be assumed to be present until proven otherwise.

C. Presentation/evaluation

   1. Patients experience pain after, and eventually during, a game. The pain may be mild at first but eventually inhibits throwing entirely.

   2. Patients typically lose the ability to achieve throwing distance and accuracy early on, followed by a loss of velocity. Eventually, most note persistent pain at rest.

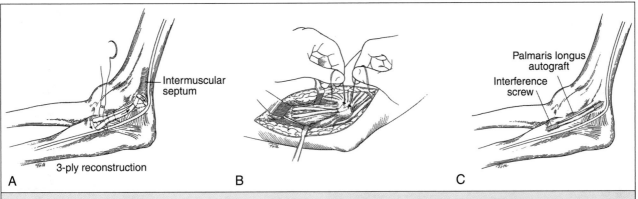

Figure 2 Medial UCL reconstruction techniques. **A**, Tendon graft passed through bone tunnels. **B**, Docking technique. **C**, Anatomic interference technique. (*Reproduced with permission from ElAttrache NS, Bast SC, David T: Medial collateral ligament reconstruction.* Tech Shoulder Elbow Surg *2001;2:38-49.*)

3. The differential diagnosis includes medial epicondylar apophysitis, posterior stress impingement, osteochondritis dissecans (OCD)/Panner disease, and instability and valgus extension overload.

4. Physical examination

   a. Examination is best done with the patient seated. Observe the arm for deformity. Chronic conditions may produce an increased carrying angle or a flexion contracture.

   b. Look for sites of maximum point tenderness. Point tenderness over the medial epicondyle and/or flexor mass could be due to muscle strain, ulnar collateral ligament (UCL) sprain, or medial epicondylitis.

   c. Apply valgus stress with the arm in varying degrees of flexion and extension.

      i. As with a UCL injury where the ligament is avulsed at its origin on the apophysis of the medial epicondyle, instability may be present.

      ii. Evaluate UCL instability with the valgus stress test, the milking maneuver, valgus stress radiographs, MRI, and/or MR arthrography.

      iii. The younger the patient, the more likely the diagnosis is to be an apophysitis or an avulsion injury rather than a UCL sprain.

5. Radiographic evaluation

   a. Compare with the normal side to determine whether an irregular appearance of the physis exists. This may also be helpful for determining degree of displacement. A radiograph of just the involved extremity is sufficient to determine whether the apophysis has closed, however.

   b. Look for fragmentation of the medial epicondyle, trochlea, olecranon, or capitellum.

   c. Medial epicondyle hypertrophy or radial head hypertrophy may be present as well.

D. Treatment

   1. Nonsurgical treatment

      a. The best treatment is prevention through education of coaches, parents, and athletes.

      b. Alteration in form/motion, playing habits, and adherence to recommended pitch/inning counts should be used first for all elbow overuse injuries.

      c. Medial epicondylitis is treated with 4 to 6 weeks of no stress on the physis.

      d. Treatment of OCD/Panner is discussed in section V, below.

      e. Valgus extension overload and posterior stress syndromes typically can be treated with activity and throwing modifications.

      f. Intra-articular steroids may be used to control inflammation.

   2. Surgical treatment

      a. Indications

         i. Failure of response to nonsurgical treatment

         ii. Instability of elbow with avulsion fracture or fragmentation of medial epicondyle

      b. Contraindications—Uncertain diagnosis with ulnar nerve symptoms.

      c. Procedures

         i. UCL reconstruction of choice when indicated for UCL insufficiency (**Figure 2**)

         ii. Open reduction and internal fixation is recommended by most surgeons for medial epicondyle avulsion fractures in serious, competitive throwers, although definitive research is lacking.

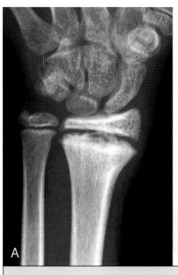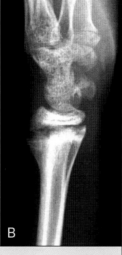

Figure 3 AP (**A**) and lateral (**B**) radiographs of the wrist of a 13-year-old girl who was an elite-level female gymnast and who presented with persistent pain and progressive deformity of the left wrist.

iii. Arthroscopic débridement of posterolateral synovium and olecranon osteophytes for recalcitrant posterior symptoms, and arthroscopic decompression of valgus-extension overload with failed prolonged nonsurgical treatment.

E. Complications

1. Ulnar nerve neuropathy

2. Loss of motion

3. Infection

4. Continued pain

5. Inability to return to play at same level

6. Aggressive débridement of the olecranon or osteophytes may lead to instability.

F. Rehabilitation

1. Rehabilitation should be tailored according to whether ligament injury is involved.

2. For injuries not involving ligaments, minimal immobilization with early range of motion, strengthening, and pain modalities is indicated.

3. For ligament reconstructions, the recommended treatment is a brief period of immobilization and then protected range of motion.

IV. Distal Radius Epiphysiolysis/Epiphysitis

A. Overview/pathoanatomy

1. Injury to the distal radial epiphysis most com-

monly occurs in adolescent athletes in sports that require weight bearing on the upper extremities, such as gymnastics or cheerleading.

2. Children of an average age of 10 to 14 years at higher skill levels spend more time in more intensive training, making these injuries more likely to occur in this age group.

3. The mechanism involves overloading of the distal radial epiphysis, causing inflammation and/or fracture of the epiphysis.

B. Evaluation

1. Diagnosis is made by history of painful wrist with weight-bearing activities and physical examination consistent with pain and swelling at the joint with or without deformity of the wrist.

2. Radiographs may show widened physis, blurred growth plate, metaphyseal changes, and fragmentation of radial and volar aspects of the plate (**Figure 3**).

C. Treatment

1. Allow the patient to participate in treatment choices.

2. Relative rest is indicated in mild to moderate cases, complete rest in severe cases. In-season athletes and less severe cases may be managed with relative rest in a splint and physical therapy.

3. Immobilization is indicated in all cases, from a splint in mild to moderate cases, to casting in more severe cases. Do not be afraid to be aggressive in immobilization.

4. In severe cases, bone stimulation can be used.

5. Surgical intervention is typically indicated only for the correction of complications.

D. Complications

1. This injury may recur even with casting for 6 to 8 weeks, particularly if the athlete goes back to full activities immediately.

2. Positive ulnar variance is a common eventual outcome with untreated athletes and may result in triangular fibrocartilage complex pathology or ulnar abutment.

E. Rehabilitation—Physical therapy is useful for regaining motion after casting and also helps to control the athlete's return to activity.

V. Osteochondritis Dissecans

A. General

1. Osteochondritis dissecans (OCD) is so named because of the tendency for the untreated lesion to

3: Pediatrics

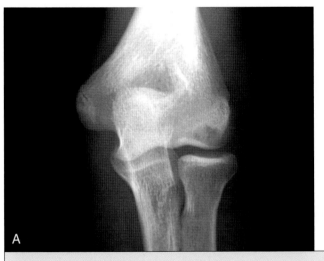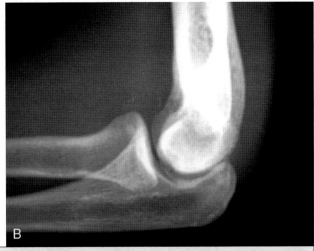

Figure 4   AP (**A**) and lateral (**B**) radiographs showing capitellar OCD in a 14-year-old gymnast.

wind up as a loose body, "dissected" free of its original location.

2. OCD is found in the elbow, knee, and ankle in asymptomatic skeletally immature individuals, but it may not be detected until early adulthood.

3. No one etiologic theory is uniformly accepted, with the origin of OCD variously thought to be traumatic (macro or micro), vascular, or hereditary/constitutional.

B. Elbow OCD

1. Overview

a. Osteonecrosis of the capitellum, which is called Panner disease and has a relatively benign course, typically occurs in the first decade of life.

b. Capitellar OCD typically occurs after the age of 10 years. It is a frequent cause of permanent disability, ranging from inability to participate in sports at the same level to long-term arthritic changes.

2. Pathoanatomy

a. Both Panner disease and capitellar OCD are considered to be the result of overuse/overload compression-type repetitive injuries, leading to insult of the blood supply of the vulnerable immature capitellum.

b. Ossification of the capitellum usually is complete by the age of 10 years, which accounts for the distinction between Panner disease and OCD.

3. Evaluation

a. Typical presentation is an insidious onset of activity-related pain with or without stiffness in the dominant arm of an overhead throwing

athlete or athlete in a sport that involves weight bearing on the upper extremity.

b. History of locking or catching may be present.

c. Physical examination typically reveals a flexion contracture, point tenderness, and possibly crepitus.

d. Staging and classification of OCD is based on both radiographic studies and arthroscopy (**Figure 4**).

i. Type I lesions—Intact cartilage with or without bony stability underneath.

ii. Type II lesions—Cartilage fracture with bony collapse or displacement.

iii. Type III lesions—Loose pieces in the joint.

4. Nonsurgical treatment

a. Panner disease and type I OCD lesions are best treated nonsurgically, which has a success rate >90%.

b. Treatment consists of rest with or without immobilization for 3 to 6 weeks, longer for OCD than Panner.

c. The patient then is allowed to slowly progress back to activities over the next 6 to 12 weeks.

5. Surgical treatment

a. Indications

i. Failure of nonsurgical management

ii. Persistent pain

iii. Symptomatic loose bodies

iv. Displacement of OCD lesions

b. Contraindications—Patients younger than 10 years without loose bodies, chondral fractures,

3: Pediatrics

or displacement of the OCD have Panner disease.

c. Procedures

    i. Extra-articular or transarticular drilling of type I lesions without bony stability or type II lesions that are not unstable arthroscopically has good clinical success.

    ii. Fixation of OCD lesions of the capitellum has variable success at best and should be reserved for large lesions with primary intact fragments that sit well or are not completely displaced.

    iii. Débridement of the base of the lesion with or without drilling of the subchondral bone and loose-body excision is frequently required in unstable type II lesions and type III lesions.

    iv. Cartilage restoration may be necessary if symptoms continue or lesion is large. Start with a high anteromedial portal.

d. Pearls

    i. Use the posterior portals and anconeus portal for most work, as nearly all of the capitellum can be visualized through this approach.

    ii. Avoid excessive cartilage débridement; only flaps or loose cartilage should be débrided.

    iii. Avoid cartilage damage when possible by drilling extra-articularly.

    iv. Large lesions may need cartilage restoration initially or if symptoms do not abate after débridement.

6. Complications include elbow stiffness, infection, progression of arthritis, continued pain, and inability to return to sport.

7. Rehabilitation

a. The rehabilitation protocol depends on the particular procedure.

    i. Débridements/loose-body excisions call for early range of motion with or without an elbow brace. Progression to strengthening can be initiated when painless range of motion is achieved, with avoidance of valgus positions, throwing, and weight bearing for 3 to 4 months.

    ii. Elbows that undergo fixation or drilling procedures need more prolonged protection, with protected early range of motion followed by strengthening at approximately 2 months, then slow return to valgus positions. Throwing and then weight bearing is begun at 4 to 6 months.

b. Overhead or weight-bearing athletes may not return to same level of play.

c. Changes in mechanics/position/sport may be necessary.

C. Knee OCD

1. Overview/epidemiology

a. The knee is the most common site of osteochondrosis in growing children, which is seen in an estimated 0.002% to 0.003% of knee radiographs.

b. The actual incidence may actually be far greater because no studies exist for a general population of asymptomatic children.

c. Often confused with irregularities of epiphyseal ossification, this entity (despite earlier beliefs) does not always get better with benign neglect.

d. Age and level of skeletal maturation at onset are considered prognostic. It is generally thought that children with closed or nearly closed growth plates at the time of onset have a worse prognosis.

2. Evaluation

a. Patients present with generalized, often anterior, knee pain and variable swelling with or without temporally related trauma.

b. Onset may also be associated with a period of relative increase of activity or change in activities.

c. Care should be taken to assess whether the symptoms include only pain or actual mechanical popping and locking. This distinction can be helpful in determining appropriate treatment.

d. In thin patients, it is not unusual for deep pressure over the medial parapatellar area to produce pain with the knee flexed but no pain when it is extended.

e. Application of varus stress throughout a similar range of motion may produce similar reports of pain and popping if the fragment is sufficiently loose.

f. A thorough provocative and ligamentous examination is necessary to identify the possibility of comorbid conditions such as meniscal tears, loose bodies, or instability.

g. Standard weight-bearing AP, lateral, tunnel, and Merchant radiographic views should be obtained.

    i. An OCD lesion in the classic position on the lateral aspect of the medial femoral condyle

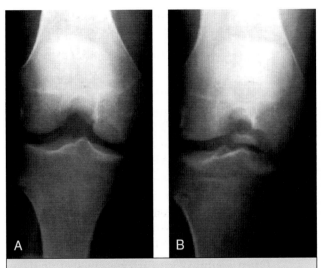

Figure 5   Tunnel views of the knee demonstrating the classic location of an OCD lesion, on the lateral aspect of the medial femoral condyle, before (**A**) and after (**B**) displacement. (*Reproduced from Crawford DC, Safran MR: Osteochondritis dissecans of the knee. J Am Acad Orthop Surg 2006;14:90-100.*)

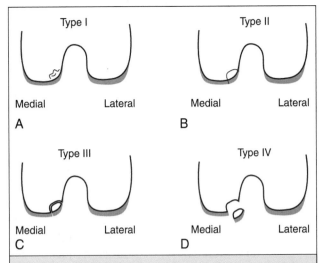

Figure 6   Guhl classification of OCD. **A**, Type I: Signal change around the lesion without bright signal. **B**, Type II: Bright signal surrounding bone portion of lesion without signs of cartilage breach. **C**, Type III: Bright signal around whole lesion including cartilage (unstable lesion). **D**, Type IV: Empty bed of the lesion with loose body. (Courtesy of Jay Albright, MD and the Children's Specialists of San Diego, CA.)

may be overlooked on the AP view in extension because of overriding bone.

ii. Classic lesions are best visualized on the tunnel view (**Figure 5**).

h. MRI and bone scans are adjunctive studies that help stage the lesions and potentially help predict prognosis.

3. Classification

a. Lesions are classified both by evaluation of radiographs and MRI and by arthroscopic evaluation, with multiple classifications in the literature.

b. Guhl MRI classification is shown in **Figure 6**.

4. Nonsurgical treatment

a. Patients with stable lesions at any age are treated with rest, activity restriction, anti-inflammatory medication, and pain modalities as needed.

b. A period of 6 weeks of protected weight bearing or immobilization may be employed as necessitated if symptoms persist.

5. Surgical treatment

a. Indications

i. Unstable lesions with or without loose bodies

ii. Older children with persistent pain despite a sufficient nonsurgical treatment period

iii. Younger patients with continued pain and swelling with or without loss of motion in whom 3 to 6 months of nonsurgical treatment has failed

b. Contraindications—Very young patients with inconsistent pain who have not failed a long course of nonsurgical treatment.

c. Procedures

i. Stable lesions are typically amenable to arthroscopic drilling of the lesion either extra-articularly or transarticularly. When drilling a stable OCD arthroscopically, pay attention to avoid slipping across the cartilage or producing excessive heat that creates cartilage damage when transarticularly perforating a lesion. Use fluoroscopy or an anterior cruciate ligament (ACL) type of drill guide when extra-articular drilling is to be performed.

ii. Unstable lesions are managed with either arthroscopic or open débridement with fixation. In young adolescents, fixation of unstable lesions should be attempted if at all possible; later procedures may be necessary, however. Bioabsorbable pins/screws work well; however, make sure appropriate length is chosen and cut flush so that no excess protrudes from the cartilage surface.

iii. A loose body that does not fit or is severely damaged should be treated with removal plus arthroplasty or a cartilage restoration

3: Pediatrics

procedure; however, every attempt should first be made to save the piece by trimming it and securing it with pins, screws, etc.

6. Complications include stiffness, infection, failure of fixation, continued pain, and arthrofibrosis.

7. Rehabilitation

   a. Crutches and touch-down weight bearing is prescribed for 6 weeks.

   b. Immediate active-assisted and passive motion is started, along with quadriceps activation and strengthening.

   c. Progression of weight bearing is allowed from 6 to 12 weeks with or without radiographic evidence of healing, as long as no pain or swelling is clinically present.

VI. Knee Ligament Injuries

A. Overview/pathoanatomy

1. Posterior cruciate ligament (PCL) and lateral collateral ligament tears are relatively rare. Medial collateral ligament tears are the most common, but ACL tears in adolescents appear to be increasing in frequency.

2. Ligaments fail when loaded at speeds and forces that lead to elongation in excess of 10% of the original length of the ligament.

3. The speed at which the load is applied determines whether the ligament fails or the bone/physis fails.

B. Evaluation/classification

1. History can be traumatic, such as a motor vehicle accident or sports-related (contact or noncontact) injury, or atraumatic. Patients present with pain and swelling acutely, with or without instability. Loss of motion is frequent as well.

2. Physical examination in the acute setting may be difficult; however, instability and point tenderness in this initial setting can be diagnostic. Repeat examination in a few days or a week may aid in the diagnosis in lieu of an MRI.

3. Radiographs taken during the initial examination can rule out physeal or other fractures about the knee. Occasionally they will demonstrate abnormalities of alignment, such as an anteriorly translated tibia seen on a lateral view, that make it possible to diagnose a ligament injury.

4. MRI is a useful tool for confirming a suspected diagnosis or when an adequate physical examination is not possible.

5. Classification—Ligament injuries are graded according to severity of injury of each ligament individually.

C. Treatment

1. General principles of ACL treatment in particular

   a. When deciding treatment, the patient needs to be considered as a whole. This includes age, growth remaining, ligament injured, severity of injury, and level of planned activity.

   b. When a patient is not within 2 years of skeletal maturity, choose treatment carefully and weigh all factors. When in doubt, repair other pathology and rehabilitate, with or without bracing.

   c. Although not common, physeal injury or arrest can occur in the hands of even the most experienced surgeon, no matter what procedure is used.

   d. Use all tools necessary to determine skeletal age when considering ligament reconstruction (growth charts, bone age, Tanner staging, etc).

   e. Partial tears of the ACL, PCL, or medial/lateral collateral ligaments without other intraarticular pathology are amenable to nonsurgical treatment.

      i. Bracing provides initial stabilization as well as support for return to sport.

      ii. Physical therapy, including strength and gait training and pain modalities, is useful to obtain full range of motion.

      iii. Anti-inflammatory medications may be used initially, but there is some question about their effect on the soft-tissue healing process.

      iv. Return to sport may be allowed when full motion, strength, and stability have returned with or without a brace.

   f. Complete tears

      i. Complete PCL injuries seem to cause fewer feelings of instability than ACL tears but probably have the same potential for long-term arthritis, although surgical intervention is more easily avoided until skeletal maturity.

      ii. Posterolateral corner injuries rarely occur by themselves, and when they are combined with PCL injuries, a more difficult circumstance is created.

   g. The obvious concern in treatment of any ligament injury is balancing the risk of iatrogenic physeal injury from surgical reconstruction or long-term disability and/or arthritis with attempts at nonsurgical treatments. The younger the patient, the greater the risk of deformity if a growth arrest ensues after a reconstructive procedure. Such cases of iatrogenic injury have been reported.

2. Nonsurgical treatment

   a. Initial treatment for all ligament tears should be nonsurgical, unless the tear is associated with meniscal damage, loose bodies, or other immediate urgent surgical indications.

   b. Activity modification, brief immobilization, physical therapy, and pain modalities are all indicated initially.

   c. Obtaining full motion and relative stability with bracing and muscle control may obviate the need for surgical intervention in a select group of individuals (copers) even when skeletally mature.

3. Surgical treatment

   a. Indications

      i. Failure to maintain stability despite physical therapy and bracing, and unwillingness to modify activities

      ii. Need to assess other pathology, such as meniscal pathology

   b. Procedures

      i. Ligament repair—Ligament reconstruction has not been shown to prevent long-term disability or arthritis in skeletally immature or mature patients.

      ii. Physeal sparing—Either all epiphyseal or extra-articular reconstructions (**Figure 7**).

      iii. Transtibial over the top of femur

      iv. Transphyseal

      v. Combination procedures

   c. Surgical pearls

      i. Avoid spanning the physis with bone or metal.

      ii. Keep transphyseal tunnels to a minimum size in a central location.

      iii. Avoid dissection or damage to the perichondral ring (ie, do not dissect subperiosteally) when going around the over-the-top position on the femur.

D. Complications include physeal arrest, either partial or complete; arthrofibrosis; infection; short/long-term ligament failure; arthritis; and atrophy.

E. Rehabilitation

   1. Immediate motion, quadriceps activation, swelling and pain control

   2. Prolonged physical therapy

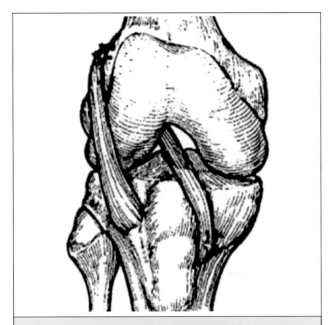

Figure 7 Extraphyseal ACL reconstruction. (*Reproduced with permission from Kocher MS, Garg S, Micheli LJ: Physeal sparing reconstruction of the anterior cruciate ligament in skeletally immature prepubescent children and adolescents. J Bone Joint Surg Am 2005;87:2371-2379.*)

   a. Slow, steady progress back to straightforward running at around 6 months

   b. No start-stop or cutting for 8 to 12 months

   c. Return to sports in 1 year with or without a brace

VII. Meniscal Injuries and Discoid Meniscus

A. Pathoanatomy

   1. Injuries to the meniscus occur as a result of twisting events during loading of the knee on either a normal or discoid meniscus.

   2. Common meniscal tears include horizontal, vertical, bucket-handle, parrot beak, radial, or combinations thereof (**Figure 8**).

   3. Meniscal injuries occur in both the vascular and avascular zones.

   4. The location and pattern of the tear have significant implications for the success of repair attempts; eg, tears occurring close to the vascular zone have higher rates of success, and parrot beak and radial tears have lower rates of success.

   5. Removing any part of the meniscus significantly decreases the effectiveness/function of the meniscus.

3: Pediatrics

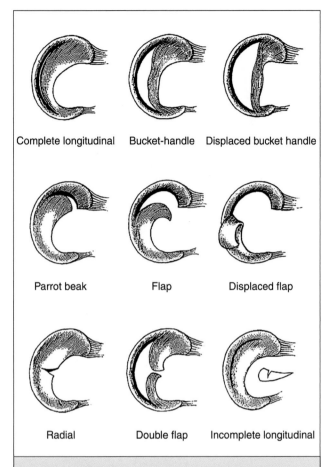

Complete longitudinal   Bucket-handle   Displaced bucket handle

Parrot beak   Flap   Displaced flap

Radial   Double flap   Incomplete longitudinal

Figure 8   Illustrations of common meniscal tear morphology. (*Reproduced with permission from Tria AJ, Klein KS: An Illustrated Guide to the Knee. New York, NY, Churchill Livingstone, 1992.*)

B. Evaluation

1. History

   a. Like ligament tears, meniscal tears either may be associated with traumatic events or may follow a nontraumatic event such as twisting, turning, or even kneeling.

   b. Young children often cannot recall when the pain began and may present with insidious onset.

2. Physical examination

   a. Point tenderness at the joint line anterior and posterior to the collateral ligament on that side is typical.

   b. Pain with deep knee flexion, loss of motion, and a positive provocative test may also be present.

3. Radiographs may indicate suspicion of discoid lateral meniscus with widened lateral joint line with or without lateral femoral condyle changes.

4. MRI should be used as a confirmatory test for discoid meniscus, tears of the meniscus, and evaluation of other confounding diagnoses. MRI has a high false-positive rate in children under 10 years of age because the vascularity can be misinterpreted.

C. Classification

1. Meniscal tears are classified descriptively.

   a. Location of tear—Red (vascular) zone, red-white, white (avascular) zone (outer third, middle third, inner third)

   b. Size

   c. Pattern—Horizontal, vertical, radial, bucket-handle, parrot beak, complex, or combination (Figure 8)

2. Discoid menisci are classified by shape and stability as complete, incomplete, and Wrisberg (**Figure 9**).

D. Nonsurgical treatment

1. The treatment of asymptomatic discoid menisci is observation.

2. Small or peripheral tears may heal with nonsurgical care, which may include activity modification, physical therapy, anti-inflammatory medication, and pain modalities.

3. Bracing may help diminish effusion but will not prevent incarceration of the tear.

E. Surgical treatment

1. Indications

   a. True mechanical symptoms, presence of a loose body, and associated ligament tears

   b. Failure of nonsurgical treatment

2. Contraindications

   a. Peripheral tears in the red-red vascular zone where the meniscus is more likely to heal without intervention, unless the patient still has pain after a prolonged period of activity modification

   b. Equivocal MRI without locking symptoms

3. Procedures

   a. Fixation methods

      i. Inside-out is the gold standard.

      ii. All-inside has gained popularity as a method of fixation of torn or unstable menisci because of its relative speed of use and because it does not require an extra incision. Meniscal healing with all-inside devices is less reliable than the inside-out technique, however, particularly in the lateral meniscus. The new

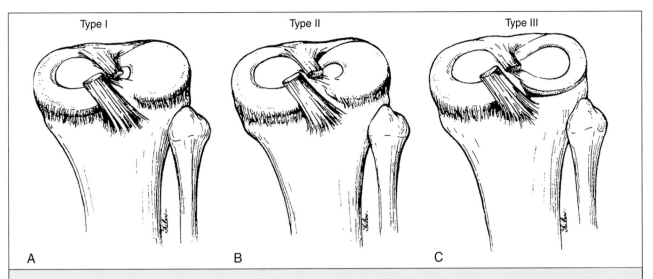

Figure 9   Classification system for lateral discoid menisci: **A,** type I (complete), **B,** type II (incomplete), and **C,** type III (Wrisberg ligament). Type III discoid menisci have no posterior attachment to the tibia. The only posterior attachment is through the ligament of Wrisberg toward the medial femoral condyle. (*Reproduced with permission from Neus-chwander DC: Discoid lateral meniscus, in Fu FH, Harner CD, Vince KG [eds]: Knee Surgery. Baltimore, MD, Williams & Wilkins, 1994, p 394.*)

lower profile devices are less likely to damage articular cartilage.

   iii. Outside-in is used less frequently than the others but may be useful for anterior horn repair.

  b. Partial meniscectomy

4. Surgical pearls

  a. It is best to leave only sutures or devices with a closely matched modulus of elasticity in the joint on the surface of the meniscus.

  b. When repairing a large tear, remember to stabilize both the superior and inferior surfaces.

  c. Vertical divergent suture pattern is the strongest.

  d. Reserve partial meniscectomy for those tears that are irreparable only—fix first, remove second.

F. Complications

1. Arthrofibrosis

2. Infection

3. Short- or long-term repair failure

4. New tears

5. Arthritis

6. Atrophy

G. Rehabilitation

1. Immediate motion, quadriceps activation, swelling and pain control

2. For repaired meniscus, 4 to 6 weeks of touchdown weight bearing depending on size and side of tear

3. Reserve longer periods of restricted weight bearing for larger and/or lateral tears.

4. Consider 3 to 4 weeks of restricted range of motion (0° to 90°).

5. When repair is not possible, weight bearing is allowed as tolerated and as return of quadriceps strength dictates.

VIII. Plica Syndrome

A. Epidemiology

1. Painful plica is a diagnosis of exclusion and its true incidence is difficult to discern.

2. Reportedly, these are medially based parapatellar bands in approximately 90% of symptomatic patients.

B. Pathoanatomy

1. A plica is a remnant of embryologic development; it consists of normal synovial tissue that causes mechanically based synovitis from repetitive motion.

2. On occasion, plicas can even cause arthroscopically visible evidence of chondromalacia of the edge of the femoral condyle.

C. Evaluation

1. Plica syndrome is a diagnosis of exclusion of other pathologies.

2. Patients report activity-related anteromedial to medial knee pain, sometimes with catching or partial giving way.

3. Physical examination reveals a painful, palpable band of tissue along the medial parapatellar area.

   a. Feel the knee while the patient performs active motion. If patellar compression is nonpainful in 45° of knee flexion but around the patellar soft tissue is painful, then plica may be present.

   b. It is often also valuable to attempt to look for an accompanying and very sensitive lateral suprapatellar soft-tissue mass that lies under the vastus lateralis.

   c. The parapatellar bands can also be occasionally palpated lateral and even inferior to the patella.

   d. MRI may miss a plica; although it is easier to see when there is a knee effusion, it is usually difficult to visualize, so a high index of suspicion is warranted.

D. Treatment

1. Nonsurgical treatment

   a. Anti-inflammatory medications, ice, activity modification, immobilization

   b. Physical therapy modalities such as ultrasound and iontophoresis of cortisone solution

   c. Cortisone injections

2. Surgical treatment

   a. Indications

      i. When the patient has pain not resolved by nonsurgical methods

      ii. When the problem is discovered at the time of surgery for another diagnosis that is

found to be erroneous with only an irritated plica for a plausible explanation

   b. Contraindications—Reflex sympathetic dystrophy or chronic regional pain syndrome, as well as saphenous neuritis, should all be ruled out before surgical intervention.

   c. Procedure

      i. Arthroscopic resection of the plica is performed in a standard two- or three-portal approach.

      ii. The inferomedial parapatellar portal or the medial/lateral suprapatellar portals are typically sufficient for excision with shaver/biter/heat probe of choice.

   d. Surgical pearls

      i. The most worrisome pitfall is a too-aggressive resection of the plica that includes the retinaculum and not just the abnormal band of synovium.

      ii. Look for denuding/irritation/deformation of the medial condylar articular surface under the contact area of the plica; if found, this is an indication that it should be resected.

      iii. Use an arthroscopic punch or heat device to create a working resection edge in the thickened yet smooth plicas that a shaver has a difficult time getting started on.

E. Complications—The standard complications that can occur after routine arthroscopy also can occur after arthroscopy for plica syndrome: arthrofibrosis, infection, nerve/vessel injury, patellar instability, unresolved pain.

F. Rehabilitation

1. Immediate motion and quadriceps activation, with quick return to weight bearing as tolerated

2. At 3 to 4 weeks the patient may be ready to return to full participation, depending on other pathology present at the time of surgery.

Top Testing Facts

1. Little Leaguer shoulder is an epiphysiolysis, or a fracture through the proximal humeral physis, that causes pain during the late cocking or deceleration phases of pitching.

2. Little Leaguer elbow occurs secondary to valgus-hyperextension overloading at the elbow during pitching. Initial treatment of apophysitis is activity modification.

3. The radiographic diagnosis of a capitellar lesion in a child younger than 10 years is Panner disease; in a child older than 10 years, it is OCD.

4. OCD of the knee classically involves the lateral aspect of the medial femoral condyle and is best visualized on a tunnel view. The stability of the lesion influences the prognosis.

5. Initial treatment of OCD in the knee is with activity modification/rest with or without immobilization, unless locking symptoms or a loose body is present.

6. A feared complication of ACL reconstruction is partial or complete physeal arrest in the skeletally immature.

7. Tears of the meniscus in the outer, vascular zone should be operated on only if locking symptoms exist or if there is no improvement after prolonged nonsurgical treatment.

8. The treatment of asymptomatic discoid menisci is observation.

9. Partial ACL tears can be treated nonsurgically, with physical therapy with or without bracing.

Bibliography

Andrish JT: Meniscal injuries in children and adolescents: Diagnosis and management. *J Am Acad Orthop Surg* 1996;4:231-237.

Cahill BR: Osteochondritis dissecans of the knee: Treatment of juvenile and adult forms. *J Am Acad Orthop Surg* 1995;3:237-247.

Cassas KJ, Cassettari-Wayhs A: Childhood and adolescent sports-related overuse injuries. *Am Fam Physician* 2006;73:1014-1022.

Chen FS, Diaz VA, Loebenberg M, Rosen JE: Shoulder and elbow injuries in the skeletally immature athlete. *J Am Acad Orthop Surg* 2005;13:172-185.

Crawford DC, Safran MR: Osteochondritis dissecans of the knee. *J Am Acad Orthop Surg* 2006;14:90-100.

Jackson RW, Marshall DJ, Fujisawa Y: The pathologic medical shelf. *Orthop Clin North Am* 1982;13:307-312.

Kobayashi K, Burton KJ, Rodner C, Smith B, Caputo AE: Lateral compression injuries in the pediatric elbow: Panner's disease and osteochondritis dissecans of the capitellum. *J Am Acad Orthop Surg* 2004;12:246-254.

Kocher MS, Saxon HS, Hovis WD, Hawkins RJ: Management and complications of anterior cruciate ligament injuries in skeletally immature patients: Survey of the Herodicus Society and the ACL Study Group. *J Pediatr Orthop* 2002;22:452-457.

Larsen MW, Garrett WE Jr, Delee JC, Moorman CT III: Surgical management of anterior cruciate ligament injuries in patients with open physes. *J Am Acad Orthop Surg* 2006;14:736-744.

National Federation of State High School Associations (NFHS): 2005-2006 High School Athletic Participation Survey. Indianapolis, IN, NHFS, 2006. Available at http://www.nfhs.org/sports.aspx.

Stanitski CL: Anterior cruciate ligament injury in the skeletally immature patient: Diagnosis and treatment. *J Am Acad Orthop Surg* 1995;3:146-158.

3: Pediatrics

Chapter 30

Pediatric Neuromuscular Disorders
M. Siobhan Murphy Zane, MD

I. Cerebral Palsy

A. Epidemiology

1. Cerebral palsy (CP) has an incidence of 1 to 3 per 1,000 live births.

2. Prematurity and low birth weight (<1,500 g) increase the incidence to 90 per 1,000.

B. Pathoanatomy

1. CP is a static encephalopathy, ie, a nonprogressive, permanent injury to the brain that is caused by injury, damage, defect, or illness.

2. CP can affect the child's motor development as well as speech, cognition, and sensation.

3. Although the brain injury is static, the peripheral manifestations (eg, contractures and bony deformities) in patients with CP often are not static.

C. Risk factors for CP are listed in **Table 1**.

D. Evaluation

1. Positive predictive factors for walking

   a. Sitting by age 2 years

   b. Pulling to stand by age 2 years

2. Poor prognostic indicators for walking

   a. Persistence of 2 or more primitive reflexes (eg, Moro) at age 1 year

   b. Not sitting by age 5 years

   c. Not walking by age 8 years

3. Computerized 3-dimensional gait analysis can aid in distinguishing abnormalities in gait pattern.

E. Classification—Several classification systems are useful in treating CP.

1. Physiologic—The location of the brain injury will cause different types of motor dysfunction.

   a. Patients with spastic-type (pyramidal) CP exhibit increased tone or rigidity with rapid stretch. This can lead to gait disturbances and contracture. These patients most often benefit from orthopaedic interventions.

   b. Patients with dyskinetic (extrapyramidal) or choreoathetoid CP exhibit involuntary movements, athetosis, and dystonia. This type is less frequently seen since Rh-immune globulin has been administered to prevent Rh incompatibility between mother and infant.

   c. Patients with ataxia (cerebellar) exhibit disturbed balance and coordination.

   d. Patients with mixed types show spasticity and dyskinesia.

2. Anatomic—The affected areas of the body are described in **Table 2**.

3. Functional—The patient is assigned a grade of functioning according to ambulation and activities (**Figure 1**).

F. Treatment

1. Physical therapy (PT) addresses development of gait and functional mobility with gait trainers, walkers or crutches, and prevention of contracture through stretching, bracing, and standing programs.

2. Occupational therapy (OT) addresses fine motor function, activities of daily living (ADLs), self-feeding, self-dressing, and communication through speech or adaptive equipment.

Table 1
Risk Factors for Cerebral Palsy
Prematurity
Low birth weight
Multiple births
TORCH infections (toxoplasmosis, other infections [syphilis, etc], rubella, cytomegalovirus, herpes)
Chorioamnionitis
Placental complications
Third trimester bleeding
Maternal epilepsy
Toxemia
Low Apgar scores
Anoxia
Intraventricular hemorrhage
Infection
Maternal drug and alcohol use
Teratogens

Table 2

Anatomic Classification of Cerebral Palsy

Type	Area Affected
Quadriplegia	4 limbs
Whole body	4 limbs and bulbar problems (eg, swallowing)
Hemiplegia	1 side of the body
Diplegia	Lower extremities, but can have some upper extremity posturing

3. Speech therapy is often requisite, particularly in children with significant bulbar involvement.

4. Splinting or serial casting may prevent or improve spasticity and contracture.

5. Bracing is often used to improve joint or limb position in stance or ambulation or to prevent deformity.

   a. Supramalleolar orthoses (SMOs) may be used to control coronal plane deformities of the foot and ankle (pronation or supination) but do not address the sagittal plane (equinus or calcaneus).

   b. Ankle-foot orthoses (AFOs) may be used to stabilize the ankle joint.

      i. Solid-ankle AFOs may be used to prevent equinus or a crouched stance due to uncontrolled dorsiflexion at the ankle. Prevention of equinus and calcaneus has been shown to improve walking speed and stride length for most children.

      ii. Hinged AFOs may be used to allow dorsiflexion while preventing equinus during gait.

      iii. Floor-reaction AFOs cause knee extension to improve crouched gait secondary to ankle plantar flexion weakness.

   c. Knee-ankle-foot orthoses (KAFOs) stabilize the knee and are useful for maintaining knee position in children who walk very limited distances or only stand.

6. Antispasticity medicines

   a. Baclofen

      i. Oral administration is common, but dosage needs to be adjusted if relaxation is accompanied by an unacceptable amount of sedation.

      ii. Intrathecal baclofen (ITB) is administered by an intrathecal pump and is associated with less sedation. ITB is considered only if oral medications (including baclofen) have failed. Potential recipients are nonambulatory pa-

tients with moderate to severe spasticity and patients with a component of dystonia.

   b. Valium is administered orally, but it also can result in significant sedation before sufficient muscle relaxation is obtained.

7. Surgical spasticity management—Selective dorsal rhizotomy (SDR) reduces spasticity by selectively cutting dorsal nerve rootlets between L1 and S1.

   a. SDR may be indicated in ambulatory patients with diplegia, age 3 to 8 years with good selective motor control and intelligence in the "normal" range.

   b. Fewer than 50% of rootlets should be cut at any given level.

   c. Cautions—SDR can increase the risk of spine and hip deformities and may increase weakness as the child reaches adolescence.

8. Botulinum toxin affects the neuromuscular junction by irreversibly binding synaptic proteins to block the presynaptic release of acetylcholine.

   a. Botulinum toxin A is the form commonly used in the United States for children with CP.

   b. In CP, intramuscular botulinum toxin injection results in 3 to 6 months of relaxation in spastic muscles; it is commonly used in conjunction with PT, stretching, casting, or bracing.

   c. Botulinum toxin is useful for dynamic spasticity only, not for fixed contractures.

   d. Botulinum toxin may be considered a temporizing measure to delay surgery.

9. Surgical intervention is generally undertaken when a patient has plateaued or worsened in regard to function and/or deformity despite nonsurgical interventions.

10. **Table 3** lists recommended surgical interventions for common gait disturbances associated with CP.

G. Spine problems specific to CP

   1. Scoliosis

      a. The incidence and severity are related to the severity of CP.

         i. Scoliosis occurs in >50% of patients with quadriplegia and in ~1% with hemiplegia.

         ii. Scoliosis progression is common after skeletal maturity in patients with quadriplegia.

      b. Treatment

         i. Bracing may not be an effective treatment of neuromuscular scoliosis in children with CP, but it may be effective in the treatment of idiopathic curves in children with mild involvement.

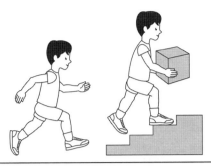

GMFCS Level I

Children walk indoors and outdoors and climb stairs without limitation. Children perform gross motor skills including running and jumping, but speed, balance and co-ordination are impaired.

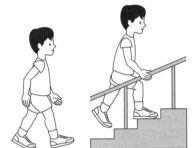

GMFCS Level II

Children walk indoors and outdoors and climb stairs holding onto a railing but experience limitations walking on uneven surfaces and inclines and walking in crowds or confined spaces.

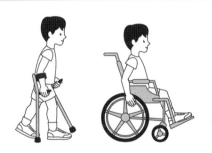

GMFCS Level III

Children walk indoors or outdoors on a level surface with an assistive mobility device. Children may climb stairs holding onto a railing. Children may propel a wheelchair manually or are transported when traveling for long distances or outdoors on uneven terrain.

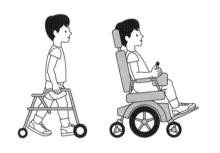

GMFCS Level IV

Children may continue to walk for short distances on a walker or rely more on wheeled mobility at home and school and in the community.

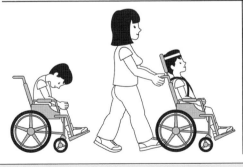

GMFCS Level V

Physical impairment restricts voluntary control of movement and the ability to maintain antigravity head and trunk postures. All areas of motor function are limited. Children have no means of independent mobility and are transported.

Figure 1   Gross motor function classification system (GMFCS) for ages 6-12 years. *(Reproduced with permission from Palisano RJ, Rosenbaum P, Walter S, Russell D, Wood E, Galuppi B: Development and reliability of a system to classify gross motor function in children with cerebral palsy. Dev Med Child Neurol 1997;45:113-120. Illustrated by Kerr Graham and Bill Reid, The Royal Children's Hospital, Melbourne.)*

3: Pediatrics

Table 3		
Surgical Treatment of Common Gait Disturbances in Cerebral Palsy		
Gait Disturbance	**Problem**	**Recommended Surgery**
Scissoring	Tight adductors	Adductor tenotomy
Toe-walking	Tight gastrocnemius-soleus (equinus deformity)	Gastrocnemius or Achilles lengthening (Do not overlengthen!)
	Apparent equinus with crouched gait because of hip and/or knee deformities (ankle is actually neutral)	Do not lengthen gastrocnemius-soleus; address hip and knee contractures!
Back-knee gait	Tight gastrocnemius-soleus (equinus deformity)	Gastrocnemius or Achilles lengthening (Do not overlengthen!)
	Iatrogenic overlengthening of the hamstrings without distal RF transfer	Distal RF transfer may be helpful
Decreased knee flexion in swing phase (even without crouched gait)	Overactive RF	Distal RF transfer (to semitendinosis if possible)
Crouched gait	Tight hip flexors	Intramuscular psoas lengthening
	Tight hamstrings	Hamstring lengthenings
	Excessively loose heel cords (which can then cause tight hip flexors and hamstrings)	None (Achilles tendon shortening and proximal calcaneal slide have mixed results) (usually need to go to solid AFOs)
	Lever arm dysfunction	See intoeing and pes valgus below.
Intoeing	Increased femoral anteversion	Femoral rotational osteotomy
	Internal tibial torsion	Tibial rotational osteotomy
	Varus foot	Varus foot correction (as described below)
Pes valgus, common in patients with diplegia and quadriplegia	Spastic gastrocnemius-soleus and peroneals with tibialis posterior weakness	Calcaneal lengthening (best after age 6 years) Calcaneal medial sliding osteotomy
Equinovarus foot	Spastic tibialis anterior and/or tibialis posterior overpower the peroneals, with gastrocnemius-soleus equinus	Treat equinus as noted above. Split anterior tendon transfer if anterior tibialis causative Posterior tibialis lengthening or split transfer if posterior tibialis causative Must add calcaneal osteotomy if hindfoot deformity is rigid

RF = rectus femoris

ii. Surgery, typically fusion that is performed from the upper thoracic spine to the pelvis in nonambulatory patients, may be indicated for large curves that cause pain and/or interfere with sitting.

2. Lumbar hyperlordosis

a. Lumbar hyperlordosis can occur.

b. It is almost always secondary to hip flexion contractures.

H. Hip problems specific to CP

1. Subluxation

a. Epidemiology/overview

i. Subluxation is uncommon in the ambulatory

patient, but it is very common in the nonambulatory patient.

ii. Subluxation (usually posterosuperior) is due to adductor and iliopsoas spasticity, and non–weight-bearing status.

iii. Hip subluxation will develop in 50% of quadriplegic CP patients.

iv. 50% to 75% of dislocated hips will become painful.

b. Treatment

i. Goals are to prevent hip subluxation and dislocation, maintain comfortable seating, and facilitate care and hygiene.

ii. Treatment is based on radiologic assessment with the Reimer migration percentage (**Figure 2**).

iii. Nonsurgical treatment consists first of PT and range of motion (ROM), hip abduction orthosis, with consideration of botulinum toxin injections to adductors.

iv. Surgical management is appropriate with progressive subluxation to ≥50% subluxation (Reimer index). Patients younger than 8 years and with <60% subluxation can be treated with adductor and iliopsoas release. Patients younger than 8 years and with >60% subluxation or older than 8 years and with >40% subluxation should be treated with proximal femoral osteotomy (varus derotational osteotomy—VDRO) and possible pelvic osteotomy (Dega or Albee-type). Older children with closed triradiate cartilage or those with recurrent subluxation may benefit from a Schanz or Chiari pelvis osteotomy. Children with failed hip reconstruction or older children with arthritis, even without previous surgery, may require resection arthroplasty (Castle procedure) for pain relief.

c. Pitfalls—The Castle procedure requires careful interposition of the hip capsule and muscle in the joint space, and the recovery time is often prolonged (6 months or more).

2. Scissoring

   a. Scissoring (due to adductor tightness) at the hip joint can interfere with gait and hygiene and is treated with proximal adductor release.

   b. Obturator neurectomy should not be performed.

3. Hip flexion contracture is treated with intramuscular iliopsoas lengthening.

I. Lever arm dysfunction associated with CP

1. Lever arm dysfunction results in posterior displacement of the ground reaction force relative to the knee and often results in crouch and power abnormalities in gait.

2. Intoeing from femoral anteversion can be treated with femoral rotational osteotomies.

3. Intoeing from internal tibial torsion can be treated with supramalleolar tibial osteotomies (concurrent fibular osteotomy is not needed).

4. Intoeing is rarely due to medial hamstring spasticity because of the small lever arm of the hamstrings.

5. Pes planus (pes valgus)

   a. Pes planus is common in patients with diplegia and quadriplegia.

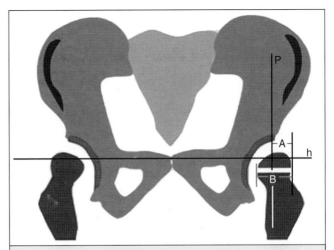

Figure 2 Schematic representation showing how the Reimer migration percentage is measured from an AP radiograph. The Hilgenreiner (h) and Perkin (P) lines are drawn. Distance A (the distance from P to the lateral border of the femoral epiphysis) is divided by distance B (the width of the femoral epiphysis) and multiplied by 100 to calculate the Reimer migration percentage (A/B × 100). *(Reproduced with permission from Miller F: Hip, in Dabney K, Alexander M (eds): Cerebral Palsy. New York, NY, Springer, 2005, p 532.)*

b. The foot is externally rotated due to spastic gastrocnemius, soleus, and peroneal muscles, with weak tibialis posterior function.

c. Patients bear weight on the medial border of the foot, on the talar head.

d. The foot is unstable in push-off.

e. Treatment

   i. Mild planovalgus feet can be treated with SMOs or AFOs.

   ii. Moderate to severe deformities can be treated with a calcaneal osteotomy. Calcaneal lengthening osteotomy (best undertaken after age 6 years) is able to restore normal anatomy and is combined with peroneus brevis lengthening and tightening of the medial talonavicular joint capsule and/or posterior tibial tendon. The peroneus longus should not routinely be lengthened, because this will exacerbate first ray dorsiflexion. A medial calcaneal sliding osteotomy enhances alignment but creates a secondary (compensatory) deformity.

   iii. Severe deformities can be treated with subtalar fusion, although this is usually only needed in very large children and/or those with extreme laxity. (Triple arthrodesis is almost never required.)

   iv. Compensatory midfoot supination can be treated with first ray plantar flexion osteot-

3: Pediatrics

Table 4

Causes of Anterior Knee Pain in Cerebral Palsy

Patella alta
Weak quadriceps
Tight hamstrings
Femoral anteversion
External tibial torsion
Pes valgus
Genu valgum
Patellar instability (may sometimes be asymptomatic)

omy, often with a peroneus brevis lengthening.

J. Knee problems specific to CP

1. Crouched gait

   a. Causes—The most common cause is tight hamstrings, although crouch may be secondary to excessive ankle dorsiflexion or ankle equinus.

   b. Treatment

      i. Nonsurgical treatment includes PT, bracing (such as knee immobilizers at night), and botulinum toxin injection.

      ii. Surgical treatment is medial (and possibly lateral) hamstring lengthening. Lengthening medial and lateral hamstrings in an ambulatory patient carries an increased risk of recurvatum.

2. Stiff-knee gait

   a. Stiff-knee gait causes difficulties with foot clearance in swing phase and tripping.

   b. The cause is often overactivity of the rectus femoris (RF) in swing phase.

   c. Treatment is with distal RF transfer. Indications for surgery are decreased magnitude and/or delayed timing of peak knee flexion in swing phase in conjunction with overactivity of the RF in swing phase.

3. Anterior knee pain—Causes of anterior knee pain in CP are listed in **Table 4**.

4. Knee contracture—In a nonambulatory patient, hamstring release may be useful to maintain leg position in a standing program.

K. Foot and ankle—Abnormal position or ROM at the foot and ankle cause gait abnormalities and decrease push-off power. Goals of treatment include a painless, plantigrade (stable) foot.

1. Equinus deformity results from gastrocnemius-soleus muscle complex spasticity. It can create toe-walking or a back-knee (genu recurvatum) gait.

   a. Nonsurgical treatment includes stretching, PT

for ROM, AFO use, and botulinum toxin injection.

   b. Surgical treatment should be considered only in patients with fixed contractures.

      i. Testing under anesthesia helps determine whether a gastrocnemius recession or Achilles tendon lengthening is appropriate. If the ankle is in equinus with the knee flexed and extended, then the soleus is also tight, and an Achilles tendon lengthening should be performed. If the ankle comes above neutral with the knee flexed (gastrocnemius relaxed), then a gastrocnemius recession should be performed.

      ii. Overlengthening the heel cord may cause crouched gait, calcaneus foot position, and poor push-off power. This is less of a problem with a gastrocnemius recession than with an Achilles tendon lengthening.

2. Equinovarus foot deformity can cause painful weight bearing over the lateral border of the foot and instability in stance phase.

   a. The anterior tibialis and/or the posterior tibialis (the invertors) overpowers the peroneals (the evertors), whereas a tight gastrocnemius-soleus muscle causes equinus.

   b. Dynamic EMG is useful in distinguishing whether the anterior tibialis and/or the posterior tibialis is causing the varus.

   c. Clinically, the tibialis anterior can be checked using the confusion test.

      i. The patient sits on the edge of the examining table and flexes the hip actively.

      ii. The tibialis anterior will fire.

      iii. If the forefoot supinates as it dorsiflexes, the varus is at least partially due to the tibialis anterior.

      iv. If the forefoot just dorsiflexes, the varus is likely not due to the tibialis anterior.

   d. Clinically, the posterior tibialis is assessed by tightness as the hindfoot is positioned in valgus.

   e. Generally, isolated forefoot supination comes from the tibialis anterior, while hindfoot varus comes from the posterior tibialis.

   f. Anterior tibialis and/or posterior tibialis split tendon transfers are recommended rather than full tendon transfers because whole tendon transfers may lead to overcorrection.

   g. Tibialis posterior lengthenings are helpful in less severe deformities that are caused by the posterior tibialis.

h. Pitfalls

  i. Rigidity of the varus must be assessed preoperatively to determine the need for calcaneal osteotomy.

  ii. A soft-tissue procedure will not be sufficient if the hindfoot deformity is rigid.

  iii. In rigid feet, soft-tissue and bone procedures are both needed.

3. Equinovalgus arises from gastrocnemius-soleus and peroneal spasticity with tibialis posterior weakness.

  a. Weight-bearing AP radiographs of the ankles must be obtained because ankle valgus may also contribute to deformity.

  b. Nonsurgical treatment includes SMO or AFO bracing and PT for ROM, and may include botulinum toxin injection.

  c. Surgical treament

    i. Calcaneal osteotomies preserve ROM and are preferred when feasible. Calcaneal lengthening with peroneus brevis lengthening is preferred because it can restore the anatomy. Avoid peroneus longus lengthening because this can cause increased first ray dorsiflexion. Calcaneal (medial) sliding osteotomy brings the calcaneus in line with the weight-bearing axis of the tibia.

    ii. Subtalar arthrodesis is rarely needed but may be necessary in the presence of marked deformity or ligamentous laxity.

    iii. Triple arthrodesis is rarely required.

4. Hallux valgus

  a. Occurs frequently with pes valgus, equinovalgus, and equinovarus feet

  b. Toe straps added to AFOs or nighttime hallux valgus splinting may be helpful.

  c. Severe hallux valgus should be treated with a fusion of the first metatarsophalangeal (MTP) joint.

  d. Pes valgus must be simultaneously corrected to avoid recurrence.

  e. Pitfalls—At the time of hallux valgus correction, consider that the patient will often also have valgus interphalangeus, which should be treated with a proximal phalanx (Akin) osteotomy.

5. Dorsal bunion

  a. Overview/etiology

    i. Dorsal bunion is a deformity in which the great toe is flexed in relation to an elevated metatarsal, causing a prominence over the uncovered metatarsal head, which can be painful with shoe wear.

    ii. Dorsal bunion may be iatrogenic, occurring after surgery to balance the foot.

    iii. The deformation may either be caused by an overpowering tibialis anterior or an overpowering flexor hallucis longus (FHL).

  b. Treatment

    i. Nonsurgical treatment is with shoes with soft, deep toe boxes.

    ii. Surgical treatment is needed in recalcitrant cases. Flexible deformities are treated with lengthening or split transfer of the anterior tibialis and transfer of the FHL to the plantar aspect of the first metatarsal head. Osteotomies of the medial column are rarely needed. Rigid deformities require fusion of the first MTP joint and lengthening or split transfer of the anterior tibialis. Osteotomies are rarely needed.

L. Upper extremity problems specific to CP

1. General information

  a. Upper extremity involvement is typical in patients with hemiplegia and quadriplegia. Commonly, the hand is fisted, the thumb is in the palm, the forearm is flexed and pronated, the wrist is flexed, and the shoulder is internally rotated.

  b. Nonsurgical treatment

    i. OT is useful in early childhood for ADL, stretching, and splinting.

    ii. Botulinum toxin is useful for dynamic deformities.

    iii. Constraint-induced therapy (splinting of the uninvolved upper extremity to encourage use of the involved arm) in patients with hemiplegia is gaining popularity but does not have a long track record.

  c. Surgical treatment

    i. Surgical treatment is undertaken primarily for functional concerns, hygiene, and sometimes for appearance.

    ii. If shoulder adduction and internal rotation contractures are interfering with hand function, they may be treated with subscapularis release and pectoralis major lengthening. A proximal humeral derotational osteotomy is rarely necessary.

    iii. Elbow flexion contractures may be treated with lacertus fibrosis resection, biceps and brachialis lengthening, and brachioradialis origin release.

3: Pediatrics

iv. Elbow pronation contractures should be treated with pronator teres release. Transfer of the pronator teres to an anterolateral position (to act as a supinator) may cause a supination deformity, which is not preferable to pronation.

v. Radial head dislocation is uncommon and, if symptomatic, may be treated with radial head excision when the patient reaches maturity.

vi. Wrist deformities usually include flexion contracture with ulnar deviation and are associated with weak wrist extension and a pronated forearm. If finger extension is good and there is little wrist flexion spasticity, the flexor carpi ulnaris (FCU) or flexor carpi radialis (FCR) should be lengthened. Releasing the wrist and finger flexors and the pronator teres from the medial epicondyle of the humerus weakens wrist and finger flexion but is nonselective. In severe spasticity, an FCU transfer is recommended. If grasp is good, release is weak, and the FCU is active in release, it should be transferred to the extensor digitorum communis (EDC). If grasp is weak with the wrist flexed, release is good, and the FCU is active in grasp, it should be transferred to the extensor carpi radialis brevis (ECRB). A concurrent FCR release should not be performed, to avoid overweakening wrist flexion.

2. Hand deformities

a. Thumb-in-palm—Caused by metacarpal adduction contracture with metacarpophalangeal (MCP) flexion or extension contracture, sometimes with interphalangeal (IP) joint flexion contracture.

b. Clawing of the fingers, with wrist flexion and MCP hyperextension, can be treated with FCR or FCU transfer to the ECRB.

c. Finger flexion contracture is treated with flexor digitorum sublimis (FDS) and flexor digitorum longus (FDL) lengthening or tenotomies.

d. Swan-neck deformities of the fingers are a result of intrinsic tightness and extrinsic overpull. These deformities are sometimes caused by wrist flexion or weak wrist extensors and can sometimes be helped by correcting the wrist flexion deformity.

M. Fractures specific to CP

1. Nonambulatory patients are at risk for fracture due to low bone mineral density.

2. Intravenous (IV) pamidronate should be considered for children with three or more fractures and a dual-energy x-ray absorptiometry (DEXA) Z-score <2 SD.

II. Myelodysplasia

A. Overview/epidemiology

1. Myelodysplasia is congenital malformation of the spinal column and spinal cord due to failure of closure of neural crests 3 to 4 weeks after fertilization, causing motor and sensory deficits.

2. Myelodysplasia is the most common major birth defect, affecting 0.9 per 1,000 live births.

3. Prenatal diagnosis via maternal serum α-fetoprotein is 60% to 95% accurate.

4. Diagnosis can also be made by ultrasound or amniocentesis.

5. Women of child-bearing age should be encouraged to have adequate folic acid intake. Supplementation with folic acid decreases the risk of myelodysplasia, but only if taken in the first weeks following conception. This has also been addressed by the addition of folic acid to many foods, such as breads and cereals.

B. Risk factors

1. History of previously affected pregnancy

2. Low folic acid intake

3. Pregestational maternal diabetes

4. In utero exposure to valproic acid or carbamazepine

C. Classification

1. Motor level and functional status are given in **Table 5**.

2. L4 level or lower (active quadriceps) is considered necessary for community ambulation.

D. Treatment—The long-term medical and skeletal issues associated with myelodysplasia are often best addressed by multidisciplinary teams.

1. Nonsurgical treatment

a. Frequent skin checks for pressure sores and well-fitting braces and wheelchairs are important because these patients often have significant sensory deficits.

b. Urologic and gastrointestinal issues, including detrusor malfunction and abnormal sphincter tone, make early catheterization and bowel regimens important. Kidney reflux and pyelonephritis cause significant morbidity and mortality.

c. Latex allergies are common, so latex precautions should be exercised for all patients with myelodysplasia.

d. Rehabilitation efforts should include early mo-

Table 5

Motor Level and Functional Status for Myelomeningocele

Group	Lesion Level	Muscle Involvement	Function	Ambulation
1	Thoracic/high lumbar	No quadriceps function	Sitter Possible household ambulatory with RGO	Some degree until age 13 years with HKAFO, RGO 95% to 99% wheelchair dependent as adults
2	Low lumbar	Quadriceps and medial hamstring function, no gluteus medius, maximus	Household/community ambulator with KAFO or AFO	Require AFO and crutches, 79% community ambulators as adults, wheelchair for long distances; significant difference between L3 and L4 level, medial hamstring needed for community ambulation
3	Sacral	Quadriceps and gluteus medius function	Community ambulator with AFO, UCBL, or none	94% retain walking ability as adults
	High sacral	No gastrosoleus strength	Community ambulator with AFO, UCBL, or none	Walk without support but require AFO, have gluteus lurch and excessive pelvic obliquity and rotation during gait
	Low sacral	Good gastrocnemius-soleus strength, normal gluteus medius, maximus		Walk without AFO, gait close to normal

RGO = reciprocating gait orthosis; UCBL = University of California/Berkeley Lab (orthosis); KAFO = knee-ankle-foot orthosis; AFO = ankle-foot orthosis; HKAFO = hip-knee-ankle-foot orthosis
(Reproduced from Sarwark JF, Aminian A, Westberry DE, Davids JR, Karol LA: Neuromuscular Disorders in Children, in Vaccaro AR (ed): Orthopaedic Knowledge Update 8. Rosemont, IL, American Academy of Orthopaedic Surgeons, 2005, p 678.)

bilization, PT, bracing, and functional wheel-chair fitting.

  e. Bracing

   i. Hip-knee-ankle-foot orthoses (HKAFOs), knee-ankle-foot orthoses (KAFOs), or AFOs are frequently used to support stance and/or to prevent contracture.

   ii. As the child grows, bracing and crutch requirements may decrease as the child gains skills or increase if the child gains weight or a deformity develops.

2. Surgical

  a. Spine—Neurosurgeons perform closure of myelomeningocele within 48 hours with a shunt for hydrocephalus. Later issues can develop with the shunt, a tethered cord, or syrinx, so diligent neurologic examinations need to be repeated and documented.

   i. Tethered cord can cause progressive scoliosis, change functional levels, or cause spasticity.

   ii. Syrinx, shunt problems, or new hydrocephalus can cause new upper extremity symptoms such as weakness or increasing spasticity.

   iii. Arnold-Chiari malformation is often addressed with shunting in infancy but may require later decompression.

   iv. Scoliosis and kyphosis may be progressive. 90% of patients with thoracic myelodysplasia may require kyphectomy and posterior fusion; 10% of patients with L4 myelodysplasia may require surgery. Prior to kyphectomy, it is important to check shunt function, because shunt failure can result in acute hydrocephalus and death when the spinal cord is tied off during the kyphectomy.

  b. Hip

   i. Flexion contractures are common but are often not severe. If the contracture is >40° in patients with lower lumbar level involvement, they may require flexor release.

   ii. Hip dysplasia and/or dislocation occur in four of five patients with midlumbar level involvement. Currently, the trend in treatment is not to reduce a dislocated hip in any child with myelodysplasia, but flexion deformity may be addressed for functional reasons. The rare exception to this may be the child with a unilateral hip dislocation who has a low-level lesion (ie, a community ambulator), but the recurrence rate is high and therefore the procedure is controversial.

  c. Knee

   i. Flexion contracture >20° should be treated with hamstring lengthening, capsular release, and/or distal femoral extension osteotomy.

3: Pediatrics

Table 6

Muscular Dystrophies

	Frequency	Inheritance	Gene Defect
Duchenne (DMD)	1/3,500 males	X-linked recessive	Xp21 dystrophin, point deletion, nonsense mutation, no dystrophin protein produced
Becker	1/30,000 males	X-linked recessive	Xp21 dystrophin in noncoding region with normal reading frame, lesser amounts of truncated dystrophin produced
Emery-Dreifuss	Uncommon	X-linked recessive, but seen mildly in females	Xq28
Limb girdle	1/14,500	Heterogeneous, mostly AR	AD 5q AR 15q
Fascioscapular humeral (FSH), adult	Rare	AD	4q35
Infantile FSH	Rare	AR	Unknown
Myotonic	13/100,000 adults (most common neuromuscular disease in adults)	AD	C9 near myotin protein kinase gene. Severity increases with amplification (number of trinucleotide repeats increases with oogenesis). Mildly affected mothers may have severely affected children.

AR = autosomal recessive; AD = autosomal dominant

There is, however, a significant rate of recurrence after extension osteotomy in growing children.

ii. Extension contracture can be treated with serial casting or V-Y quadriceps lengthening.

iii. Knee valgus, often with associated external tibial torsion and femoral anteversion, is common in patients with midlumbar level involvement because they lack functional hip abductors and have a significant trunk shift when walking with AFOs. This can be addressed by the use of KAFOs or crutches with AFOs.

iv. External tibial torsion can be addressed with a distal tibial derotational osteotomy.

d. Foot

i. About 30% of children with myelodysplasia have a rigid clubfoot.

ii. With surgical treatment, a portion of the tendons (eg, Achilles, posterior tibialis, FHL, flexor digitorum communis [FDC]) may be resected rather than lengthened to decrease the risk of recurrence.

iii. Equinus contracture is common in patients with thoracic and high lumbar level involvement.

iv. Calcaneus foot position can occur with unopposed tibialis anterior (L3-L4 level).

v. Equinovarus, equinus, and calcaneal foot deformities often are best treated with simple tenotomy rather than tendon transfer, achieving a flail but braceable foot.

vi. Valgus foot deformities are common in L4-L5 level patients. If surgery is necessary to achieve a plantigrade foot, fusion should

Diagnostic Features	EMG/Biopsy	Clinical Course
2/3 diagnosed by DNA, CPK 10 to 200 × normal Delayed walking, waddling gait, toe walking, Gower sign, calf pseudohypertrophy Present deep tendon reflexes, lumbar hyperlordosis, often with static encephalopathy	EMG: myopathic, decreased amplitude, short duration, polyphasic motor Biopsy: fibrofatty muscle replacement	Decreasing ambulation by age 6 to 8 years, transitions to wheelchair about age 12 years. Progressive scoliosis and respiratory illness, cardiac failure, death toward end of second decade
CPK less elevated than in DMD, similar physical findings but later onset and less progressive	Similar to DMD, but some dystrophin present by biopsy	Onset after age 7 years, slower progression Walks into teens Cardiac and pulmonary symptoms present but less severe Equinus frequent
Mildly elevated CPK, toe-walking Distinctive clinical contractures of Achilles, elbows, and neck extension occur in late childhood.	Myopathic	Slowly progressive, walks into sixth decade
CPK mildly elevated, mild DMD symptoms, muscle weakness in the muscles around the shoulder and hip	Dystrophic muscle biopsy	Begins in second or third decade, death before age 40 years
CPK normal Face, shoulder, upper arm affected		Weak shoulder flexion and abduction Normal life expectancy
Face, shoulder, upper arm affected, and weak gluteus maximus muscle leading to significant lumbar lordosis		Lumbar lordosis leads to wheelchair dependency and fixed hip flexion contractures
Often severe hypotonia at birth Weakness is worse distally than proximally (unlike DMD)	EMG demonstrates classic "dive bomber" response	75% survive at birth, growing stronger with age, walk by age 5 years Equinus deformities and distal weakness are common. "Drooping face" appearance Cardiomyopathy and conduction problems frequent, very sensitive to anesthesia

be avoided to maintain foot flexibility and to decrease the risk of pressure sores.

E. Fractures in children with myelodysplasia

1. In these children, fractures often present with erythema, warmth, and swelling in insensate patients.

2. A child with myelodysplasia who presents with a red, hot, swollen leg should be assumed to have a fracture until proven otherwise.

III. Muscular Dystrophies

A. Overview

1. Muscular dystrophies are genetically based mus-cle diseases causing progressive weakness (**Table 6**).

2. Pseudohypertrophy of the calf is classic for DMD, although it is present in only approximately 85% of patients (**Figure 3**).

3. Although genetically based, new mutations are frequent; for example, one third of cases of Duchenne muscular dystrophy (DMD) are the result of new mutations that arise during spermatogenesis on the patient's mother's paternal side.

B. Treatment of DMD

1. Nonsurgical

a. Corticosteroid therapy

i. Prolongs ambulation, slows progression of scoliosis, and slows the deterioration of forced vital capacity (FVC).

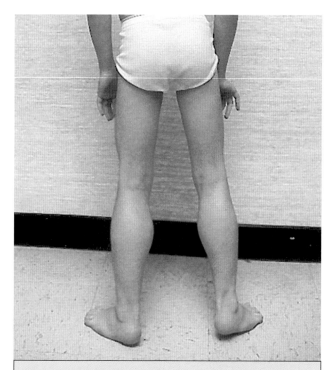

Figure 3 Clinical photograph of a 5-year-old boy with Duchenne muscular dystrophy. The marked pseudohypertrophy of the calves is a common physical finding. *(Reproduced from Sussman M: Duchenne muscular dystrophy. J Am Acad Orthop Surg 2002;10:138-151.)*

ii. The optimum age for beginning therapy is 5 to 7 years.

iii. Treatment carries a high risk of complications and side effects including osteonecrosis, weight gain, cushingoid appearance, GI symptoms, mood swings, headaches, short stature, and cataracts.

 b. Nighttime ventilation significantly prolongs survival.

 c. Rehabilitation includes PT for ROM, adaptive equipment, power wheelchairs, and nighttime bracing.

2. Surgical

 a. Lower extremity surgery is controversial in children with DMD.

  i. If surgery is performed, the focus should be on early postoperative mobilization and ambulation to prevent deconditioning and deterioration.

  ii. If performed, contracture release surgery (in the form of hip abductor, hamstring, Achilles tendon, posterior tibialis lengthening) should be performed while the child is still ambulatory.

 b. Spine—Scoliosis develops in 95% of patients

after they transition to a wheelchair (usually around age 12 years).

  i. Bracing is contraindicated because in most patients progression occurs relentlessly after 20°. Bracing can also interfere with respiration.

  ii. Early posterior instrumented fusion (at 20°) is recommended before loss of FVC occurs due to respiratory muscle weakness and progressively decreasing cardiac output.

  iii. Stiff curves may require anterior and posterior fusion.

 c. Malignant hyperthermia is common intraoperatively and is pretreated with dantrolene at surgery.

IV. Spinal Muscle Atrophy

A. Overview

1. Spinal muscle atrophy (SMA) is the most common genetic disease resulting in death during childhood, with an incidence of 1 in 10,000 live births.

2. The inheritance pattern of SMA is autosomal recessive.

3. Progressive weakness starts proximally and moves distally.

B. Classification

1. SMA I (Werdnig-Hoffmann) has onset at birth with severe involvement. Death occurs from respiratory failure by age 2 years.

2. SMA II has onset at age 6 to 18 months, and function diminishes with time.

 a. Hip dislocations, scoliosis, and joint contractures are common.

 b. Life expectancy is 15+ years.

3. SMA III has onset at age >18 months with physical manifestations similar to SMA II, but patients can stand independently. Life expectancy is normal.

C. Pathoanatomy

1. C5 mutations cause deficient survival motor neuron (SMN) protein resulting in progressive loss of α-motor neurons in the anterior horn of the spinal cord and progressive weakness.

2. There are two genes—SMN-I and SMN-II.

 a. All patients with SMA lack both copies of SMN-I.

 b. Severity is determined by the number of functional copies of SMN-II. (Patients with SMA I have one copy, patients with less severe forms have more than one.)

D. Treatment—No effective medical treatment (such as steroids) is available.

1. Scoliosis is very common, occurs by age 2 to 3 years, and is progressive.

   a. A thoracolumbosacral orthosis (TLSO) improves sitting balance but does not stop progression.

   b. Flexible curves; often can be fused posteriorly only

   c. The patient should be evaluated for lower extremity contractures to ensure seating balance.

   d. A vertical expandable prosthetic titanium rib (VEPTR) for thoracic insufficiency in young patients with SMA II with curves >50° has had good results.

   e. Fusion may cause an ambulatory child to lose the ability to walk (and may cause temporary loss of upper extremity function) because of loss of trunk motion.

2. Hip dislocation

   a. May be unilateral or bilateral

   b. Rarely symptomatic and surgery rarely indicated

3. Lower extremity contractures occur commonly.

   a. Hip and knee contractures >30° to 40° are not generally treated surgically. In lesser contractures, hamstring lengthening may sometimes be considered in patients who are strong enough with a strong motivation to walk.

   b. Foot deformities such as equinovarus occur commonly. Rarely, if the patient is ambulatory and retains strength, then gastrocnemius-soleus, posterior tibialis, FDL, and FHL tenotomy may be performed to maintain standing and walking.

V. Hereditary Motor Sensory Neuropathies

A. Overview/pathoanatomy/types

1. Hereditary motor sensory neuropathies (HMSNs) are chronic progressive peripheral neuropathies. They are common causes of cavus feet in children, but they may not be diagnosed before age 10 years.

2. HMSN I (myelinopathy Charcot-Marie-Tooth disease)

   a. HMSN I is the most common HMSN (1 in 2,500 children).

b. Peripheral myelin degeneration occurs with decreased motor nerve conduction.

   c. HMSN I is commonly caused by a mutation in 17p11 (*PMP-22*) or X-linked connexin 32.

   d. Autosomal dominant inheritance is most common, but can also be autosomal recessive, X-linked, or sporadic.

   e. The age at onset is the first to second decade of life.

   f. EMG is slow (<38 mm/s).

3. HMSN II (neuropathy Charcot-Marie-Tooth disease)

   a. The myelin sheath is intact, but wallerian axonal degeneration, with decreased motor and sensory conduction, occurs.

   b. Autosomal dominant inheritance is most common, but it can also be autosomal recessive, X-linked, or sporadic.

   c. The age at onset is the second decade of life or later.

   d. EMG is normal or slightly prolonged.

4. HMSN III (Dejerine-Sottas disease)

   a. HMSN III is characterized by peripheral nerve demyelination with severely decreased motor nerve conduction.

   b. Autosomal recessive inheritance is common, with the mutation in the *MPZ* gene.

   c. HMSN III presents in infancy.

   d. It is characterized by enlarged peripheral nerves, ataxia, and nystagmus. The patient stops walking by maturity.

5. Other peripheral nerve abnormalities include polyneuritis and small muscle atrophy.

B. Treatment

1. HMSN commonly presents as distal weakness, affecting intrinsic and extrinsic muscles.

2. Decreased sensation and areflexia may also be present.

3. Hip dysplasia (5% to 10%) develops from weak hip abductors and extensors.

   a. Hip dysplasia requires treatment, even if it is not symptomatic.

   b. Acetabular reconstruction is usually performed before VDRO.

4. Cavus foot (**Figure 4**)

   a. Cavus foot develops from contracted plantar fascia, weak tibialis anterior, weak peroneals, and tight foot intrinsic muscles with normal FDL and FHL.

3: Pediatrics

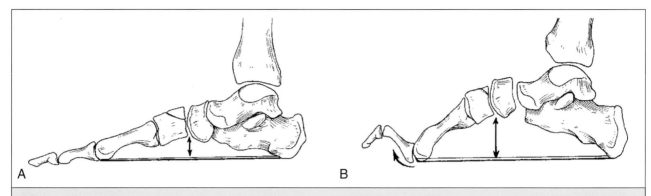

Figure 4 Drawings contrasting a normal and a cavus foot. **A,** Normal foot with normal height of the arch (double arrow) during standing. **B,** Cavus foot with increased height of the arch (double arrow) as a result of metatarsophalangeal joint hyperextension (curved arrow), such as occurs at toe-off and as seen in the windlass effect of the plantar fascia. *(Adapted with permission from Sabir M, Lyttle D: Pathogenesis of pes cavus in Charcot-Marie-Tooth disease. Clin Orthop Relat Res 1983;175:173-178.)*

b. The peroneus longus is generally somewhat stronger than the peroneus brevis and anterior tibialis.

c. Surgery for cavus feet aims to balance the muscle forces and maintain flexibility.

   i. Surgery typically involves plantar release and posterior tibial tendon transfer to the dorsum or split posterior tibial tendon transfer.

   ii. Forefoot equinus should be corrected with plantar release and possibly midfoot osteotomies.

   iii. Achilles tendon lengthening is occasionally needed, but only if there is true hindfoot equinus.

   iv. Osteotomies to correct bony deformities in adolescence include a calcaneal osteotomy (Dwyer) for fixed hindfoot varus (determined by Coleman block test).

   v. Fusions should be avoided to maintain flexibility.

5. Claw toes may become rigid and require treatment, such as IP fusion, often in conjunction with Jones transfers of the extensor tendons to the metatarsal heads.

6. Scoliosis or kyphoscoliosis is seen in 15% to 37% of children with HMSN and up to 50% of patients with HMSN who are skeletally mature—more commonly in HMSN I and girls.

   a. Bracing arrests progression in the minority of cases.

   b. Surgery with posterior fusion is effective.

   c. Intraoperative somatosensory cortical-evoked potentials may show no signal transmission because of the underlying disease.

7. Hand intrinsics, thenar, and hypothenar muscles

may also show wasting, creating clawing of the thenar and hypothenar eminences, limiting thumb abduction, and compromising pinch power. Surgically, sometimes transfer of the FDS, nerve decompression, contracture releases, and joint arthrodesis may be helpful.

VI. Neurofibromatosis

A. Overview

1. Two forms of neurofibromatosis (NF)—NF1 and NF2

2. NF1 is the most common single gene disorder (1 in 3,000 births).

B. Pathoanatomy

1. The mutation in NF is in the neurofibromin gene.

2. Neurofibromin regulates cell growth by modulating Ras signaling

3. Malignant transformation to neurofibrosarcoma is possible if there is a second mutation in the remaining normal gene.

C. Evaluation (**Table 7**)

D. Treatment

1. Anterolateral bowing of the tibia (**Figure 5**) is often treated with prophylactic bracing with total contact orthosis to prevent pseudarthrosis. 50% of patients with anterolateral bowing have NF, but only 10% of children with NF have anterolateral bowing.

2. Pseudarthrosis may be treated with bone graft and intramedullary rodding and sometimes later will require vascularized bone graft or bone transport by distraction osteogenesis. Amputation is rarely necessary.

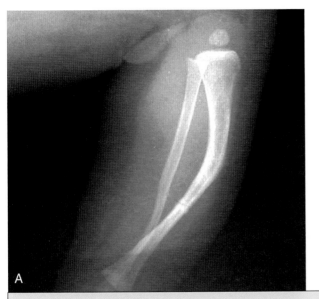
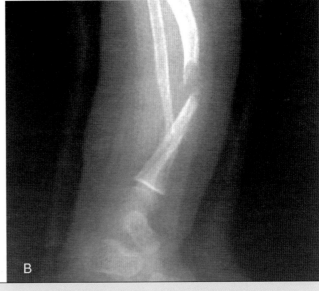

Figure 5   Congenital pseudarthrosis of the tibia. **A,** Lateral radiograph of the tibia and fibula in a child with neurofibromatosis demonstrating anterolateral bowing of a dystrophic tibia. **B,** Lateral radiograph of the same child after the tibia has progressed to a true pseudarthrosis. *(Reproduced from Mackenzie WG, Ballock RT: Genetic diseases and skeletal dysplasias, in Vaccaro AR (ed):* Orthopaedic Knowledge Update 8. *Rosemont, IL, American Academy of Orthopaedic Surgeons, 2005, pp 663-675.)*

3. Plexiform neurofibromas (in 40% of patients with NF1) may cause limb overgrowth. Limb equalization procedures are indicated for children with projected limb-length discrepancies >2 cm.

4. Scoliosis

   a. Scoliosis is common in patients with NF.

   b. Nondystrophic scoliosis in NF is treated like adolescent idiopathic scoliosis.

   c. Dystrophic scoliosis is short (4 to 6 levels), with sharp curves, and often occurs in children younger than age 6 years.

      i. It is characterized by scalloping end plates, foraminal enlargement, and penciling of ribs.

      ii. 87% of curves rapidly progress when three or more ribs are penciled.

      iii. Dystrophic scoliosis in NF is resistant to brace treatment.

      iv. Dystrophic scoliosis in NF is treated with early anterior and posterior fusion.

      v. A preoperative MRI scan should be obtained to rule out dural ectasia and intraspinal neurofibromas.

VII. Friedrich Ataxia

A. Overview

   1. Friedrich ataxia (FA) is the most common form of

Table 7

Diagnostic Criteria for Neurofibromatosis 1

Six or more café-au-lait spots, with greatest diameter 5 mm in prepubertal and 15 mm in postpubertal patients
Two or more neurofibromas of any type or one plexiform neurofibroma
Axillary freckling
Optic glioma
Two or more Lisch nodules (iris hamartomas)
A distinctive osseous lesion
A first-degree relative with NF1

(Reproduced from Mackenzie WG, Ballock RT: Genetic diseases and skeletal dysplasias, in Vaccaro AR (ed): Orthopaedic Knowledge Update 8. *Rosemont, IL, American Academy of Orthopaedic Surgeons, 2005, pp 663-675.)*

the uncommon spinocerebellar degenerative diseases. It occurs in 1 in 50,000 births.

   2. Onset is before age 25 years, with ataxia, areflexia, positive plantar response, and weakness. Often the gluteus maximus is the first muscle involved.

   3. Death usually occurs by the fourth or fifth decade of life.

   4. Nerve conduction velocity studies are decreased in the upper extremities.

B. Pathoanatomy

   1. The FA mutation is GAA repeats in 9q13, causing a lack of the frataxin protein.

   2. The age of onset of the disease is related to the number of GAA repeats.

C. Treatment

1. Pes cavovarus is progressive and rigid, resistant to bracing.

    a. Ambulatory patients may be treated with lengthenings and transfers.

    b. For rigid deformities, arthrodesis is needed to achieve a plantigrade foot.

2. Scoliosis occurs frequently and will usually progress if onset of the disease occurred before age 10 years and scoliosis occurred before age 15.

3. Posterior instrumented fusion is effective and does not need to be to the pelvis.

Top Testing Facts

Cerebral Palsy

1. The CNS lesion in cerebral palsy is static, but the peripheral manifestations of CP often change over time.

2. Botulinum toxin blocks the presynaptic release of acetylcholine and generally relaxes the muscle(s) into which it is injected for 3 to 6 months.

3. Scoliosis occurs in >50% of patients with quadriplegia and ~1% of patients with hemiplegia.

4. The most common causes of intoeing in children with CP are femoral anteversion and internal tibial torsion. Varus foot deformities commonly cause intoeing in patients with hemiplegia but not in patients with diplegia or quadriplegia.

5. Varus foot deformities are due to overactivity of the anterior tibialis, posterior tibialis, or both. Dynamic electromyography (EMG) is helpful in distinguishing the etiology.

6. Soft-tissue transfers alone will not suffice to correct a rigid foot deformity. Bone surgery will be needed in such cases as well.

Myelodysplasia

1. Supplementation with folic acid decreases the risk of myelodysplasia, but only if taken in the first weeks following conception.

2. Serial neurologic examinations are critical. Changes in strength and/or spasticity are early signs of a tethered cord.

3. Prior to kyphectomy surgery, ventriculoperitoneal (VP) shunt function must be checked. If the VP shunt is not working, tying off the spinal cord at the time of surgery can cause death due to acute hydrocephalus.

4. Hip dislocations in children with myelodysplasia rarely require treatment.

5. Fusions should be avoided during foot surgery to decrease the risk of pressure sores.

6. A child with myelodysplasia who presents with a red, hot, swollen leg should be assumed to have a fracture until proven otherwise.

Muscular Dystrophies

1. Pseudohypertrophy of the calf is classic for DMD, although present in only about 85% of patients.

2. Steroids, when tolerated, slow the progression of DMD. Unfortunately, they are often poorly tolerated because of their significant side effects.

3. Early posterior instrumented fusion (curves ≥ 20°) is recommended in DMD because 95% of such curves are progressive and because of progressive cardiopulmonary deterioration as children age.

4. Malignant hyperthermia is common in children with muscular dystrophy and should be treated with dantrolene.

Spinal Muscle Atrophy

1. The course and prognosis of SMA are directly related to the age at onset.

2. Scoliosis progression is not impacted by use of a TLSO.

3. Spine fusion may cause an ambulatory child to lose the ability to walk (and may cause temporary decrease of upper extremity function) because of loss of trunk motion.

4. Hip dislocation rarely requires treatment.

Hereditary Motor Sensory Neuropathies

1. The most common cause of bilateral cavus feet is Charcot-Marie-Tooth disease.

2. If foot surgery is required, soft-tissue balancing and avoidance of fusions are important.

3. Scoliosis is very common and often does not respond to brace treatment.

Neurofibromatosis

1. Many patients have café-au-lait spots. Six or more (of the noted size) are required as a criterion for NF.

2. Although 50% of congenital pseudarthroses of the tibia cases are due to NF, only 10% of patients with NF have congenital pseudarthrosis of the tibia.

3. Scoliosis in patients with NF is often dystrophic (short and sharply angular curve). Surgical success is much higher with combined anterior and posterior fusions.

4. 87% of curves rapidly progress when three or more ribs are penciled.

5. A preoperative MRI scan should be obtained to rule out dural ectasia and intraspinal neurofibromas.

Bibliography

Alman BA, Raza S, Biggar W: Steroid treatment and the development of scoliosis in males with Duchenne muscular dystrophy. *J Bone Joint Surg Am* 2004;86:519-524.

Beaty JH, Canale ST: Orthopaedic aspects of myelomeningocele. *J Bone Joint Surg Am* 1990;72:626-630.

Chan G, Bowen JR, Kumar SJ: Evaluation and treatment of hip dysplasia in Charcot-Marie-Tooth disease. *Orthop Clin North Am* 2006;37:203-209.

Dabney KW, Miller F: Cerebral palsy, in Abel MF (ed): *Orthopaedic Knowledge Update: Pediatrics 3*. Rosemont, IL, American Academy of Orthopaedic Surgeons, 2006, pp 93-109.

Flynn JM, Miller F: Management of hip disorders in patients with cerebral palsy. *J Am Acad Orthop Surg* 2002;10:198-209.

Gabrieli AP, Vankoski SJ, Dias LS, et al: Gait analysis in low lumbar myelomeningocele patients with unilateral hip dislocation or subluxation. *J Pediatr Orthop* 2003;23:330-336.

Hensinger RN, MacEwan GD: Spinal deformity associated with heritable neurological conditions: Spinal muscle atrophy, Friedrich's ataxia, familial dysautonomia, and Charcot-Marie-Tooth disease. *J Bone Joint Surg Am* 1976;58:13-24.

Kerr GH, Selber P: Musculoskeletal aspects of cerebral palsy. *J Bone Joint Surg Br* 2003;85:157-166.

Sarwark JF, Aminian A, Westberry DE, Davids JR, Karol LA, Neuromuscular disorders in children, in Vaccaro AR (ed): *Orthopaedic Knowledge Update 8*. Rosemont, IL, American Academy of Orthopaedic Surgeons, 2005, pp 677-689.

Scher DM, Mubarak SJ: Surgical prevention of foot deformity in patients with Duchenne muscular dystrophy. *J Pediatr Orthop* 2002;22:384-391.

Schwend RM, Drennan JC: Cavus foot deformity in children. *J Am Acad Orthop Surg* 2003;11:201-211.

Smucker JD, Miller F: Crankshaft effect after posterior spinal fusion and unit rod instrumentation in children with cerebral palsy. *J Pediatr Orthop* 2001;21:108-112.

Sussman M: Progressive neuromuscular diseases, in Abel MF (ed): *Orthopaedic Knowledge Update: Pediatrics 3*. Rosemont, IL, American Academy of Orthopaedic Surgeons, 2006, pp 123-135.

Sussman M: Duchenne muscular dystrophy. *J Am Acad Orthop Surg* 2002;10:138-151.

Thompson GH, Bereson FR: Other neuromuscular diseases, in Morrissy RT, Weinstein SL (eds): *Lovell and Winter's Pediatric Orthopaedics*, ed 5. Philadelphia, PA, Lippincott Williams & Wilkins, 2001, pp 634-676.

Thompson JD: Myelomeningocele, in Abel MF (ed): *Orthopaedic Knowledge Update: Pediatrics 3*. Rosemont, IL, American Academy of Orthopaedic Surgeons, 2006, pp 111-122.

3: Pediatrics

Chapter 31

Congenital Hand and Wrist Anomalies and Brachial Plexus Palsies

Donald S. Bae, MD

I. Embryology, Development, and Classification

A. Embryology

1. The limb bud first appears during the fourth week of gestation; the upper limb develops during the fifth to eighth week of gestation.

2. Several signaling centers are critical for upper limb development

   a. The apical ectodermal ridge guides proximal-to-distal development and mediates interdigital necrosis.

   b. The zone of polarizing activity guides radio-ulnar development.

   c. The Wnt signaling center guides dorsoventral development.

3. Joint motion is required for joint development in utero.

B. Developmental milestones—Although these are highly variable, general guidelines are listed in **Table 1**.

C. Radiographic appearance of secondary centers of ossification

1. Carpal bones ossify in a predictable sequence:

   a. Capitate (3 to 4 months)

   b. Hamate (4 to 8 months)

   c. Triquetrum (2 to 3 years)

   d. Lunate (4 years)

   e. Scaphoid (4 to 5 years)

   f. Trapezium (5 years)

   g. Trapezoid (6 years)

   h. Pisiform (6 to 8 years)

2. Most common carpal coalition: lunotriquetral.

D. Classification of congenital hand differences—Classification based on embryologic development is currently accepted by the International Federation of Societies for Surgery of the Hand (IFSSH) (**Table 2**).

Table 1

General Developmental Milestones for Hand and Upper Limb Function

Age	Function
4-6 months	Bimanual reach in midline
6 months	Grasp
6-8 months	Independent sitting
9-12 months	Thumb-index pinch
18 months	Voluntary digital release
2-3 years	Fine motor patterns established
3-4 years	Hand dominance established

Table 2

Embryologic Classification of Congenital Anomalies

Category	Example(s)
Failure of formation	Congenital transradial amputation, radial dysplasia
Failure of differentiation	Syndactyly
Duplication	Pre- and postaxial polydactyly
Overgrowth	Macrodactyly
Undergrowth	Poland's syndrome
Congenital constriction band	Amniotic band syndrome
Generalized skeletal abnormalities	

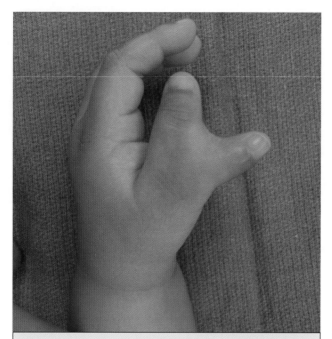

Figure 1 Clinical photograph of the hand of a child with preaxial polydactyly. *(Reproduced with permission from Children's Orthopaedic Surgery Foundation.)*

II. Duplications

A. Preaxial polydactyly (**Figure 1**)

1. Also referred to as thumb duplication, thumb polydactyly, or "split thumb"

2. Incidence reported to be approximately 1 per 1,000 to 10,000 live births

   a. Males more commonly affected than females; whites more commonly affected than blacks

   b. Typically sporadic; associated congenital anomalies rare (except type VII)

3. Classification

   a. Wassel classification most commonly used (**Figure 2**)

   b. Wassel type IV (43%) and type II (15%) most common

4. Pathoanatomy

   a. Both the radial and ulnar components have structures that must be preserved and reconstructed to provide a stable, mobile, and functional thumb.

   b. In Wassel type II, the radial digit has the radial collateral ligament insertion and the ulnar digit has the ulnar collateral ligament insertion of the interphalangeal (IP) joint.

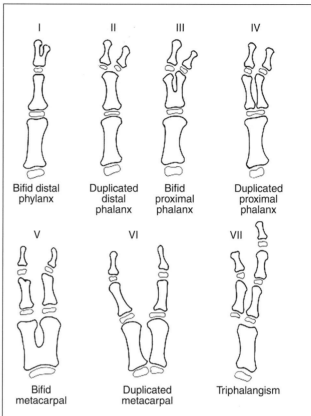

Figure 2 Wassel classification of preaxial polydactyly. *(Reproduced with permission from Wassel HD: The results of surgery for polydactyly of the thumb. Clin Orthop 1969;64:179.)*

c. In Wassel type IV, the thenar muscles insert on the more radial digit and the adductor pollicis inserts on the more ulnar digit.

d. Pollex abductus is an abnormal connection between the extensor pollicis longus (EPL) and flexor pollicis longus (FPL) tendons, seen in approximately 20% of hypoplastic and duplicated thumbs; presence of a pollex abductus is suggested by abduction of the affected digit and absence of IP joint creases.

5. Surgical treatment

   a. Typically involves ablation of the bony elements of the more underdeveloped (usually radial) thumb and reconstruction of the (radial) collateral ligament and, in Wassel type IV thumbs, transfer of the thenar muscles from the ablated proximal phalanx to the preserved (ulnar) proximal phalanx.

   b. Chondroplasty of the metacarpal head and/or corrective osteotomy of an abnormally shaped phalanx or metacarpal may need to be performed to restore the longitudinal alignment of the thumb.

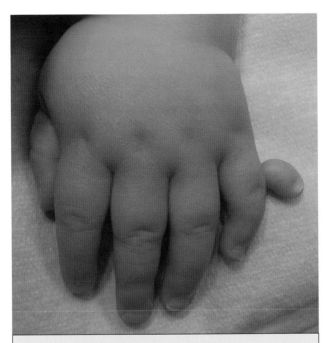

Figure 3   Clinical photograph of the hand of a child with postaxial polydactyly. *(Reproduced with permission from the Children's Orthopaedic Surgery Foundation.)*

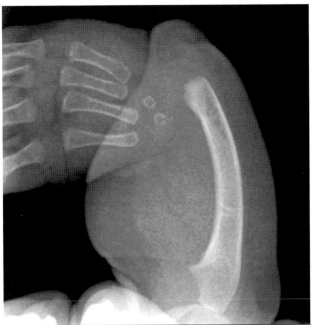

Figure 4   PA radiograph of the arm of a child with radial longitudinal deficiency. Note the absent radius, bowed ulna, and radially deviated wrist. *(Reproduced with permission from Children's Orthopaedic Surgery Foundation.)*

c. The Bilhaut-Cloquet procedure is technically difficult and often results in an aesthetically unpleasing thumb with physeal mismatch and articular incongruity.

d. Pollicization is recommended for unrecontructable or triphalangeal thumbs.

e. Approximately 15% to 20% of patients develop late deformity following surgery. Causes include failure to recognize a pollex abductus, inadequate correction of the longitudinal thumb alignment, inadequate reconstruction of the collateral ligament, and failure to centralize the extensor and/or flexor tendons.

B. Postaxial polydactyly (**Figure 3**)

1. Refers to duplication of ulnarmost digit

2. Inheritance is autosomal dominant (AD) with variable penetrance; affects blacks more than whites or Asians.

3. Classification

a. Type A: extra digit fully developed

b. Type B: extra digit is rudimentary and pedunculated

4. Treatment is surgical excision of extra digit.

a. In type A, reconstruction of collateral ligament and hypothenar muscle insertions may be needed (akin to thumb duplication).

b. Type B postaxial polydactyly may be treated with suture ligature of the base of the pedicle in the newborn nursery.

III. Deficiencies

A. Radial longitudinal deficiency (RLD)—Also known as radial dysplasia, radial clubhand.

1. Longitudinal failure of formation of the radial side of the forearm, wrist, and hand (**Figure 4**)

2. RLD is associated with several congenital conditions and syndromes:

a. Thrombocytopenia-absent radius (TAR)—Low platelet count that normalizes over time.

b. Fanconi anemia—Platelet and blood cell counts normal at birth but decrease dramatically during first few years of life; diagnosed with mitomycin-C chromosomal challenge test; treated with bone marrow transplantation.

c. Holt-Oram syndrome—RLD with congenital heart disease, typically atrial or ventricular septal defects.

d. VACTERL—Constellation of anomalies including *v*ertebral, *a*nal, *c*ardiac, *t*racheal, *e*sophageal, *r*enal, and *l*imb.

3: Pediatrics

3. Clinical features

   a. Elbow flexion contracture

   b. Shortened and/or bowed forearm

   c. Radial deviation of the wrist

   d. Aplasia or hypoplasia of the thumb

4. In addition to skeletal deficiencies, there are similar deficiencies of soft-tissue structures (eg, radial artery, median nerve, flexor carpi radialis).

5. Bayne classification

   a. I: delayed appearance of distal epiphysis, slightly shortened radius

   b. II: deficient growth proximal and distal, considerably shortened radius

   c. III: partial absence of the radius (distal and middle thirds most common)

   d. IV: completely absent radius (most common)

6. Treatment

   a. Splinting and/or serial casting are initiated early to stretch the tight radial soft tissues.

   b. Surgical procedures include centralization (axis of the ulna realigned with long metacarpal) or radialization (ulna is realigned with index metacarpal).

   c. Surgery is not recommended in the setting of elbow stiffness or in older patients who have compensated/adjusted to their deficiency.

B. Ulnar longitudinal deficiency (ULD)—Also known as ulnar dysplasia, ulnar clubhand.

   1. Longitudinal failure of formation of the ulnar forearm, wrist, and hand

   2. 5 to 10 times less common than RLD; usually sporadic with rare AD inheritance patterns

   3. Associated congenital anomalies occur less commonly than with RLD and include syndactyly, thumb duplication or hypoplasia, elbow instability, radial head dislocation, and synostosis.

   4. Clinical features

      a. Shortened and bowed forearm

      b. Typically, the wrist is stable but elbow function is compromised.

   5. Bayne classification

      a. I: hypoplastic ulna with proximal and distal physes

      b. II: absent distal ulna (most common)

      c. III: completely absent ulna

      d. IV: absent ulna with proximal radius fused to the distal humerus

6. Surgical options

   a. Excision of the ulnar anlage

   b. Corrective radial osteotomy

   c. Corrective humeral osteotomy

   d. Creation of a single-bone forearm

C. Thumb hypoplasia

   1. Within spectrum of RLD, but classified as "undergrowth" by IFSSH classification

   2. Often bilateral; males and females equally affected

   3. Associated conditions include Holt-Oram, TAR, Fanconi anemia, and VACTERL

   4. Classification

      a. Buck-Gramcko modification of Blauth classification (**Figure 5**)

      b. Type V most common (30% to 35% of cases), followed by type IV and type III

   5. Clinical features of types I through IIIA

      a. Tight first web space

      b. IP joint stiffness

      c. Metacarpophalangeal (MCP) instability

      d. Absence of thenar musculature

   6. Treatment—depends on type

      a. I: no treatment

      b. II through IIIA: surgical reconstruction (first web deepening, MCP stabilization, and opponensplasty)

      c. IIIB through V: index pollicization with or without ablation of thumb. In the treatment of thumb hypoplasia, pollicization is recommended in the setting of an underdeveloped or unstable carpometacarpal (CMC) joint (Blauth types IIIB through V).

      d. Principles of pollicization

         i. Use of local skin flaps to reconstitute first web space

         ii. Bony reduction to recreate metacarpal and phalanges of pollex (**Figure 6**) in appropriate position (120° to 140° pronation, 15° extension, 40° palmar abduction)

         iii. Transfer of index finger on neurovascular pedicles to new position

         iv. Tendon transfers (extensor digitorum communis [EDC] to abductor pollicis longus [APL], extensor indicis proprius [EIP] to EPL, first dorsal interosseous [DIO] to abductor pollicis brevis [APB], first volar interosseous [VIO] to adductor pollicis [AdP])

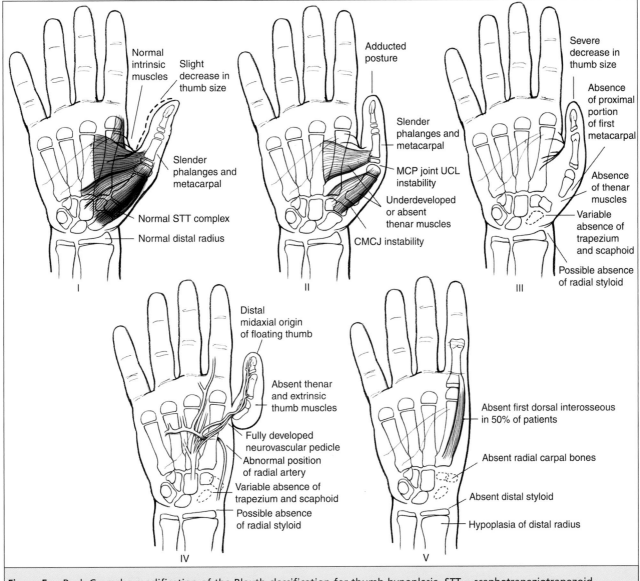

Figure 5 Buck-Gramcko modification of the Blauth classification for thumb hypoplasia. STT = scaphotrapeziotrapezoid, MCP = metacarpophalangeal, UCL = ulnar collateral ligament, CMCJ = carpometacarpal joint. *(Adapted with permission from Kleinman WB: Management of thumb hypoplasia. Hand Clin 1990;6:617-641.)*

D. Aphalangia

1. Nonvascularized toe phalanx transfer useful

2. Prerequisite is appropriate soft-tissue pocket at recipient site

3. Best if performed at young age (<12 to 18 months)

4. Presence of open physis after transfer is 94% if performed before 1 year of age, 71% between 1 and 2 years, and 48% after 2 years of age.

E. Transverse deficiencies (congenital amputations)

1. Typically sporadic, unilateral, and not associated with other conditions

2. Transradial amputation most common

3. Fitting with a passive terminal prosthesis recommended at 6 months ("sit to fit")

4. Free vascularized toe transfer(s) may be considered for congenital amputations at the level of the hand.

IV. Hypertrophy

A. Macrodactyly

1. "Overgrowth" according to IFSSH classification

2. Typically unilateral, involving radial digits

3: Pediatrics

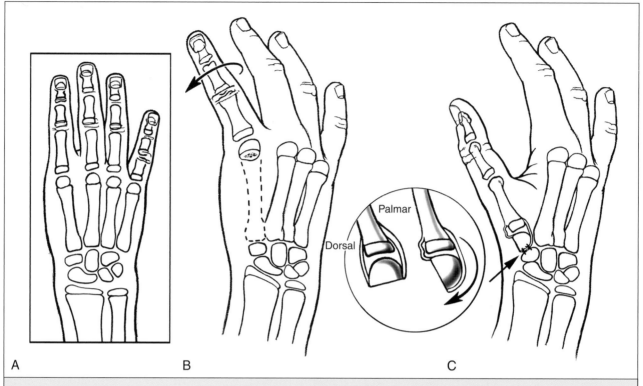

Figure 6 Drawings showing index finger pollicization for thumb aplasia. **A,** Blauth grade V hypoplasia of the thumb. **B,** The index finger is reduced and rotated. The inset demonstrates the turning of the metacarpal head for prevention of hyperextension deformity. **C,** The metacarpal head is anchored down (*arrow*). *(Adapted with permission from Buck-Gramcko D: Pollicization of the index finger. J Bone Joint Surg Am 1971;53:1605-1617.)*

3. Usually isolated, but may occur in setting of neurofibromatosis, Proteus syndrome, or Klippel-Trenaunay-Weber syndrome

4. May be static or progressive; with asymmetric digital nerve involvement, may result in radio-ulnar or flexion deformity

5. Classification

   a. Type I: macrodactyly and lipofibromatosis; most common type, associated with fibrofatty proliferation in the distribution of a digital or peripheral nerve, which is typically enlarged and tortuous

   b. Type II: macrodactyly and neurofibromatosis

   c. Type III: macrodactyly and hyperostosis

   d. Type IV: macrodactyly and hemihypertrophy

6. Surgical options

   a. Include soft-tissue debulking, epiphysiodesis of affected phalanges, bony and soft-tissue reduction procedures, and amputation

   b. Individualized according to the anatomic distribution, degree of deformity, and skeletal growth remaining

V. Amniotic Band Syndrome

A. Overview

   1. Also referred to as constriction ring syndrome or amniotic disruption sequence

   2. Reported incidence: 1 in 15,000 live births

   3. Sporadic, not hereditary

   4. Commonly associated with other anomalies (eg, clubfoot, cleft lip/palate, craniofacial defects)

B. Etiology

   1. Unknown

   2. Endogenous and exogenous theories of causation have been proposed.

   3. Prevailing theory is that amniotic disruption releases strands of membrane that circumferentially wrap around the developing upper limb.

C. Clinical presentation—Bands typically lie perpendicular to longitudinal axis of the affected digit/limb (**Figure 7**).

   1. More than 90% occur distal to wrist.

   2. Central digits more commonly affected

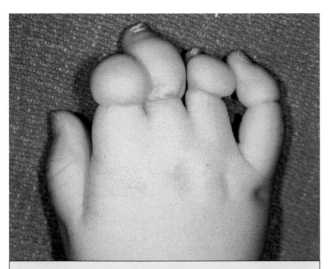

Figure 7 Clinical photograph of the hand of a child with amniotic band syndrome. *(Courtesy of Dr. Peter M. Waters, Children's Orthopaedic Surgery Foundation.)*

3. Varying depths of constriction

4. If no amputation, secondary syndactyly or bony fusions may occur with proximal epithelialized sinus tracts

5. Key: normal anatomy proximal to constriction ring

D. Classification—Patterson, 1961

1. I: simple constriction ring

2. II: deformity distal to ring (lymphedema, hypoplasia)

3. III: fusion of distal parts

4. IV: amputation

E. Treatment

1. Type I: observation versus excision/release of constriction ring

2. Type II: excision of constriction ring with local flaps (Z-plasty)

3. Type III: syndactyly release

4. Type IV: Function may be improved with reconstructive procedures, including bony lengthenings, web deepenings, "on top" plasties, nonvascularized toe phalanx transfers, or free vascularized toe transfers.

VI. Syndactyly

A. Overview

1. Failure of differentiation resulting in webbed fingers.

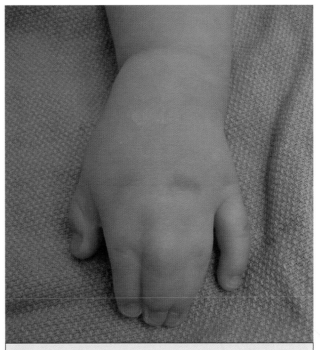

Figure 8 Clinical photograph of the hand of a child with complete syndactyly of the second and third web spaces. *(Reproduced with permission from the Children's Orthopaedic Surgery Foundation.)*

2. Most common congenital hand difference, occurring in 1 per 2,000 to 2,500 live births

3. Males affected more commonly than females; whites affected more commonly than blacks

4. Inheritance: AD with variable penetrance

B. Associated conditions

1. Poland syndrome: congenital absence of the sternocostal head of the pectoralis major, limb hypoplasia, synbrachydactyly

2. Apert syndrome (also known as acrocephalosyndactyly): mental retardation; premature fusion of cranial sutures resulting in high, broad forehead, occipital flattening, and bulging low-set eyes; and acrosyndactyly (spadelike hand)

3. Carpenter syndrome: acrocephalopolysyndactyly

C. Classification

1. Simple syndactyly defined by web formed by soft tissue only (**Figure 8**).

2. Complex syndactyly denotes fusion of adjacent phalanges.

3. Complicated syndactyly refers to interposition of accessory phalanges or abnormal bones.

4. Complete syndactyly refers to webbing that extends to the tips of the involved digits.

5. Incomplete syndactyly does not extend to the digital tips.

3: Pediatrics

6. The third web is most commonly affected, followed by the fourth, second, and first web spaces.

D. Treatment principles

1. Release digits of differing sizes first to avoid growth disturbance.

2. Do not operate on both sides of the digit at the same time to avoid vascular embarrassment.

3. Use local skin flaps to reconstitute the web commissure to avoid scar contracture and "web creep."

4. Use zigzag lateral flaps to avoid longitudinal scar contracture.

5. Use full-thickness skin grafts to cover bare areas.

E. Symphalangism

1. Failure of differentiation of the IP joint, usually of ulnar digits

2. Characterized by absence of flexion/extension creases and digital stiffness

3. Joint space may appear narrow on radiographs.

4. Capsulectomies/arthroplasties have met with limited success.

5. Osteotomy or arthrodesis may be considered at maturity, although rarely needed due to adequate digital function.

VII. Camptodactyly

A. Overview

1. Refers to flexion contracture/deformity of finger

2. True incidence is unknown; it is estimated that 1% of the population is affected.

3. Little finger and proximal interphalangeal (PIP) joint most commonly affected

4. Usually sporadic, but some exhibit AD inheritance with variable penetrance

B. Classification

1. Type I: presents in infancy

2. Type II: presents in adolescence

3. Type III: occurs in setting of underlying syndrome

C. Pathoanatomy

1. Nearly every structure about the base of the finger has been implicated as causal.

2. Abnormal lumbrical insertion and adherent or hypoplastic flexor digitorum sublimis (FDS) most commonly cited

3. Other causes theorized

a. Skin contracture

b. Absent central slip/extensor tendon

c. Articular incongruity

d. Abnormal volar plate

e. Abnormal oblique retinacular ligament

D. Treatment principles

1. Splinting and stretching exercises may be attempted, but these often have mixed results.

2. Surgical treatment is indicated for significant flexion contracture with functional impairment, but this often has limited results.

a. All identifiable pathology should be addressed (eg, anomalous lubrical insertion).

b. For passive deformity, consider FDS tenotomy or transfer to the radial lateral band.

c. For fixed deformity, consider osteotomy versus arthrodesis.

E. Kirner deformity (**Figure 9**)

1. Progressive, nonpainful volar-radial curvature of little finger distal phalanx

2. Typically affects preadolescent females, usually bilaterally

3. Sporadic or AD

4. Unknown etiology, but likely due to disturbance of distal phalangeal physis

5. Usually an aesthetic concern, but not functionally limiting

6. Corrective osteotomy can be considered at the completion of growth.

F. Trigger thumb

1. Caused by constriction of FPL tendon at A1 pulley

2. Not thought to be congenital

3. Likelihood of spontaneous resolution 30% if younger than 1 year, <10% if older than 1 year

4. Surgical treatment: A1 pulley release

G. Trigger finger

1. Much less common than trigger thumb

2. Caused by anomalous anatomy, including abnormal lumbrical insertion and/or proximal decussation of FDS tendon

3. Association with other conditions, including mucopolysaccharidoses

4. Surgical treatment

a. Release of A1 pulley alone may not suffice; recurrence rates up to 50%

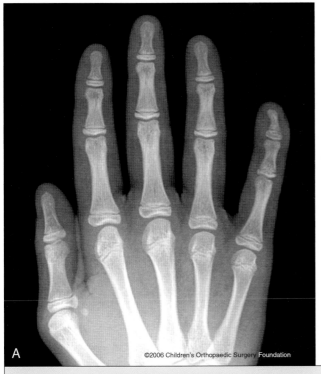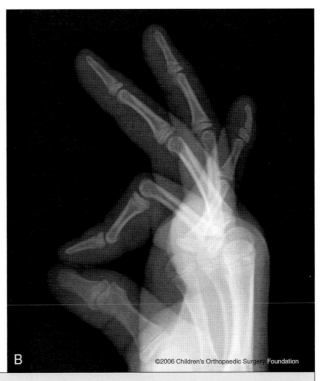

Figure 9 PA **(A)** and lateral **(B)** radiographs of the hand of a child with Kirner deformity. *(Reproduced with permission from Children's Orthopaedic Surgery Foundation.)*

b. Requires extensile exposure, release of A1 pulley, and addressing anomalous anatomy (release of lumbrical; A1, partial A2, A3 release; excision of single slip of FDS)

VIII. Clinodactyly

A. Overview

1. Refers to angular deformity of digit in the radioulnar plane.

2. True incidence unknown; estimated between 1% and 10% of population

3. Typically bilateral, little finger most commonly affected

4. AD inheritance

5. Many syndromic associations (including trisomy 21)

B. Classification (Cooney)

1. Simple (bony deformity alone) versus complex (soft-tissue involvement)

2. Uncomplicated (15° to 45° angulation) versus complicated (>45° angulation with rotation)

C. Treatment

1. Clinodactyly is usually more of an aesthetic concern than a functional problem.

2. Splinting/stretching may be initiated, although it is often ineffective.

3. Surgery is indicated for severe deformity with functional compromise (eg, digital overlap).

D. Delta phalanx

1. If the proximal physis is not oriented perpendicular to the long axis of the phalanx, this may result in triangular- or trapezoidal-shaped bone with progressive angular deformity—the so-called delta phalanx.

2. The shortened side of phalanx contains the longitudinal epiphyseal bracket.

3. For significant deformity and functional limitations, surgical options include physiolysis or corrective osteotomy.

IX. Brachial Plexus Birth Palsy

A. Overview

1. Definition: Brachial plexus birth palsy (BPBP) is a traction or compression injury sustained to the brachial plexus during birth.

2. Incidence reported to be 0.1% to 0.4% of live births

3: Pediatrics

3. Risk factors include macrosomia, shoulder dystocia/difficult delivery, prior BPBP.

B. Classification

1. Anatomic: upper trunk, lower trunk, total plexus

2. Neurologic: avulsion, rupture, neurapraxia

C. Natural history

1. Few long-term prospective data are available.

2. 80% to 90% of patients demonstrate spontaneous recovery.

3. If antigravity biceps function recovers by 2 months, full recovery is anticipated.

4. If biceps function recovers at or after 5 months, incomplete recovery is likely.

5. Presence of Horner syndrome portends worse prognosis.

D. Indications—Indications for microsurgery remain controversial.

1. Absent return of biceps function at 3 to 6 months

2. Flail extremity (total plexus injury) in setting of Horner syndrome at 3 months

E. Microsurgical treatment

1. Avulsion injuries: consider nerve transfers/neurotizations

2. Nerve ruptures: excision of neuroma, nerve grafting

F. Glenohumeral dysplasia—In setting of persistent muscular imbalance across the developing shoulder, there is progressive dysplasia of the glenohumeral joint, with posterior subluxation of the humeral head, humeral head flattening, and increased glenoid retroversion.

G. Secondary procedures

1. Tendon transfers: latissimus dorsi and teres major tendon transfers to rotator cuff (Sever-L'Episcopo procedure), often combined with releases of the pectoralis major, subscapularis, and coracobrachialis muscles, to improve shoulder abduction and external rotation

2. Humeral osteotomy: external rotation osteotomy of the distal humeral segment; recommended in setting of advanced glenohumeral joint dysplasia

Top Testing Facts

1. RLD is commonly associated with other congenital anomalies, including TAR, Fanconi anemia, Holt-Oram syndrome, and VACTERL association.

2. In the treatment of thumb hypoplasia, pollicization is recommended in the setting of an underdeveloped or unstable CMC joint (Blauth types IIIB through V).

3. Amniotic band syndrome usually occurs distal to the wrist and typically involves the central digits.

4. When performing syndactyly release, only one side of an affected digit should be operated on at a time to avoid vascular embarrassment.

5. Failure of antigravity biceps recovery by 3 to 6 months is an indication for microsurgery in BPBP.

Bibliography

Dao KD, Shin AY, Billings A, Oberg KC, Wood VE: Surgical treatment of congenital syndactyly of the hand. *J Am Acad Orthop Surg* 2004;12:39-48.

Kozin SH: Upper extremity congenital anomalies. *J Bone Joint Surg Am* 2003;85:1564-1576.

Light TR: Treatment of preaxial polydactyly. *Hand Clin* 1992;8:161-175.

Tay SC, Moran SL, Shin AY, Cooney WP: The hypoplastic thumb. *J Am Acad Orthop Surg* 2006;14:354-366.

Waters PM: Obstetrical brachial plexus injuries: Evaluation and management. *J Am Acad Orthop Surg* 1997;5:205-214.

Chapter 32

Pediatric Hip Conditions

Paul D. Choi, MD

I. Developmental Dysplasia of the Hip

A. Overview

1. Definition

   a. Developmental dysplasia of the hip (DDH) refers to the complete spectrum of pathologic conditions involving the developing hip, ranging from acetabular dysplasia to hip subluxation to irreducible hip dislocation.

   b. Teratologic dislocation of the hip occurs in utero and is irreducible on neonatal examination.

      i. Pseudoacetabulum usually is present.

      ii. This condition always accompanies other congenital anomalies or neuromuscular conditions, most frequently arthrogryposis and myelomeningocele.

2. Epidemiology

   a. DDH is the most common disorder of the hip in children. One in 1,000 children (0.1%) is born with a dislocated hip; 10 in 1,000 children (1%) are born with hip subluxation or dysplasia.

   b. 80% of affected children are female.

   c. The left hip is more commonly involved (60%).

   d. DDH occurs more commonly in Native Americans and Laplanders; DDH is rarely seen in African-Americans.

B. Pathoanatomy

1. Etiology—The exact cause is largely unknown but is thought to be multifactorial (genetic, hormonal, and mechanical).

2. Risk factors

   a. DDH occurs more commonly in females and firstborns, and with breech presentation (30% to 50%).

   b. DDH is commonly associated with intrauterine "packaging" problems, such as prematurity, oligohydramnios, congenital dislocation of the knee, congenital muscular torticollis (8% to 17% coexistence), and metatarsus adductus (0% to 10% coexistence).

   c. Family history is a strong risk factor.

      i. No parent involvement: 6% risk for DDH

      ii. At least one parent involved: 12% risk

      iii. Parent and sibling involved: 36% risk

C. Evaluation

1. Clinical presentation—The clinical presentation varies with age.

   a. In the neonatal period, instability of the hip is the key clinical finding.

   b. Hip clicks are nonspecific physical findings.

   c. Because asymmetric skin folds are common in children with normal hips, children with such asymmetry have a high rate of false positives.

   d. In infants older than 6 months, limitation of motion and apparent limb shortening are common findings.

   e. In toddlers, in addition to restricted motion and limb-length inequalities, a limp or waddling gait may be appreciated.

   f. In adolescents, all the above findings may be present in addition to fatigue and pain in the hip, thigh, or knee.

2. Physical examination—Accuracy of the physical examination requires that the child be relaxed.

   a. The Galeazzi (or Allis) test is positive only in unilateral severe subluxations or dislocations. In the Galeazzi test, the hips are flexed to 90°; the test is positive if one knee (the involved side) is lower than the other.

   b. The Barlow test is performed by applying a posterolateral force to the extremity with the hip in a flexed and adducted position (**Figure 1**). The test is positive if the hip subluxates or even dislocates.

   c. The Ortolani test is performed by abducting and lifting the proximal femur anteriorly (**Fig-**

3: Pediatrics

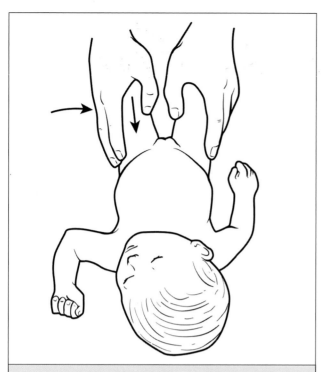

Figure 1 The Barlow test is positive if the hip subluxates or dislocates. *(Reproduced from Griffin LY (ed): Essentials of Musculoskeletal Care, ed. 3. Rosemont, IL, American Academy of Orthopaedic Surgeons, 2005, p 850.)*

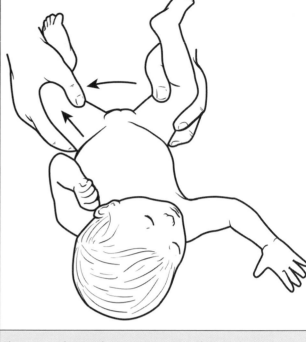

Figure 2 The Ortolani test is positive if the dislocated hip is reducible. *(Reproduced from Griffin LY (ed): Essentials of Musculoskeletal Care, ed. 3. Rosemont, IL, American Academy of Orthopaedic Surgeons, 2005, p 850.)*

ure 2). The test is positive if the dislocated hip is reducible.

    d. Range of motion (ROM) testing of the hip is important, with decrease in abduction as the most sensitive test for DDH. Remember, however, that ROM will be normal in children younger than 6 months because contractures will not yet have developed.

3. Diagnostic tests

    a. Ultrasonography

       i. In the first 4 months of life, plain radiographic evaluation is unreliable because the femoral epiphysis has not yet ossified.

      ii. Ultrasonography of the infant hip (before the appearance of the proximal femoral ossific center) is useful in confirming a diagnosis of DDH and also in documenting reducibility and stability of the hip in an infant undergoing treatment with a Pavlik harness or brace.

     iii. Reference parameters (**Figure 3**)

        (a) At age 4 to 6 weeks, a normal α angle is >60°; a normal β angle is <55°. (The α angle is the angle formed by a vertical reference line through the iliac bone and tangential to the osseous roof of the ac-

etabulum; the β angle is the angle formed by a line drawn through the labrum intersecting the iliac reference line—ie, it represents the cartilaginous roof of the acetabulum.)

        (b) The amount of femoral head coverage should be >50%.

    b. Plain radiographs—**Figure 4** shows reference lines and angles for the AP view of the pelvis (**Figure 5**).

       i. The Hilgenreiner line is a line drawn horizontally through each triradiate cartilage of the pelvis.

      ii. The Perkin line is drawn perpendicular to the Hilgenreiner line at the lateral edge of the acetabulum.

     iii. The Shenton line is a continuous arch drawn along the medial border of the femoral neck and superior border of the obturator foramen.

     iv. The acetabular index is the angle formed by an oblique line (through the outer edge of the acetabulum and triradiate cartilage) and the Hilgenreiner line.

        (a) In the newborn, a normal value averages 27.5°.

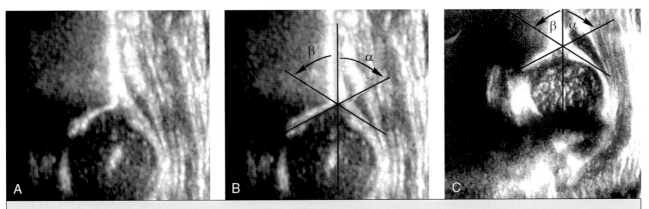

Figure 3   Ultrasound images of a normal hip and a hip with DDH. **A,** Ultrasound image of a normal hip. **B,** The same ultrasound image with the α and β angles drawn. In a normal hip, femoral head coverage should be greater than 50%. The α angle should be greater than 60°. **C,** Ultrasound image of a dysplastic hip reveals approximately 30% femoral head coverage, an α angle of 50°, a β angle of 90°, and an echogenic labrum. *(Reproduced from Abel MF (ed): Orthopaedic Knowledge Update: Pediatrics 3. Rosemont, IL, American Academy of Orthopaedic Surgeons, 2006, p. 181.)*

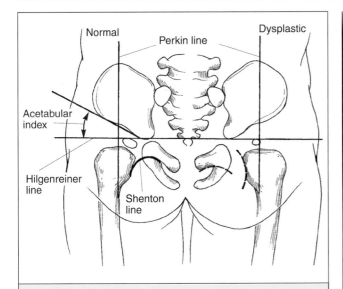

Figure 4   Reference lines and angles used in the evaluation of DDH.

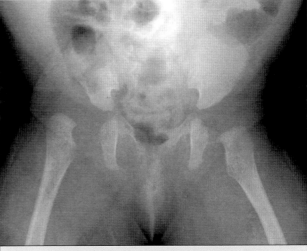

Figure 5   AP plain radiograph of the pelvis demonstrates a dislocated right hip. The proximal femoral ossific nucleus is not yet present. Also note that the Shenton line is disrupted.

(b) By 24 months of age, the acetabular index decreases to 21°.

v. The center-edge angle of Wiberg is the angle formed by a vertical line through the center of the femoral head and perpendicular to the Hilgenreiner line and an oblique line through the outer edge of the acetabulum and center of the femoral head (**Figure 6**).

(a) The center-edge angle is reliable only in patients older than 5 years.

(b) A center-edge angle <20° is considered abnormal.

c. Arthrography of the hip—Useful in confirming the acceptability of a closed reduction and in diagnosing the blocks to reduction, such as

capsular narrowing and labral hypertrophy.

d. CT—The standard for confirming acceptable reduction for a patient in a spica cast following closed or open procedures.

e. Magnetic resonance imaging

i. MRI can also be used to confirm acceptable reduction of the hip following closed or open procedures.

ii. MRI can also be useful in an older patient with suspected labral pathology.

4. Neonatal screening

a. Clinical screening (thorough history taking and physical examination) of all newborn infants is necessary.

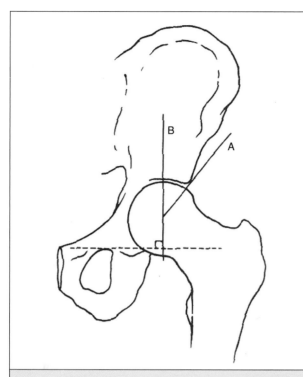

Figure 6   The center-edge angle of Wiberg is formed between two lines passing through the center of the femoral head; one extends to the lateral edge of the sourcil (A), and the other is a perpendicular to the interteardrop line (B). (*Reproduced with permission from MacDonald SJ, Hersche O, Ganz R: Periacetabular osteotomy in the treatment of neurogenic acetabular dysplasia. J Bone Joint Surg Br 1999;81:975-978.*)

Table 1		
Management of Developmental Dysplasia of the Hip		
Age (months)	**Hip Status**	**Initial Treatment**
0-6	Dysplastic	Pavlik harness
6-18	Dislocated	Closed or open reduction (Closed reduction is preferred if the hip has a small medial dye pool and is stable with < 60° of abduction.)
> 18*	Dislocated	Open reduction Femoral shortening osteotomy is indicated in high-riding dislocations (typically, in children ≥ 2 years old) Pelvic osteotomy is indicated for significant dysplasia (often in children ≥ 18-24 months old)

*Open treatment is generally indicated for children with unilateral dislocations up to 8 years old at the time of initial presentation and for those with bilateral dislocations presenting at up to 5-6 years of age.

b. Ultrasound screening of all newborn hips appears unnecessary.

  i. Routine ultrasound screening should be performed for infants with risk factors for the condition.

  ii. Screening by ultrasound should be delayed until age 4 to 6 weeks (or corrected age for premature infants) because ultrasononography is associated with poor specificity in the initial newborn period (4 to 6 weeks).

D. Treatment—Based on the age of the child, stability of the hip (unstable versus dislocated hip), and severity of acetabular dysplasia (**Table 1**).

1. Dysplastic hip in neonate through 6 months of age

  a. In a child with an abnormal abnormal α angle on ultrasound or with an unstable hip (subluxatable hip on examination), initial treatment usually includes a Pavlik harness.

    i. Proper positioning of the Pavlik harness is critical.

      (a) The hips should be flexed to 100° with mild abduction (two to three finger breadths between knees when knees are flexed and adducted).

      (b) Excessive flexion should be avoided to lower the risk of femoral nerve palsy.

      (c) Excessive abduction should be avoided to lower the risk of osteonecrosis; osteonecrosis can occur in both the normal and dysplastic hip.

    ii. The child can be weaned from the Pavlik harness over a 3- to 4-week period when ultrasound parameters become normal.

    iii. Success rates for Pavlik harness treatment in this setting have been reported at >90%.

    iv. The recurrence rate is 10%; therefore, follow-up evaluation until maturity is necessary.

  b. In a relatively large child or in a child older than age 6 months with a dysplastic hip or with hip subluxation, a fixed abduction orthosis or spica casting is an option. Pavlik harness treatment is ineffective in this setting because the child generally "overpowers" the brace.

2. Dislocated hip in neonate through 6 months of age

  a. If the hip is Ortolani-positive, Pavlik harness treatment is initiated.

i. Frequent (every 1 to 2 weeks) reexamination (clinical plus ultrasound) is necessary to ensure that the hip is reduced.

ii. Once the hip becomes stable, treatment is the same as the protocol described above for treatment of dysplastic hip.

iii. Success rate (ie, hip becomes reduced) is reported to be 85%.

iv. The risk of osteonecrosis is low (<5%), especially if treatment is initiated early (ie, in the first 3 months of life).

b. If the hip is Ortolani-negative, initial treatment still includes a Pavlik harness. If reduction is not achieved by 3 to 4 weeks (confirmed by ultrasound), however, Pavlik harness treatment is abandoned, and closed reduction is necessary.

i. Pavlik harness treatment should be discontinued if the dislocated hip does not relocate within 3 to 4 weeks, to avoid Pavlik harness disease.

ii. In Pavlik harness disease, the femoral head sits up against the edge of the acetabulum and worsens the acetabular dysplasia, particularly the posterolateral rim.

3. Dislocated hip in children 6 to 18 months of age

a. Closed reduction is the preferred method of treatment in children age 18 months or younger.

b. Secondary femoral or acetabular procedures are rarely necessary in this age group.

c. The evidence for preliminary traction is equivocal. Given this and the possible complications of skin slough and leg ischemia, most centers have abandoned preliminary traction.

d. Closed reduction is performed under general anesthesia.

i. Adductor tenotomy frequently is necessary.

ii. Hip arthrography is used intraoperatively to confirm adequacy of reduction.

iii. There should be <5 mm of medial contrast pooling between the femoral head and acetabulum.

iv. The safe and stable zones for abduction/adduction, flexion/extension, and internal/external rotation should be established.

v. A spica cast is applied with the hip maintained in the "human position" (hip flexion of 90° to 100° and abduction). Hip abduction should be <60° to minimize the risk of osteonecrosis.

vi. The reduction of the hip in the cast must be confirmed.

(a) Presently, CT is the standard.

(b) MRI is used in some centers to confirm adequacy of reduction of the hip.

vii. Cast immobilization is continued for 3 to 4 months.

(a) Cast change is sometimes necessary.

(b) Removable abduction brace is used afterwards until the acetabulum normalizes.

4. Dislocated hip in children >18 months of age

a. Open reduction is the preferred treatment.

i. Unilateral dislocation: Surgical treatment is generally indicated in children up to 8 years of age with a unilateral dislocation. After 8 years of age, the risks of surgery are felt to outweigh the benefits.

ii. Bilateral dislocation: The upper age limit for surgical treatment in these children is typically 5 to 6 years.

b. Femoral shortening is indicated in children with significantly high-riding dislocations.

i. This is necessary in most, but not all, children ≥ 2 years of age.

ii. Pelvic osteotomy is needed for significant acetabular dysplasia (typical in children > 18 to 24 months old). If a pelvic osteotomy is performed in this age group at the time of initial surgery, the rate of reoperation is reduced significantly.

5. Open reduction

a. Open reduction is indicated if concentric closed reduction cannot be achieved or when excessive abduction (>60°) is required to maintain reduction.

b. The goal of open reduction is to remove the obstacles to reduction and/or safely increase its stability (**Table 2**)

i. Impediments to congruent reduction are the iliopsoas, hip adductors, capsule, ligamentum teres, pulvinar, and transverse acetabular ligament. An infolded labrum may be an impediment in some cases.

ii. The most commonly used approaches are anterior, anteromedial, and medial (**Table 3**).

6. Secondary procedures

a. Secondary femoral and/or pelvic procedures are frequently necessary in children older than

3: Pediatrics

2 years of age to achieve and maintain concentric reduction and minimize the risk of osteonecrosis.

b. Femoral osteotomy

  i. Femoral osteotomy provides shortening (to decrease pressure on the femoral head, thereby minimizing the risk of osteonecrosis), derotation (external rotation to address the abnormally high femoral anteversion in DDH), and varus.

  ii. Avoid excessive varus, because the greater trochanter can impinge against the acetabulum and prevent concentric reduction.

c. Pelvic osteotomy

  i. Indications for pelvic osteotomy include persistent acetabular dysplasia and hip instability.

  ii. There is considerable variability in clinical practice with regard to pelvic osteotomy in children > 2 years of age.

  iii. The two general types of pelvic osteotomy are reconstructive and salvage (Table 4).

    (a) Reconstructive osteotomies redirect or reshape the roof of the acetabulum with its normal hyaline cartilage into a more appropriate weight-bearing position. A prerequisite to a reconstructive pelvic osteotomy is a hip that can be reduced concentrically and congruently. The hip must also have near-normal ROM. Redirectional osteotomies include single innominate (Salter), triple innominate (Steel), and peri-acetabular (Ganz) (Figure 7). Reshaping osteotomies include Pemberton and Dega (Figure 8).

    (b) Salvage procedures are typically indicated in adolescents with severe dysplasia in whom acetabular deficiency precludes the use of a redirectional osteotomy. In salvage procedures, weight-bearing coverage is increased by using the joint capsule as an interposition between the femoral head and bone above it. The intent of these osteotomies is to reduce point loading at the edge of the acetabulum. These osteotomies rely on fibrocartilaginous metaplasia of the interposed joint capsule to provide an increased articulating surface. Salvage osteotomies include Chiari (Figure 9) and shelf osteotomies.

Table 2

Obstacles to a Concentric Reduction of the Hip in DDH

Extra-articular	Intra-articular
Tight psoas tendon	Constricted joint capsule
Tight adductor muscles	Pulvinar
	Hypertrophied ligamentum teres
	Infolded labrum
	Hypertrophied transverse acetabulum ligament

(Adapted from Vitale MG, Skaggs DL: Developmental dysplasia of the hip from six months to four years of age. J Am Acad Orthop Surg 2001;9:401-411.)

Table 3

Advantages and Disadvantages of Anterior Versus Medial or Anteromedial Approaches

Approach	Advantages	Disadvantages
Anterior	1. Capsulorrhaphy and pelvic osteotomy possible through same incision 2. Acetabulum (including labrum) directly accessible 3. Lower reported risk of osteonecrosis 4. Shorter duration of spica casting (6 weeks) 5. Familiar surgical approach.	1. Postoperative stiffness 2. Potential blood loss 3. Potential injury to lateral femoral cutaneous nerve
Medial or anteromedial	1. Allows direct access to medial structures blocking reduction (pulvinar, ligamentum teres, transverse acetabular ligament) 2. Avoids splitting iliac crest apophysis 3. Avoids damage to hip abductors 4. Less invasive, minimal dissection 5. Cosmetically acceptable scar	1. Capsulorrhaphy and pelvic osteotomy not possible through this incision 2. Poor visualization of acetabulum; labrum not accessible 3. Higher risk of osteonecrosis 4. Longer duration of cast immobilization (3 to 4 months)

Table 4

Pelvic Osteotomies for the Treatment of DDH

Reconstructive		Salvage
Redirectional	**Reshaping**	
Single innominate (Salter)	Pemberton	Chiari osteotomy
Triple innominate (Steel)	Dega	Shelf arthroplasty
Periacetabular (eg, Ganz)		

(Adapted from Gillingham BL, Sanchez AA, Wenger DR: Pelvic osteotomies for the treatment of hip dysplasia in children and young adults. J Am Acad Orthop Surg 1999;7:325-337.)

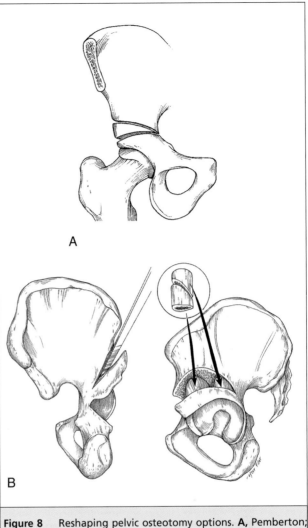

B

Figure 8 Reshaping pelvic osteotomy options. **A,** Pemberton; **B,** Dega.

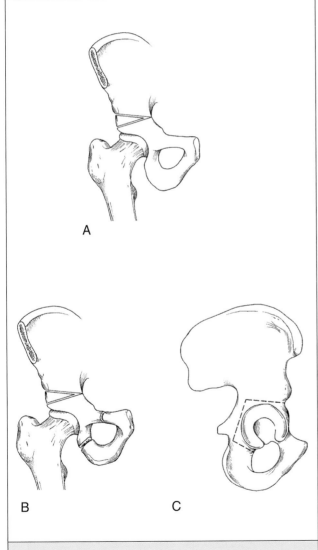

Figure 7 Redirectional pelvic osteotomy options. **A,** Single innominate (Salter); **B,** triple innominate; **C,** periacetabular.

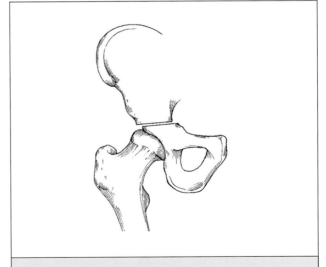

Figure 9 Salvage pelvic osteotomy—Chiari medial displacement osteotomy.

3: Pediatrics

II. Legg-Calvé-Perthes Disease

A. Overview

1. Definition—Legg-Calvé-Perthes disease (LCPD) is an idiopathic osteonecrosis of the capital femoral epiphysis in children.

2. Epidemiology

   a. LCPD affects 1 in 1,200 children.

   b. The disease more commonly affects boys than girls (4:1 to 5:1).

   c. The hips are involved bilaterally in 10% to 12% of cases.

   d. LCPD is more commonly diagnosed in urban than rural communities.

   e. There appears to be a predilection in certain populations, with a higher incidence in Asians, Eskimos, and central Europeans. Incidence is lower in native Australians, Native Americans, Polynesians, and African-Americans.

B. Pathoanatomy

1. Etiology

   a. The exact etiology of LCPD is unknown.

   b. Historically, the cause was thought to be inflammatory or infectious in nature, with transient synovitis as a possible precursor. Trauma was also thought to be causative at one time.

   c. Current theories propose that a disruption of the vascularity of the capital femoral epiphysis occurs, resulting in necrosis and subsequent revascularization.

      i. Deficient vascularity may be due to interruption of the blood supply to the femoral head.

      ii. The vascularity of the capital femoral epiphysis may also be threatened by thrombophilia and/or various coagulopathies (protein C and S deficiency, activated protein C resistance).

         (a) Thrombophilia has been reported to be a possible causative factor in 50% of children with LCPD.

         (b) As many as 75% of patients with LCPD will have a coagulopathy.

2. Risk factors

   a. Family history is positive in 1.6% to 20% of cases.

   b. LCPD is associated with attention-deficit hyperactivity disorder (33%).

   c. Patients are commonly skeletally immature, with bone age delayed in 89% of cases.

3. Pathology—The capital epiphysis and physis are abnormal histologically, with disorganized cartilaginous areas of hypercellularity and fibrillation.

C. Evaluation

1. Clinical presentation

   a. LCPD occurs most commonly in children from age 4 to 8 years (range, 2 years to late teens).

   b. Onset is insidious, and children with LCPD will commonly have a limp and pain in the groin, hip, thigh, or knee regions.

   c. Occasionally, children with LCPD will have a history of recent or remote viral illness.

2. Physical examination

   a. Examination of the child with LCPD may reveal an abnormal gait (antalgic and/or Trendelenburg).

   b. ROM testing will often reveal decreased abduction and internal rotation. Hip flexion contractures are seen rarely.

   c. Limb-length inequality, if present, is mild secondary to femoral head collapse. The presence of hip contractures may make the limb-length inequality appear greater than it actually is.

3. Diagnostic tests

   a. Plain radiographs

      i. Standard AP and frog-leg lateral views of the pelvis are critical in making the initial diagnosis and assessing the subsequent clinical course.

      ii. LCPD typically proceeds through four radiographic stages.

         (a) Initial stage—Early radiographic findings are a sclerotic, smaller proximal femoral ossific nucleus (due to failure of the epiphysis to increase in size) and widened medial clear space (distance between teardrop and femoral head).

         (b) Fragmentation stage—Segmental collapse (resorption) of the capital femoral epiphysis follows, with increased density of the epiphysis.

         (c) Reossification or reparative stage—Necrotic bone is resorbed with subsequent reossification of the capital femoral epiphysis.

         (d) Remodeling stage—Remodeling begins when the capital femoral epiphysis is completely reossified.

   b. Other imaging studies—Other imaging modalities, including bone scans, MRI, and arthrography, are not routinely necessary.

i. Bone scan—Can confirm a suspected diagnosis of LCPD (and the extent of femoral head involvement). Decreased uptake in the capital femoral epiphysis ("cold" lesion, suggesting decreased blood flow) is one of the earliest findings in LCPD and can predate changes on plain radiographs.

ii. MRI—Can also aid in the early diagnosis of LCPD, revealing areas of decreased signal intensity in the capital femoral epiphysis and alterations in the physis.

iii. Arthrography (especially dynamic)—A useful modality to assess coverage and containment of the femoral head. Arthrography is often used at the time of surgery and confirms the degree of correction needed for femoral and/or pelvic osteotomies.

D. Classification

1. The Herring (lateral pillar) classification is based on the height of the lateral pillar of the capital epiphysis on AP view of the pelvis (**Figure 10**).

   a. Group A—No involvement of the lateral pillar, with no density changes and no loss of height of the lateral pillar.

   b. Group B—More than 50% of the lateral pillar height is maintained.

   c. Group C—Less than 50% of the lateral pillar height is maintained.

   d. B/C border group—This group has been added more recently to increase the consistency of readings and to increase prognostic accuracy of the lateral pillar classification. In this group, the lateral pillar is narrow (2 to 3 mm wide) or poorly ossified, or exactly 50% of lateral pillar height is maintained.

   e. The Herring classification is the most reliable classification scheme and is related to prognosis. Its limitation is that the final classification cannot be determined at the time of initial presentation.

2. The Catterall classification is based on the amount of epiphyseal involvement (**Figure 11**). Although commonly used in the past, it has more recently been criticized for its poor interobserver reliability.

   a. Group I—Involvement is limited to the anterior part of the capital epiphysis.

   b. Group II—The anterior and central parts of the capital epiphysis are involved.

   c. Group III—Most of the capital epiphysis is involved, with sparing of the medial and lateral parts of the epiphysis.

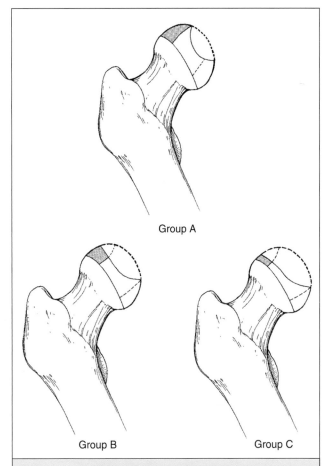

Group A

Group B   Group C

Figure 10   Herring lateral pillar classification for LCPD. Group A hips have no evident involvement of the lateral pillar (lateral third of epiphysis; shaded area) and the lateral pillar height is normal. Group B hips have loss of lateral pillar height < 50%. Type C hips have lost > 50% of the lateral pillar height.

   d. Group IV—The entire epiphysis is involved.

   e. Catterall also described four at-risk signs, which indicate a more severe disease course.

      i. Gage sign (radiolucency in the shape of a V in the lateral portion of the epiphysis)

      ii. Calcification lateral to the epiphysis

      iii. Lateral subluxation of the femoral head

      iv. A horizontal physis

E. Treatment

1. Principles

   a. Treatment is controversial.

   b. Most patients (60%) with LCPD will not require treatment.

   c. Patients with a good prognosis will not usually require treatment.

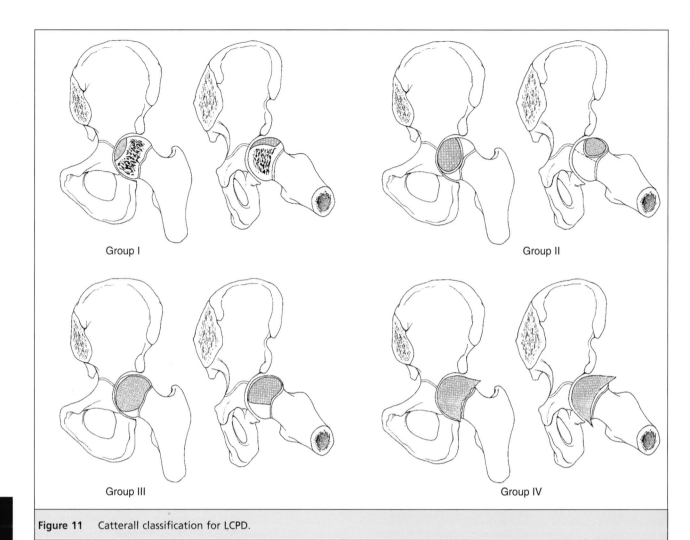

Group I

Group II

Group III

Group IV

Figure 11 Catterall classification for LCPD.

i. Good prognosis is expected for patients with Catterall type I and Herring group A disease.

ii. Young age (<8 years) at onset of disease is also a good prognostic factor.

d. Patients with a poor prognosis will usually need treatment.

i. Prognosis is poor for patients with Catterall types III and IV and Herring groups B and C disease.

ii. Children older than 8 years at onset of disease have a guarded prognosis.

e. All patients require careful periodic clinical and radiographic assessments.

2. Indications

a. For patients with a good prognosis, including younger patients (<8 years of age at initial presentation) with containable hips (ie, femoral heads that are seated well in the acetabulum), symptomatic and supportive measures are usually adequate.

i. Preservation of ROM is essential.

ii. Protected weight bearing has also been recommended, especially before the reossification stage.

b. For patients with a poor prognosis or for patients with progressive deformity and/or progressive loss of motion, particularly abduction, the basis for treatment is containment.

i. The aim of containment is to ensure that the femoral head remains well seated in the acetabulum.

ii. In the long term, the goal of treatment is to prevent deformity and thereby prevent degenerative joint disease.

3. Containment treatment

a. Nonsurgical

i. Containment may be achieved by nonsurgical means, specifically by casting or bracing in an abducted and internally rotated position.

ii. Petrie casts and a variety of abduction orthoses have been used.

iii. The long-term benefit of casting and bracing has been called into question.

b. Surgical

i. Several surgical methods (described below) have been recommended to preserve containment. The results of these methods are comparable.

ii. For these methods to be effective, the hips must be "containable," ie, relatively full ROM with congruency between the femoral head and acetabulum.

iii. Surgical containment may be approached from the femoral side, the acetabular side, or both sides of the hip joint, according to surgeon preference.

(a) On the femoral side, a proximal femoral varus osteotomy is an option.

(b) On the acetabular side, a pelvic osteotomy (Salter, triple innominate, Dega, or Pemberton) may be performed.

(c) A shelf arthroplasty can also be performed to prevent subluxation and lateral overgrowth of the capital epiphysis.

(d) An arthrodiastasis (hip distraction) for 4 to 5 months has also been advocated in some centers, although this is more complicated and cumbersome for the patient.

iv. Once the hip is no longer containable, or for patients presenting late with deformity, treatment strategy focuses on salvage procedures, and the goals of treatment are relief of symptoms and restoration of stability.

(a) These patients are at risk for hinge abduction, ie, lateral extrusion of the femoral head resulting in the femoral head impinging on the edge of the acetabulum with abduction.

(b) An abduction-extension proximal femoral osteotomy should be considered.

(c) Pelvic osteotomy procedures such as a Chiari osteotomy and shelf arthroplasty may be beneficial.

4. Complications

a. The wide range of complications includes femoral head deformity, premature physeal arrest patterns, osteochondritis dissecans, labral injury, and late arthritis.

b. The most important prognostic factors are the shape of the femoral head and its congruency

at skeletal maturity and patient age at onset of disease. Stulberg correlated worse long-term outcomes to greater deformities in the femoral head at maturity.

c. Long-term follow-up studies indicate that most patients with LCPD do well until the fifth or sixth decade of life, at which time degenerative changes in the hip joint are common.

III. Slipped Capital Femoral Epiphysis

A. Overview

1. Definition

a. Slipped capital femoral epiphysis (SCFE) is a disorder of the hip in which the femoral neck displaces anteriorly and superiorly relative to the femoral epiphysis.

b. Displacement occurs through the proximal femoral physis.

2. Epidemiology

a. SCFE is the most common disorder of the hip in adolescents. It occurs in 1 to 61 per 100,000 children annually.

b. Males are more commonly affected than females (2:1). The cumulative risk in males is 1 per 1,000 to 2,000; in females, 1 per 2,000 to 3,000.

c. The left hip is more commonly involved.

d. Unilateral involvement at time of presentation is more common (80%). Ultimately, the hips are involved bilaterally in 10% to 60% of cases.

e. SCFE occurs more commonly in Polynesians and African-Americans.

B. Pathoanatomy

1. Etiology

a. The precise etiology is unknown.

b. In general, SCFE is thought to be the result of mechanical insufficiency of the proximal femoral physis to resist load. This can occur because of either physiologic loads across an abnormally weak physis or abnormally high loads across a normal physis.

i. Conditions that weaken the physis include endocrinopathies such as hypothyroidism, panhypopituitarism, growth hormone abnormalities, hypogonadism, and hyper- or hypoparathyroidism; systemic diseases such as renal osteodystropy; and a history of previous radiation therapy to the femoral head region.

3: Pediatrics

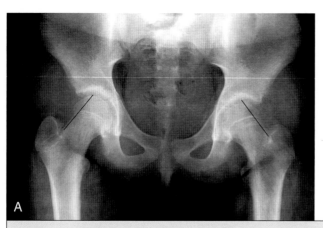 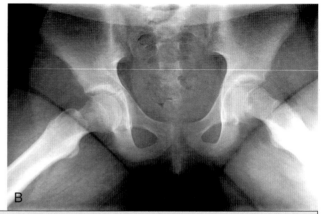

Figure 12 Radiographs of a 10-year old girl with a stable SCFE on the left. **A**, AP view demonstrates that the Klein line intersects the epiphysis bilaterally. **B**, Frog-leg lateral view of the same patient, however, more clearly demonstrates the left SCFE.

ii. Several mechanical factors that can increase the load across the physis are associated with SCFE.

(a) SCFE occurs more commonly in overweight children, with 50% of patients at or above the 90th percentile for weight and 70% of patients above the 80th percentile for weight.

(b) Decreased femoral anteversion and decreased femoral neck-shaft angle are also associated with SCFE.

2. Pathology—The physis is abnormally widened with irregular organization. The slip occurs through the proliferative and hypertropic zones of the physis.

C. Evaluation

1. Clinical presentation

a. SCFE occurs most commonly in children 10 to 16 years of age.

i. In boys, age of presentation is between 12 and 16 years (average, 13.5 years).

ii. In girls, age of presentation is between 10 and 14 years (average, 11.5 years).

b. Children with SCFE commonly have a limp and pain in the groin, hip, thigh, or knee region.

i. Pain is localized to the distal thigh and/or knee region in 23% to 46% of cases.

ii. Symptoms are usually present for weeks to several months before a diagnosis is made.

2. Physical examination

a. Common physical findings include an abnormal gait (antalgic and/or Trendelenburg) and decreased ROM (in particular, decreased hip flexion and decreased internal rotation).

b. ROM testing may also reveal obligate external rotation, ie, external rotation of the hip as the hip is brought into flexion.

c. The foot and knee progression angles are usually externally rotated.

3. Diagnostic tests

a. Plain radiographs—Standard AP and frog-leg lateral views of the pelvis are recommended.

i. The Klein line, a line tangential to the superior border of the femoral neck on the AP view, intersects the proximal femoral epiphysis in a normal hip. The Klein line may fail to intersect the proximal femoral epiphysis in a hip involved with SCFE or will be asymmetric in the two hips (**Figure 12, A**).

ii. Lateral radiographs are more sensitive in detecting a SCFE (**Figure 12, B**).

iii. Radiographic findings also include the metaphyseal blanch sign—superimposition of the posteriorly displaced epiphysis on the femoral neck (seen on AP view).

b. Other imaging studies

i. MRI may be useful in diagnosing "pre-slip" hips. An abnormally widened physis with surrounding edematous changes on MRI are suggestive of pre-slip hips.

ii. Although usually not necessary for the diagnosis of SCFE, MRI may be helpful in the evaluation of osteonecrosis afterward.

iii. CT can be useful in characterizing the proximal femoral deformity—especially during preoperative planning for reconstructive procedures—although it is generally not needed.

D. Classification

1. The Loder classification is the most widely used classification and is based on SCFE stability (Table 5).

   a. The SCFE is stable if the patient is able to weight bear on the involved extremity (with or without crutches).

   b. The SCFE is unstable if the patient is unable to weight bear on the involved extremity.

      i. The value of the Loder classification is its superior ability to predict osteonecrosis.

      ii. Based on a single study, the risk of osteonecrosis in unstable hips was reported as 47%; in stable hips, 0%.

2. The traditional classification is temporal and based on duration of symptoms but has largely been replaced by the Loder classification because of the superior prognostic value of the latter.

   a. The SCFE is chronic when symptoms have been present for >3 weeks.

   b. The SCFE is acute when symptoms have been present for <3 weeks.

   c. The SCFE is acute-on-chronic when there is an acute exacerbation of symptoms following a prodrome of at least 3 weeks.

3. Radiographic classifications

   a. Depending on the amount of slip (percentage of epiphyseal displacement relative to metaphyseal width of femoral neck [on AP or lateral radiographs]), the SCFE is mild (0% to 33%), moderate (33% to 50%), or severe (>50%).

   b. Depending on the difference in Southwick angle between the involved and uninvolved sides, the SCFE is mild (<30° difference), moderate (30° to 50°), or severe (>50°). The Southwick angle, or the head-shaft angle, is the angle formed by the proximal femoral physis and femoral shaft on lateral radiographs.

E. Treatment

1. Nonsurgical—Nonsurgical management, including spica casting, is no longer recommended. Complication rates were high and included chondrolysis, further slip, and osteonecrosis.

2. Surgical

   a. Procedures

      i. In situ screw fixation is the preferred initial treatment of SCFE (Figure 13).

         (a) Forceful manipulation is never indicated because it is associated with an increased risk of complications, including osteonecrosis.

Table 5

Classification of SCFE

Type of SCFE	Able to Bear Weight?	Risk of Osteonecrosis
Stable	Yes	0%
Unstable	No	47%

(Adapted with permission from Loder RT: Unstable slipped capital femoral epiphysis. J Pediatr Orthop 2001;21:694-699.)

         (b) Serendipitous or gentle reduction does not appear to negatively affect patient outcomes.

         (c) For a stable SCFE, a single-screw construct is usually adequate. For an unstable SCFE, use of two screws should be considered, though this entails an increased risk of implant penetration.

         (d) Technical points—Cannulated screw systems are convenient. There are two reasons for starting the screw(s) on the anterior femoral neck: First, because the femoral head has slipped posteriorly, an anterior starting point allows the screw to be targeted to the center position of the femoral head and perpendicular to the physis on both AP and lateral views. Second, a lateral entry point (particularly at or below the lesser trochanter) increases the risk of postoperative fracture. Because of the "blind spot," screws in the center-center position must be at least 5 mm from subchondral bone in all views, and screws in any other position must be at least 10 mm from subchondral bone.

      ii. Bone peg epiphysiodesis is an alternative treatment option. Given its increased complexity and high complication rates (including blood loss), bone peg epiphysiodesis has fallen out of favor in most centers.

      iii. For severe deformities, a proximal femoral osteotomy at the subcapital, femoral neck, intertrochanteric, or subtrochanteric level can be performed. Osteotomy at the subcapital and femoral neck levels can provide the most correction but in general should be avoided because the complication rates are highest among all osteotomies.

      iv. Indications for prophylactic fixation of the contralateral hip include age younger than 10 years and associated at-risk conditions

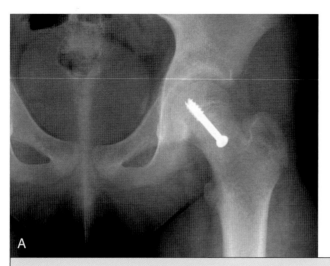 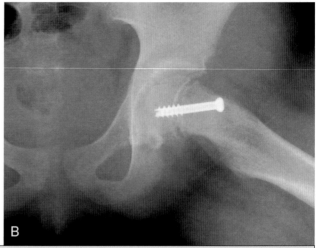

Figure 13 Postoperative AP **(A)** and frog-leg lateral **(B)** views after in situ screw fixation of a stable SCFE.

such as endocrinopathies, renal osteodystrophy, and a previous history of radiation therapy.

  b. Complications

    i. Osteonecrosis (ON)—The most accurate predictor of ON is the stability of the slip, with up to 47% risk of ON for unstable slips. However, hardware placement in the posterior and superior femoral neck can disrupt the interosseous blood supply and also cause osteonecrosis.

    ii. Chondrolysis—Chondrolysis is due to unrecognized implant penetration of the articular surface. If penetration is recognized at the time of surgery and corrected, chondrolysis does not occur. Chondrolysis was a common complication of spica casting in children with SCFE before casting fell out of favor.

    iii. Slip progression—Slip progression occurs in 1% to 2% of cases following in situ single-screw fixation.

    iv. Fracture—The risk of fracture is increased with entry sites through the lateral cortex and those at or distal to the lesser trochanter.

3. Rehabilitation—Weight bearing is usually protected postoperatively.

  a. With an unstable SCFE, 4 to 6 weeks of non-weight-bearing precautions is recommended.

  b. With a stable SCFE, recommendations for weight bearing are variable but usually involve a brief period of partial weight-bearing precautions.

IV. Coxa Vara

A. Overview

1. Definition—Coxa vara is defined as an abnormally low femoral neck-shaft angle (<120°).

  a. Types

    i. Congenital—Congenital coxa vara is characterized by a primary cartilaginous defect in the femoral neck. It commonly is associated with congenital short femur, congenital bowed femur, and proximal femoral focal deficiency (PFFD; also known as partial longitudinal deficiency of the femur).

    ii. Acquired—Coxa vara can be secondary to numerous conditions including trauma, infection, pathologic bone disorders (eg, osteopetrosis), SCFE, LCPD, and skeletal dysplasias.

    iii. Developmental—Developmental coxa vara occurs in early childhood, with classic radiographic changes (including the inverted Y sign) and no other skeletal manifestations. The remainder of the coxa vara section focuses on developmental coxa vara.

2. Epidemiology

  a. Coxa vara occurs in 1 in 25,000 live births worldwide.

  b. Boys and girls are affected equally.

  c. The right and left sides are affected equally.

  d. Bilateral involvement occurs in 30% to 50% of cases.

e. There is no major variation in incidence by race.

B. Etiology

1. The exact cause of coxa vara remains unknown.

2. There appears to be a genetic predisposition, with an autosomal dominant pattern and incomplete penetrance.

3. The most widely accepted theory attributes the deformity in the proximal femur to a primary defect in endochondral ossification in the medial part of the femoral neck.

   a. The eventual dystrophic bone along the medial inferior aspect of the femoral neck fatigues with weight bearing, resulting in a progressive varus deformity.

   b. The vertical orientation of the proximal femoral physis converts normal compressive forces across the physis to a greater shear force. In addition, compressive forces across the medial femoral neck are increased.

C. Evaluation

1. Clinical presentation

   a. The child usually presents after walking is started and before 6 years of age.

   b. Pain is uncommon.

   c. An apparent limb shortening or painless limp may be present in unilateral cases. A waddling gait is more characteristic in bilateral cases.

2. Physical examination

   a. Physical findings include a prominent greater trochanter, which also may be more proximal relative to the contralateral side.

   b. With unilateral involvement, limb-length inequality (usually minor, <3 cm) may be present.

   c. Abductor muscle weakness is common. Consequently, Trendelenburg gait may be present and the Trendelenburg sign may be positive.

   d. ROM testing may demonstrate decrease in abduction and internal rotation.

   e. With bilateral involvement, lumbar lordosis may be increased.

3. Plain radiographs—AP and frog-leg lateral views of the pelvis are recommended. Radiographic findings include:

   a. A decreased femoral neck-shaft angle

   b. The inverted Y sign (resulting from a triangular metaphyseal fragment in the inferior femoral neck), which is pathognomic (**Figure 14**)

   c. Vertical orientation of the physis, a shortened

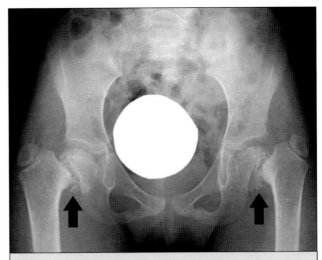

| Figure 14 | The inverted Y sign (arrows), a triangular metaphyseal fragment in the inferior femoral neck, is pathognomic for coxa vara. |

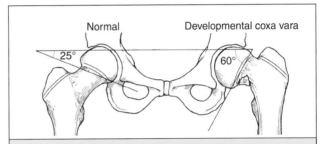

| Figure 15 | The Hilgenreiner-epiphyseal angle is formed by a line through the physis and the Hilgenreiner line. The normal angle is about 25°. |

femoral neck, and decreased femoral anteversion

   d. Abnormal Hilgenreiner-epiphyseal angle, the angle formed by the physis and Hilgenreiner's line. This angle correlates with the risk of disease progression (**Figure 15**).

D. Treatment—Treatment recommendations are based on the severity of the Hilgenreiner-epiphyseal angle and presence of symptoms.

1. Nonsurgical

   a. Asymptomatic patients with a Hilgenreiner-epiphyseal angle <45° should be observed.

   b. Asymptomatic patients with a Hilgenreiner-epiphyseal angle between 45° and 59° can also be observed. Serial radiographs are critical to assess for progression.

2. Surgical

   a. Indications

      i. Patients with a Trendelenburg gait and/or fatigue pain in the hip abductors and a Hilgenreiner angle between 45° and 59° or those with evidence of progression

3: Pediatrics

ii. Patients with a Hilgenreiner-epiphyseal angle >60°

iii. Patients with a progressive decrease in the femoral neck-shaft angle to 90° or 100° or less

b. Procedures

i. The standard procedure is a proximal femoral valgus derotational osteotomy

(a) The osteotomy can occur at the intertrochanteric or subtrochanteric level as described by Langenskiold (intertrochanteric), Pauwel (Y-shaped intertrochanteric), and Borden (subtrochanteric).

(b) Osteotomy at the femoral neck level should be avoided because higher morbidity rates and poorer clinical results have been reported.

ii. The ultimate goal of surgery is to provide valgus overcorrection of the femoral neck-shaft angle (Hilgenreiner-epiphyseal angle <38°).

iii. Adductor tenotomy is frequently necessary.

3. Complications

a. Varus deformity recurs following valgus osteotomy in up to 50% of cases. The risk of recurrence may be decreased by valgus overcorrection.

b. Premature closure of the proximal femoral physis has been reported in up to 89% of cases.

i. Premature closure is usually noted within the first 12-24 months after surgery.

ii. Premature closure may lead to limb-length inequality and/or trochanteric overgrowth.

4. Rehabilitation—Spica cast immobilization is recommended for 6 to 8 weeks after surgery.

Bibliography

Beals RK: Coxa vara in childhood: Evaluation and management. *J Am Acad Orthop Surg* 1998;6:93-99.

Carney BT, Weinstein SL, Noble J: Long-term follow-up with slipped capital femoral epiphysis. *J Bone Joint Surg Am* 1991;73:667-674.

Carroll K, Coleman S, Stevens PM: Coxa vara: Surgical outcomes of valgus osteotomies. *J Pediatr Orthop* 1997;17:220-224.

Gillingham BL, Sanchez AA, Wenger DR: Pelvic osteotomies for the treatment of hip dysplasia in children and young adults. *J Am Acad Orthop Surg* 1999;7:325-337.

Herring JA, Hui K, Browne R: Legg-Calve-Perthes disease: Classification of radiographs with use of the modified lateral pillar and Stulberg classifications. *J Bone Joint Surg Am* 2004;86:2103-2120.

Herring JA, Hui K, Browne R: Legg-Calve-Perthes disease: Prospective multicenter study of the effect of the treatment on outcome. *J Bone Joint Surg Am* 2004;86:2121-2133.

Kocher MS, Bishop JA, Weed B, et al: Delay in diagnosis of slipped capital femoral epiphysis. *Pediatrics* 2004;113:e322-e325.

Loder RT: Unstable slipped capital femoral epiphysis. *J Pediatr Orthop* 2001;21:694-699.

McAndrew MP, Weinstein SL: A long-term follow-up of Legg-Calve-Perthes disease. *J Bone Joint Surg Am* 1984;66:860-869.

Schultz WR, Weinstein JN, Weinstein SL, Smith BG: Prophylactic pinning of the contralateral hip in slipped capital femoral epiphysis: Evaluation of long-term outcome for the contralateral hip with use of decision analysis. *J Bone Joint Surg Am* 2002;84:1305-1314.

Skaggs DL, Tolo VT: Legg-Calve-Perthes disease. *J Am Acad Orthop Surg* 1996;4:9-16.

Staheli LT: Surgical management of acetabular dysplasia. *Clin Orthop Relat Res* 1991;264:111-121.

Vitale MG, Skaggs DL: Developmental dysplasia of the hip from six months to four years of age. *J Am Acad Orthop Surg* 2001;9:401-411.

Weinstein JN, Kuo KN, Millar EA: Congenital coxa vara: A retrospective review. *J Pediatr Orthop* 1984;4:70-77.

Weinstein SL, Mubarak SJ, Wenger DR: Developmental hip dysplasia and dislocation: Part I. *J Bone Joint Surg Am* 2003;85:1824-1832.

Weinstein SL, Mubarak SJ, Wenger DR: Developmental hip dysplasia and dislocation: Part II. *J Bone Joint Surg Am* 2003;85:2024-2035.

Wientroub S, Grill F: Ultrasonography in developmental dysplasia of the hip. *J Bone Joint Surg Am* 2000;82:1004-1018.

Top Testing Facts

Developmental Dysplasia of the Hip

1. Because the ossific nucleus of the femoral head does not appear until 4 to 6 months of age, ultrasound is a better test than plain radiographs in the first 4 to 6 months of life.

2. Routine ultrasound screening should be performed for infants with risk factors for the condition.

3. Because of the poor specificity of ultrasonography in children younger than 1 month, hip ultrasonography should be deferred until after 1 month of life.

4. Pavlik harness treatment should be discontinued if the dislocated hip does not relocate within 3 to 4 weeks, to avoid Pavlik harness disease.

5. Excessive hip flexion in the Pavlik harness results in an increased risk of femoral nerve palsy.

6. Excessive hip abduction in the Pavlik harness results in an increased risk of osteonecrosis of the femoral head.

7. The Galeazzi (or Allis) test is positive in unilateral dislocation but not bilateral dislocations.

8. Because asymmetric skin folds are common in children with normal hips, children with such asymmetry have a high rate of false positives.

9. Hip abduction does not become limited in DDH until approximately 6 months of age.

Legg-Calvé-Perthes Disease

1. The most important prognostic factors are the shape of the femoral head and its congruency at skeletal maturity and patient age at onset of disease. Stulberg correlated worse long-term outcomes to greater deformities in the femoral head at maturity.

2. The Herring lateral pillar classification, based on preservation of the height and integrity of the lateral pillar of the femoral head, is the most reliable classification scheme and is related to prognosis. Its limitation is that a final staging cannot be accurately determined at the time of presentation.

3. Most hips (60%) will not require treatment other than symptomatic and supportive measures.

4. Most patients with LCPD will do well until the 5th to 6th decades of life.

5. Treatment continues to be controversial. For surgical containment methods, the results of proximal femoral osteotomy, pelvic osteotomy, and shelf arthroplasty procedures appear comparable.

Slipped Capital Femoral Epiphysis

1. The frog-leg lateral radiograph is the most sensitive for detecting SCFE.

2. During in situ screw fixation, the starting point should be positioned anteriorly because the femoral epiphysis is posterior relative to the femoral neck.

3. Because of an increased risk of fracture, a lateral entry point should be avoided, especially when at or distal to the lesser trochanter.

4. Because of the "blind spot," screws in the center-center position must be at least 5 mm from subchondral bone on all views—at least 10 mm when the screw is not in the center-center position.

5. The most accurate predictor of osteonecrosis is the stability of the hip at presentation; up to 47% risk of osteonecrosis is associated with unstable slips.

6. Chondrolysis is a consequence of unrecognized permanent screw penetration. If screw penetration is noted at time of surgery and corrected, there is no increased risk of chondrolysis. Before casting fell out of favor, chondrolysis was commonly seen after cast treatment of SCFE as well.

Coxa Vara

1. The inverted Y sign on radiographs is pathognomic for the diagnosis of coxa vara.

2. The Hilgenreiner-epiphyseal angle is prognostic and critical in treatment decision making. Surgery is indicated for an angle >60° and observation for an angle <45°. Those with angles between 45° and 59° require observation for potential progression.

3. A successful outcome following surgery is dependent on valgus overcorrection of the proximal femoral deformity.

Chapter 33
Pediatric Conditions Affecting the Lower Extremity

Anthony Scaduto, MD

I. Limb-Length Discrepancy

A. Epidemiology—Small (up to 2 cm) limb-length discrepancies (LLDs) are common, occurring in up to two thirds of the general population.

B. Secondary problems from LLD

1. The prevalence of back pain may be higher with large discrepancies (>2 cm), but the evidence is limited.

2. During double-limb stance, the hip on the long side is relatively less covered by the acetabulum. Osteoarthritis is seen more commonly (84% of the time) on the long-leg side.

3. LLD increases the incidence of structural scoliosis to the short side. In up to one third of cases, the scoliosis is in a noncompensatory direction.

C. Evaluation

1. Measure the discrepancy by placing blocks under the short leg to level the pelvis.

2. Hip, knee, and ankle contractures will affect the apparent limb length and must be ruled out. A hip adduction contracture causes an apparent shortening of the adducted side.

3. The advantages and disadvantages of various imaging techniques are listed in **Table 1**.

4. Up to 6% of patients with LLD from hemihypertrophy develop embryonal cancers (eg, Wilms tumor). Routine abdominal ultrasounds are recommended until age 6 years.

D. Prediction methods

1. Rule of thumb method

a. Assumes growth ends at age 14 years for girls and 16 years for boys

b. Estimates the annual contribution to leg length of each physis near skeletal maturity (during the last 4 years of growth)

i. Proximal femoral physis—4 mm

ii. Distal femoral physis—10 mm

iii. Proximal tibial physis—6 mm

iv. Distal tibial physis—5 mm

2. Growth remaining method—LLD prediction based on Green and Anderson tables of extremity length for a given age.

Table 1

Assessment of Limb-Length Discrepancy Using Imaging Techniques

Technique	Description	Advantages	Disadvantages
Teleoradiograph	Single exposure of entire leg on a long cassette	Can assess angular deformity	Magnification error
Orthoradiograph	Three separate exposures (hip, knee and ankle) on a long cassette	Eliminates magnification error	Cannot assess angular deformity Movement error may occur
Scanogram	Three separate exposures on a small cassette	Eliminates magnification error Small cassette	Cannot assess angular deformity Movement error may occur
CT scanogram	CT scan through hip, knee, and ankle to assess length	Accurate length measurement possible in the presence of joint contractures	Cannot assess angular deformity

---

Table 2

Treatment Algorithm for Limb-Length Discrepancy

Discrepancy	Treatment Options
0 to 2 cm	No treatment if asymptomatic. May use shoe lift if symptomatic.
2 to 5 cm	Shoe lift, epiphysiodesis, shortening, lengthening
5 to 15 cm	Lengthening(s). May be combined with epiphysiodesis/shortening procedure(s).
>15 cm	Lengthenings plus epiphysiodesis/shortening versus prosthesis

3. Moseley straight line graph method

    a. This method improves the accuracy of Green and Anderson prediction by reformatting the data in graph form.

    b. It accounts for differences between skeletal age and chronologic age.

    c. It minimizes errors of arithmetic or interpretation by averaging serial measurements.

4. Multiplier method

    a. This method predicts final limb length by multiplying the current discrepancy by a sex- and age-specific factor. It is most accurate for discrepancies that are constantly proportional (eg, congenital).

    b. Girls have one half of their final leg length at age 3 years and boys at 4 years.

E. Classification

1. There are many causes of LLD including congenital conditions, infection, paralytic conditions, tumors, trauma, and osteonecrosis.

    a. In congenital conditions, the absolute discrepancy increases but the relative percentage remains constant (eg, a short limb that is 70% of the long side at birth will be 70% of the long side at maturity).

        i. Average female leg length at maturity: 80 cm

        ii. Average male leg length at maturity: 85 cm

    b. Children with paralysis usually have shortening of the more severely affected side.

2. Static discrepancies (eg, a malunion of the femur in a shortened position) must be differentiated from progressive discrepancies (eg, physeal growth arrest).

F. Treatment

1. Physeal bar excision

    a. Physeal bars following trauma tend to be more discrete (and more amenable to excision) than are bars resulting from infection or ischemia.

    b. Bridge resection is indicated if the bony bridge involves <50% of the physis in patients with at least 2 years of growth remaining.

2. Discrepancy correction (**Table 2**)

    a. Nonsurgical—Any size discrepancy can be corrected with a shoe lift, but shoe lifts >5 cm are poorly tolerated because they are heavy and may result in subtalar and ankle inversion injuries.

    b. Surgical

        i. General principles

            (a) The surgical correction must address the anticipated final LLD, not just the current discrepancy.

            (b) In paralytic conditions (such as myelodysplasia, cerebral palsy, or polio), it is often best to leave the LLD undercorrected to facilitate foot clearance of the weak leg. This is especially important if the patients walks with a brace that locks the knee in extension.

        ii. Shortening techniques

            (a) Epiphysiodesis is the treatment of choice for discrepancies of 2 to 5 cm because of the very low complication rate. If proximal tibial epiphysiodesis is performed, concomitant proximal fibular epiphysiodesis should also be performed if more than 2 to 3 years of growth remain (to prevent proximal fibular overgrowth and prominence).

            (b) Acute osseous shortening is typically used for discrepancies of 2 to 5 cm after skeletal maturity.

                (1) Fewer complications occur with femoral shortening than with tibial shortening.

                (2) Shortening is best tolerated when limited to <5 cm.

        iii. Lengthening techniques

            (a) Methods

                (1) Uniplanar or multiplanar external fixation

                (2) External fixation with intramedullary nail

                (3) Intramedullary distraction

3: Pediatrics

(b) Pearls

(1) Lengthen at metaphyseal level whenever possible.

(2) Delay the onset of distraction by 5 to 7 days after the corticotomy is performed.

(3) Lengthen at a rate of 1 mm/day (0.25 mm four times/day).

(4) Limit the lengthening goal to <20% of the individual bone length per lengthening period.

iv. Complications

(a) Incomplete arrest or angular deformity can result from either open or percutaneous epiphysiodesis techniques.

(b) Common complications of lengthening include pin site infection, pin or wire failure, regenerate deformity or fracture, delayed union, premature cessation of lengthening, and joint subluxation/dislocation.

II. Angular Deformities

A. Overview

1. Normal physiologic knee alignment includes periods of "knock knees" and "bowed legs" (Figure 1).

2. Children with bowed legs after age 2 years may require further evaluation.

B. Blount disease (tibia vara)

1. Epidemiology

a. The most common cause of pathologic genu varum is Blount disease.

b. Progressive tibia vara can occur in infants and adolescents (Table 3).

2. Pathoanatomy

a. Excess medial pressure (eg, heavy, early walkers who are in physiologic varus alignment) produces an osteochondrosis of the physis and adjacent epiphysis that can progress to a complete physeal bar.

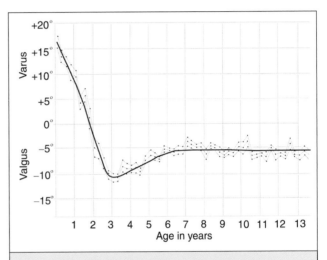

Figure 1   Graph illustrating the development of the tibiofemoral angle in children during growth, based on measurements from 1,480 examinations of 979 children. Of the lighter lines, the middle one represents the mean value at a given point in time, and the other two represent the deviation from the mean. The darker line represents the general trend. *(Adapted with permission from Salenius P, Vankka E: The development of the tibiofemoral angle in children. J Bone Joint Surg Am 1975;57:259-261.)*

Table 3						

Infantile Versus Adolescent Blount Disease

Condition	Age (Years)	Typical History	Location of Deformity	Other Angular Deformities	Laterality	Treatment
Infantile Blount	1 to 3	Early walker, obese	Epiphysis/physis; joint depression in advanced stages	None	Often bilateral	Bracing (limited effectiveness) Proximal tibia/fibula osteotomy
Adolescent Blount	9 to 11	Morbid obesity	Proximal tibia; no joint depression	Distal femur and distal tibia common	Unilateral more common	Bracing not effective Hemiepiphysiodesis if growth remaining Proximal tibia/fibula osteotomy ± femoral and distal tibia osteotomies

3: Pediatrics

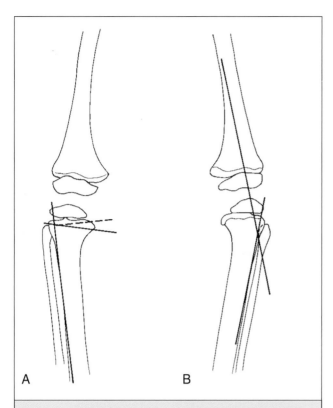

Figure 2   Assessment of the metaphyseal-diaphyseal **(A)** and tibial-femoral **(B)** angles. *(Reproduced from Brooks WC, Gross RH: Genu varum in children: Diagnosis and treatment.* J Am Acad Orthop Surg *1995;3:326-336.)*

b. In adolescent Blount disease, a varus moment at the knee during the stance phase of gait inhibits medial physeal growth according to the Heuter-Volkmann principle.

3. Evaluation

   a. Physiologic bowing versus Blount

   b. Clinical findings suggestive of pathologic bowing

      i. Proximal tibial location of bowing

      ii. Sharply angular deformity

      iii. Asymmetric bowing of the two legs

      iv. Progressive deformity on serial examinations

      v. Lateral thrust during gait

      vi. Very severe deformity

   c. Radiographs

      i. Indications

         (a) Children older than 18 months of age with clinical deformity >20°

         (b) Less than 5th percentile for height, or a family history of metabolic bone disease

         (c) Findings suggestive of pathologic bowing (as noted above)

      ii. Because of internal tibial torsion, it is essential to obtain the radiographs with the patellae directed anteriorly.

      iii. When the metaphyseal-diaphyseal (MD) angle (**Figure 2**) is <10°, there is 95% chance the bowing will resolve.

      iv. If the MD angle is >16°, there is 95% chance of progression. For MD angles between 11° and 16°, there is considerable overlap between physiologic genu varum and Blount disease.

4. Classification—Langenskiold described six radiographic stages that can develop over 4 to 5 years.

   a. Early changes include metaphyseal beaking and sloping.

   b. Advanced changes include articular depression and medial physeal closure.

5. Treatment

   a. Nonsurgical

      i. Bracing efficacy is controversial.

      ii. Bracing is indicated only in patients 2 to 3 years of age with mild disease (stage 1 to 2).

      iii. Poor results are associated with obesity and bilaterality.

      iv. Improvement should occur within 1 year.

      v. Bracing must be continued until the bony changes resolve, which usually takes 1.5 to 2 years.

   b. Surgical

      i. General surgical principles

         (a) To avoid undercorrection, the distal fragment is fixed in slight valgus, lateral translation, and external rotation.

         (b) Performing an anterior compartment fasciotomy at the time of surgery decreases the postoperative risk of compartment syndrome.

         (c) The mechanical axis can be confirmed intraoperatively by holding the bovie cord directly over the center of the femoral head and ankle. The cord should pass over the lateral tibial plateau.

      ii. Infantile Blount disease

         (a) Patients older than 3 years require proximal tibial valgus and rotational osteotomy.

Table 4

Common Causes of Genu Valgum

Bilateral
Physiologic genu valgum
Rickets
Skeletal dysplasia (eg, chondroctodermal dysplasia, spondyloepiphyseal, Morquio syndrome)

Unilateral
Physeal injury (trauma, infection, or vascular)
Proximal tibial metaphyseal (Cozen) fracture
Benign tumors (eg, fibrous dysplasia, Ollier disease, osteochondroma)

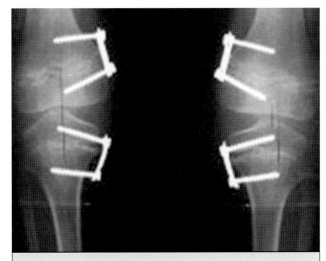

Figure 3 Radiographs demonstrate hemiphyseal tethering with a plate-screw construct. *(Courtesy of Ortho-fix, McKinney, TX.)*

(1) 1 or 2 pins and a cast provide fixation.

(2) Fibular osteotomy is needed to allow for sufficient correction.

(3) The risk of recurrence is much less if the surgery is performed before age 4 years.

(b) If a bony bar is present, a bar resection with interposition of methylmethacry-late (epiphysiolysis) is performed concomitantly.

(c) If significant depression of the medial tibial plateau exists, a medial tibial plateau elevation and realignment osteotomy may be necessary.

iii. Adolescent Blount disease

(a) Temporary or permanent epiphysiodesis prevents deformity progression and may allow some correction in adolescents with mild to moderate Blount in whom at least 15 to 18 months of growth remain.

(b) Severe deformities require proximal tibial osteotomy and occasionally a femoral osteotomy (if distal femoral varus exceeds 7° to 10°).

(c) Fixation is generally with a plate or external fixation.

C. Genu valgum

1. Epidemiology

a. Typically, developing children aged 3 to 4 years have up to 20° of genu valgum.

b. Genu valgum should not increase after 7 years of age.

c. After age 7 years, valgus should not exceed 12° with an intermalleolar distance <8 cm.

2. Pathoanatomy

a. The deformity is usually in the distal femur but may also arise in the proximal tibia.

b. The degree of deformity necessary to lead to degenerative changes in the knee is not known.

3. Causes (**Table 4**)

4. Treatment

a. Nonsurgical

i. Bracing is unnecessary for physiologic valgus and often ineffective in pathologic valgus.

ii. Genu valgum following proximal tibial metaphyseal (Cozen) fractures almost universally spontaneously remodels and should be observed.

b. Surgical

i. Indications—Correction is indicated if a line drawn from the center of the head of the femur to the center of the ankle falls in the outer quadrant of the tibial plateau (or beyond) in children older than 10 years.

ii. Procedures

(a) Hemiepiphysiodesis or temporary physeal tethering

(1) Tethering options include staples, screws across the physis, or newer plate/screw devices (**Figure 3**). The hardware must be placed extraperiosteally in order to avoid unintended physeal injury and growth arrest.

3: Pediatrics

(2) Close follow-up is necessary to avoid overcorrection.

(3) Growth can resume with tether removal by 24 months.

(4) Nomograms are available to determine the timing for permanent hemiepiphysiodesis or the anticipated time to correction for temporary hemiepiphysiodesis.

(b) Osteotomies are necessary when insufficient growth remains or the site of the deformity is away from the physis.

5. Complications—To reduce the risk of peroneal injury with varus osteotomy, consider either gradual correction, preemptive peroneal nerve release, or a closing-wedge technique.

III. Rotational Deformities

A. Intoeing

1. Rotational profiles not only change during childhood, but they also vary widely among healthy children of the same age.

2. Femoral anteversion

   a. Epidemiology

      i. Intoeing from femoral anteversion is most evident between 3 and 6 years of age.

      ii. Anteversion is 30° to 40° at birth. It decreases to 15° by skeletal maturity.

      iii. Anteversion occurs more commonly in girls than boys (2:1) and often is hereditary.

   b. Pathoanatomy

      i. Rotation variations have not been directly correlated to degenerative changes of the hip or knee.

      ii. Patellofemoral pain can arise with increasing femoral anteversion, but a pathologic threshold has not been identified.

      (a) Brace-dependent ambulators (such as those with cerebral palsy or myelodysplasia) tolerate less tibial torsion because the compensatory gait mechanisms (knee and subtalar motion) are unavailable.

      (b) Lever-arm dysfunction in children with neuromuscular disorders is the reason osteotomies are frequently indicated in such children. (See chapter 27, Neuromuscular Disorders.)

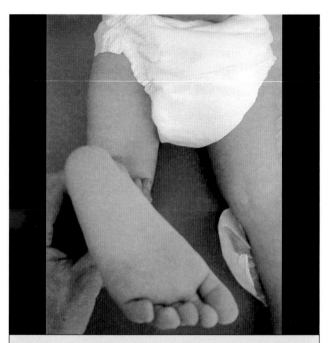

Figure 4   The thigh-foot axis is best measured with the child in the prone position. *(Reproduced from Lincoln TL, Suen PW: Common rotational variations in children. J Am Acad Orthop Surg 2003; 11:312-320.)*

   c. Evaluation

      i. Intoeing gait with medially rotated patellae is indicative of femoral anteversion.

      ii. Rotational profile assessment should include the knee- and foot-progression angles during gait, the thigh-foot angle, and maximum hip internal and external rotation (**Figure 4**). Estimate femoral anteversion by measuring the degree of internal hip rotation necessary to make the greater trochanter most prominent laterally (trochanteric prominence angle test).

      iii. CT or MRI can quantify anteversion most accurately, but they are unnecessary in most cases.

   d. Differential

      i. Other common causes of intoeing include internal tibial torsion and metatarsus adductus.

      ii. After age 10 years, internal rotation >70° and external rotation <20° suggests excessive femoral anteversion.

   e. Treatment

      i. Shoes, orthoses, and braces are ineffective.

      ii. For able-bodied children older than 8 years with unacceptable awkward gait or pain and <10° external hip rotation, a derotation osteotomy is indicated. The amount of rotation needed to correct excessive anteversion = (prone internal rotation – prone external rotation)/2.

3. Tibial torsion

   a. Epidemiology

      i. Most evident between ages 1 and 2 years

      ii. Usually resolves by age 6 years

   b. Evaluation—Tibial torsion is the angular difference between the bimalleolar axis at the ankle and the bicondylar axis of the knee (normal is 20° external rotation).

   c. Treatment

      i. Parent education is the primary treatment.

      ii. Special shoes and braces do not change the natural history.

      iii. Derotation osteotomy is rarely needed in able-bodied children.

      iv. If an isolated distal tibial rotational osteotomy is performed, rotation >30° generally results in translation of the distal fragment. This is not clinically significant and will remodel quickly in growing children.

IV. Tibial Bowing

A. Overview—Three types of tibial bowing exist in children, with considerable differences in prognosis and treatment (**Table 5**).

B. Anterolateral bowing

   1. Epidemiology

      a. 50% of patients with anterolateral bowing have neurofibromatosis.

      b. 10% of patients with neurofibromatosis have anterolateral bowing.

2. Classification—The presence of sclerosis, cysts, fibular dysplasia, and narrowing are the basis of the Boyd and Crawford classifications (**Figure 5**). Neither is predictive of prognosis.

3. Natural history—Spontaneous resolution is unusual. Good prognostic signs include:

   a. Duplicated hallux

   b. Delta-shaped osseous segment in the concavity of the bow

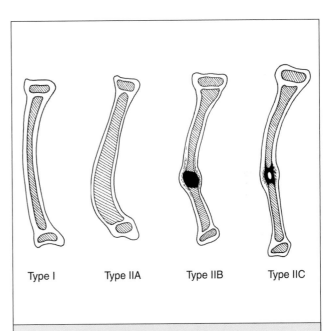

Type I   Type IIA   Type IIB   Type IIC

Figure 5   Classification of congenital tibial dysplasia. Type I is characterized by anterior lateral bowing with increased cortical density and a narrow but normal medullary canal; type IIA, by anterior lateral bowing with failure of tubularization and a widened medullary canal; type IIB, by anterior lateral bowing with a cystic lesion before fracture or canal enlargement from a previous fracture; and type IIC, by frank pseudarthrosis and bone atrophy with "sucked candy" narrowing of the ends of the two fragments. *(Reproduced from Crawford AH, Schorry EK: Neurofibromatosis in children: The role of the orthopaedist. J Am Acad Orthop Surg 1999;7:217-230.)*

Table 5

Types of Tibial Bowing

	Anterolateral Bowing	Posteromedial Bowing	Anteromedial Bowing
Associated Conditions	Neurofibromatosis	Calcaneal valgus foot	Fibular deficiency
Prognosis	1. Progressive bowing 2. Pseudarthrosis	1. Spontaneous improvement in bowing (rarely complete) 2. Limb-length discrepancy	Varies with severity of shortening and foot function
Treatment	1. Bracing to prevent fracture 2. Osteotomy contraindicated	Observation	Osteotomy with lengthening versus amputation

3: Pediatrics

4. Treatment

a. The primary goal of treatment is prevention of pseudarthrosis.

 i. A clam-shell total contact brace is used.

 ii. Osteotomies to correct bowing are contra-indicated because of the risk of pseudarthrosis of the osteotomy site.

 iii. Fracture risk decreases at skeletal maturity.

b. Pseudarthrosis

 i. All treatment options have limited success.

 (a) Intramedullary rod and bone grafting

 (b) Circular fixator with bone transport

 (c) Vascularized fibular graft

 ii. Amputation is indicated for persistent pseudarthrosis (usually after 2 or 3 failed surgeries).

C. Posteromedial bowing

1. Congenital posteromedial bowing is often confused with a calcaneal valgus foot. Dorsum of the foot may be in contact with the anterior tibia (**Figure 6**).

2. The bow improves in the first years of life, but it rarely resolves completely.

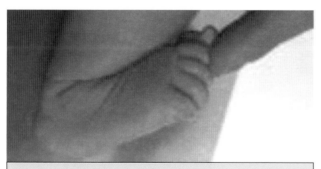

Figure 6   A calcaneus foot is easily dorsiflexed against the tibia. A posteromedial bow of the tibia can be confused with a calcaneus foot. *(Reproduced from Sullivan JA: Pediatric flatfoot: Evaluation and management. J Am Acad Orthop Surg 1999;7:44-53.)*

3. Must monitor for LLD—LLDs at maturity are usually in the 3 to 8 cm range (average 4 cm) and are treated as noted above in section I.

D. Anteromedial bowing—See proximal femoral focal deficiency, section V.B, below.

V. Limb Deficiencies

A. General principles for amputation, when indicated

1. Optimal age for amputation for limb deficiency is 10 months to 2 years.

2. Avoid early amputation if severe upper extremity deficiencies may require use of the feet for activities of daily living (ADLs).

3. Syme versus Boyd amputation:

a. The Syme amputation (ankle disarticulation) is simple and accommodates a tapered prosthesis at the ankle for optimal cosmesis.

b. The Boyd amputation (the calcaneus is retained and is fused to the distal tibia) prevents heel pad migration, aids prosthesis suspension, and may provide better end bearing. However, it also may limit prosthetic foot options because of its greater length.

B. Proximal femoral focal deficiency (PFFD; also called partial longitudinal deficiency of the femur) and congenital short femur

1. Overview (epidemiology)

a. The spectrum of femoral hypoplasia includes congenital short femur on the mild end to complete absence of the proximal femur on the severe end.

b. Bilateral involvement is seen in 15% of cases. Other limb anomalies are present 50% of the time.

c. There is no genetic link except in a rare autosomal dominant form with dysmorphic facies.

2. Pathoanatomy (**Table 6**)

a. Associated clinical problems are quite variable.

Table 6

Spectrum of Problems Associated With Proximal Femoral Focal Deficiency (PFFD)

Condition	Acetabulum	Proximal Femur	Knee	Lower Leg
Mild PFFD	Normal	Delayed ossification and varus	Anterior-posterior laxity	Normal
Moderate PFFD	Dysplastic	Pseudarthrosis	Cruciate deficiency	Fibular deficiency
Severe PFFD	Absent	Complete absence	Flexion contracture	Severe fibular and foot deficiency

b. The lower leg can appear normal despite severe upper leg involvement.

3. Evaluation

a. The thigh is short, flexed, abducted, and externally rotated (**Figure 7**).

b. Fibular deficiency occurs in 70% of PFFD patients.

4. Treatment

a. Nonsurgical

  i. "Extension" prosthesis

    (a) Initial treatment is provided when the patient is pulling to stand.

    (b) The bulbous segment necessary to accommodate the foot makes the prosthesis less attractive.

b. Surgical

  i. Surgery is best delayed until the patient is 2.5 to 3 years of age.

  ii. Lengthening

    (a) Indications include a predicted discrepancy at maturity <20 cm, a stable hip joint, and a functional foot.

    (b) Any varus, proximal pseudarthrosis, or acetabular dysplasia is addressed before lengthening.

  iii. Knee arthrodesis and foot ablation

    (a) Indications—Foot on the affected side is at the level of the contralateral knee or higher.

    (b) The procedure creates a single long lever arm that is aligned with the weight-bearing line of the body, which improves prosthetic fit, function, and appearance.

    (c) Ideally, the short limb should be short enough that the prosthetic knee is not below the level of the contralateral knee (about 7 cm shorter) at maturity.

  iv. van Ness rotationplasty

    (a) This procedure converts the ankle joint into a functional knee joint by rotating the foot 180°.

    (b) Modified below-knee (transtibial) prosthesis improves gait pattern and efficiency.

    (c) Indications: The foot of the affected limb lies around the level of contralateral knee, and the ankle is stable with >60° of motion.

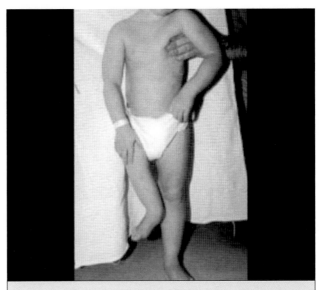

Figure 7 In this child with PFFD, the ankle of the affected extremity is almost at the level of the contralateral knee. The foot on the affected side is almost normal. This child would be a good candidate for knee fusion and rotationplasty. *(Reproduced from Krajbich JI: Lower-limb deficiencies and amputations in children. J Am Acad Orthop Surg 1998;6:358-367.)*

B. Fibular deficiency

1. Overview (epidemiology)

a. Previously known as fibular hemimelia

b. The most common long-bone deficiency

c. No known inheritance pattern

2. Pathoanatomy

a. It is best to think of fibular deficiency as an abnormality involving the entire limb (**Figure 8**).

b. Associated anomalies

  i. Shortening of the femur and tibia

  ii. Genu valgum from hypoplasia of the lateral femoral condyle

  iii. Cruciate ligament deficiency

  iv. Anteromedial bow of the tibia

  v. Ball-and-socket ankle

  vi. Equinovalgus foot deformity

  vii. Tarsal coalition

  viii. Absent lateral rays

3. Evaluation

a. Classically there is a short limb with an equinovalgus foot and skin dimpling over the midanterior tibia.

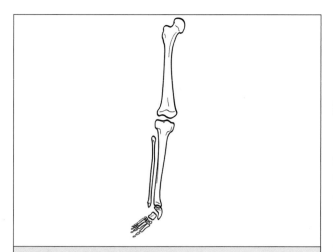

Figure 8   Osseous anatomy of fibular deficiency. *(Reproduced from Kayes KJ, Spiegel DA: Knee and leg: Pediatrics, in Vaccaro AR (ed):* Orthopaedic Knowledge Update 8. *Rosemont, IL, 2005, p 751.)*

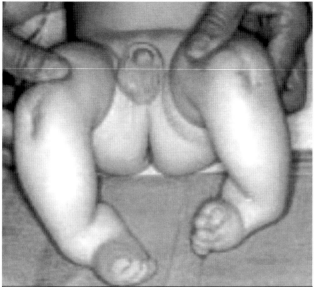

Figure 9   Typical clinical appearance of tibial deficiency. *(Reproduced from Krajbich JI: Lower-limb deficiencies and amputations in children.* J Am Acad Orthop Surg *1998;6:358-367.)*

Table 7

Treatment Guidelines for Fibular Deficiency

Findings	Treatment
Nonfunctional foot	Amputation (Syme or Boyd)
Functional foot plus:	
LLD <10%	Lengthening
LLD 10% to 30%	Lengthening or amputation
LLD >30%	Amputation

LLD = limb-length discrepancy

b. Radiographs

   i. Fibula is short or absent (partial or complete hemimelia).

   ii. The intercondylar notch of the femur is typically shallow and the tibial spines are small.

4. Classification

   a. Achterman and Kalamchi classification—Based on the amount of fibula present.

   b. Birch classification—Treatment guidelines based on limb length and foot function.

5. Treatment (**Table 7**)

   a. The level or extent of fibular deficiency does not determine treatment.

   b. Severity of discrepancy and foot function guide treatment.

C. Tibial deficiency

   1. Overview

      a. Tibial deficiency was previously known as tibial hemimelia.

   b. It has an autosomal dominant inheritance pattern. Formal genetic counseling is recommended.

   c. Other musculoskeletal anomalies occur in 75% of patients.

2. Evaluation

   a. Typical appearance includes a short tibial segment with a flexed knee and prominent proximal fibula. Commonly the foot is in rigid equinovarus and supination (**Figure 9**).

   b. The presence or absence of active knee extension must be determined.

   c. A proximal tibia anlage may be present but not apparent on early radiographs because of delayed ossification. An early clue to the absence of the proximal tibia is a small and minimally ossified distal femoral epiphysis.

   d. Associated limb anomalies include preaxial polydactyly and lobster clawhand deformity.

3. Classification (Jones)

   a. The Jones classification distinguishes partial from complete absence.

   b. Partial absence is further categorized as proximal, distal, or ankle diastasis.

4. Treatment (**Table 8**)

   a. Presence of active knee extension determines treatment.

   b. The proximal tibia can be present without active extension.

Table 8

Treatment Algorithm for Tibial Deficiency

Deformity/Findings	Treatment
No active knee extension	Knee disarticulation
Active knee extension	Synostosis of fibula to partial tibia plus Syme amputation
Ankle diastasis	Syme/Boyd amputation

c. The Brown procedure (centralization of the fibula under the femur to treat complete tibial absence) has a high failure rate.

d. A tibiofibular synostosis is effective at extending a short proximal tibial segment.

VI. Congenital Dislocation of the Knee

A. Overview

1. Congenital dislocation of the knee is a rare disorder that is commonly sporadic but occasionally occurs within families.

2. Conditions producing muscle imbalance or laxity (myelodysplasia, arthrogryposis, Larsen syndrome) are also associated with congenital dislocation of the knee.

B. Pathoanatomy—Abnormal fetal position (breech position with feet locked under the mandible), congenital absence of the cruciate ligaments, and fibrosis/contracture of the quadriceps have all been proposed as etiologic factors.

C. Evaluation

1. The knee can be hyperextended and the foot is easily placed against the baby's face. Minimal or no flexion of the knee is possible.

2. A dimple or skin crease is seen at the anterior knee.

3. Hip examination is important because an ipsilateral hip dislocation is very common (70% to 100%).

D. Classification—The spectrum has been classified from severe genu recurvatum (grade I), subluxation (grade II), and complete dislocation (grade III).

E. Treatment—The treatment of a knee dislocation takes priority over treatment of ipsilateral hip dysplasia or clubfoot. The Pavlik harness and clubfoot casts both require knee flexion.

1. Nonsurgical

a. Initial treatment begins with stretching followed by serial casting.

b. Flexion should be attempted only after the tibia is reduced on the end of the femur (must confirm with lateral radiograph or ultrasound). Distal femoral physeal separation or plastic deformity of the tibia is possible.

c. Prognosis is generally excellent if reduction is achieved nonsurgically.

2. Surgical

a. Surgical treatment is indicated if nonsurgical treatment fails to reduce the tibia on the end of the femur.

b. The release always includes quadriceps lengthening.

c. Best results are seen when performed before 6 months of age.

VII. Foot Problems

A. Clubfoot (talipes equinovarus)

1. Overview (epidemiology)

a. Clubfoot is a congenital foot deformity consisting of hindfoot equinus and varus as well as midfoot and forefoot adduction and cavus.

b. It is more common in males and is the most common birth defect (1 in 750 live births).

c. Half the cases are bilateral.

d. Unaffected parents with an affected child have a 2.5% to 6.5% chance of having another child with clubfoot.

2. Pathoanatomy

a. Potential etiologies include abnormal fibrosis, neurologic abnormalities, and arrested embryologic development.

b. Key components of the deformity are medial and plantar subluxation of the navicular on the talar head, a medially rotated calcaneus, and a shortened talar neck with medial angulation.

3. Evaluation

a. Common clinical findings are a small foot, small calf, slightly shortened tibia, and skin creases medially and posteriorly.

b. Nonidiopathic clubfeet must be identified. Clubfeet associated with arthrogryposis, myelodysplasia, diastrophic dysplasia, and amniotic

Table 9

Treatment of Residual Clubfoot Deformity

Residual/Recurrent Deformity	Corrective Surgery
Supination	Whole or split transfer of tibialis anterior tendon
Varus	Revision posteromedial release versus calcaneal osteotomy. (Osteotomy is needed for rigid deformity.)
Adductus	Medial column lengthening/lateral column shortening osteotomies
Internal rotation of foot	Supramalleolar tibial osteotomy
Planovalgus	Calcaneal neck lengthening or medial calcaneal slide
Severe multiplanar residual clubfoot deformity	Multiplanar osteotomies of midfoot and/or hindfoot Triple arthrodesis if not amenable to joint-sparing osteotomies

band syndrome are resistant to casting treatment.

   c. Radiographs

     i. Minimal ossification of the foot in the newborn limits the utility of radiographs.

     ii. In both the AP and lateral views of a clubfoot, the talus and calcaneus are less divergent and more parallel (smaller talocalcaneal angle) than normal.

     iii. Radiographic appearance has poor correlation with clinical outcome.

  4. Classification

   a. The two most commonly used classification systems are those described by Dimeglio and Pirani.

   b. Both classifications assign points based on the severity of clinical findings and the correctability of the deformity.

  5. Treatment

   a. Nonsurgical—Ponseti serial casting.

     i. Outcome is much better than with historical casting techniques (80% to 90% success versus 10% to 50%).

     ii. Sequence of deformity correction is *c*avus, *a*dductus, *v*arus, and finally *e*quinus (CAVE).

     iii. Important Ponseti casting concepts

       (a) Forefoot is supinated, not pronated.

       (b) Lateral pressure is applied to neck of talus only.

       (c) Long leg casts

       (d) Weekly cast changes

       (e) Percutaneous Achilles tenotomy is frequently done before final cast application to address residual equinus (up to 90% of feet).

     iv. The most common cause of failure after initial correction with Ponseti casting is poor compliance with the Denis-Brown brace. Recommended use is 23 hr/day for 3 months after casting and then at night for 2 to 3 years.

     v. Anterior tibial tendon transfer (split or whole transfer) is needed in one third to one half of clubfeet treated with the Ponseti method.

   b. Surgical

     i. Complete posteromedial release indications: persistent deformity after casting, syndrome-associated clubfoot, and delayed presentation (older than 1 to 2 years of age).

     ii. Secondary or residual deformities may require surgical intervention (**Table 9**).

B. Congenital vertical talus

  1. Overview

   a. Congenital vertical talus is an irreducible dorsal dislocation of the navicular on the talus.

   b. Rare condition (1 in 150,000 births) commonly (~50%) associated with neuromuscular disease (myelodysplasia, arthrogryposis, diastematomyelia) or chromosomal abnormalities.

  2. Pathoanatomy

   a. The navicular is dislocated dorsolaterally.

   b. The deformity also includes eversion of the calcaneus, contracture of the dorsolateral muscles and Achilles tendon, and attenuation of the spring ligament.

  3. Evaluation

   a. Clinically, the foot has a rigid convex plantar surface with a prominent talar head (rocker-bottom).

   b. Unlike flexible flatfoot, the arch will not reconstitute upon standing on the toes or hyperextending the great toe.

   c. An awkward, calcaneal-type gait pattern results from limited push-off power, limited (if any) forefoot contact, and excessive heel contact.

d. Radiographs—The radiographic view that is diagnostic for a vertical talus is a lateral view in forced plantar flexion (**Figure 10**).

   i. The navicular remains dorsally dislocated in this view. This differs from oblique talus, in which the navicular reduces on this view.

   ii. Prior to ossification of the navicular (age 3 years), the first metatarsal is used as a proxy for the dorsal alignment of the navicular on the lateral view.

4. Differential and prognosis

a. Untreated congenital vertical talus causes significant disability.

b. Physiologic flatfoot and oblique talus are benign conditions that are easily distinguished from a vertical talus.

5. Treatment

a. Nonsurgical

   i. Initial treatment begins with casting.

   ii. Casting is usually insufficient to correct a vertical talus but may help stretch the tight dorsolateral soft tissues.

b. Surgical

   i. Surgery is usually performed between 12 and 18 months of age.

   ii. Surgical treatment includes extensive talar release with lengthening of the Achilles, toe extensors, and peroneal tendons and pinning of the talonavicular joint. The anterior tibialis is generally transferred to the talar neck.

   iii. Outcome of reconstruction after age 3 years is less predictable. Triple arthrodesis is rarely needed as a salvage procedure.

C. Calcaneovalgus foot

1. Overview (epidemiology)

a. Calcaneovalgus foot is a positional deformity seen at birth. The foot is hyperdorsiflexed due to intrauterine positioning (**Figure 6**).

b. It is more common in girls who are first-born children.

2. Pathoanatomy

a. A calcaneovalgus foot in newborns is a soft-tissue contracture problem.

b. No dislocation or bony deformity of the foot exists.

3. Evaluation

a. Should be passively correctable to neutral

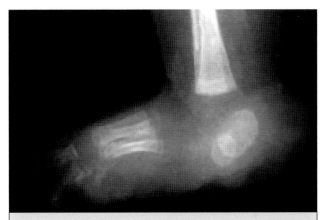

Figure 10   Lateral forced plantar flexion view of foot with congenital vertical talus. The first metatarsal (and unossified navicular) remain dorsally dislocated relative to the talus. *(Reproduced from Sullivan JA: Pediatric flatfoot: Evaluation and management.* J Am Acad Orthop Surg *1999;7:44-53.)*

b. Posteromedial bow of the tibia may also be present. In fact, an isolated posteromedial tibial bow is often confused with a calcaneovalgus foot.

4. Treatment

a. Typically, the deformity will resolve without intervention.

b. Stretching may expedite the resolution of the deformity.

D. Pes cavus (cavus foot)

1. Overview

a. A cavus foot has an elevated longitudinal arch from medial forefoot equinus or, less frequently, from excessive calcaneal dorsiflexion.

b. Two thirds of patients with a cavus foot have a neurologic problem (most commonly Charcot-Marie-Tooth disease).

2. Pathoanatomy

a. The primary structural problem is forefoot plantar flexion, particularly of the first ray.

b. For the lateral half of the foot to be in contact with the ground, the hindfoot must deviate into varus (**Figure 11**).

c. First ray plantar flexion may result from a weak tibialis anterior relative to the peroneus longus, but it is more commonly due to intrinsic weakness and contracture.

d. Over time, the plantar fascia contracts and the hindfoot varus deformity becomes more rigid.

3. Evaluation

a. Patients may report instability (ankle sprains).

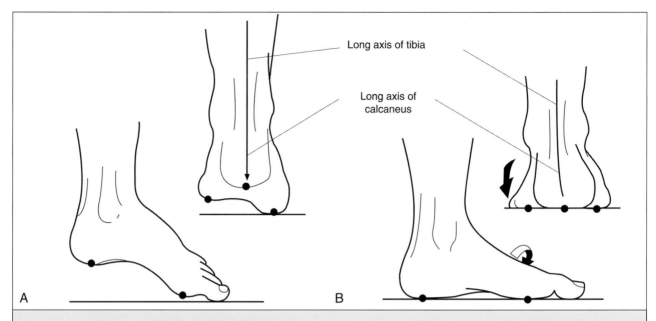

Figure 11   Tripod effect in a cavus foot. **A,** Posterior and lateral views of a cavus foot in non–weight-bearing position. The long axes of the tibia and the calcaneus are parallel and the first metatarsal is pronated. Dots indicate the three major weight-bearing plantar areas (heel and first and fifth metatarsals). **B,** Posterior and lateral views of a cavus foot in weight-bearing position. The long axes of the tibia and the calcaneus are not parallel. With weight bearing, a rigid equinus forefoot deformity forces the flexible hindfoot into varus. This is the tripod effect. *(Adapted with permission from Paulos L, Coleman SS, Samuelson KM: Pes cavovarus: Review of a surgical approach using selective soft-tissue procedures.* J Bone Joint Surg Am *1980;62:942-953.)*

b. A neurologic examination and family history are essential.

   i. Unilateral involvement suggests a focal diagnosis (eg, spinal cord anomaly or nerve injury).

   ii. Bilateral involvement and a positive family history are common with Charcot-Marie-Tooth disease. Despite bilateral involvement, asymmetry may be seen in children with Charcot-Marie-Tooth.

c. Hindfoot flexibility is assessed by placing a 1-inch block under the lateral border of the foot (Coleman block test).

d. Radiographs

   i. The long axis of the talus will intersect the long axis of the first metatarsal dorsally on the lateral view of the foot (normally collinear).

   ii. MRI of the spine is indicated with unilateral involvement.

4. Treatment

   a. Joint-sparing procedures are preferred whenever possible.

   b. A key to surgical decision making is the flexibility of the hindfoot. Some general guidelines exist (**Table 10**).

c. Percutaneous plantar fascia release is insufficient to correct a cavus foot. At minimum, an open release and soft tissue rebalancing are needed.

d. Achilles tendon lengthening should not be performed concomitantly with plantar fasciotomy. An intact Achilles tendon provides the resistance necessary to stretch the contracted plantar tissues and correct the cavus deformity.

E. Pes planovalgus (flexible flatfoot)

   1. Overview

   a. Flexible flatfoot is a physiologic variation of normal.

   b. It is defined by a decreased longitudinal arch and a valgus hindfoot during weight bearing.

   c. It is rarely symptomatic, is common in childhood, and resolves spontaneously in most cases.

   d. Flexible flatfoot is present in 20% to 25% of adults.

   2. Pathoanatomy

   a. Generalized ligamentous laxity is common.

   b. Approximately one fourth of flexible flatfeet have a contracture of the gastrocnemius-soleus complex. Only these cases are associated with disability.

Table 10		
Treatment of Pes Cavus		
Severity of Deformity	**Examination and History**	**Corrective Treatment**
Mild	Flexible, painless	Heel cord stretching, eversion/dorsiflexion strengthening program
Mild	Progressive or symptomatic	Plantar release ± peroneus longus to brevis transfer
	Varus due to peroneal weakness	Add anterior and/or posterior tibial tendon transfer to the peroneals
Moderate	Rigid medial cavus	Dorsiflexion osteotomy of either first metatarsal or cuneiform
	Rigid medial and lateral cavus	Dorsiflexion osteotomies of the cuboid and cuneiforms
	Rigid hindfoot varus	Closing/sliding calcaneal osteotomy
	Clawing of hallux	Add EHL transfer to first metatarsal (Jones)
Severe	Not correctable to plantigrade with other procedures	Triple arthrodesis is rarely needed and should be avoided whenever possible

EHL = extensor hallucis longus

3. Evaluation

   a. An arch should be evident when toe-standing, dorsiflexing the hallux, or not weight bearing.

   b. Subtalar motion should be full and painless.

   c. On a lateral radiograph, the talus is plantar flexed relative to the first metatarsal (Meary angle has a plantar apex).

   d. Apparent hindfoot valgus may actually be due to ankle valgus (particularly in children with myelodysplasia). If there is any suspicion of ankle valgus, ankle radiographs should be obtained.

4. Classification and differential diagnosis

   a. Flatfoot should be categorized into three groups

      i. Flexible flatfoot without tight heel cord

      ii. Flexible flatfoot with tight heel cord

      iii. Rigid flatfoot

   b. The differential of flatfoot includes tarsal coalition, congenital vertical talus, and accessory navicular.

5. Treatment

   a. No treatment is indicated for asymptomatic patients.

   b. Nonsurgical

      i. Shoes or orthoses do not promote arch development.

      ii. Use of athletic shoes with arch and heel support can help relieve pain.

      iii. The University of California Biomechanics Lab (UCBL) orthosis is a rigid orthotic insert designed to support the arch and control the hindfoot. The rigid material may be poorly tolerated. A soft molded insert is an alternative but may be inadequate to control hindfoot valgus.

      iv. Stretching exercises are recommended if the patient is symptomatic and an Achilles contracture is present.

   c. Surgical

      i. Surgery is reserved for rare cases in which pain is recalcitrant to nonsurgical treatment.

      ii. A calcaneal neck lengthening with soft-tissue balancing is the treatment of choice. It corrects deformity while preserving motion and growth. Arthrodesis and arthroeisis are rarely, if ever, indicated.

F. Metatarsus adductus

   1. Overview

      a. Metatarsus adductus is a medial deviation of the forefoot with normal alignment of the hindfoot.

      b. It occurs in up to 12% of newborns.

   2. Pathoanatomy—Intrauterine positioning of the foot is thought to be one possible cause.

3: Pediatrics

3. Evaluation

   a. The foot has a kidney-bean shape (convex lateral border) and the hindfoot is in a neutral position.

   b. Assess the amount of active correction by tickling the foot.

4. Classification—Bleck graded the severity of the metatarsus adductus based on flexibility. Another classification uses the heel bisector line.

5. Differential diagnosis—The differential diagnosis includes clubfoot, skewfoot (severe forefoot adductus combined with hindfoot valgus), and atavistic great toe (congenital hallux varus).

6. Prognosis and treatment

   a. Nonsurgical

      i. Spontaneous resolution of metatarsus adductus occurs in 90% of children by age 4 years.

      ii. Passive stretching is recommended for mild deformity but does not improve final outcome.

      iii. Serial casting is useful in children between 6 and 12 months of age with moderate deformity.

   b. Surgical

      i. Surgery is indicated only in older children (older than 7 years) with severe residual deformity that produces problems with shoe wear and pain.

      ii. A medial column lengthening (opening wedge osteotomy of cuneiform) and lateral column shortening (closing wedge of the cuboid) produces good results with fewer complications than historical techniques.

      vi. If the child has a skewfoot (hindfoot valgus in addition to the metatarsus adductus), then hindfoot osteotomy is required in addition to the midfoot osteotomy(ies).

G. Tarsal coalition

1. Overview (epidemiology)

   a. Tarsal coalition is an osseous, cartilaginous, or fibrous connection between bones of the hindfoot and midfoot.

   b. It occurs in 1% to 6% of the population.

   c. Most tarsal coalitions are asymptomatic.

   d. 10% to 20% of patients with tarsal coalitions have two coalitions. 50% are bilateral.

   e. Calcaneonavicular coalitions are the most common, followed by talocalcaneal coalitions.

Table 11

Radiographic Evaluation of Tarsal Coalitions

Type of Coalition	Radiographic View	Findings Suggestive of Coalition
Calcaneonavicular	Oblique	Elongated dorsal process of calcaneus (anteater's nose)
Talocalcaneal	Lateral	C-shaped line that extends from talar dome to sustentaculum tali (C sign of Lefleur)
	CT scan	Absent or vertically oriented middle facet

2. Pathoanatomy

   a. The onset of symptoms usually coincides with the transition of a cartilaginous coalition to bone during late childhood and early adolescence.

      i. Age 8 to 12 years for calcaneonavicular coalitions

      ii. Age 12 to 15 years for talocalcaneal coalitions

   b. Coalitions of the talus to the calcaneus can occur at any of the three facets. A middle facet coalition is most common.

3. Evaluation

   a. Pain and limited subtalar motion are the hallmarks of a tarsal coalition.

      i. Pain is typically in the tarsal sinus or the longitudinal arch.

      ii. Patients have difficulty with uneven ground and frequent ankle sprains.

   b. Radiographs

      i. Plain radiographs should include AP, lateral oblique, and Harris views (**Table 11 and Figure 12**).

      ii. Dorsal talar beaking is a nonspecific finding associated with a variety of coalitions. It is not a sign of degenerative arthrosis.

      iii. Harris axial radiographs have a high false-positive rate for tarsal coalition. If the view is slightly oblique to the posterior or middle facet, it will appear as if a coalition is present when it is not.

      iv. A CT scan helps delineate the coalition and will clarify whether the child has multiple coalitions in the foot.

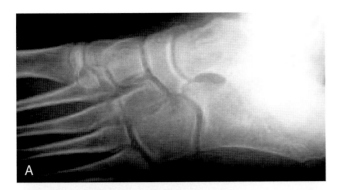

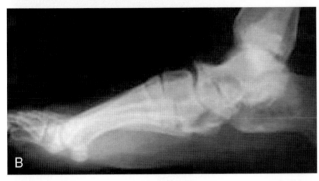

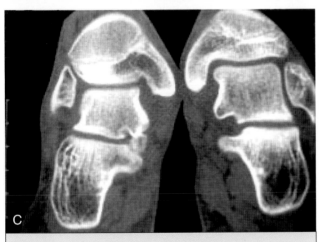

Figure 12 Images demonstrating calcaneonavicular and talocalcaneal coalitions. **A,** This 45° oblique view demonstrates a calcaneonavicular coalition. **B,** Non–weight-bearing lateral radiograph depicts a talocalcaneal coalition. There is beaking of the talus and loss of definition of the subtalar joint space. **C,** CT scan illustrates a talocalcaneal coalition in the left foot as viewed from the posterior. *(Reproduced from Sullivan JA: Pediatric flatfoot: Evaluation and management.* J Am Acad Orthop Surg *1999;7:44-53.)*

4. Associated syndromes—Multiple coalitions are common with fibular deficiency and with Apert syndrome.

5. Treatment

   a. No treatment is indicated for asymptomatic coalitions.

b. Nonsurgical

   i. Management includes NSAIDs, activity modification, shoe orthoses, and cast immobilization.

   ii. Not all symptomatic coalitions require surgery. 30% percent of patients remain pain free after nonsurgical cast immobilization.

c. Surgical

   i. A preoperative CT scan is helpful to rule out multiple coalitions and assess bar size.

   ii. Calcaneonavicular coalition

      (a) Coalition resection and interposition of extensor digitorum brevis or fat is effective in most cases.

      (b) Contraindications to resection are advanced degenerative changes in adjacent joints or multiple coalitions.

   iii. Talocalcaneal coalition

      (a) Resection has traditionally been limited to small coalitions (<50% of middle facet) with minimal hindfoot valgus (<20°) and no degenerative arthrosis. More recent studies call these recommendations into question.

      (b) Adequate excision typically involves complete excision of sustentaculum tali.

      (c) If severe valgus is present at the time of coalition excision, a calcaneal osteotomy (either a calcaneal neck lengthening or medial slide) generally improves clinical outcome and decreases the risk of recurrent symptoms.

   iv. A triple arthrodesis or limited subtalar arthrodesis may be indicated when there is degenerative arthrosis, multiple coalitions, or coalition resection fails to relieve symptoms.

H. Accessory navicular

   1. Overview

      a. Accessory navicular is an enlargement of the plantar medial aspect of the navicular.

      b. The extra bone may be completely separate or in continuity with the true navicular.

      c. It occurs in up to 12% of the population, with most being asymptomatic.

   2. Pathoanatomy

      a. The accessory navicular usually does not ossify until after age 8 years. The ossicle will often fuse to the true navicular.

3: Pediatrics

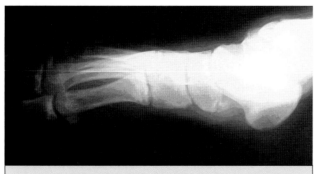

Figure 13   External oblique view of foot with accessory navicular.

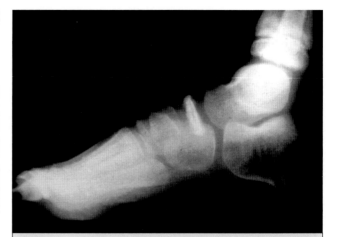

Figure 14   Lateral radiograph of the foot of a child with Köhler bone disease. Note the sclerosis and flattening of the navicular bone. *(Reproduced from Olney BW: Conditions of the foot, in Abel MF (ed): Orthopaedic Knowledge Update: Pediatrics 3. Rosemont, IL, American Academy of Orthopaedic Surgeons, 2006, p 239.)*

   b. Pain is secondary to repeated microfracture or inflammatory response.

3. Evaluation

   a. A firm and tender prominence on the plantar medial midfoot (distal to the talar head)

   b. Often the ossicle is evident on weight-bearing AP radiographs. An external oblique view (not the commonly used internal oblique) may show the accessory navicular best (**Figure 13**).

4. Treatment

   a. Doughnut-shaped pads and orthotic devices that reduce direct pressure on the prominence are often effective.

   b. A short-leg cast may also be effective.

   c. Simple excision of the ossicle and any navicular prominence via a tendon-splitting approach (without tendon advancement) has been shown to be effective 90% of the time.

I. Köhler bone disease

   1. Overview

      a. Köhler bone disease is a self-limiting painful condition of the navicular in young children.

      b. It occurs more commonly in boys than girls (4:1) and is frequently bilateral.

   2. Pathoanatomy—The navicular is the last tarsal bone to ossify. It is more susceptible to direct mechanical compression injury.

   3. Evaluation

      a. Children with Köhler bone disease typically walk with an antalgic gait on the lateral border of the foot.

      b. Radiographs confirm the diagnosis with flattening, sclerosis, and fragmentation of the navicular (**Figure 14**).

      c. Irregular ossification of the navicular is common during early ossification. The diagnosis of

Köhler bone disease requires clinical findings as well.

   4. Prognosis and treatment

      a. Symptoms resolve spontaneously within 6 to 15 months.

      b. The navicular reconstitutes over 6 to 48 months.

      c. No residual deformity or disability occurs in adulthood.

      d. Casting for 4 to 8 weeks with a short-leg walking cast will decrease the duration of symptoms.

      e. Surgery is never indicated.

J. Overlapping fifth toe

   1. A dorsal adduction deformity of the fifth toe

   2. It is typically familial and bilateral.

   3. The extensor digitorum longus (EDL) tendon is contracted.

   4. Treatment indicated when pain or shoe-wear problems arise. The Butler procedure involves a double racket-handle incision and release of the EDL.

K. Curly toes

   1. A malrotation and flexion deformity of one or more toes

   2. A contracture of the flexor digitorum longus (FDL) or flexor digitorum brevis (FDB) is the most common cause.

3. Treatment involves FDL tenotomy around age 3 to 4 years.

L. Polydactyly

1. Polydactyly occurs in 1 in 500 births.

2. Postaxial polydactyly is most common and has an autosomal dominant inheritance pattern in some families.

3. Surgery is indicated to facilitate shoe wear and prevent toe deformities.

Top Testing Facts

Limb-Length Discrepancy

1. Estimates of the yearly growth contribution of the distal femur and proximal tibia physes (eg, 10 mm/year for distal femur) are valid for only the last 4 years of growth.

2. Limb equalization procedures must take into account the final projected LLD, not the LLD present at the time of surgery. If the current LLD is used, the LLD will be undercorrected.

3. Undercorrection of an LLD associated with paralysis facilitates the foot clearing the floor during the swing phase of gait and is especially important if the patient walks with a brace in which the knee is locked in extension.

4. A proximal fibular epiphysiodesis should be included with proximal tibial epiphysiodesis if more than 2 to 3 years of growth remain.

Tibia Vara (Blount Disease)

1. Beware of internal tibial torsion with tibia vara. The patella should be pointed directly anterior on all weight-bearing lower extremity radiographs.

2. To avoid undercorrection, fix the distal fragment in slight valgus, lateral translation, and external rotation.

3. The risk of postoperative compartment syndrome is decreased if an anterior compartment fasciotomy is performed at the time of surgery.

4. Confirm the new mechanical alignment on the surgical table with bovie cord. A cord held directly over the center of the femoral head and ankle should pass over the lateral tibial plateau.

5. One or two pins and a cast is all the fixation necessary for infantile cases. Plate or external fixation is necessary for fixation in adolescent Blount disease.

6. Recurrence is less when the osteotomy is done before age 4 years.

Tibial Bowing

1. Anterolateral bowing is typical of congenital pseudarthrosis of the tibia and is often associated with neurofibromatosis.

2. Posteromedial bowing is often associated with development of a limb-length discrepancy.

Genu Valgum

1. Unilateral genu valgum following a Cozen fracture almost always resolves spontaneously.

2. Physeal tethers must be placed extraperiostally to avoid unintended arrest.

3. Physeal tethers (staples or eight-plate systems) must be placed in the midcoronal plane to prevent recurvatum or procurvatum deformities.

4. Nomograms are available to appropriately time a permanent hemiepiphysiodesis (or predict the duration necessary for correction with a temporary physeal tethering).

Rotational Deformities

1. Brace-dependent ambulators (eg, patients with cerebral palsy or myelodysplasia) tolerate less tibial torsion because the compensatory mechanisms (knee and subtalar joint motion) are unavailable.

2. Lever-arm dysfunction in children with neuromuscular disorders is the reason osteotomies are frequently indicated in such children.

3. Estimate anteversion clinically by measuring the degree of internal rotation of the hip necessary to make the greater trochanter maximally prominent laterally (trochanteric prominence angle test).

4. Amount of rotation to correct excess anteversion = (prone internal rotation – prone external rotation)/2.

5. If an isolated distal tibial osteotomy is performed, rotation of >30° generally results in translation of the distal fragment. This is of no clinical consequence and will remodel rapidly in growing children.

Limb Deficiencies

1. Optimal age range to perform amputation for limb deficiency is age 10 months to 2 years.

2. Avoid early amputation if severe upper extremity deformities may require the use of the feet for activities of daily living.

3. The Syme amputation is simple and accommodates a tapered prosthesis at the ankle for optimal cosmesis.

4. The Boyd amputation prevents heel pad migration, aids prosthesis suspension, and may provide better end bearing; however, it also may limit prosthetic foot options because of excessive length.

5. In tibial deficiency, a good early radiographic clue to the absence of the proximal tibia is a small and minimally ossified distal femoral epiphysis.

6. The Brown procedure has a high failure rate. In contrast, a tibiofibular synostosis is effective at extending a short proximal tibia segment.

3: Pediatrics

Top Testing Facts (cont.)

Foot Problems

1. The sequence of deformity correction with the Ponseti technique is cavus, adductus, varus, equinus (CAVE).

2. The most common cause of a late failure after initial clubfoot correction with Ponseti casts is poor compliance with the Denis-Brown brace.

3. Most clubfeet treated with the Ponseti method (up to 90%) require percutaneous Achilles tenotomy at the time the final cast is applied.

4. Anterior tibial tendon transfer (split or whole transfer) is needed in one third to one half of clubfeet treated with the Ponseti method.

5. Percutaneous plantar fascia release is insufficient to correct a cavus foot.

6. Congenital vertical talus is associated with neuromuscular disease and/or genetic syndromes in up to 50% of children.

7. The diagnostic radiographic view for congenital vertical talus is the forced plantar flexion lateral view.

8. Unless proven otherwise, a child with pes cavus should be assumed to have an underlying neurologic condition causing the deformity. Charcot-Marie-Tooth disease is the most common etiology of pes cavus in children.

9. Simultaneous plantar fascia release should be avoided with an Achilles tendon lengthening. An intact Achilles tendon provides the resistance necessary to stretch the divided plantar tissues.

10. Preoperative CT assessment is helpful before tarsal coalition excision because multiple coalitions are present in 10% to 20% of feet with tarsal coalition. A calcaneonavicular coalition is most common.

11. Apparent hindfoot valgus may actually be the result of ankle valgus. If there is any suspicion of ankle valgus, radiographic views of the ankle should be obtained.

12. Severe forefoot adductus combined with hindfoot valgus is a condition known as skewfoot. Although rare, it is important to recognize because correction requires both hindfoot and midfoot osteotomies.

13. An iatrogenic skewfoot deformity is possible when correcting adductus with serial casts. The hindfoot must be maintained in a neutral or slight varus position.

14. Harris axial radiographs have a high false-positive rate for tarsal coalition. If the view is slightly oblique to the posterior or middle facet, it will appear as if a coalition is present when it is not.

15. Beware of interpreting irregular ossification of the navicular as indicative of Köhler bone disease. Irregular ossification is common during early ossification. Clinical findings are always present with Köhler bone disease.

Bibliography

Bowen JR, Leahey JL, Zhang ZH, MacEwen GD: Partial epiphysiodesis at the knee to correct angular deformity. *Clin Orthop Relat Res* 1985;198:184-190.

Brooks WC, Gross RH: Genu varum in children: Diagnosis and treatment. *J Am Acad Orthop Surg* 1995;3:326-335.

Crawford AH, Schorry EK: Neurofibromatosis in children: The role of the orthopaedist. *J Am Acad Orthop Surg* 1999;7:217-230.

Herzenberg JE, Nogueira MP: Idiopathic clubfoot, in Abel MF (ed): *Orthopaedic Knowledge Update: Pediatrics 3*. Rosemont, IL, American Academy of Orthopaedic Surgeons, 2006, pp 227-233.

Krajbich JI: Lower-limb deficiencies and amputations in children. *J Am Acad Orthop Surg* 1998;6:358-367.

Lincoln TL, Suen PW: Common rotational variations in children. *J Am Acad Orthop Surg* 2003;11:312-320.

Olney BW: Conditions of the foot, in Abel MF (ed): *Orthopaedic Knowledge Update: Pediatrics 3*. Rosemont, IL, American Academy of Orthopaedic Surgeons, 2006, pp 235-245.

Romness MJ: Limb-length discrepancy and lower limb deformity, in Abel MF (ed): *Orthopaedic Knowledge Update: Pediatrics 3*. Rosemont, IL, American Academy of Orthopaedic Surgeons, 2006, pp 199-214.

Schwend RM, Drennan JC: Cavus foot deformity in children. *J Am Acad Orthop Surg* 2003;11:201-211.

Staheli LT: Motor development in orthopaedics, in Abel MF (ed): *Orthopaedic Knowledge Update: Pediatrics 3*. Rosemont, IL, American Academy of Orthopaedic Surgeons, 2006, pp 3-12.

Sullivan JA: Pediatric flatfoot: Evaluation and management. *J Am Acad Orthop Surg* 1999;7:44-53.

Chapter 34
Normal and Abnormal Growth

Samantha A. Spencer, MD

I. Normal Growth

A. Anatomy

1. Long-bone growth/fracture healing is endochondral.

   a. Vessel invades cartilage in the primary ossification center and growth occurs longitudinally at either end as chondrocytes proliferate, hypertrophy, die, and are replaced by calcified matrix and osteoblasts.

   b. Widening of the bone is achieved by osteoblasts differentiating from stem cells from the ring of Lacroix/node of Ranvier.

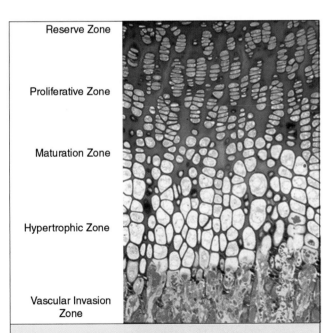

Figure 1   Photomicrograph showing the structure and zones of the growth plate, x220. *(Adapted with permission from Farnum CE, Nixon A, Lee AO, Kwan DT, Belanger L, Wilsman NJ: Quantitative three-dimensional analysis of chondrocytic kinetic responses to short-term stapling of the rat proximal tibial growth plate. Cells Tissues Organs 2000;167:247-258.)*

2. Flat bone growth/distraction osteogenesis is intramembranous.

   a. The skull is formed by neural crest cells invading a connective tissue scaffold.

   b. The clavicle has both intramembranous and endochondral ossification.

   c. The scapula has seven ossification centers.

B. Physiology

1. An endochondral growth plate is divided into four main zones (**Figure 1**).

   a. Reserve zone—Gaucher disease and other storage diseases affect this zone.

   b. Proliferative zone—Achondroplasia and spondyloepiphyseal dysplasia (SED) affect this zone.

   c. Hypertrophic zone—Fractures occur in this zone.

   d. Zone of calcification—Type X collagen is present, but type II collagen is still predominant.

2. Calcifying fracture callus has some type IV collagen.

II. Skeletal Dysplasias

A. Achondroplasia (**Table 1**)

1. Overview

   a. Short-limbed dwarfism with abnormal facial features

   b. The most common skeletal dysplasia

   c. Autosomal dominant, but 90% are new mutations

2. Pathoanatomy

   a. Mutation affects a single protein in fibroblast growth factor receptor-3 (*FGFR-3*) gene, changing glycine to arginine at position 380.

Table 1

Skeletal Dysplasias: Genetics and Features

Name	Genetics	Features
Achondroplasia	*FGFR-3*; autosomal dominant; 90% sporadic mutations; affects proliferative zone of physis	Rhizomelic shortening with normal trunk, frontal bossing, button nose, trident hands (cannot approximate long and ring fingers), thoracolumbar kyphosis (usually resolves with sitting), lumbar stenosis and lordosis, radial head subluxations, champagne glass pelvic outlet, genu varum
Hypochondroplasia	*FGFR-3* in a different area than achondroplasia; autosomal dominant	Milder than achondroplasia; short stature, lumbar stenosis, genu varum
Thantophoric dysplasia	*FGFR-3*	Rhizomelic shortening, platyspondyly, protuberant abdomen, small thoracic cavity Death by age 2 years
SED congenita	Type II collagen mutation in *COL2A1* gene; autosomal dominant but usually sporadic mutation; affects proliferative zone of physis	Short stature, trunk, and limbs, abnormal epiphyses including spine, atlantoaxial instability/odontoid hypoplasia, coxa vara and DDH, genu valgum, early OA, retinal detachment/myopia, sensorineural hearing loss
SED tarda	Unidentified mutation likely in type II collagen, X-linked recessive	Late onset (age 8 to 10 years), premature OA, associated with DDH but not lower extremity bowing
Kniest dysplasia	Type II collagen mutation in *COL2A1* gene, autosomal dominant	Joint contractures (treat with early physical therapy), kyphosis/scoliosis, dumbbell-shaped femurs, respiratory problems, cleft palate, retinal detachment/myopia, otitis media/hearing loss, early OA
Cleidocranial dyplasia	Defect in CBFA-1, a transcription factor that activates osteoblast differentiation; autosomal dominant; affects intramembranous ossification	Aplasia/hypoplasia of clavicles (no need to treat), delayed skull suture closure, frontal bossing, coxa vara (osteotomy if neck-shaft angle <100°), delayed ossification pubis, genu valgum, shortened middle phalanges of third through fifth fingers
Nail-patella syndrome (osteoonychodysplasia)	Mutation in LIM homeobox transcription factor 1-β also expressed in eyes/kidneys; autosomal dominant	Aplasia/hypoplasia of the patella and condyles, dysplastic nails, iliac horns, posterior dislocation of the radial head; 30% will get renal failure and glaucoma as adults
Diastrophic dysplasia	Mutation in sulfate transporter gene affects proteoglycan sulfate groups in cartilage. Autosomal recessive. 1 in 70 mutated sulfate transporter gene in Finland; very rare elsewhere.	Short stature; rhizomelic shortening, cervical kyphosis, kyphoscoliosis, hitchhiker thumbs, cauliflower ears, rigid clubfeet, skewfoot, severe OA, joint contractures
Mucopolysaccharidoses	All defects in enzymes that degrade glycosaminoglycans in lysosomes. The incomplete degradation products accumulate in various organs and cause dysfunction. All autosomal recessive except Hunter syndrome (X-linked recessive).	Visceromegaly, corneal clouding, cardiac disease, deafness, short stature, mental retardation (except Morquio syndrome, which has normal intelligence). C1-C2 instability is common, as is hip dysplasia and abnormal epiphyses. Hurler syndrome is the most severe; bone marrow transplant improves life expectancy but does not alter orthopaedic manifestations.
Metaphyseal dysplasia: Schmid type	Type X collagen mutation in *COL10A1* gene; autosomal dominant; affects proliferative/hypertrophic zones	Milder; coxa vara, genu varum
Metaphyseal dyplasia: Jansen type	Mutation in parathyroid hormone receptor (affects parathyroid hormone-related protein), which regulates chondrocyte differentiation; affects proliferative/hypertrophic zones; autosomal dominant	Wide eyes, squatting stance, hypercalcemia, bulbous metaphyseal expansion of long bones and extremity malalignment

3: Pediatrics

Table 1

Skeletal Dysplasias: Genetics and Features (continued)

Name	Genetics	Features
Metaphyseal dysplasia: McKusick type	Mutation in *RMRP* gene (ribosomal nucleic acid component of mitochondrial ribosomal nucleic acid processing endoribonuclease); affects proliferative/hypertrophic zones	C1-C2 instability, hypoplasia of cartilage, small-diameter "fine" hair, intestinal malabsorbtion and megacolon, increased risk of viral infections and malignancies (immune dysfunction), ligamentous laxity, pectus abnormalities, genu varum and ankle deformities due to fibular overgrowth
Pseudoachondroplasia	Mutation in *COMP* on chromosome 19, which is an extracellular matrix glycoprotein in cartilage; autosomal dominant	C1-C2 instability due to odontoid hypoplasia, normal facies, metaphyseal flaring, delayed epiphyses, lower extremity malalignment, DDH, scoliosis, early OA
MED	Mutations in *COMP*, *COL9A2*, or *COL9A3* genes (collagen IX, which is a linker for collagen II in cartilage); autosomal dominant	Short stature, epiphyseal dysplasia, genu valgum, hip osteonecrosis and dysplasia, early OA. Spine not involved. Short metacarpals/metatarsals, double-layer patella.
Ellis-van Creveld (EVC) syndrome/ chondroectodermal dysplasia	Mutation in the *EVC* gene; autosomal recessive	Acromesomelic shortening (distal and middle limb segments), postaxial polydactyly, genu valgum, dysplastic nails/teeth, medial iliac spikes, fused capitate/hamate, 60% congenital heart disease
Diaphyseal dysplasia (also known as Camurati-Engelmann syndrome)	Autosomal dominant	Symmetric cortical thickening of long bones most commonly seen in tibia, femur, humerus. Treat with NSAIDs, watch for limb-length discrepancy.
Leri-Weil dyschondrosteosis	*SHOX* gene tip of sex chromosome; autosomal dominant	Mild short stature, mesomelic shortening, Madelung deformity
Menke syndrome and occipital horn syndrome	Both are copper transporter defects; Menke syndrome is X-linked recessive	Menke syndrome: kinky hair Occipital horn syndrome: bony projections from the occiput

OA = osteoarthritis, DDH = developmental dysplasia of the hip, MED = multiple epiphyseal dysplasia

b. Result is growth retardation of the proliferative zone of the growth plate, resulting in short limbs.

c. The growth plates with the most growth (proximal humerus/distal femur) are most affected, resulting in rhizomelic (proximal more than distal) short stature.

3. Evaluation

a. Features include rhizomelic shortening with a normal trunk, frontal bossing, button nose, trident hands (cannot approximate middle and ring fingers), thoracolumbar kyphosis (usually resolves with ambulation), lumbar stenosis with lordosis and short pedicles, posterior radial head dislocation, "champagne glass" pelvic outlet, and genu varum (**Figure 2**).

b. Foramen magnum stenosis and upper cervical stenosis may be present and cause central apnea and weakness in the first few years of life.

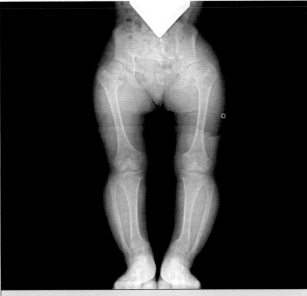

Figure 2 Weight-bearing hip-to-ankle AP radiograph of a child with achondroplasia demonstrates the classic lower extremity features of a champagne glass pelvic outlet and genu varum.

3: Pediatrics

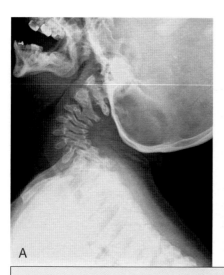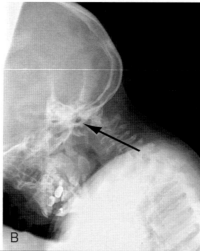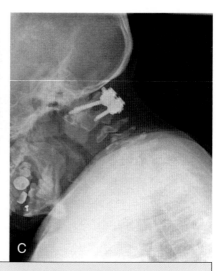

Figure 3   Radiographs of the cervical spine of a patient with Hurler syndrome who had cervical instability that was corrected surgically. **A,** Extension lateral view demonstrates cervical instability. **B,** Flexion lateral view shows the widened atlanto-dens interval (arrow). **C,** Postoperative flexion lateral view shows a stable atlanto-dens interval.

4. Treatment

   a. Nonsurgical treatment is usual for the thoracolumbar kyphosis present early on. Avoidance of unsupported sitting may help prevent it.

   b. Genu varum is treated with osteotomies if symptomatic.

   c. Foramen magnum/upper cervical stenosis may require urgent decompression if cord compression is present; this area does grow bigger in later life.

   d. The main issue in adult life is lumbar stenosis requiring decompression and/or fusion.

   e. Limb lengthening is controversial and does not treat the other dysmorphic features; if lower limb lengthening is done, humeral lengthening is indicated too.

   f. Growth hormone is not effective at increasing stature.

B. Pseudoachondroplasia (**Table 1**)

   1. Overview

      a. Short-limbed rhizomelic dwarfism with normal facial features

      b. Normal development up to age 2 years

   2. Pathoanatomy

      a. Autosomal dominant

      b. Mutation is in cartilage oligomeric matrix protein (*COMP*) on chromosome 19.

      c. Epiphyses are delayed and abnormal, metaphyseal flaring is present, and early onset osteoarthritis (OA) is common.

3. Evaluation

   a. Cervical instability is common and must be looked for (**Figure 3,** *A* **and** *B*).

   b. Lower extremity bowing may be valgus, varus, or windswept.

   c. Joints may be hyperlax in early life but later develop flexion contractures and early OA.

   d. Platyspondyly is always present, but spinal stenosis is not present.

4. Treatment

   a. Cervical instability should be stabilized (**Figure 3,** *C*).

   b. Symptomatic limb bowing should be surgically corrected, but recurrence is common and OA progressive.

C. Diastrophic dysplasia (**Table 1**)

   1. Overview—Short-limbed dwarfism apparent from birth. Other common findings include cleft palate and hitchhiker thumbs (**Figure 4**).

   2. Pathoanatomy

      a. Autosomal recessive

      b. Mutation in sulfate transport protein that primarily affects cartilage matrix. Present in 1 in 70 Finnish citizens.

   3. Evaluation

      a. Cleft palate is present in 60%.

      b. Cauliflower ears are present in 80% and develop after birth from cystic swellings in the ear cartilage (**Figure 5,** *A*).

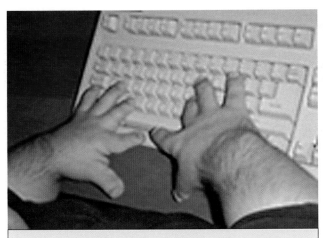

Figure 4 Photograph of the hands of a child with diastrophic dysplasia. Note the hitchhiker thumbs. *(Courtesy of Ms. Vita Gagne, from the 2004 Diastrophic Dysplasia booklet.)*

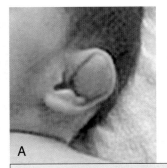 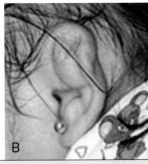

Figure 5 Clinical photographs of the ear of a child with diastrophic dysplasia. **A,** The classic cauliflower ear appearance is observed in the neonate. **B,** The same ear several years later, after early treatment with compressive bandages. *(Courtesy of Ms. Vita Gagne, from the 2004 Diastrophic Dysplasia booklet.)*

   c. Cervical kyphosis and thoracolumbar scoliosis are often present.

   d. Joint contractures (hip flexion, genu valgum with dislocated patellae) and rigid clubfeet or skewfeet are often present.

  4. Treatment

   a. Surgery is indicated for progressive spinal deformity or cord compromise; note that cervical kyphosis often resolves spontaneously.

   b. Surgery is also indicated for progressive, symptomatic lower extremity deformity; recurrence is common.

   c. Compressive wrapping is used for cystic swelling of the ears (**Figure 5,** *B*).

D. Cleidocranial dysostosis (**Table 1**)

  1. Overview—Proportionate dwarfism characterized by mildly short stature, a broad forehead, and absent clavicles.

  2. Pathoanatomy

   a. Autosomal dominant

   b. Defect in core-binding factor alpha 1 (CBFA-1), which is a transcription factor for osteocalcin

   c. Affects intramembranous ossification: skull, clavicles, pelvis

  3. Evaluation

   a. Delayed skull suture closure with frontal bossing is present, and delayed eruption of the permanent teeth is found.

   b. Aplasia of the clavicles with ability to appose the shoulders in front of the chest is present.

   c. Symphysis pubis is widened.

   d. Coxa vara may be present.

   e. Shortening of the middle phalanges of the long, ring, and little fingers is seen.

  4. Treatment

   a. Progressive and/or symptomatic coxa vara is treated with intertrochanteric osteotomy.

   b. The other features are treated supportively.

E. Mucopolysaccharidoses (**Table 2**)

  1. Overview—All patients are short statured; additional features vary but often include corneal clouding, enlarged skull, bullet-shaped phalanges, mental retardation, visceromegaly, cervical instability, genu valgum, and developmental dysplasia of the hip (DDH) that is later in onset.

  2. Pathoanatomy

   a. Mucopolysaccharidoses are lysosomal storage diseases that result in the intracellular accumulation of mucopolysaccharides in multiple organs.

   b. All are autosomal recessive except Hunter syndrome type II, which is X-linked recessive.

  3. Evaluation

   a. Urine test to see which mucopolysaccharide breakdown products are present

   b. Testing enzyme activity in skin fibroblast culture

   c. Chorionic villous sampling

  4. Treatment

   a. Hurler syndrome is now treated with a bone marrow transplant in the first year of life; intelligence is normal in some affected individu-

Table 2		
Mucopolysaccharidoses Subtypes		
Subtype	**Cause**	**Prognosis**
Type I H (Hurler syndrome) Type I HS (Hurler-Scheie syndrome) Type I S (Scheie syndrome)	Alpha-L-iduronidase deficiency	Type I H: death in first decade of life Type I HS: death in third decade of life Type I S: good survival
Type II (Hunter syndrome)	Sulpho-iduronate-sulphatase deficiency	Death in second decade of life
Type III (Sanfilippo syndrome)	Multiple enzyme deficiency	Death in second decade of life
Type IV (Morquio syndrome)	Type A (galactosamine-6-sulfate-sulphatase deficiency) Type B (beta-galactosidase deficiency)	More severe involvement in patients with type IV A than in those with type IV B; survival into adulthood is possible
Type VI (Maroteaux-Lamy syndrome)	Arylsulphatase B deficiency	Poor survival with severe form
Type VII (Sly syndrome)	Beta-glycuronidase deficiency	Poor survival

(Reproduced from Mackenzie WG, Ballock RT: Genetic diseases and skeletal dysplasias, in Vaccaro AR (ed): Orthopaedic Knowledge Update 8. Rosemont, IL American Academy of Orthopaedic Surgeons, 2005, pp 663-675.)

als, but short stature and orthopaedic deformities are always present.

b. Surgery is indicated for cervical instability (often atlantoaxial—assess with dynamic MRI) and progressive lower extremity deformity (**Figure 3**, *C*).

F. Multiple epiphyseal dysplasia (MED) (**Table 1**)

1. Overview

a. Proportionate dwarfisim with multiple epiphyses involved but no spinal involvement.

b. Often diagnosed in midchildhood

2. Pathoanatomy

a. Autosomal dominant

b. Genes identified causing this phenotype include *COMP*; *COL9A2*, which encodes a chain for type IX collagen (a link protein for type II collagen); and, recently, a similar gene, *COL9A3*.

3. Evaluation

a. Multiple abnormal epiphyses

b. Shortened metacarpals and metatarsals are present.

c. Valgus knees with a double-layer patella are found (**Figure 6**, *A*).

d. May be mild to severe involvement of epiphyses; long-term prognosis ranges from mild joint problems to end-stage OA with severe joint contractures at a young age.

e. No spinal involvement

f. For any bilateral Legg-Calvé-Perthes patients, rule out MED.

4. Treatment

a. Progressive genu valgum can be managed by staple hemiepiphysiodesis or osteotomy (**Figure 6**, *B*).

b. Painful, stiff joints are managed with therapy and nonsteroidal anti-inflammatory drugs; end-stage OA with joint arthroplasty.

G. Spondyloepiphyseal dysplasia (SED) (**Table 1**)

1. Overview—Proportionate dwarfism with spinal involvement and a barrel chest.

2. Pathoanatomy

a. Most common autosomal dominant form is SED congenital, which is apparent from birth and caused by mutations in *COL2A1,* which encodes type II collagen found in articular cartilage and vitreous humor of the eyes. The proliferative zone of the growth plates is affected.

b. Rarer, X-linked recessive form is SED tarda, which is milder, with later onset from age 8 to 10 years and is thought to involve the *SEDL* gene.

3. Evaluation

a. Cervical instability is common in both forms.

b. Platyspondyly and delayed epiphyseal ossification are present in both, as is premature OA.

c. SED congenita—Coxa vara, genu valgum, planovalgus feet, retinal detachment, myopia, and hearing loss also present.

d. SED tarda—No lower limb bowing, but dislocated hips are sometimes seen.

4. Treatment

   a. Cervical instability should be stabilized.

b. Progressive, symptomatic lower extremity deformity should be corrected with osteotomies, being careful to assess the whole limb for deformities in joints above and below, and recognizing that early OA and joint arthroplasty is still likely.

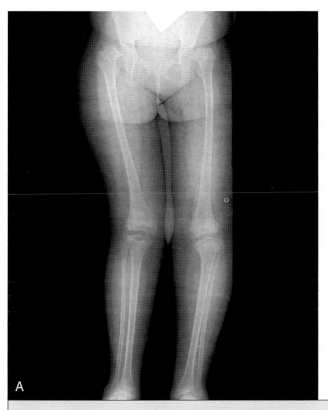 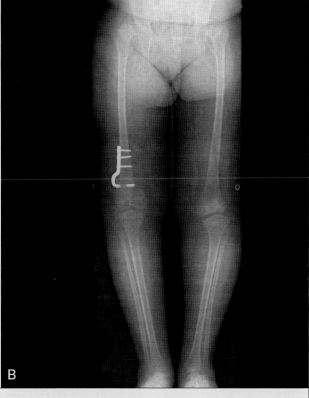

Figure 6 Radiographs of a patient with SED. **A,** Preoperative weight-bearing hip-to-ankle AP radiograph demonstrates classic epiphyseal irregularities and significant right genu valgum. **B,** Postoperative weight-bearing hip-to-ankle AP radiograph of the same patient after varus distal femoral osteotomy.

Top Testing Facts

1. Achondroplasia affects the proliferative zone of the growth plate.

2. Achondroplasia is the most common skeletal dysplasia.

3. Achondroplasia is caused by an autosomal dominant mutation in *FGFR-3;* 90% are sporadic mutations.

4. Subluxation of the radial head is common in achondroplasia and nail-patella syndrome.

5. Diastrophic dysplasia is associated with a mutation in the sulfate transporter gene, which affects proteoglycan sulfate groups in cartilage.

6. Cauliflower ears and hitchhiker thumbs are characteristic of diastrophic dysplasia.

7. Atlantoaxial instability is common in pseudoachondroplasia, SED, mucopolysaccharidoses, trisomy 21, and McKusick type metaphyseal dysplasia.

8. The most serious complications of achondroplasia in the infant and toddler are cervical spine and foramen magnum stenosis, which may cause apnea, weakness, and sudden death.

9. The most common disabling feature of achondroplasia in the adult is lumbar stenosis due to decreased interpedicular distance and shortened pedicles.

10. Pseudochondroplasia is associated with a mutation in *COMP*.

11. Cleidocranial dysplasia is caused by a defect in CBFA-1, which is a transcription factor important in osteoblast differentiation that regulates osteocalcin gene expression.

12. The mucopolysaccharidoses are all autosomal recessive except for Hunter syndrome, which is X-linked recessive.

Bibliography

Ain MC, Chaichana KL, Schkrohowsky JG: Retrospective study of cervical arthrodesis in patients with various types of skeletal dysplasia. *Spine* 2006;31:E169-E174.

Aldegheri R, Dall'Oca C: Limb lengthening in short stature patients. *J Pediatr Orthop B* 2001;10:238-247.

Beguiristain JL, de Rada PD, Barriga A: Nail-patella syndrome: Long term evolution. *J Pediatr Orthop B* 2003;12:13-16.

Bethem D, Winter RB, Lutter L, et al: Spinal disorders of dwarfism: Review of the literature and report of eighty cases. *J Bone Joint Surg Am* 1981;63:1412-1425.

Cooper SC, Flaitz CM, Johnston DA, Lee B, Hecht JT: A natural history of cleidocranial dysplasia. *Am J Med Genet* 2001;104:1-6.

Carten M, Gagne V: *Diastrophic Dysplasia.* http://www.pixelscapes.com/ddhelp/DD-booklet/. Accessed June 29, 2007.

Fassier F, Hamdy RC: Arthogrypotic syndromes and osteochondrodysplasias, in Abel MF (ed): *Orthopaedic Knowledge Update: Pediatrics,* ed 3. Rosemont, IL, American Academy of Orthopaedic Surgeons, 2006, pp 137-151.

Goldberg MJ: *The Dysmorphic Child: An Orthopedic Perspective.* New York, NY, Raven Press, 1987.

Sponseller PD, Ain MC: The skeletal dysplasias, in Morrissy RT, Weinstein SL (eds): *Lovell and Winter's Pediatric Orthopaedics,* ed 6. Philadelphia, PA, Lippincott Williams & Wilkins, 2006, pp 205-250.

Taybi H, Lachman RS: *Radiology of Syndromes, Metabolic Disorders, and Skeletal Dyplasias,* ed 4. St. Louis, MO, Mosby-Year Book Inc, 1996.

Unger S: A genetic approach to the diagnosis of skeletal dysplasia. *Clin Orthop Relat Res* 2002;401:32-38.

Vaccaro AR (ed): *Orthopaedic Knowledge Update 8.* Rosemont, IL, American Academy of Orthopaedic Surgeons, 2005, pp 663-675.

Chapter 35

Connective Tissue Diseases, Arthritides, and Other Diseases

Samantha A. Spencer, MD

I. Connective Tissue Diseases

A. Marfan syndrome (**Table 1**)

1. Overview

    a. Marfan syndrome is a connective tissue disorder affecting elasticity that results in joint laxity, scoliosis, and cardiac valve and aortic dilatation, among others.

    b. Incidence is 1 in 10,000, with no ethnic or gender predilections.

2. Pathoanatomy

    a. Autosomal dominant; 25% new mutations

Table 1

Marfan Syndrome

System	Major Criteria	Minor Criteria
Musculoskeletal*	Pectus carinatum; pectus excavatum requiring surgery; dolichostenomelia; wrist and thumb signs; scoliosis > 20° or spondylolisthesis; reduced elbow extension; pes planus; protrusio acetabuli	Moderately severe pectus excavatum; joint hypermobility; highly arched palate with crowding of teeth; facies (dolichocephaly, malar hypoplasia, enophthalmos, retrognathia, downslanting palpebral fissures)
Ocular†	Ectopia lentis	Abnormally flat cornea; increased axial length of globe; hypoplastic iris or hypoplastic ciliary muscle causing decreased miosis
Cardiovascular‡	Dilatation of ascending aorta ± aortic regurgitation, involving sinuses of Valsalva; or dissection of ascending aorta	Mitral valve prolapse ± regurgitation
Family/Genetic history§	Parent, child, or sibling meets diagnostic criteria; mutation in *FBN1* known to cause Marfan syndrome; or inherited haplotype around *FBN1* associated with Marfan syndrome in family	None
Skin and integument‖	None	Stretch marks not associated with pregnancy, weight gain, or repetitive stress; or recurrent incisional hernias
Dura§	Lumbosacral dural ectasia	None
Pulmonary‖	None	Spontaneous pneumothorax or apical blebs

*Two or more major or one major plus two minor criteria required for involvement
†At least two minor criteria required for involvement
‡One major or minor criterion required for involvement
§One major criterion required for involvement
‖One minor criterion required for involvement
(Adapted from Miller NH: Connective tissue disorders, in Koval KJ (ed): Orthopaedic Knowledge Update 7. Rosemont, IL, American Academy of Orthopaedic Surgeons, 2002, pp 201-207.)

3: Pediatrics

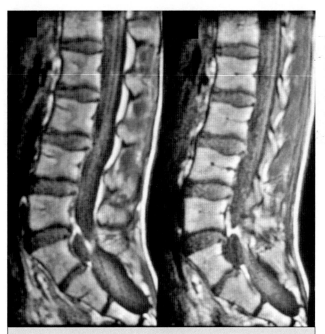

Figure 1   MRI of the lower spine in a patient with Marfan syndrome demonstrates dural ectasia of the lumbosacral junction. (*Courtesy of Dr. M. Timothy Hresko.*)

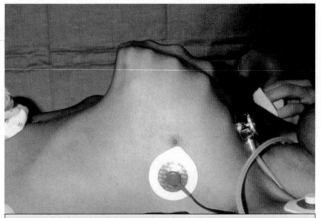

Figure 2   Pectus deformity in a patient with Marfan syndrome. (*Courtesy of Dr. M. Timothy Hresko.*)

b. Mutation is in fibrillin-1 gene on chromosome 15q21; multiple mutations have been identified.

3. Evaluation

a. Affected individuals often are tall and thin with long limbs (dolichostenomelia) and spider-like fingers (arachnodactyly) and joint hypermobility.

b. Positive wrist sign (Walker sign)—The thumb and little finger overlap when used to encircle the opposite wrist.

c. Positive thumb sign (Steinberg sign)—When the thumb is adducted across the hand and the fingers are closed in a fist over it, the thumb protrudes out the other side of the hand.

d. Arm span–to-height ratio >1.05

e. Cardiac defects, especially aortic root dilatation and later dissection, are common; accordingly, if Marfan is suspected, an echocardiogram and a cardiology consultation should be ordered.

f. Scoliosis is seen in 60% to 70% of patients with Marfan and is hard to brace. Because dural ectasia is common (>60%), an MRI should be obtained before surgery (**Figure 1**).

g. Pectus excavatum and spontaneous pneumothoraces can occur in the chest (**Figure 2**).

h. Superior lens dislocation (ectopia lentis) and myopia are common. (Remember inferior lens dislocation is seen in homocysteinuria.)

i. Protrusio acetabuli and severe pes planovalgus are seen in the lower extremity.

4. Classification

a. Ghent system requires one major criterion in each of two different organ systems and involvement in a third system.

b. MASS (mitral valve prolapse, aortic root diameter at upper limits of normal, stretch marks, skeletal manifestations of Marfan) phenotype—These patients do not have ectopia lentis or aortic dissections and have a better prognosis.

5. Treatment

a. Nonsurgical

i. Beta blockers for mitral valve prolapse, aortic dilatation

ii. Bracing for early scoliosis, pes planovalgus

b. Surgical

i. For progressive scoliosis, long scoliosis fusion is indicated to correct junctional problems (with mandatory preoperative cardiac workup and preoperative MRI to assess dural ectasia); this surgery has a high pseudarthrosis rate.

ii. For progressive protrusio acetabuli, closure of the triradiate cartilage is indicated.

iii. For progressive pes planovalgus, corrective surgery is indicated.

B. Ehlers-Danlos syndrome (EDS) (**Table 2**)

1. EDS is a connective tissue disorder with skin and joint hypermobility.

Table 2

Ehlers-Danlos Syndrome Classification

Villefranche Classification (1998)	Berlin Classification (1988)	Genetics	Major Symptomatic Criteria	Biochemical Defects (Minor Criteria)
Classic	Type I (gravis) Type II (mitis)	AD	Hyperextensible skin, atrophic scars, joint hypermobility	COL5A1, COL5A2 mutations (40% to 50% of families) Mutations in type V collagen
Hypermobility	Type III (hypermobile)	AD	Velvety soft skin, small and large joint hypermobility, and tendency for dislocation, chronic pain, scoliosis	Unknown
Vascular	Type IV (vascular)	AD (rarely) AR	Arterial, intestinal and uterine fragility, rupture, thin translucent skin, extensive bruising	COL3A1 mutation, abnormal type III collagen structure of synthesis
Kyphoscoliosis	Type VI (ocular scoliotic)	AR	Severe hypotonia at birth, progressive infantile scoliosis, generalized joint laxity, scleral fragility, globe rupture	Lysyl hydroxylase deficiency, mutations in PLOD gene
Arthrochalasis	Type VIIA, VIIB	AD	Congenital bilateral hip dislocation, hypermobility, soft skin	Deletion of type I collagen exons that encode for N-terminal pro-peptide (COL1A1, COL1A2)
Dermatosparaxis	Type VIIIC	AR	Severe sagging or redundant skin	Mutations in type I collagen N peptidase

AD = autosomal dominant; AR = autosomal recessive.
(Reproduced from D'Astous JL, Carroll KL: Connective tissue disorders, in Vaccaro AR (ed): Orthopaedic Knowledge Update 8, Rosemont, IL, American Academy of Orthopaedic Surgeons, 2005, p 246.)

2. Pathoanatomy

a. 40% to 50% of patients have a mutation in *COL5A1* or *COL5A2*, the gene for type V collagen (type V collagen is important in the assembly of proper skin matrix collagen fibrils and of the basement membrane); this classic form is autosomal dominant.

b. Type VI, autosomal recessive, is a mutation in lysyl hydroxylase, an enzyme important in collagen cross-linking. Severe kyphoscoliosis is characteristic.

c. Type IV, autosomal dominant, is a mutation in *COL3A1* resulting in abnormal collagen III; arterial, intestinal, and uterine rupture are seen.

3. Evaluation

a. Skin is velvety and fragile. Severe scarring with minor trauma is common.

b. Joints are hypermobile, particularly the shoulders, patellae, and ankles.

c. Up to one third of patients have aortic root dilatation; therefore, an echocardiogram and a cardiac evaluation are mandatory.

d. The vascular subtype can have spontaneous visceral or arterial ruptures.

4. Treatment

a. Avoid surgery for lax joints; soft-tissue procedures are unlikely to work.

b. Scoliosis is most common in type VI EDS (**Figure 3**) and usually is progressive. Surgery is indicated for progressive curves, and longer fusions are necessary to prevent junctional problems.

c. Chronic musculoskeletal pain is present in more than 50% of these patients; treat supportively if at all possible.

3: Pediatrics

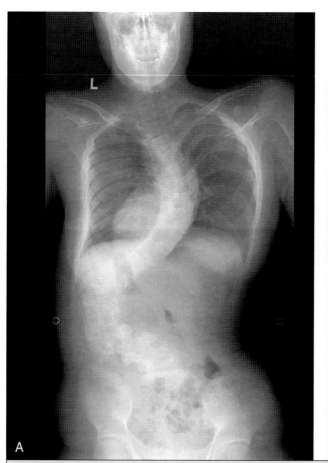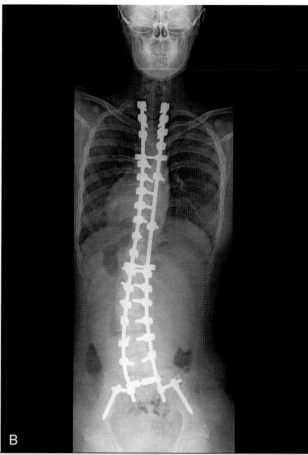

Figure 3   PA spine views of a patient with EDS type VI. **A,** Preoperative view demonstrates severe scoliosis. **B,** Postoperative view demonstrates the long fusion needed in connective tissue syndromes.

II. Arthritides

A. Rheumatoid (seropositive) arthritis (RA) (**Table 3**)

   1. Overview—RA is an inflammatory autoimmune arthritis that causes joint destruction at a younger age than does osteoarthritis (OA).

   2. Pathoanatomy

     a. The synovium thickens and fills with B-cells, T-cells, and macrophages, which erode the cartilage.

     b. The process is autoimmune and systemic.

   3. Evaluation

     a. Rheumatoid factor is found in only half of patients with RA and in 5% of the general population; however, it may help identify more aggressive cases.

     b. Prevalence is 1% in the general population; it is higher in aboriginal North Americans. Twin concordance is only 12% to 15% for monozygotic twins.

     c. Physical examination demonstrates multiple hot, swollen, stiff joints. Subcutaneous calcified nodules and iridis may be present.

     d. Radiographic findings include symmetric joint space narrowing, periarticular erosions, and osteopenia.

   4. Treatment

     a. Nonsurgical—Most treatment is now medical, by rheumatologists, with a combination of NSAIDs and disease-modifying antirheumatic drugs (DMARDs). Most DMARDs are immunosuppressive and must be stopped before orthopaedic procedures and the cell count checked to avoid neutropenia.

     b. Surgical—involves synovectomy and joint realignment early and joint arthroplasty in the later stages.

B. Juvenile idiopathic arthritis (JIA) (previously known as juvenile rheumatoid arthritis, or JRA)

   1. Definition—JIA is an autoimmune inflammatory arthritis of joints in children lasting more than 6 weeks.

Table 3

Differentiating Osteoarthritis from Rheumatoid Arthritis

	Osteoarthritis	Rheumatoid Arthritis
Age	Older	Younger
Physical findings	IP joints affected in hands, gradual stiffness/loss of motion in affected joints (most common in knees/hips), oligoarticular	MCP joints affected in hands with ulnar deviation, polyarticular, joint effusions, warmth; rheumatoid nodules on extensor surfaces
Pathology	Cartilage fibrillation, increased water content of the cartilage, increased collagen I/II ratio, higher friction and lower elasticity	Thickened synovial pannus that cascades over the joint surface; numerous T-cells and B-cells and some plasma cells seen
Radiographic findings	Osteophytes, subchondral sclerosis, subchondral cyst formation; superolateral joint-space narrowing in the hip and medial compartment of the knee commonly seen	Symmetric joint space narrowing with osteopenia and periarticular erosions; protrusio in the hip
Pathophysiology	Chondrocytes release matrix metalloproteinases that degrade the extracellular matrix; cytokines such as IL-1 and TNF-α are also found in the joint fluid. These cause prostaglandin release, which may cause pain.	Autoimmune arthritis in which the joint synovium triggers a T-cell-mediated attack leading to release of IL-1 and TNF-α, which degrade cartilage
Associated findings	Obesity is associated with an increased risk of knee (but not hip) and hand OA, particularly in women.	Basilar invagination, eye involvement, entrapment neuropathies, pleural/pericardial effusions

IP = interphalangeal; MCP = metacarpophalangeal; IL = interleukin; TNF = tumor necrosis factor

2. Pathoanatomy

   a. As in adult RA, autoimmune erosion of cartilage occurs.

   b. Positive rheumatoid factor and antinuclear antibody (ANA) may indicate a more aggressive course.

3. Types of JIA

   a. Systemic JIA/JRA (Still disease)

      i. Rash, high fever, multiple inflamed joints, and acute presentation are typical.

      ii. Anemia and/or a high white blood cell (WBC) count may occur.

      iii. Serositis, hepatosplenomegaly, lymphadenopathy, pericarditis may be present.

      iv. Infection must be ruled out.

      v. Usually presents at age 5 to 10 years; girls and boys affected equally

      vi. Poorest long-term prognosis

      vii. Least common type of JIA (accounts for 20%)

   b. Oligoarticular JIA (previously known as pauciarticular JRA)

      i. Most common type of JIA (accounts for 30% to 40%)

      ii. Four or fewer joints are involved; usually large joints, commonly knees and ankles, are affected.

      iii. Peak age 2 to 3 years; four times as common in girls as in boys.

      iv. A limp that improves during the day is typical.

      v. 20% have uveitis. Ophthalmology evaluation needed every 4 months if ANA-positive, every 6 months if ANA-negative

      vi. Limb-length discrepancy with the affected side often longer is another sequela.

      vii. Best prognosis for long-term remission (70%)

   c. Polyarticular JIA/polyarticular JRA

      i. Five or more joints are involved; often, small joints (hand/wrist) are affected.

      ii. Uveitis sometimes present, but less common than in oligoarticular JIA

      iii. More common in girls

      iv. Prognosis is good (60% remission).

4. Treatment

   a. Limb-length discrepancy may require epiphysiodesis; arthroplasty may be needed in adulthood for destroyed joints.

b. Medical management with NSAIDs or DMARDs by a rheumatologist is usual.

c. An arthrocentesis or synovial biopsy may be needed for diagnosis.

d. Steroid injections and synovectomy may help if medical management fails.

C. Seronegative spondyloarthopathies

1. Definition—Autoimmune arthropathies with a negative rheumatoid factor.

2. Types of seronegative spondyloarthropathies

a. Ankylosing spondylitis

i. Onset age 15 to 35 years; affects males more commonly than females; characterized by morning stiffness, low back pain

ii. Sacroiliitis and progressive fusion of the spine ("bamboo spine") are typical.

iii. Peripheral joint arthritis, usually unilateral, is common.

iv. Uveitis is common in up to 40% of patients; cardiac and pulmonary disease can also occur. Aphthous mouth ulcers and fatigue are common.

v. Aggressive physical therapy and NSAIDs are indicated.

vi. Spinal fractures are highly unstable and have high rates of neurologic injury.

vii. 95% of whites and 50% of blacks with ankylosing spondylitis are HLA-B27-positive, although < 5% of all HLA-B27-positive individuals have ankylosing spondylitis.

b. Psoriatic arthritis

i. The typical psoriatic skin plaques (scaly extensor surface, silvery plaques) usually precede the arthritis, but in 20% of patients, the arthritis occurs first.

ii. Common radiographic finding is "pencil-in-cup" deformity of hand; X-linked recessive.

iii. Nail pitting and dactylitis are common.

c. Reactive arthritis/Reiter syndrome

i. Reactive arthritis is triggered by an infectious disease such as *Chlamydia, Yersinia, Salmonella, Campylobacter,* or *Shigella* that causes an autoimmune complex deposition in the joints (commonly the knee), which leads to painful swelling.

ii. The mnemonic "Can't see, can't pee, can't climb a tree" is useful to remember the associated conjunctivitis and dysuria. Mouth ulcers and a rash on the hands and feet can occur.

iii. The underlying condition should be treated, and the arthritis should be managed supportively.

d. Enteropathic arthropathies—Arthritis associated with inflammatory bowel disease such as Crohn or ulcerative colitis.

i. These arthropathies occur in 20% of patients with inflammatory bowel disease.

ii. They should be managed supportively.

III. Other Conditions With Musculoskeletal Involvement

A. Rickets

1. Overview

a. Defective mineralization in growing bone is due to a variety of causes.

b. The most common form of rickets in North America is hypophosphatemic rickets.

2. Pathoanatomy

a. Calcium/phosphate homeostasis is disturbed, leading to poor calcification of the cartilage matrix of growing long bones.

b. Radiographic features (**Figure 4**) include widened osteoid seams, metaphyseal cupping, prominence of the rib heads (osteochondral junction [ie, rachitic rosary]), bowing (particularly genu varum), fractures.

c. Microscopically, the zone of proliferation is disordered and elongated in the growth plate.

3. Evaluation

a. Serum Ca^{2+}, phosphorus, alkaline phosphatase, parathyroid hormone (PTH), 25 hydroxyvitamin D, and 1,25 dihydroxyvitamin D must be checked to assess the cause.

b. A history of breast-feeding with little sun exposure is the most likely scenario for vitamin D-deficient rickets.

4. Classification/treatment (**Table 4**)

5. Surgery is indicated for lower limb bowing that does not resolve after medical treatment of the rickets; hemiepiphysiodesis or osteotomy may be indicated.

B. Trisomy 21 (Down syndrome)

1. Trisomy 21 is the most common chromosomal abnormality, with an incidence of 1 in 800 to 1,000 live births. Incidence increases with advanced maternal age.

2. Pathoanatomy—Usually a duplication of mater-

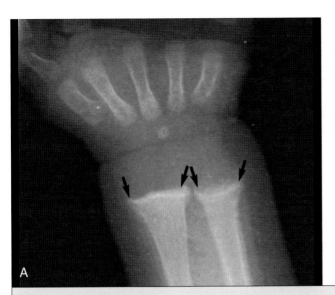 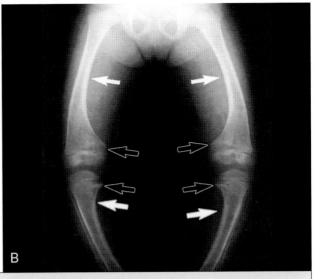

Figure 4   Radiographic features of rickets. **A,** PA view of the wrist in a child with rickets shows radial and ulnar metaphyseal fraying and cupping (arrows). **B,** AP view of the lower extremities in a child with rickets demonstrates bowing of the femurs and tibias (white arrows) as well as metaphyseal widening and irregularity (black arrows). *(Reproduced from Johnson TR: General orthopaedics, in Johnson TR, Steinbach LS (eds): Essentials of Musculoskeletal Imaging. Rosemont, IL, American Academy of Orthopaedic Surgeons, 2004, p 78.)*

Table 4

Most Common Types of Rickets With Associated Genetics, Features, and Treatment

Condition	Genetics	Serum Values	Associated Features	Treatment
Hypophosphatemic rickets	X-linked dominant, impaired renal phosphate absorption	Decreased phosphate; normal calcium, PTH, and vitamin D; increased alkaline phosphatase	Most common type in North America	No established medical therapy
Vitamin D-deficient rickets	Nutritional	Decreased vitamin D, calcium, and phosphate; increased PTH and alkaline phosphate		Vitamin D replacement
Vitamin D-dependent rickets, type 1	Autosomal recessive; defect in renal 25-hydroxyvitamin D 1-α-hydroxylase	Low calcium and phosphate; normal 25-hydroxyvitamin D, very low 1,25-dihydroxyvitamin D; high alkaline phosphatase and PTH		1,25-dihyroxyvitamin D replacement
Vitamin D-dependent rickets, type 2	Defect in the intracellular receptor for 1,25-dihydroxyvitamin D	Low calcium and phosphate; high alkaline phosphatase and PTH; very high 1,25-dihydroxyvitamin D levels	Alopecia	High-dose 1,25-dihydroxy-vitamin calcium
Hypophosphatasia	Autosomal recessive, deficient or nonfunctional alkaline phosphatase	Increased calcium and phosphate levels; very low alkaline phosphatase levels; normal PTH/vitamin D levels	Early loss of teeth	No established medical therapy

nal chromosome 21, ie, three copies of chromosome 21.

3. Evaluation

   a. Phenotypic features include flattened face, upward slanting eyes with epicanthal folds, single palmar crease, mental retardation (varies), congenital heart disease (endocardial cushion defects 50%), duodenal atresia, hypothyroidism, hearing loss, ligamentous laxity, high incidence of leukemia/lymphoma, diabetes and Alzheimer's in later adult life.

Table 5

Clinical Classification of Osteogenesis Imperfecta

Type	Features	Inheritance
I (dominant, blue sclerae)	IA: bone fragility, blue sclerae, and normal teeth IB: same as IA but with dentinogenesis imperfecta IC: more severe than IB but with normal teeth	Autosomal dominant
II (lethal perinatal)	IIA: broad crumpled long bones and beaded rib; generally perinatal death IIB: broad crumpled long bones but ribs show minimal or no beading; death variable from perinatal to several years IIC: thin fractured cylindrical, dysplastic long bones, and thin beaded ribs; very low birth rate; stillbirth or perinatal death IID: severely ostepenic with generally well-formed skeleton; normally shaped vertebrae and pelvis; perinatal death	Autosomal dominant
III (progressive deforming)	Multiple fractures at birth with progressive deformities, normal sclerae, and dentinogenesis imperfecta	Autosomal recessive
IV (dominant, white sclerae)	IVA: bone fragility, white sclerae, and normal teeth IVB: similar to IVA but with dentinogenesis imperfecta	Autosomal dominant

(Reproduced with permission from Cole WG: The molecular pathology of osteogenesis imperfecta. Clin Orthop 1997;343:235-248.)

Table 6

Biochemical Classification of Type I Collagen Mutations in Osteogenesis Imperfecta

Protein Feature	Category of Mutation	Clinical Phenotype
Moderate reduction of normal type I collagen in tissues	Haploinsufficiency	OI-IA
Mixture of normal and mutant type I collagen molecules in tissues	Dominant negative	OI-IB:IIA-IIC:III:IVB
Severe reduction of normal type I collagen in tissues	Dominant negative	OI-IC
Very severe reduction of normal type I collagen in tissues	Dominant negative	OI-IID

(Reproduced with permission from Cole WG: The molecular pathology of osteogenesis imperfecta. Clin Orthop 1997;343:235-248.)

b. Spine

   i. Atlantoaxial instability is present in 9% to 22%; it is controversial if flexion-extension views are needed before participation in sports.

   ii. Scoliosis in present in up to 50%.

   iii. Spondylolisthesis is present in up to 6%.

c. Metatarsus primus varus/pes planovalgus/hallux valgus are seen.

d. Patellar dislocation, pain, and instability are common.

e. Hip instability (often late) is common, sometimes with only mild bony abnormality.

4. Treatment

a. Supportive bracing is indicated for feet (supramalleolar or University of California at Berkeley Laboratory orthoses for pes planovalgus) and knees (patellar stabilizing braces) and for hips (hip abduction braces) in children younger than 6 years.

b. Atlanto-dens interval (ADI) of ≤5 mm is normal.

c. Treatment of asymptomatic ADI of 5 to 10 mm is controversial; many watch and obtain an MRI to look for cord compromise.

d. Fusion is indicated if cord compromise is seen on MRI or if there is ADI >5 and the patient has symptoms; however, fusion has a high (up to 50%) complication rate.

e. Soft-tissue surgeries fail due to ligamentous laxity and hypotonia; therefore, if surgery is done, bony realignment is indicated (ie, periacetabular osteotomy for hip dislocation, tibial tubercle osteotomy for lateral patellar dislocation).

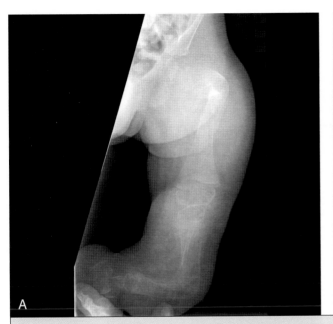
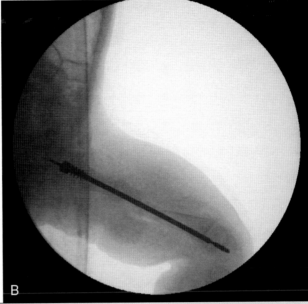

Figure 5   Images of the femur of a patient with type III OI. **A,** Preoperative frog-lateral hip-to-ankle radiograph demonstrates femoral deformity. **B,** Postoperative frog-lateral fluoroscopic radiograph shows osteotomies and fixation with a telescoping rod.

C. Osteogenesis imperfecta (OI) (**Tables 5 and 6**)

1. Overview

   a. Weak organic bone matrix causes frequent fractures and severe bowing and deformity in the more severe types.

   b. Intelligence is normal.

2. Pathoanatomy

   a. Types I through IV are a mutation in the *COL1A1* and *COL1A2* genes that encode type I collagen, the mainstay of the organic bone matrix.

      i. The result is bone that has a decreased number of trabeculae and decreased cortical thickness (wormian bone).

      ii. Specific mutation is identified by DNA analysis of blood.

   b. Types V through VII have no collagen I mutation but have a similar phenotype and abnormal bone on microscopy.

3. Evaluation

   a. Child abuse should not be ruled out in OI patients; conversely, OI should not be ruled out in a child abuse workup.

   b. Particularly in types II and III, basilar invagination and severe scoliosis may occur.

   c. Olecranon apophyseal avulsion fractures are characteristic; children presenting with these should be evaluated for OI.

   d. Associated dentinogenesis imperfecta, hearing loss, blue sclerae, joint hyperlaxity, and wormian skull bones (puzzle piece appearance to the skull after fontanelle closure) are seen.

4. Treatment

   a. Manage fractures with light splints.

   b. Bisphosphonates and growth hormone are used; bisphosphonates inhibit osteoclasts, yielding increased cortical thickness with decreased fracture rates and pain.

   c. For severe bowing of the limbs or recurrent fracture, intramedullary fixation is indicated with or without osteotomy. Newer devices have telescoping rods to allow growth (**Figure 5**).

   d. Progressive scoliosis/basilar invagination is treated with spinal fusion.

D. Gaucher disease

1. Overview—An enzymatic defect leads to overaccumulation of glucocerebrosides (lipids) in many organ systems, including the bone marrow and the spleen.

2. Pathoanatomy

   a. Defect in the gene encoding beta glucocerebrosidase, which breaks down glucocerebrosides, leads to accumulation of glucocerebrosides in macrophages in many organ systems.

   b. Always autosomal recessive

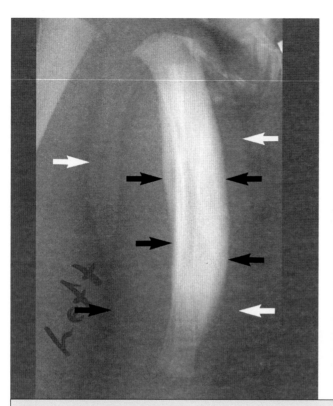 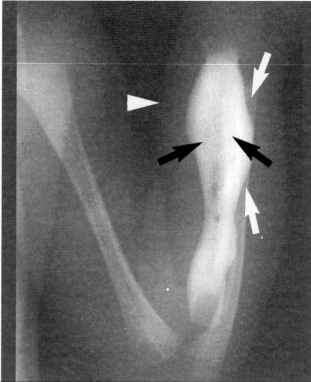

Figure 6 Radiographic features of Caffey disease. **A,** Lateral view of the tibia shows increased bone formation throughout the diaphysis (black arrows) with increased diameter and soft-tissue swelling (white arrows). **B,** Lateral view of the forearm shows increased diameter of the diaphysis in the radius (black arrows), extensive periosteal reaction (white arrows), and soft-tissue swelling (arrowhead). (*Reproduced from Sarwark JF, Shore RM: Pediatric orthopaedics, in Johnson TR, Steinbach LS (eds): Essentials of Musculoskeletal Imaging. Rosemont, IL, American Academy of Orthopaedic Surgeons, 2004, p. 814.*)

3. Evaluation

  a. A WBC examination for enzyme activity is diagnostic.

  b. Three forms are identified, based on age of onset.

    i. Type 1 (adult): easy bruising (thrombocytopenia), anemia, enlarged liver/spleen, bone pain/fractures

    ii. Type 2 (infantile): enlarged spleen/liver by age 3 months; brain involvement; lethal by age 2 years

    iii. Type 3 (juvenile): onset in teen years; (thrombocytopenia), anemia, enlarged liver/spleen, bone pain/fractures; gradual and mild brain involvement

  c. Radiographic findings include Erlenmeyer flask appearance of distal femurs (also seen in osteopetrosis), osteonecrosis of hips/femoral condyles, cortical thinning.

4. Treatment

  a. Enzyme replacement therapy is now available and works well for all but neurologic symptoms.

  b. Bone marrow transplant performed early can be curative.

E. Caffey disease

  1. Definition—A cortical hyperostosis of infancy (average age of onset <9 weeks) that is self-resolving and is a diagnosis of exclusion.

  2. Pathoanatomy

    a. The erythrocyte sedimentation rate (ESR) and alkaline phosphatase are elevated, but cultures are negative.

    b. Pathology shows hyperplasia of collagen fibers and fibrinoid degeneration.

  3. Evaluation

    a. Bones of the jaw (mandible) and forearm (ulna) are most commonly affected, with diffuse cortical thickening present, but any bone except the vertebrae and phalanges may be affected (**Figure 6**).

    b. Febrile illness with hyperirritability, swelling of soft tissues, and cortical thickening of the bone

  4. Treatment is supportive, with occasional glucocorticoid use.

Top Testing Facts

1. Dural ectasia is commonly seen in Marfan syndrome and may cause back pain and complicate scoliosis surgery; preoperative MRI is mandatory.

2. Ectopia lentis associated with Marfan syndrome is a superior dislocation; with homocysteinuria, the lens dislocation is inferior.

3. MASS phenotype patients never have ectopia lentis or aortic dissections.

4. Marfan syndrome is caused by a mutation in the fibrillin-1 gene.

5. JIA is commonly associated with uveitis, which should be screened for. JIA may be associated with limb-length discrepancy.

6. The most common form of rickets in North America is hypophosphatemic rickets, which is X-linked dominant.

7. The most common chromosomal abnormality is trisomy 21.

8. Olecranon apophyseal avulsion fractures are characteristic of OI.

9. Erlenmyer flask deformities of the femurs are seen in Gaucher disease and osteopetrosis.

10. Gaucher disease is associated with a defect in the gene encoding beta glucocerebrosidase.

Bibliography

Aldegheri R, Dall'Oca C: Limb lengthening in short stature patients. *J Pediatr Orthop B* 2001;10:238-247.

D'Astous JL, Carroll KL: Connective tissue diseases, in *Orthopaedic Knowledge Update 8*. Rosemont, IL, American Academy of Orthopaedic Surgeons, 2005, pp 245-254.

Fassier F, Hamdy RC: Arthogrypotic syndromes and osteochondrodysplasias, in Abel MF (ed): *Orthopaedic Knowledge Update: Pediatrics 3*. Rosemont, IL, American Academy of Orthopaedic Surgeons, 2006, pp 137-151.

Goldberg MJ: *The Dysmorphic Child: An Orthopedic Perspective*. New York, NY, Raven Press, 1987.

Judge DP, Dietz HC: Marfan's syndrome. *Lancet* 2005;366: 1965-1976.

Morris CD, Einhorn TA: Bisphosphonates in orthopaedic surgery. *J Bone Joint Surg Am* 2005;87:1609-1618.

Sponseller PD, Ain MC: The skeletal dysplasias, in Morrissy RT, Weinstein SL (eds): *Lovell and Winter's Pediatric Orthopaedics*, ed 6. Philadelphia, PA, Lippincott Williams & Wilkins, 2006, pp 205-250.

Stanitski DF, Nadjarian R, Stanitski CL, Bawle E, Tsipouras P: Orthopaedic manifestations of Ehlers-Danlos syndrome. *Clin Orthop Relat Res* 2000;376:213-221.

Taybi H, Lachman RS: *Radiology of Syndromes, Metabolic Disorders, and Skeletal Dyplasias*, ed 4. St. Louis, MO, Mosby-Year Book Inc., 1996.

Unger S: A genetic approach to the diagnosis of skeletal dysplasia. *Clin Orthop Relat Res* 2002;401:32-38.

Zeitlin L, Fassier F, Glorieux F: Modern approach to children with osteogenesis imperfecta. *J Pediatr Orthop B* 2003;12: 77-87.

3: Pediatrics

Section 4

Orthopaedic Oncology and Systemic Disease

Section Editors

Kristy Weber, MD

Frank J. Frassica, MD

Chapter 36

Overview of Orthopaedic Oncology and Systemic Disease

*Frank J. Frassica, MD

I. General Information and Terminology

A. Each year in the United States there are approximately 2,700 new bone sarcomas and 9,000 new soft-tissue sarcomas. Most of these sarcomas are high-grade malignancies with a high propensity to metastasize to the lungs.

B. Benign bone conditions

1. Developmental processes

2. Reactive processes (osteomyelitis, stress fractures)

3. Benign tumors (giant cell tumor, chondroblastoma)

C. Malignant bone conditions

1. Malignancies that arise from mesenchymal derivatives are called sarcomas.

2. Primary bone sarcomas include osteosarcoma and chondrosarcoma.

3. Bone malignancies that are not sarcomas include metastatic bone disease, multiple myeloma, and lymphoma.

D. Soft-tissue masses

1. Most common soft-tissue tumors

a. Benign: lipoma

b. Malignant: malignant fibrous histiocytoma, liposarcoma

2. Nonneoplastic reactive conditions include hematomas and heterotopic ossification.

II. Bone Tumors

A. Classification/staging systems

1. Lichtenstein system—Modified by Dahlin to

Frank J. Frassica, MD, is a consultant or employee for SLACK Inc.

group conditions together based on the type of proliferating cell and whether the lesion is benign or malignant (**Table 1**).

2. Bone tumors can be classified according to whether the process involves intramedullary bone or surface bone.

a. Common intramedullary tumors

i. Enchondroma

ii. Osteosarcoma

iii. Chondrosarcoma

b. Common surface tumors

i. Osteochondroma

ii. Periosteal chondroma

iii. Parosteal osteosarcoma

3. Bone sarcomas also can be characterized as being primary or secondary.

a. Common primary bone sarcomas

i. Osteosarcoma

ii. Ewing sarcoma

iii. Chondrosarcoma

b. Common secondary sarcomas

i. Chondrosarcoma arising in an osteochondroma

ii. Malignant fibrous histiocytoma arising in a bone infarct

4. Bone tumor grade

a. Grade 1 (G1): low grade (well differentiated)

i. Parosteal osteosarcoma

ii. Low-grade intramedullary osteosarcoma (rare)

iii. Adamantinoma

iv. Intramedullary chondrosarcoma

v. Chordoma

Table 1

Dahlin Modification of Lichtenstein Classification System

Cell Type	Benign	Malignant
Bone	Osteoid osteoma Osteoblastoma	Osteosarcoma Parosteal osteosarcoma Periosteal osteosarcoma High-grade surface osteosarcoma
Cartilage	Enchondroma Periosteal chondroma Osteochondroma Chondroblastoma Chondromyxoid fibroma	Chondrosarcoma Dedifferentiated chondrosarcoma Periosteal chondrosarcoma Mesenchymal chondrosarcoma Clear cell chondrosarcoma
Fibrous	Nonossifying fibroma	Fibrosarcoma Malignant fibrous histiocytoma
Vascular	Hemangioma	Hemangioendothelioma Hemangiopericytoma
Hematopoietic		Myeloma Lymphoma
Nerve	Neurilemmoma	Malignant peripheral nerve-sheath tumor
Lipogenic	Lipoma	Liposarcoma
Notochordal	Notochordal rest	Chordoma
Unknown	Giant cell tumor	Ewing sarcoma Adamantinoma

Table 2

Enneking Classification of Benign Bone Tumors

Stage	Description	Tumor Examples
1	Inactive (latent)	Nonossifying fibroma Enchondroma
2	Active	Giant cell tumor* Aneurysmal bone cyst* Chondroblastoma Chondromyxoid fibroma Unicameral bone cyst
3	Aggressive	Giant cell tumor* Aneurysmal bone cyst*

*Giant cell tumor and aneurysmal bone cyst can be either stage 2 active or stage 3 aggressive lesions, depending on the amount of bone destruction, soft-tissue masses, or joint involvement.

Table 3

Enneking Classification of Malignant Bone Tumors

Stage	Description
IA	Low grade, intracompartmental
IB	Low grade, extracompartmental
IIA	High grade, intracompartmental
IIB	High grade, extracompartmental
III	Metastatic disease

Suffix A = intracompartmental (confined to bone, no soft-tissue involvement); suffix B = extracompartmental (penetration of the cortex with a soft-tissue mass)

b. Grade 2 (G2): intermediate grade (moderately differentiated)

   i. Periosteal osteosarcoma

   ii. Grade 2 chondrosarcoma of bone

c. Grades 3 (G3) and 4 (G4): high grade (poorly differentiated or undifferentiated)

   i. Osteosarcoma

   ii. Ewing sarcoma

   iii. Malignant fibrous histiocytoma

5. Enneking system—Enneking and associates developed a staging system for benign and malignant musculoskeletal tumors.

a. Benign lesions—Classified into stages 1, 2, and 3 (Table 2).

b. Malignant bone tumors—Classified into stages I, II, and III (Table 3).

6. American Joint Commission for Cancer (AJCC) classification system

a. Based on the tumor grade, size, and presence or absence of discontinuous tumor or regional/systemic metastases (Table 4).

b. In this system, the order of importance of prognostic factors is:

   i. Presence of metastasis (stage IV)

   ii. Discontinuous tumor (stage III)

   iii. Grade (I—low, II—high)

   iv. Size

      (a) T1 ≤ 8 cm

      (b) T2 > 8 cm

B. Patient presentation of malignant bone tumors

1. Pain—Patients with high-grade malignant bone tumors present with bone pain.

Table 4

AJCC Classification System for Bone Tumors

Stage	Grade	Size of Tumor	Regional Nodes	Metastasis
IA	G1-G2	T1	N0	M0
IB	G1-G2	T2	N0	M0
IIA	G3-G4	T1	N0	M0
IIB	G3-G4	T2	N0	M0
III	Any	T3	N0	M0
IVA	Any	Any	N1	M0
IVB	Any	Any	Any nodal status	M1

Grades: G1 = well differentiated; G2 = moderately differentiated; G3 = poorly differentiated; G4 = undifferentiated
Size: T1 ≤8 cm; T2 >8 cm; T3 = discontinuous tumor or skip metastasis
Nodal status: N0 = no nodal metastasis; N1 = nodal metastasis
Metastases: M0 = no distant metastasis; M1 = distant metastasis

a. The pain begins as intermittent and progresses to constant pain that does not respond to nonsteroidal anti-inflammatory drugs or weak narcotic medications.

b. A common presentation is severe pain that occurs at rest and with activity.

c. Night pain is often present.

2. Mass—Patients present with a hard, fixed, soft-tissue mass adjacent to the bone lesion that is often tender on deep palpation.

3. Range of motion—The range of motion of the affected joint is often diminished, and muscle atrophy is common.

4. Fractures

a. Fractures occur in 5% to 10% of patients with malignant bone tumors.

b. A history of antecedent pain is common.

c. These fractures generally occur with minor trauma or following activities of daily living.

C. Evaluation

1. Imaging strategy

a. Primary lesion—Radiographs and MRI (occasionally thin cut CT if osteoid osteoma suspected).

b. Pulmonary staging

i. Chest radiograph is used for initial screening.

ii. CT is used as a baseline to detect pulmonary metastases not seen on chest radiographs and to use for future comparison.

2. Plain radiographs—AP/lateral views of the lesion.

a. Inspect cortices for bone destruction.

b. Assess if lesion is mineralized.

i. Rings/stipples suggest cartilage lesion.

ii. Cloud, ivory-like suggests bone formation.

c. Check for evidence of periosteal reaction.

3. Technetium Tc 99m bone scan

a. Technetium Tc 99m forms chemical adducts to sites of new bone formation.

b. Detects multiple sites of bone involvement

c. Very sensitive but not specific

d. High false-negative rate in multiple myeloma

4. Magnetic resonance imaging

a. Sensitive and specific for detecting bone marrow involvement

b. Defines anatomic features (T1-weighted sequences)

5. Computed tomography

a. Determines the mineral distribution in normal and abnormal bone

b. Helpful in evaluating pelvic and spine lesions

III. Soft-Tissue Tumors

A. Classification

1. Soft-tissue tumors are classified histologically, according to the predominant cell type.

2. This system encompasses benign and malignant neoplasms and reactive conditions.

3. There are hundreds of different soft-tissue tumors; some of the most significant are listed in **Table 5**.

B. Staging—The most common system is the AJCC system (**Table 6**). The order of importance of prognostic factors is:

1. Presence of metastasis (stage IV)

2. Grade

a. Low—stage I

b. High—stage II

3. Size (>5 cm)

4. Location (superficial or deep)

Table 5

Histologic Classification of Soft-Tissue Tumors

Type	Benign	Malignant
Fibrous	Nodular fasciitis Proliferative fasciitis Elastofibroma Infantile fibromatosis Adult fibromatosis	Fibrosarcoma Infantile fibrosarcoma
Fibrohistiocytic	Fibrous histiocytoma	DFSP Malignant fibrous histiocytoma
Lipomatous	Lipoma Angiolipoma Hibernoma Atypical lipoma	Well-differentiated liposarcoma Myxoid round cell liposarcoma Pleomorphic liposarcoma Dedifferentiated liposarcoma
Smooth muscle	Leiomyoma	Leiomyosarcoma
Skeletal muscle	Rhabdomyoma	Rhabdomyosarcoma
Blood vessels	Hemangioma Lymphangioma	Angiosarcoma Kaposi sarcoma
Perivascular	Glomus tumor	Hemangiopericytoma
Synovial	Focal PVNS Diffuse PVNS	Malignant PVNS
Nerve sheath	Neuroma Neurofibroma Neurofibromatosis Schwannoma	MPNST
Neuroectodermal	Ganglioneuroma	Neuroblastoma Ewing sarcoma PNET
Cartilage	Chondroma Synovial chondromatosis	Extraskeletal chondrosarcoma
Bone	FOP	Extraskeletal osteosarcoma
Miscellaneous	Tumoral calcinosis Myxoma	Synovial sarcoma Alveolar soft-part sarcoma Epithelioid sarcoma

DFSP = dermatofibrosarcoma protuberans; PVNS = pigmented villonodular synovitis; MPNST = malignant peripheral nerve sheath tumor; PNET = primitive neuroectodermal tumor; FOP = fibrodysplasia ossificans progressiva

Table 6

AJCC Staging System for Soft-Tissue Sarcomas

Stage	Grade	Size/Depth	Regional Node	Metastasis
IA	G1, G2	T1a	N0	M0
		T1b	N0	M0
IB	G1, G2	T2a	N0	M0
IIA	G1, G2	T2b	N0	M0
IIB	G3, G4	T1a	N0	M0
		T1b	N0	M0
IIC	G3, G4	T2a	N0	M0
III	G3, G4	T2b	N0	M0
IV	Any	Any	N1	M1

Grades: G1 = well differentiated; G2 = moderately differentiated; G3 = poorly differentiated; G4 = undifferentiated
Size/depth: T1 ≤5 cm; T2 >5 cm; a = superficial; b = deep
N0 = no nodal metastasis; N1 = nodal metastasis
M0 = no distant metastasis; M1 = distant metastasis

2. Significant problems can occur when a biopsy is not done correctly.

   a. Altered treatment

   b. Major errors in diagnosis

   c. Complications (infection, nerve, injury, etc)

   d. Nonrepresentative tissue

   e. Adverse outcome (local recurrence etc)

   f. Unnecessary amputation

B. Major types of biopsy

  1. Needle biopsy—Most common method of establishing a diagnosis, but requires an experienced cytopathologist and surgical pathologist.

   a. Fine needle aspiration (FNA)—Needle aspiration of cells from the tumor.

   b. Core needle biopsy—A larger bore needle is placed into the tumor and a core of tissue is extracted.

  2. Open incisional biopsy—Surgical procedure to obtain tissue.

   a. The entire biopsy tract should be designed to be excised at the time of the definitive resection if the tumor is malignant.

     i. The incision should be small and usually is oriented longitudinally.

     ii. Occasionally, a nonlongitudinal incision is used

       (a) A transverse incision is used for the clavicle.

IV. Biopsy

A. General

  1. Biopsy is a key step in the evaluation and treatment of patients with bone or soft-tissue lesions.

(b) An oblique incision is used for the scapular body.

b. Soft-tissue flaps are not elevated; the biopsy is performed directly onto the tumor mass.

c. A frozen section analysis is often performed to ensure that diagnostic tissue has been obtained.

3. Excisional biopsy

a. Indicated only when the surgeon is sure that the lesion is benign or when the tumor can be removed with a wide margin (eg, if the radiographic appearance suggests a superficial, small soft-tissue malignancy)

b. Two low-grade malignancies for which an excisional biopsy is sometimes performed are parosteal osteosarcoma and low-grade chondrosarcoma.

V. Molecular Markers/Genetic Considerations

A. Tumor suppressor genes—Tumor suppressor genes and associated conditions are listed in **Table 7**.

B. Chromosomal alterations

1. Chromosomal alterations in malignant tumors are generally translocations (**Table 8**).

2. Alterations often produce unique gene products that may affect prognosis.

Table 7

Tumor Suppressor Genes

Gene	Syndrome	Tumor Examples
RB	Hereditary neuroblastoma	Retinoblastoma, osteosarcoma
P53	Li-Fraumeni syndrome	Sarcomas, breast cancer
P16INK4a	Familial melanoma	Chondrosarcoma, osteosarcoma, melanoma
APC	Familial adenomatous polyposis	Colon adenomas, desmoids
NF1	Neurofibromatosis	Neurofibroma, sarcomas
EXT1/EXT2	Hereditary multiple exostosis	Osteochondromas, chondrosarcomas

Table 8

Chromosomal Alterations

Tumor	Translocation	Genes
Ewing sarcoma, PNET	t(11;22)(q24;q12)	EWS, FLI1
Synovial sarcoma	t(X;18)(p11;q11)	SYT, SSX
Clear cell sarcoma	t(12;22)(q13;a12)	EWS, ATF1
Alveolar rhabdomyo-sarcoma	t(2;13)(q35;q14)	PAX3, FKHR
Myxoid liposarcoma	t(12;16)(q13;p11)	CHOP, TLS

PNET = primitive neuroectodermal tumor

4: Orthopaedic Oncology and Systemic Disease

Top Testing Facts

1. The most common site of metastases from bone and soft-tissue sarcomas is the pulmonary system.

2. The most common low-grade bone sarcomas are chondrosarcoma, parosteal osteosarcoma, adamantinoma, and chordoma.

3. The most common high-grade sarcomas are osteosarcoma, Ewing sarcoma, and malignant fibrous histiocytoma.

4. The order of importance of prognostic factors in bone tumor staging is presence of metastases, discontinuous tumor, grade, and size.

5. A high rate of false-negative results occur with technetium Tc 99m bone scanning in multiple myeloma.

6. The order of importance of prognostic factors in soft-tissue tumor staging is presence of metastases, grade, size, and depth.

7. The retinoblastoma gene is the tumor suppressor gene associated with osteosarcoma.

8. *EXT1/EXT2* are the tumor suppressor genes associated with multiple exostoses.

9. Ewing sarcoma and primitive neuroectodermal tumor (PNET) have a characteristic chromosomal translocation t(11;22).

10. Synovial sarcoma has a characteristic chromosomal translocation t(X;18).

Bibliography

Enneking WF: A system of staging musculoskeletal neoplasms. *Clin Orthop Relat Res* 1986;204:9-24.

Enneking WF, Spanier SS, Goodman MA: A system for the surgical staging of musculoskeletal sarcoma. *Clin Orthop Relat Res* 1980;153:106-120.

Greene FL, Page DL, Fleming ID, Balch CM, Haller DG, Morrow M: *AJCC Cancer Staging Manual*, ed 6. New York, NY, Springer, 2002, pp 221-228.

Jemal A, Siegel R, Ward E, et al. Cancer statistics, 2006. *CA Cancer J Clin* 2006;56:106-130.

Hopyan S, Wunder JS, Randall RL: Molecular biology in musculoskeletal neoplasia, in Schwartz HS (ed): *Orthopaedic Knowledge Update: Musculoskeletal Tumors 2*. Rosemont, IL, American Academy of Orthopaedic Surgeons, 2007, pp 13-21.

Mankin HJ, Lange TA, Spanier SS: The hazards of biopsy in patients with malignant primary bone and soft-tissue tumors. *Clin Orthop Relat Res* 2006;450:4-10.

Unni KK: Introduction and scope of study, in Unni KK (ed): *Dahlin's Bone Tumors: General Aspects and Data on 11,087 Cases*, ed 5. Philadelphia, PA, Lipppincott-Raven, 1996.

Weiss SW, Goldblum JR, eds: General considerations, in *Enzinger and Weiss's Soft Tissue Tumors*, ed 5. St Louis, MO, Mosby, 2007, pp 1-20.

Chapter 37

Principles of Treatment of Musculoskeletal Tumors

*Frank J. Frassica, MD

I. Overview

A. Biologic activity and potential morbidity

  1. The treatment of musculoskeletal tumors is based on the biologic activity and potential morbidity of each lesion.

  2. The important biologic aspects are the risk of local recurrence and metastasis.

B. Surgical margins are designed to reduce the risk of local recurrence.

  1. Intralesional—The plane of dissection enters into the tumor.

  2. Marginal—The plane of dissection is through the reactive zone at the edge of the tumor.

  3. Wide—The entire tumor is removed with a cuff of normal tissue.

  4. Radical—The entire compartment that the tumor occupies is removed.

C. Chemotherapy—Common mechanism is to induce programmed cell death (apoptosis). Chemotherapeutic agents achieve apoptosis in various ways:

  1. Directly damage DNA—alkylating agents, platinum compounds, anthracyclines

  2. Deplete cellular building blocks—antifolates, cytidine analogs, 5-fluoropyrimidines

  3. Interfere with microtubule function—vinca alkaloids, taxanes

D. Radiation therapy—Mechanism is to cause DNA damage through production of free radicals.

*Frank J. Frassica, MD, is a consultant for or an employee for SLACK, Inc.

II. Treatment of Bone Tumors

A. Benign processes/tumors

  1. Observation—For asymptomatic inactive lesions.

  2. Aspiration and injection

    a. Injection materials for unicameral bone cysts of the humerus

      i. Methylprednisolone acetate

      ii. Bone marrow

      iii. Synthetic bone grafts

    b. Eosinophilic granuloma—Injection material used is methylprednisolone acetate.

  3. Curettage (exposing the lesion and scraping it out with hand and power tools as necessary)

    a. The margin is always intralesional.

    b. Hand curettage is often extended with a power burr, especially for giant cell tumor and aneurysmal bone cyst.

    c. Surgical adjuvants are used for tumors (ie, giant cell tumor) prone to recurrence (controversial value).

      i. Phenol

        (a) Strong base that coagulates proteins

        (b) Potential soft-tissue injury with spillage

      ii. Liquid nitrogen

        (a) Freezes up to 1 cm of tissue

        (b) High stress-fracture rate (at least 25%)

    d. Materials used for reconstruction of the defect

      i. Methylmethacrylate—Often used for giant cell tumors.

      ii. Bone graft (freeze-dried allograft, synthetic graft, autogenous graft)

4: Orthopaedic Oncology and Systemic Disease

e. Benign tumors commonly treated with curettage/grafting

   i. Giant cell tumor

   ii. Chondroblastoma

   iii. Chondromyxoid fibroma

   iv. Osteoblastoma

   v. Aneurysmal bone cyst

   vi. Unicameral bone cyst of the proximal femur

f. Benign processes *occasionally* treated with curettage and grafting

   i. Enchondroma

   ii. Unicameral bone cyst of the humerus

   iii. Nonossifying fibroma

4. Resection—Removal of the bone (or a major portion) with the intent to definitively remove all tumor.

a. Reserved for aggressive lesions with major bone destruction, soft-tissue extension, cartilage loss, or fracture

b. Benign processes that are treated by resection with a marginal or intralesional margin

   i. Osteochondroma

   ii. Periosteal chondroma

c. Methods used for reconstruction of the defect

   i. Prosthetic device

   ii. Allograft

   iii. Allograft-prosthetic reconstruction

B. Malignant bone tumors (sarcomas)

1. Overview

a. Malignant bone tumors must be removed with satisfactory margin to prevent local recurrence.

b. Marked propensity to recur locally if not completely removed

c. High risk of systemic metastases

2. Surgery

a. Limb salvage versus amputation

   i. Limb salvage—Removal of the malignant tumor with a satisfactory margin and preservation of the limb.

   ii. Amputation—Removal of the tumor with a wide or radical margin and removal of the extremity.

b. Wide resection alone, with no role for chemotherapy or radiation therapy, is the only effective modality for some tumors.

   i. Chondrosarcoma

   ii. Adamantinoma

   iii. Parosteal osteosarcoma

   iv. Low-grade intramedullary osteosarcoma

c. Chemotherapy

   i. Used to kill micrometastases present in the pulmonary parenchyma and other sites

   ii. An integral component of treatment, along with surgery, in the following malignancies:

     (a) Osteosarcoma

     (b) Ewing sarcoma/primitive neuroectodermal tumor

     (c) Malignant fibrous histiocytoma

d. Radiation therapy—External beam irradiation can be used for definitive control of the tumor in the following primary malignant bone tumors:

   i. Ewing sarcoma/primitive neuroectodermal tumor

   ii. Primary lymphoma of bone

   iii. Hemangioendothelioma

   iv. Solitary plasmacytoma of bone

III. Treatment of Soft-Tissue Tumors

A. Treatment is based on the biologic behavior and potential morbidity after removal of individual lesions.

B. Benign soft-tissue tumors

1. Observation—For inactive latent lesions. Many subcutaneous and deep lipomas are asymptomatic and require no treatment.

2. Simple excision—For active lesions with minimal risk for local recurrence.

a. Lipoma—for symptomatic superficial or deep lesions.

b. Schwannoma—Careful dissection of the tumor from the nerve fibers with an intralesional or marginal margin.

3. Wide excision—for lesions prone to local recurrence, such as extra-abdominal desmoid tumor (a benign, aggressive tumor). Extra-abdominal desmoid tumors should be removed with a wide margin.

C. Malignant soft-tissue tumors

1. Wide resection alone—Reserved for superficial low- or high-grade sarcomas that can be removed with a sufficient cuff of normal tissue.

2. Wide resection and external beam irradiation

 a. Used to minimize the risk of local failure. (Local recurrence is 5% to 10% if both wide resection and external beam irradiation are used.)

 b. The modalities below have equivalent local control rates but differing short- and long-term morbidities.

 i. Preoperative external beam irradiation followed by wide surgical resection

 (a) Higher risk of wound-healing complications (often prevented by soft-tissue reconstruction at the time of resection)

 (b) Lowest risk of long-term fibrosis

 (c) Lower total dose of irradiation (5,200 cGy)

 ii. Wide surgical resection with postoperative external beam irradiation

 (a) Lowest risk of wound-healing complications

 (b) Higher risk of long-term fibrosis

 (c) Higher dose of irradiation (6,200 to 6,600 cGy)

 iii. Wide surgical resection followed by brachytherapy (irradiation by radioactive seeds placed into plastic tubes implanted at the time of surgical resection)

 (a) Advantage: delivers all the irradiation during the hospital stay

 (b) Disadvantage: longer hospital stay

IV. Amputation

A. Amputation is sometimes indicated for malignant bone and soft-tissue tumors.

B. Indications for amputation

 1. The tumor cannot be completely removed by a limb-salvage procedure.

 2. The morbidity of the planned procedure is too high.

 3. Limb salvage will not result in a functional limb.

 4. The tumor continues to grow after preoperative chemotherapy or radiation.

 5. A major neurovascular bundle is involved. (This is a relative indication.)

Top Testing Facts

1. Chemotherapy drugs induce programmed cell death (apoptosis).

2. Radiation therapy induces DNA damage by the creation of free radicals.

3. Aspiration and injection is used for selected benign bone lesions—unicameral bone cyst of the humerus (methylprednisolone, bone marrow, or synthetic graft) and eosiniphilic granuloma (methylprednisolone).

4. Curettage and methylmethacrylate or bone graft for reconstruction is used for most benign bone tumors—giant cell tumor, chondroblastoma, osteoblastoma, chondromyxoid fibroma, and unicameral bone cyst of the proximal femur.

5. Wide surgical margins alone are used for sarcomas without effective adjuvant therapy—chondrosarcoma, adamantinoma, parosteal osteosarcoma.

6. The major benefit of chemotherapy in osteosarcoma and Ewing sarcoma is to reduce the risk of pulmonary metastases.

7. Radiation can be used as the definitive method for local control of primary lymphoma of bone, solitary plasmacytoma, hemangioendothelioma of bone, and Ewing sarcoma.

8. Simple excision is chosen for most benign soft-tissue tumors, with the exception of desmoid tumor (requires wide margins).

9. Preoperative irradiation for soft-tissue sarcomas results in less fibrosis but a higher risk of early wound complications compared to postoperative irradiation.

10. Amputation surgery criteria: (1) an adequate surgical margin cannot be achieved, (2) the morbidity is not acceptable, (3) the resulting limb will not be functional, (4) tumor growth continues after preoperative chemotherapy or irradiation, (5) the tumor involves major neurovascular bundles.

Bibliography

Kirsch DG, Hornicek FJ: Radiation therapy for soft-tissue sarcomas, in *Orthopaedic Knowledge Update: Musculoskeletal Tumors 2*. Rosemont, IL, American Academy of Orthopaedic Surgeons, 2007, pp 313-320.

Tuy BE: Adjuvant therapy for malignant bone tumors, in *Orthopaedic Knowledge Update: Musculoskeletal Tumors 2*. Rosemont, IL, American Academy of Orthopaedic Surgeons, 2007, pp 205-218.

4: Orthopaedic Oncology and Systemic Disease

Chapter 38

Benign Bone Tumors and Reactive Lesions

Kristy Weber, MD

I. Bone

A. Osteoid osteoma—A distinctive, painful, benign osteoblastic bone tumor.

1. Demographics

   a. Male to female ratio = 2:1

   b. The vast majority of patients are between 5 and 30 years of age.

2. Genetics/etiology

   a. Etiology is unclear, but nerve fibers associated with blood vessels within the nidus likely play a role in producing pain.

   b. High prostaglandin and cyclooxygenase levels within the lesion

3. Clinical presentation (**Table 1**)

   a. Classic symptom is night pain relieved by aspirin or nonsteroidal anti-inflammatory drugs (NSAIDs).

   b. The pain is progressive in its severity, can be referred to an adjacent joint, and may be present for months to years prior to diagnosis.

   c. Most common locations include femur, tibia, vertebral arch, humerus, and fingers; the proximal femur is the most common site, and the hip is the most common intra-articular location.

   d. Usually occurs in the diaphyseal or metaphyseal regions of long bones

   e. When an osteoid osteoma is the cause of a painful scoliosis, the lesion is usually at the center of the concavity of the curve.

   f. Osteoid osteomas cause extensive inflammatory symptoms in the adjacent tissues (joint effusions, contractures, limp, muscle atrophy).

4. Imaging appearance (**Figure 1**)

   a. Round, well-circumscribed intracortical lesion with radiolucent nidus

   b. Lesions usually <1 cm in diameter

   c. Extensive periosteal reaction may obscure the nidus (**Figure 1,** *A*).

   d. Lesions are occasionally intra-articular, subperiosteal, or medullary, and these cause less surrounding periosteal reaction.

   e. Radiographic differential diagnosis includes osteomyelitis and Ewing sarcoma.

   f. Intense and focal increased tracer uptake on technetium Tc 99m bone scans

   g. Thin-cut CT scan is often the key to diagnosis because it frequently identifies the small radiolucent nidus (**Figure 1,** *B*).

   h. MRI may show extensive surrounding edema (**Figure 1,** *C* and *D*).

5. Pathology

   a. Microscopic appearance consists of uniform, thin osteoid seams and immature trabeculae (**Figure 1,** *E* and *F*).

   b. Trabeculae are lined with uniform plump osteoblasts.

Table 1		

Factors Differentiating Osteoid Osteoma From Osteoblastoma

	Osteoid Osteoma	Osteoblastoma
Site	Diaphysis of long bone	Posterior elements of spine, metaphysis of long bone
Size	5-15 mm	>1.5 cm
Growth characteristics	Self-limited	Progressive
Symptoms	Exquisite pain, worse at night, relieved by aspirin	Dull ache

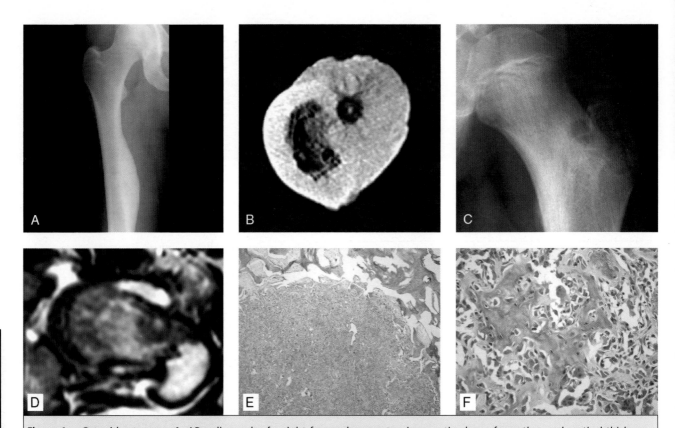

Figure 1 Osteoid osteomas. **A,** AP radiograph of a right femur shows extensive reactive bone formation and cortical thickening along the medial diaphysis. **B,** Axial thin-cut CT of the same patient shown in **A** reveals a clear radiolucent nidus with a central density that is classic for an osteoid osteoma. **C,** AP radiograph of a left femoral neck reveals a well-circumscribed subcortical lucency surrounded by sclerosis. **D,** MRI of the same patient shown in **C** reveals a nidus near the lateral cortex with surrounding edema. **E,** At low-power magnification, an osteoid osteoma has the histologic appearance of a sharply demarcated lesion (nidus) encased by dense cortical bone. **F,** High-power magnification shows osteoblastic rimming similar to that found in an osteoblastoma. The nuclei appear active but there is no pleomorphism. Marked vascularity is present within the stroma. *(Parts E and F reproduced from Schwartz HS [ed]:* Orthopaedic Knowledge Update: Musculoskeletal Tumors 2. *Rosemont, IL, American Academy of Orthopaedic Surgeons, 2007, p 95.)*

c. 1- to 2-mm fibrovascular rim surrounds the sharply demarcated nidus.

d. No pleomorphic cells, and the lesion does not infiltrate the surrounding bone

e. Similar in appearance to osteoblastoma but smaller in size (**Table 1**)

6. Treatment/outcome

a. Standard of care is percutaneous radiofrequency ablation (RFA) of the lesion. A CT-guided probe is inserted into the lesion with the temperature raised to 90°C for 4 to 6 minutes to produce a 1-cm zone of necrosis.

   i. Recurrence rates after RFA are <10%.

   ii. Contraindications include lesions close to the spinal cord or nerve roots.

b. Other surgical treatments have included surgical resection or burring, although the lesion must be localized preoperatively to identify its exact location.

c. In lesions around the hip, patients often require internal fixation, sometimes with bone grafting, if a large portion of cortex is removed with the lesion.

d. Long-term medical management with aspirin or NSAIDs can relieve symptoms after an average of 3 years because these lesions have self-limited growth.

e. Depending on the age of the child and duration of symptoms, removal of an osteoid osteoma associated with a painful scoliosis will allow resolution of the curve without further treatment.

B. Osteoblastoma—A rare, aggressive, benign osteoblastic tumor.

1. Demographics

a. Male to female ratio = 2:1

b. Osteoblastomas are much less common than osteoid osteomas.

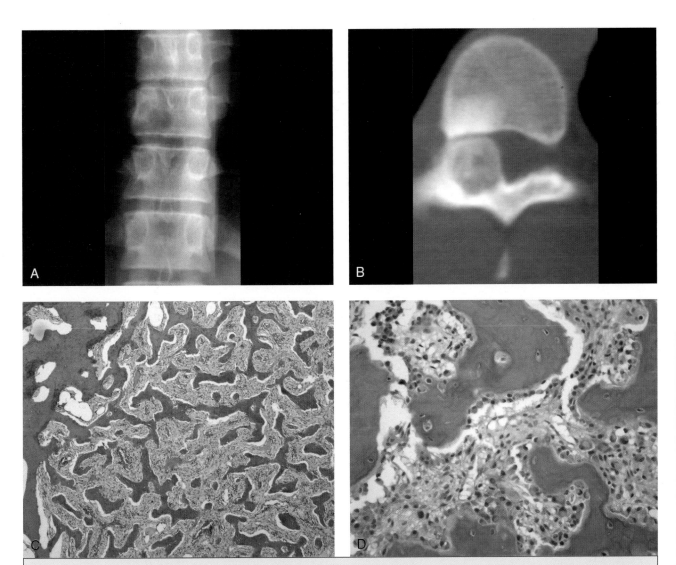

Figure 2   Osteoblastomas. **A,** AP radiograph of the lower portion of the thoracic spine of a 17-year-old boy shows a possible lesion on the right side of the T10 vertebra. **B,** A CT scan of the same patient shown in **A** better shows the location of the osteoblastoma in the pedicle of T10. **C,** The histologic appearance of an osteoblastoma shows interlacing trabeculae surrounded by fibrovascular connective tissue. The tumor merges into the normal bone at the periphery of the lesion. **D,** Higher power magnification shows osteoblastic rimming around the trabecular bone. The osteoblasts can appear plasmacytoid. (*Reproduced from Schwartz HS [ed]*: Orthopaedic Knowledge Update: Musculoskeletal Tumors 2. *Rosemont, IL, American Academy of Orthopaedic Surgeons, 2007, pp 87-102.*)

c. The vast majority of affected patients are between 10 and 30 years of age.

2. Genetics/etiology: unknown

3. Clinical presentation (**Table 1**)

   a. Slowly progressive dull, aching pain of long duration that is less severe than that from an osteoid osteoma

   b. Night pain is not typical, and aspirin does not classically relieve the symptoms.

   c. Neurologic symptoms can occur because the spine is the most common location for osteoblastoma (posterior elements) (**Figure 2,** *A* and *B*).

   d. Other locations include the diaphysis or metaphysis of long bones (tibia and femur) and the mandible.

   e. Related swelling, muscle atrophy, and a limp may occur because the lesions are large and present for a prolonged period of time.

   f. Osteoblastomas may be associated with oncogenic osteomalacia.

4. Imaging appearance

   a. Radiolucent lesion 2 to 10 cm in size with occasional intralesional densities

   b. Cortically based (two thirds) more often than medullary (one third)

4: Orthopaedic Oncology and Systemic Disease

c. Expansile with extension into the surrounding soft tissues and a rim of reactive bone around the lesion

d. 25% of the lesions have an extremely aggressive appearance and are mistaken for a malignancy.

e. Radiographic differential diagnosis includes osteosarcoma, aneurysmal bone cyst (ABC), osteomyelitis, and osteoid osteoma.

f. Three-dimensional imaging (CT, MRI) is necessary to fully evaluate the extent of the lesion prior to surgical treatment.

5. Pathology

a. Histology is similar to an osteoid osteoma but with increased giant cells.

b. Irregular seams of osteoid separated by loose fibrovascular stroma (**Figure 2**, *C*)

c. Osteoid is rimmed by prominent osteoblasts that are occasionally large and epithelioid (**Figure 2**, *D*).

d. Most commonly there is a sharp demarcation from the surrounding bone.

e. 10% to 40% are associated with secondary ABC formation.

f. Numerous mitotic figures may be present but are not atypical.

g. It is important to differentiate osteoblastoma from osteosarcoma, although giant cell tumor and ABC are also similar in appearance.

6. Treatment/outcome

a. Osteoblastoma is not self-limited and requires surgical treatment.

b. In most cases, curettage and bone grafting is adequate to achieve local control.

c. Nerve roots should be maintained when treating spinal lesions.

d. Occasionally, en bloc resection is required for lesions in the spine.

C. Parosteal osteoma—A rare, self-limited deposition of reactive bone on the surface of the cortex.

1. Demographics: adults, most commonly in their 30s or 40s

2. Genetics/etiology: no known cause, but often a history of trauma is reported

3. Clinical presentation

a. Long history of gradual swelling or dull pain

b. Occasionally, incidental radiographic findings are present.

c. Classically, osteomas are found in the craniofacial bones, but rare presentations in other parts of the skeleton include the long bones (tibia, femur), pelvis, and vertebrae.

d. Multiple osteomas are associated with Gardner syndrome (autosomal dominant), which also includes colonic polyps, fibromatosis, cutaneous lesions, and subcutaneous lesions.

4. Imaging appearance

a. Uniform radiodense lesion attached to the bone cortex with a broad base ranging from 1 to 8 cm in size (**Figure 3**, *A*)

b. Well-defined with smooth, lobulated borders

c. No cortical or medullary invasion (best noted on CT scan) (**Figure 3**, *B*)

d. Radiographic differential diagnosis includes parosteal osteosarcoma, healed stress fracture, and osteoid osteoma.

5. Pathology

a. Histologic appearance is of mature, hypocellular lamellar bone with intact Haversian systems.

b. No atypical cells are present.

6. Treatment/outcome

a. Nonsurgical treatment is preferred for incidental or minimally symptomatic lesions.

b. Biopsy should be performed if the diagnosis is unclear.

c. Local recurrence of the lesion suggests it was initially not recognized as a parosteal osteosarcoma.

D. Bone island (enostosis)—A usually small (but occasionally large) deposit of dense, compact bone within the medullary cavity.

1. Demographics: Bone islands occur frequently in adults, but their true incidence is unknown because they are usually found incidentally.

2. Genetics/etiology: Possible arrested resorption of mature bone during endochondral ossification

3. Clinical presentation

a. This nontumorous lesion is asymptomatic and found incidentally.

b. Any bone can be involved, but the pelvis and femur are most common.

c. Osteopoikilosis is a hereditary syndrome that manifests as hundreds of bone islands throughout the skeleton, usually centered about joints.

4. Radiographic appearance

a. Well-defined, round focus of dense bone

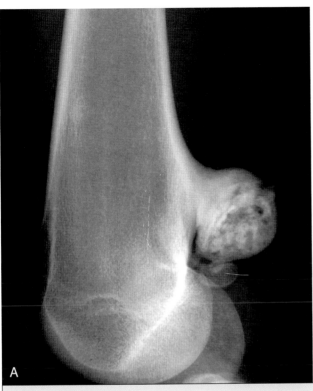 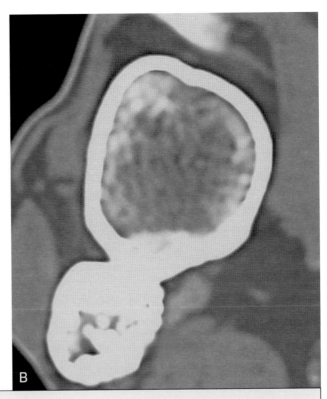

Figure 3 Parosteal osteoma. **A,** Lateral radiograph of the distal femur in a 37-year-old man reveals a heavily ossified surface lesion attached to the posterior femoral cortex. **B,** CT scan of the same patient reveals the relationship of the lesion to the cortex and differentiates it from myositis ossificans. An excisional biopsy revealed a parosteal osteoma.

within the medullary cavity usually measuring 2 to 20 mm in diameter (**Figure 4**)

b. Occasionally, radiating spicules of bone around the lesion that blend with the surrounding medullary cavity are present.

c. Approximately one third of lesions show increased activity on a bone scan.

d. No surrounding bony reaction or edema on T2-weighted MRI

e. Low intensity on T1- and T2-weighted MRI

f. Radiographic differential diagnosis includes well-differentiated osteosarcoma, osteoblastic metastasis, and bone infarct.

5. Pathology

a. Bone islands appear histologically as cortical bone with a well-defined lamellar structure and haversian systems.

b. Border between the lesion and surrounding medullary bone shows no endochondral ossification.

6. Treatment/outcome—No treatment is required, but follow-up radiographs should be taken if there is any question about the diagnosis.

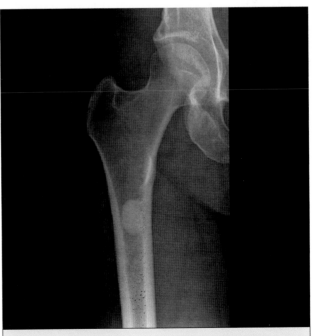

Figure 4 AP radiograph of the hip of an asymptomatic 45-year-old woman with a benign-appearing lesion in the proximal femur consistent with a bone island. (*Reproduced from Schwartz HS [ed]: Orthopaedic Knowledge Update: Musculoskeletal Tumors 2. Rosemont, IL, American Academy of Orthopaedic Surgeons, 2007, p 98.*)

4: Orthopaedic Oncology and Systemic Disease

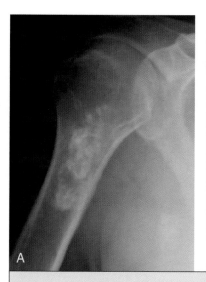
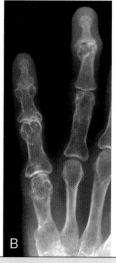
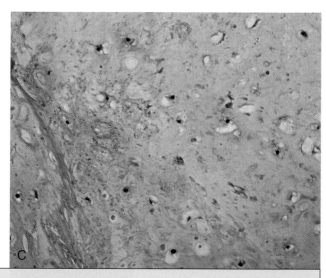

Figure 5   Enchondromas. **A,** AP radiograph of the right proximal humerus in a 49-year-old woman with shoulder pain reveals a calcified lesion in the metaphysis that is centrally located within the bone. The ring-like or stippled calcifications are consistent with an enchondroma. There is no endosteal erosion or cortical thickening. **B,** Radiograph demonstrating enchondromas in the hand of a patient with Ollier disease. Note the multiple expansile lytic lesions affecting the metacarpals and phalanges. Areas of calcified cartilage are evident within the lucent areas. **C,** Histologic appearance of an enchondroma. Note the normal chondrocytes in lacunar spaces with no mitotic figures. (*Part C reproduced from Schwartz HS [ed]:* Orthopaedic Knowledge Update: Musculoskeletal Tumors 2. *Rosemont, IL, American Academy of Orthopaedic Surgeons, 2007, p 111.*)

II. Cartilage

A. Enchondroma—A benign tumor comprised of mature hyaline cartilage and located in the medullary cavity.

1. Demographics

   a. Enchondromas can occur at all ages; most common in patients age 20 to 50 years.

   b. The incidence is unclear because most lesions are found incidentally.

2. Genetics/etiology—Enchondromas are thought to be related to incomplete endochondral ossification, where fragments of epiphyseal cartilage displace into the metaphysis during skeletal growth.

3. Clinical presentation

   a. Most enchondromas are asymptomatic and are noted incidentally when radiographs are taken for other reasons.

   b. Lesions in the small bones of the hands and feet can be painful, especially after pathologic fracture.

   c. When a patient presents with an enchondroma and pain in the adjacent joint, the pain often has a cause that is unrelated to the tumor.

   d. If the patient has pain and the radiographic appearance is suspicious, low-grade chondrosarcoma must be considered.

   e. Half of all enchondromas occur in the small tubular bones, with the vast majority in the hands; enchondromas are the most common bone tumor in the hand.

   f. Other common locations include the metaphysis or diaphysis of long bones (proximal humerus, distal femur, tibia); enchondromas are rare in the spine and pelvis.

   g. Enchondromas are classified by Enneking as inactive or latent bone lesions.

   h. The incidence of malignant transformation is <1%.

   i. A dedifferentiated chondrosarcoma rarely develops from an enchondroma.

4. Imaging appearance

   a. Enchondromas begin as well-defined, lucent, central medullary lesions that calcify over time; they appear more diaphyseal as the long bone grows.

   b. The classic radiographic appearance involves rings and stippled calcifications within the lesion (**Figure 5,** *A*).

   c. Lesions can be 1 to 10 cm in size.

   d. Small endosteal erosion (<50% width of the cortex) or cortical expansion may be present.

   e. The cortices in hand enchondromas may be thinned and expanded (**Figure 5,** *B*).

f. Cortical thickening or destruction suggests a chondrosarcoma.

g. The radiographic differential diagnosis includes a bone infarct and low-grade chondrosarcoma.

h. The radiographic appearance is more important than the pathologic appearance in differentiating an enchondroma from a low-grade chondrosarcoma.

i. Enchondromas frequently have increased uptake on bone scans due to continual remodeling of the endochondral bone within the lesion.

j. MRI is not necessary for diagnosis but shows the lesion as lobular and bright on T2-weighted images, with no bone marrow edema or periosteal reaction.

5. Pathology

a. The gross appearance is of blue-gray, lobulated hyaline cartilage with a variable amount of calcifications throughout the tumor.

b. The low-power histologic appearance is of mature hyaline cartilage lobules separated by normal marrow, which is key to differentiating an enchondroma from a chondrosarcoma.

c. Endochondral ossification encases the cartilage lobules with lamellar bone.

d. Lesions in the small tubular bones and proximal fibula are more hypercellular than lesions in other locations.

e. Enchondromas in long bones have abundant extracellular matrix but no myxoid component.

f. The cells are bland, with uniform, dark-stained nuclei; they have no pleomorphism, necrosis, mitoses, or multinucleate cells (**Figure 5**, C).

6. Treatment/outcome

a. Asymptomatic lesions require no treatment but should be followed with serial radiographs to ensure inactivity.

b. Rarely, when pain due to other causes is excluded, symptomatic enchondromas can be treated with curettage and bone grafting.

c. Pathologic fractures through enchondromas in small, tubular bones should be allowed to heal prior to curettage and bone grafting.

d. If radiographs are suspicious for a chondrosarcoma, then surgery is necessary.

e. A needle biopsy is not reliable to differentiate enchondroma from low-grade chondrosarcoma and should be used only if confirmation of tissue type is needed.

7. Related conditions: Ollier disease/Maffucci syndrome

a. Ollier disease is characterized by multiple enchondromas with a tendency toward unilateral involvement of the skeleton (sporadic inheritance).

b. Multiple enchondromas are thought to indicate a skeletal dysplasia with failure of normal endochondral ossification throughout the metaphyses of the affected bones.

c. Patients with multiple lesions have growth abnormalities causing shortening and bowing deformities.

d. Maffucci syndrome involves multiple enchondromas and soft-tissue angiomas.

e. Radiographically, the enchondromas have variable mineralization and often markedly expand the bone.

f. The angiomas in Maffucci syndrome can be identified on radiographs due to phleboliths (small, round calcified bodies).

g. The histologic appearance of lesions in a patient with multiple enchondromas is similar to solitary lesions in small tubular bones (hypercellular with mild chondrocytic atypia).

h. Patients with multiple enchondromas may require surgical correction of skeletal deformities at a young age.

i. There is an increased risk of malignant transformation of an enchondroma to a low-grade chondrosarcoma in patients with Ollier disease (25% to 30%).

j. Patients with Maffucci syndrome have an increased risk of malignant transformation of an enchondroma (23% to 100%) to a low-grade chondrosarcoma, as well as a high risk of developing a fatal visceral malignancy.

k. Patients with these syndromes need to be followed long-term because of the increased chance of malignancy.

B. Periosteal chondroma—A benign hyaline cartilage tumor located on the surface of the bone.

1. Demographics: Periosteal chondromas occur in patients from 10 to 30 years of age.

2. Genetics/etiology: These are rare lesions thought to arise from pluripotential cells deep in the periosteum that differentiate into chondroblasts instead of osteoblasts.

3. Clinical presentation

a. Patients present with pain, or sometimes the lesions are found incidentally in asymptomatic patients.

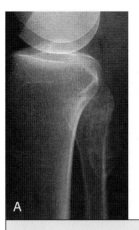 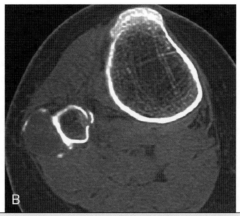 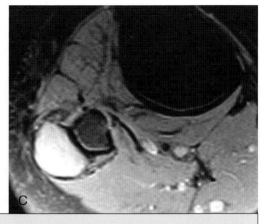

Figure 6 Periosteal chondroma. **A,** Lateral view of the right knee in a 28-year-old woman with lateral calf pain. Extraosseous calcification is seen around the proximal fibula. **B,** Axial CT reveals a surface lesion with a calcified rim and nondisplaced pathologic fracture in the fibula. **C,** MRI reveals bright signal on T2-weighted imaging and defines that this is a surface lesion without medullary involvement. A biopsy revealed a periosteal chondroma.

b. Any bone can be involved, but the proximal humerus, the femur, and the small bones of the hand are the most common locations.

c. The lesions can grow slowly after patients reach skeletal maturity but have no malignant potential.

4. Imaging appearance

a. The classic appearance is a well-defined surface lesion that creates a saucerized defect in the underlying cortex (**Figure 6**).

b. The lesion ranges from 1 to 5 cm in size and is metaphyseal or diaphyseal.

c. There is a rim of sclerosis in the underlying bone.

d. The edges of the lesion often have a mature buttress of bone.

e. The amount of calcification is variable, and soft-tissue swelling may be present because of the surface location.

f. The radiographic differential diagnosis includes periosteal chondrosarcoma and periosteal osteosarcoma.

5. Pathology

a. The low-power appearance is of well-circumscribed hyaline cartilage lobules.

b. The histologic appearance is similar to that of enchondroma, with mildly increased cellularity, binucleated cells, and occasional mild pleomorphism.

6. Treatment/outcome

a. No treatment is needed for asymptomatic patients.

b. Symptomatic patients are treated with excision with a marginal margin.

c. Local recurrence is rare.

C. Osteochondroma—A benign cartilage tumor arising from the surface of the bone.

1. Demographics

a. Osteochondromas are the most common benign bone tumor.

b. The true incidence of osteochondromas is unknown because most lesions are asymptomatic.

c. Most lesions are identified in the first two decades of life.

2. Genetics/etiology

a. Osteochondromas are hamartomatous proliferations of bone and cartilage.

b. They are thought to arise from trapped growth-plate cartilage that herniates through the cortex and grows via endochondral ossification beneath the periosteum.

c. A defect in the perichondrial node of Ranvier may allow the physeal growth to extend from the surface; as the cartilage ossifies, it forms cortical and cancellous bone that is the stalk of the lesion.

3. Clinical presentation

a. Most lesions are solitary and asymptomatic.

b. Most are <3 cm in size, but they can be as large as 15 cm.

c. Depending on size and location, patients can have pain from an inflamed overlying bursa, fracture of the stalk, or nerve compression.

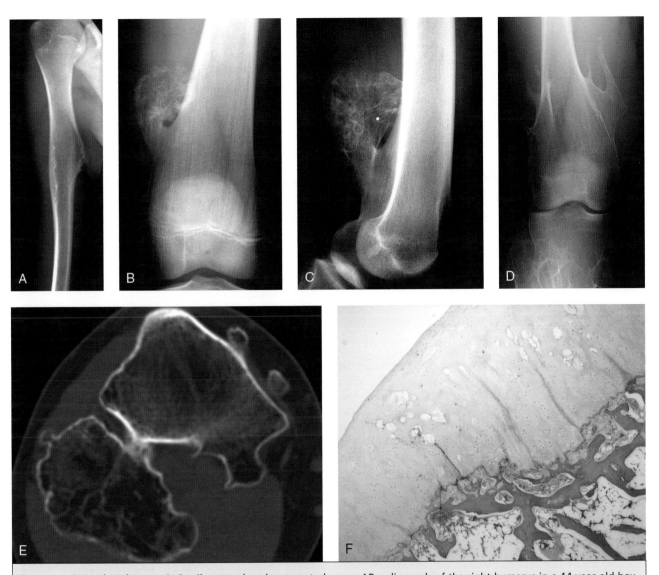

Figure 7 Osteochondromas. **A,** Sessile osteochondroma noted on an AP radiograph of the right humerus in a 14-year-old boy. AP (**B**) and lateral (**C**) radiographs of the distal femur in an 11-year-old boy reveal a pedunculated osteochondroma of the medial distal femur. The medullary portion of the lesional stalk is continuous with the medullary cavity of the distal femur. There is cortical sharing. **D,** AP radiograph of the right knee in an 18-year-old man with multiple hereditary osteochondromas. Note the multiple small lesions and the widened metaphysis. **E,** Axial CT scan of the same patient shown in **E** shows the posteromedial extension of a lesion in the proximal fibula. **F,** At low-power magnification, the histologic appearance of an osteochondroma shows the cartilage cap with the cartilage cells arranged in columns similar to a growth plate. (*Part F reproduced from Schwartz HS [ed]:* Orthopaedic Knowledge Update: Musculoskeletal Tumors 2. *Rosemont, IL, American Academy of Orthopaedic Surgeons, 2007, p 106.*)

d. When close to the skin surface, they are firm, immobile masses.

e. Osteochondromas continue to grow until the patient reaches skeletal maturity.

f. The lesions most commonly occur around the knee (distal femur, proximal tibia), proximal humerus, and pelvis; spinal lesions (posterior elements) are rare.

g. Subungual exostosis arises from beneath the nail in the distal phalanx; this is a posttraumatic lesion and not a true osteochondroma.

h. Patients can present with multiple lesions (multiple hereditary exostosis).

i. The risk of malignant degeneration of a solitary osteochondroma to a chondrosarcoma is <1%.

j. Rarely, a dedifferentiated chondrosarcoma can develop from a solitary osteochondroma.

4. Imaging appearance

a. Osteochondromas can be sessile or pedunculated on the bone surface (**Figure 7, A**).

b. There is a higher risk of malignant degeneration in sessile lesions.

c. Lesions arise near the growth plate and appear to become more diaphyseal with time.

d. Pedunculated lesions grow away from the adjacent joint (**Figure 7**, *B* and *C*).

e. The medullary cavity of the bone is continuous with the stalk of the lesion.

f. The cortex of the underlying bone is continuous with the cortex of the stalk.

g. The affected bony metaphysis is often flared or widened.

h. The cartilage cap is usually radiolucent and involutes at skeletal maturity.

i. Metaplastic cartilage nodules can occur within a bursa over the cartilage cap.

j. The radiographic differential diagnosis includes parosteal osteosarcoma and myositis ossificans.

k. CT or MRI scans can better evaluate the cartilage cap and are useful when malignant degeneration is a concern.

5. Pathology

a. The gross appearance of a pedunculated lesion is similar to a cauliflower, with cancellous bone beneath the cartilage cap.

b. Histologically, the cartilage cap consists of hyaline cartilage and is organized like a growth plate with maturation to bony trabeculae (**Figure 7**, *F*).

c. There is a well-defined perichondrium around the cartilage cap.

d. The stalk consists of cortical and trabecular bone with spaces between the bone filled with marrow.

e. The chondrocytes within the lesion are uniform, without pleomorphism or multiple nuclei.

f. Thick cartilage caps imply growth but are not a reliable indicator of malignant degeneration.

6. Treatment/outcome

a. For asymptomatic or minimally symptomatic patients who are still growing, nonsurgical treatment is preferred.

b. Relative indications for surgical excision of an osteochondroma (performed by excision at the base of the stalk)

i. Symptoms secondary to soft-tissue inflammation (bursae, muscles, joint capsule, tendons)

ii. Symptoms secondary to frequent traumatic injury

iii. Significant cosmetic deformity

iv. Symptoms secondary to nerve or vascular irritation

v. Concern for malignant transformation

c. The perichondrium over the cartilage cap must be removed to decrease the likelihood of local recurrence.

d. Delaying surgical excision until skeletal maturity allows a higher chance of local control.

e. Patients with osteochondromas extending into the popliteal fossa can have pseudoaneurysms and are subject to vascular injury during excision.

7. Related condition: multiple hereditary exostoses

a. This is a skeletal dysplasia that is inherited with an autosomal dominant pattern.

b. Patients may have up to 30 osteochondromas throughout the skeleton.

c. The *EXT1*, *EXT2*, and *EXT3* are three genetic loci associated with this disorder.

d. Mutations in these genes are found in most affected patients, and they are considered tumor-suppressor genes.

e. Clinically, the patients have skeletal deformities and short stature.

f. The lesions are similar radiographically and histologically to solitary osteochondromas.

g. Radiographs reveal primarily sessile lesions that may grow to a very large size.

h. Metaphyseal widening is present in affected patients (**Figure 7**, *D* and *E*).

i. Deformities occur due to disorganized endochondral ossification in the growth plate and may require surgical correction, especially in the paired bones (radius/ulna, tibia/fibula).

j. The risk of malignant transformation is higher (~5% to 10%) in patients with this condition.

k. The most common location of a secondary chondrosarcoma is the pelvis. Usually the malignant tumors are low grade.

D. Chondroblastoma—A rare, benign bone tumor differentiated from giant cell tumor by its chondroid matrix.

1. Demographics

a. Male to female ratio = 2:1

b. 80% of patients are younger than 25 years.

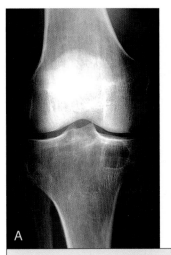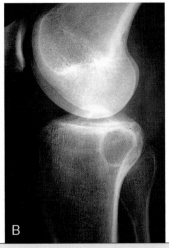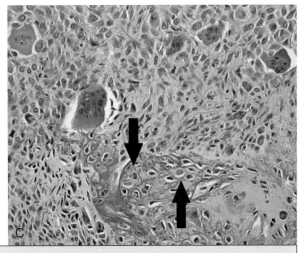

Figure 8 Chondroblastoma. AP (**A**) and lateral (**B**) views of the right knee in a 19-year-old man show a well-circumscribed round lesion in the proximal tibial epiphysis extending slightly into the metaphysis. Note the sclerotic rim. **C**, Histologic appearance of a chondroblastoma. Note the round or oval chondroblasts (arrows). On higher power, areas of dystrophic calcification are visible around the individual cells in a "chicken-wire" pattern. (*Part C reproduced from Schwartz HS [ed]:* Orthopaedic Knowledge Update: Musculoskeletal Tumors 2. *Rosemont, IL, American Academy of Orthopaedic Surgeons, 2007, p 116.*)

2. Genetics/etiology

   a. Chondroblastoma has been categorized as a cartilage tumor due to its areas of chondroid matrix, but type II collagen is not expressed by the tumor cells.

   b. It is thought to arise from the cartilaginous epiphyseal plate.

3. Clinical presentation

   a. Patients present with pain that is progressive at the site of the tumor.

   b. As these tumors often occur adjacent to a joint, there can be decreased range of motion, a limp, muscle atrophy, and tenderness over the affected bone.

   c. Most chondroblastomas are found in the distal femur and proximal tibia, followed by proximal humerus, proximal femur, calcaneus, and flat bones.

   d. <1% develop benign pulmonary metastasis from chondroblastoma.

4. Imaging appearance

   a. Chondroblastomas are small, round tumors that occur in the epiphysis or apophysis; they often extend into the metaphysis (**Figure 8,** *A* and *B*).

   b. Most are 1 to 4 cm in size and have a sclerotic rim.

   c. Most are centrally located in the epiphysis, with a small subset having a more aggressive appearance due to secondary ABC formation.

   d. Cortical expansion of the bone may be present, but soft-tissue extension is rare.

   e. 25% to 40% of chondroblastomas have stippled calcifications within the lesion.

   f. The differential diagnosis includes giant cell tumor, osteomyelitis, and clear cell chondrosarcoma.

   g. Three-dimensional imaging is not required, but a CT scan defines the bony extent of the lesion.

   h. MRI shows extensive edema surrounding the lesion.

5. Pathology

   a. The tumor consists of a background of mononuclear cells, scattered multinucleated giant cells, and focal areas of chondroid matrix.

   b. The mononuclear stromal cells are distinct, round, S100+ cells with large central nuclei that can appear similar to histiocytes; the nuclei have a longitudinal groove resembling a coffee bean (**Figure 8,** *C*).

   c. Chicken-wire calcifications are present in a lace-like pattern throughout the tumor.

   d. Mitotic figures are present but not atypical.

   e. One third of chondroblastomas have areas of secondary ABC.

6. Treatment/outcome

   a. Curettage and bone grafting is indicated for the treatment of chondroblastoma.

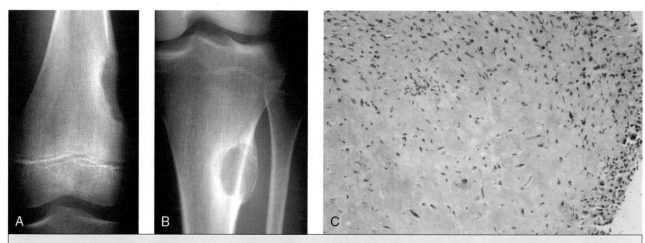

Figure 9   Chondromyxoid fibromas. **A**, AP radiograph of the right distal femur in a 12-year-old boy with knee pain shows an eccentric lytic lesion with a well-defined intramedullary border. A periosteal shell that is not easily seen is consistent with a chondromyxoid fibroma. **B,** AP radiograph of the proximal tibia in a 22-year-old woman with an eccentric lesion expanding the cortex with a visible rim. **C,** The histologic appearance of a chondromyxoid fibroma shows hypercellular regions at the periphery of the lobules. Note the spindled, stellate cells and myxoid stroma.

b. Adjuvants such as phenol or liquid nitrogen are often used to decrease local recurrence.

c. The local recurrence rate is 10% to 15%.

d. Surgical resection is indicated for rare benign pulmonary metastasis.

E. Chondromyxoid fibroma (CMF)—A rare, benign cartilage tumor containing chondroid, fibrous, and myxoid tissue.

1. Demographics

   a. Most CMFs occur in the second and third decades of life, but they may be seen in patients up to 75 years of age.

   b. There is a slight male predominance.

2. Genetics/etiology—CMF is thought to arise from remnants of the growth plate.

3. Clinical presentation

   a. Most patients present with pain and mild swelling of the affected area.

   b. Occasionally the lesions are noted incidentally.

   c. The most common locations are the long bones of the lower extremities (proximal tibia) and pelvis. Small bones in the hands and feet are also affected.

4. Imaging appearance

   a. CMF is a lucent, eccentric lesion found in the metaphysis of long bones (**Figure 9**, *A*).

   b. It can cause thinning and expansion of the adjacent cortical bone (**Figure 9**, *B*).

   c. It often has a sharp, scalloped sclerotic rim.

d. Radiographic calcifications within the lesion are rare.

e. CMF ranges in size from 2 to 10 cm.

f. The radiographic differential diagnosis includes ABC, chondroblastoma, and nonossifying fibroma.

g. There is increased tracer uptake within the lesion on bone scan.

5. Pathology

   a. On low power, the lesion is lobulated with peripheral hypercellularity.

   b. Within the lobules, the cells are spindled or stellate with hyperchromatic nuclei.

   c. Between the lobules are multinucleated giant cells and fibrovascular tissue.

   d. Areas of myxoid stroma are present, but hyaline cartilage is rare (**Figure 9**, *C*).

   e. The cellular areas may resemble chondroblastoma.

   f. Areas with pleomorphic cells with bizarre nuclei are common.

   g. The histologic differential diagnosis includes chondroblastoma, enchondroma, and chondrosarcoma.

6. Treatment/outcome

   a. CMF is treated with curettage and bone grafting.

   b. The local recurrence rate is 10% to 20%.

III. Fibrous/Histiocytic

A. Nonossifying fibroma (NOF)—A developmental abnormality related to faulty ossification rather than a true neoplasm.

1. Demographics

   a. Very common skeletal lesions

   b. Occur in children and adolescents (age 5 to 15 years)

   c. 30% of children with open physes have nonossifying fibromas.

   d. Also frequently called fibrous cortical defect or metaphyseal fibrous defect

2. Genetics/etiology—Possibly caused by abnormal subperiosteal osteoclastic resorption during remodeling of the metaphysis.

3. Clinical presentation

   a. Usually an incidental finding

   b. May be multifocal

      i. Familial multifocal

      ii. Neurofibromatosis

      iii. Jaffe-Campanacci syndrome (congenital with café au lait pigmentation, mental retardation, and nonskeletal abnormalities involving heart, eyes, gonads)

   c. Most common in long bones of lower extremity (80%)

   d. Patients occasionally present with a pathologic fracture.

4. Radiographic appearance

   a. Eccentric, lytic, cortically based lesions with a sclerotic rim (**Figure 10,** A and B)

   b. Occur in the metaphysis and appear to migrate to diaphysis as bone grows

   c. May thin the overlying cortex with expansion of the bone

   d. Lesions enlarge (1 to 7 cm) as patient grows.

   e. As patient reaches skeletal maturity, the lesions ossify and become sclerotic.

   f. Occasionally associated with secondary ABC

   g. Plain radiographs are diagnostic.

   h. A lesion similar in appearance to a nonossifying fibroma on the posteromedial aspect of the distal femur is an avulsive cortical irregularity, which is the result of an avulsion injury at the insertion of the adductor magnus muscle.

5. Pathology

   a. Prominent storiform pattern of fibrohistiocytic cells (**Figure 10,** C and D)

   b. Variable numbers of giant cells

   c. May have areas of xanthomatous reaction with foamy histiocytes

   d. Prominent hemosiderin

   e. Occasional secondary ABC component

6. Treatment/outcome

   a. Most treated with observation; will spontaneously regress

   b. Monitor along with skeletal growth if they are large lesions.

   c. When symptomatic and large, curettage and bone grafting is often necessary

   d. For pathologic fractures, often allow to heal, then observe or curettage/graft

   e. Internal fixation rarely needed, depending on anatomic location

B. Fibrous dysplasia—A common developmental abnormality characterized by hamartomatous proliferation of fibro-osseous tissue within the bone.

1. Demographics

   a. Can be found in any age, but ~75% in patients <30 years

   b. Affects females more than males

2. Genetics/etiology

   a. Solitary focal or generalized multifocal inability to produce mature lamellar bone

   b. Areas of the skeleton remain indefinitely as immature, poorly mineralized trabeculae.

   c. Not inherited

   d. Monostotic and polyostotic forms associated with activating mutations of GSα on chromosome 20q13, which produce a sustained activation of adenylate cyclase cAMP.

   e. Fibrous dysplasia tissue has high expression of fibroblast growth factor (FGF)-23, which may be the cause of hypophosphatemia in patients with McCune-Albright syndrome or oncogenic osteomalacia.

3. Clinical presentation

   a. Usually asymptomatic and found incidentally

   b. Can be monostotic or polyostotic

   c. Affects any bone, but predilection for proximal femur, rib, maxilla, tibia

4: Orthopaedic Oncology and Systemic Disease

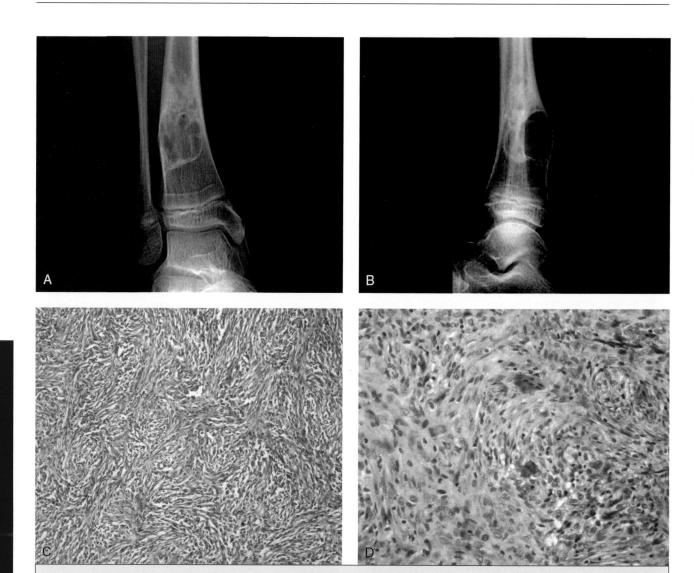

Figure 10 Nonossifying fibromas. AP (**A**) and lateral (**B**) radiographs of the distal tibia in an 11-year-old boy reveal a nonossifying fibroma that has healed after a minimally displaced pathologic fracture. It is an eccentric, scalloped lesion with a sclerotic rim. Anteriorly, the lesion is filling in with bone. **C,** Histologic appearance of a nonossifying fibroma. Bands of collagen fibers and fibroblasts can be seen coursing throughout the lesion. **D,** High-power magnification of the same specimen shown in **C** reveals multinucleated giant cells and hemosiderin-laden histiocytes that are characteristic of an NOF. (*Parts C and D reproduced from Schwartz HS [ed]:* Orthopaedic Knowledge Update: Musculoskeletal Tumors 2. *Rosemont, IL, American Academy of Orthopaedic Surgeons, 2007, p 122.*)

d. Fatigue fractures through lesion can cause pain.

e. May have swelling around lesion

f. Severe cranial deformities, blindness with craniofacial involvement

g. Patients occasionally present with pathologic fracture

h. McCune-Albright syndrome

　i. Triad of polyostotic fibrous dysplasia, precocious puberty, and pigmented skin lesions (coast of Maine)

　ii. Unilateral bone lesions

　iii. Skin lesions usually on same side as bone lesions

　iv. 3% of patients with polyostotic fibrous dysplasia

i. Myriad endocrine abnormalities with polyostotic forms

j. Most common entity causing oncogenic osteomalacia (renal phosphate wasting due to FGF-23)

k. Mazabraud syndrome is fibrous dysplasia (usually polyostotic) associated with soft-tissue intramuscular myxomas.

4. Radiographic appearance

   a. Central lytic lesions within the medullary canal—usually diaphysis/metaphysis

   b. Sclerotic rim

   c. May be expansile with cortical thinning

   d. "Ground glass" or "shower-door glass" appearance (**Figure 11**, *A*)

   e. Bowing deformity in proximal femur (shepherd's crook) or tibia

   f. Can see vertebral collapse and kyphoscoliosis

   g. Long lesion in a long bone (**Figure 11**, *B*)

   h. Increased activity on bone scan, but plain radiographs usually diagnostic

5. Pathology

   a. Gross: yellow-white gritty tissue

   b. Histology: poorly mineralized immature fibrous tissue surrounding islands of irregular, often poorly mineralized trabeculae of woven bone (**Figure 11**, *C*)

   c. "Chinese letters" or "alphabet soup" appearance

   d. Metaplastic bone arises from fibrous tissue without osteoblastic rimming.

   e. Common mitoses

   f. May have metaplastic cartilage present or areas of cystic degeneration

   g. Can be associated with secondary ABC

   h. Differential diagnosis includes low-grade intramedullary osteosarcoma.

6. Treatment/outcome

   a. Asymptomatic patients may be observed.

   b. Surgical indications include painful lesions, impending/actual pathologic fracture, severe deformity, neurologic compromise (spine).

   c. Curettage and bone-graft the lesion. (Use cortical allograft, not cancellous autograft!)

   d. Cancellous autografts are replaced by dysplastic bone.

   e. Usually requires internal fixation to achieve pain control (intramedullary device more effective than plate) in the lower extremity

   f. Osteotomies for deformity

   g. Medical treatment with bisphosphonates provided good pain relief in small series.

   h. In ~1% of lesions, malignant transformation to osteosarcoma, fibrosarcoma, or malignant

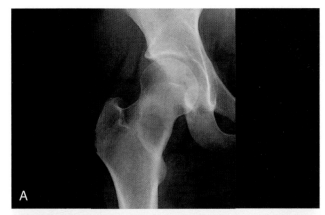

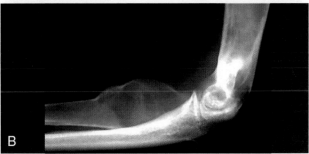

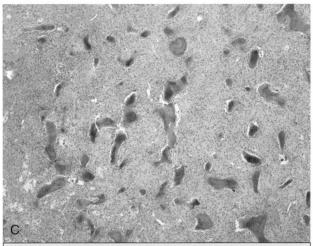

Figure 11 Fibrous dysplasia. **A,** AP radiograph of the right proximal femur in an 18-year-old woman with groin pain. A central, lytic bone lesion with a ground glass appearance fills the femoral neck, consistent with fibrous dysplasia. **B,** A lateral radiograph of an elbow reveals an expansile lesion in the proximal radius with a ground glass appearance. There is no evidence of cortical destruction. **C,** Histologic appearance on intermediate magnification. Metaplastic bone spicules can be seen scattered haphazardly; this pattern produces the characteristic radiographic ground glass appearance of fibrous dysplasia. *(Part B reproduced from Prichard DJ [ed]:* 1999 Musculoskeletal Tumors and Diseases Self-Assessment Examination. *Rosemont, IL, American Academy of Orthopaedic Surgeons, 1999 question 91, figure 66b. Part C reproduced from Schwartz HS [ed]:* Orthopaedic Knowledge Update: Musculoskeletal Tumors 2. *Rosemont, IL, American Academy of Orthopaedic Surgeons, 2007, p 125.)*

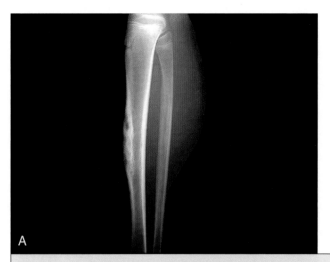
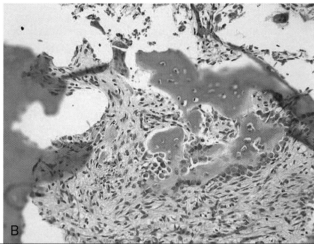

Figure 12   Osteofibrous dysplasia. **A,** Lateral radiograph of the tibia in a skeletally immature patient reveals a cortically based lytic lesion. There are multiple lucencies surrounded by dense sclerosis consistent with osteofibrous dysplasia. There is no periosteal reaction. **B,** A high-power histologic section reveals woven bone arising from a fibrous stroma. The new bone is prominently rimmed by osteoblasts, thereby differentiating this from fibrous dysplasia. *(Reproduced with permission from Scarborough MT [ed]: 2005 Musculoskeletal Tumors and Diseases Self-Assessment Examination. Rosemont, IL, American Academy of Orthopaedic Surgeons, 2005, question 64, figures 35b and 35c.)*

fibrous histiocytoma occurs, with extremely poor prognosis.

C. Osteofibrous dysplasia—A nonneoplastic fibro-osseous lesion affecting the long bones of young children.

   1. Demographics

      a. Affects males more than females

      b. Usually noted in first decade of life

   2. Genetics/etiology: Trisomy 7, 8, 12, and 22 have been reported.

   3. Clinical presentation

      a. Unique predilection for the tibia

      b. Can have anterior or anterolateral bowing deformity

      c. Pseudarthrosis develops in 10% to 30% of patients.

      d. Patients usually present with painless swelling over anterior border of tibia.

   4. Radiographic appearance

      a. Eccentric, well-defined anterior tibial lytic lesions (**Figure 12,** *A*)

      b. Usually diaphyseal

      c. Single or multiple lucent areas surrounded by dense sclerosis

      d. Confined to the anterior cortex; may expand

      e. No periosteal reaction

      f. Differential diagnosis: adamantinoma (radiographic appearance can be identical)

   5. Pathology

      a. Moderately cellular fibroblastic stroma

      b. Islands of woven bone with prominent osteoblastic rimming (**Figure 12,** *B*)

      c. No cellular atypia

      d. May have giant cells

      e. Differential diagnosis: fibrous dysplasia

   6. Treatment/outcome

      a. Avoid surgery if possible; brace when necessary.

      b. Lesions may spontaneously regress or stabilize at skeletal maturity.

      c. May need deformity correction

      d. Controversy whether there is a continuum from osteofibrous dysplasia to adamantinoma, but the exact nature of this relationship is uncertain

D. Desmoplastic fibroma—An extremely rare benign bone tumor composed of dense bundles of fibrous connective tissue.

   1. Demographics—Most common in patients age 10 to 30 years.

   2. Genetics/etiology

      a. Bone counterpart of the aggressive fibromatosis (desmoid) in soft tissue; may originate from myofibroblasts

b. Loss of 5q21-22 (gene location for familial adenomatous polyposis and Gardner syndrome) has been reported.

c. Loss of 4p and rearrangement of 12q12-13, and trisomy 8 (0%-33%), trisomy 20 (2%-25%), or both (0%-16%)

3. Clinical presentation

   a. Can occur in any bone

   b. Intermittent pain unrelated to activity

   c. Palpable mass/swelling

4. Imaging appearance

   a. Lytic lesion centrally located in metaphysis

   b. Honeycomb/trabeculated appearance (**Figure 13**)

   c. Usually no periosteal reaction unless a fracture is present (12%)

   d. May appear aggressive with cortical destruction and soft-tissue extension

   e. No calcification within lesion

   f. Increased activity on bone scan

5. Pathology

   a. Gross: dense, white, scarlike tissue

   b. Histology: abundant collagen fibrils with intermixed spindle cells

   c. Appearance is hypocellular and similar to scar tissue.

   d. Monotonous uniform nuclei

   e. Infiltrative growth pattern—trapping native trabeculae

   f. Differential diagnosis includes low-grade fibrosarcoma.

6. Treatment/outcome

   a. Surgical treatment is the standard of care.

   b. Thorough curettage allows good results.

   c. Wide resection for expendable bones or locally recurrent lesions

   d. Desmoplastic fibromas do not metastasize, but they often recur locally.

E. Langerhans cell histiocytosis—A clonal proliferation of Langerhans-type histiocytes that can have multiple clinical presentations.

   1. Demographics

      a. Most common in children (80% < 20 years of age)

      b. Male to female ratio = 2:1

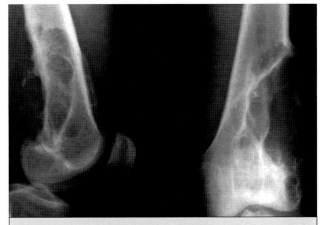

Figure 13   Lateral (left) and AP (right) radiographs of the distal femur reveal a lytic lesion expanding the posterolateral cortex and having an internal honeycomb appearance. This is consistent with the aggressive behavior of a desmoplastic fibroma.

2. Genetics/etiology: N/A

3. Clinical presentation

   a. Previously categorized as eosinophilic granuloma, Hand-Schuller-Christian disease (chronic, disseminated), and Letterer-Siwe disease (infantile, acute)

   b. Now believed to be three scenarios

      i. Solitary disease (eosinophilic granuloma)

      ii. Multiple bony sites

      iii. Multiple bony sites with visceral involvement (lungs, liver, spleen, skin, lymph nodes)

   c. Rarely, bone lesions are asymptomatic; usually, they cause localized pain/swelling/limp.

   d. Can occur in any bone but most commonly skull, ribs, clavicle, scapula, vertebrae (thoracic > lumbar > cervical), long bones, pelvis

4. Radiographic appearance

   a. Classic appearance is a "punched-out" lytic lesion (**Figure 14, A**).

   b. May have thick periosteal reaction

   c. Can appear well-demarcated or permeative (**Figure 14, B**)

   d. Commonly causes vertebral collapse (vertebra plana) when affecting the spine (**Figure 14, C**)

   e. Great mimicker of other lesions (osteomyelitis, Ewing sarcoma, leukemia)

5. Pathology

   a. The characteristic tumor cell is the Langerhans cell or histiocyte (**Figure 14, D**).

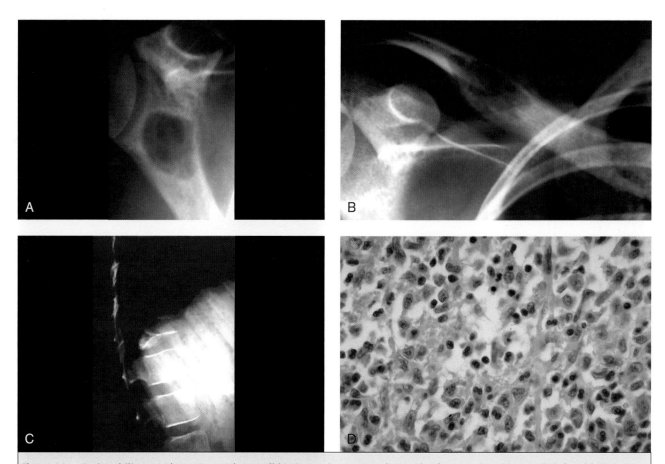

Figure 14 Eosinophilic granulomas/Langerhans cell histiocytosis. **A,** AP radiograph of a scapula with a well-defined lytic lesion having a classic "punched-out" appearance of an eosinophilic granuloma. **B,** AP radiograph of a lytic lesion in the right clavicle of a child demonstrates cortical expansion, periosteal reaction, and no sclerotic edges. This is an eosinophilic granuloma, but the radiographic appearance can also be consistent with osteomyelitis or Ewing sarcoma. **C,** A lateral radiograph of the thoracic spine shows the classic appearance of vertebra plana in a patient with eosinophilic granuloma. **D,** Histologic appearance of an eosinophilic granuloma shows a mixed inflammatory infiltrate with Langerhans histiocytes having large indented nuclei, lymphocytes, and eosinophils. *(Part C reproduced from Prichard DJ [ed]: 1999 Musculoskeletal Tumors and Diseases Self-Assessment Examination. Rosemont, IL, American Academy of Orthopaedic Surgeons, 1999, question 57, figure 44b.)*

b. Histiocytes have indented nuclei (coffee bean) with eosinophilic cytoplasm.

c. Histiocytes stain with CD1A.

d. Giant cells are present.

e. Eosinophils are variable in number.

f. Mixed inflammatory cell infiltrate

g. Birbeck granules on electron microscopy (tennis rackets)

6. Treatment/outcome

a. Solitary lesions can be treated effectively with an intralesional injection of methylprednisolone acetate.

b. Curettage/bone grafting if open biopsy is being performed for diagnosis

c. In 90% of patients with vertebra plana due to Langerhans cell histiocytosis, bracing alone will correct the deformity; 10% will need corrective surgery.

d. Low-dose radiation is used in rare cases (spinal cord compression).

e. Patients with disseminated disease and visceral involvement can die of the disease. The prognosis is improving with more effective chemotherapy but worsens with increasing number of extraosseous sites of disease.

IV. Cystic

A. Unicameral bone cyst (UBC)—A common, serous fluid–filled bone lesion.

1. Demographics—Most cases occur in patients younger than 20 years.

Table 2

Comparison of Clinical Presentation of Unicameral Bone Cysts and Aneurysmal Bone Cysts

	Unicameral Bone Cyst	Aneurysmal Bone Cyst
Presentation	Pathologic fracture	Pain, swelling
Common locations	Proximal humerus Proximal femur	Distal femur, proximal tibia Pelvis Posterior elements of spine
Radiographic characteristics	Central, lytic lesion Metaphyseal Symmetric expansion less than width of growth plate	Eccentric, lytic lesion Metaphyseal Can expand wider than growth plate Extends into soft tissues with a thin periosteal rim
Treatment	Intralesional steroid injection Curettage/grafting/internal fixation (proximal femur)	Curettage and bone grafting Embolization (spine, pelvis, etc)

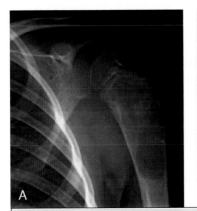
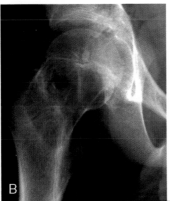
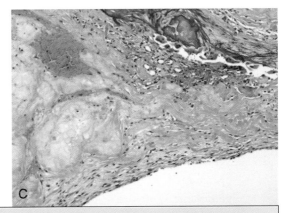

Figure 15 Unicameral bone cysts. **A,** AP radiograph of the proximal humerus in a 5-year-old girl shows a lytic lesion centrally located in the medullary canal of the metaphysis consistent with a unicameral bone cyst. The lesion does not expand the bone wider than the epiphyseal plate. The girl had had a prior pathologic fracture through the lesion. **B,** AP radiograph of a proximal femur demonstrates a lytic lesion in the metaphysis abutting the proximal femoral epiphyseal plate. The lesion is central in location and will likely require surgical treatment because of the high risk of fracture. **C,** Histologic appearance. A thin cyst lining consisting of fibroblasts is seen. Cementum is noted in the wall and no cellular atypia is present. (*Part C reproduced from Schwartz HS [ed]:* Orthopaedic Knowledge Update: Musculoskeletal Tumors 2. *Rosemont, IL, American Academy of Orthopaedic Surgeons, 2007, p 91.*)

4: Orthopaedic Oncology and Systemic Disease

2. Genetics/etiology

   a. Thought to result from a temporary failure of medullary bone formation near the epiphyseal plate during skeletal growth

   b. The cyst is active initially when adjacent to the growth plate. When medullary bone formation resumes, the cyst appears to move into the diaphysis.

   c. Possible causes and precursor lesions include lymphatic/venous obstruction, intraosseous hematoma, or intraosseous synovial rest.

3. Clinical presentation (**Table 2**)

   a. Most common presentation is a pathologic fracture after minor trauma.

   b. Painful symptoms resolve when fracture heals.

   c. Most common locations include the proximal humerus and proximal femur, but UBCs can occur in the ilium and calcaneus.

4. Imaging appearance

   a. Purely lytic lesion located centrally in the medullary canal

   b. UBCs start metaphyseal, adjacent to the growth plate, and appear to progress toward the diaphysis with bone growth (**Figure 15**, *A*).

   c. Narrow zone of transition between cyst and normal bone

   d. Cortical thinning but no soft-tissue extension (**Figure 15**, *B*)

   e. Bone expansion does not exceed width of the physis.

f. Trabeculations occur after multiple fractures.

g. "Fallen leaf" sign is pathognomonic (fallen cortical fragment into base of empty lesion).

h. Plain radiographs are usually diagnostic, but MRI shows a well-defined zone of bright uniform signal on T2-weighted images.

5. Pathology

a. Lining of the cyst is a thin fibrous membrane: no true endothelial cells (**Figure 15, C**).

b. Giant cells, inflammatory cells, hemosiderin within lining

c. Clear or serous fluid within cavity (bloody after fracture)

d. 10% contain cementum spherules (calcified eosinophilic fibrinous material) in the lining.

6. Treatment/outcome

a. Natural history is to fill in with bone as the patient reaches skeletal maturity.

b. After acute fractures, the lesion will occasionally fill in with native bone (15%).

c. Standard treatment is intralesional injection of methylprednisolone acetate.

d. May require multiple injections, especially in very young children

e. Proximal femoral lesions with or without a pathologic fracture often treated with curettage/bone grafting/internal fixation

B. Aneurysmal bone cyst (ABC)—A destructive, expansile reactive bone lesion filled with multiple blood-filled cavities.

1. Demographics—75% of patients are <20 years of age.

2. Genetics/etiology

a. Reactive, nonneoplastic process of unknown etiology

b. Possibilities include a traumatic origin or a circulatory disturbance leading to increased venous pressure and hemorrhage.

c. Can arise de novo or be associated with an underlying lesion that is identifiable in 30% of cases (most commonly chondroblastoma, giant cell tumor, chondromyxoid fibroma, nonossifying fibroma, osteoblastoma, and fibrous dysplasia)

3. Clinical presentation (**Table 2**)

a. Pain and swelling are the most common symptoms.

b. Pathologic fracture as a presenting symptom is rare.

c. Neurologic symptoms are possible with lesions in the spine.

d. Most common locations are distal femur, proximal tibia, pelvis, spine (posterior elements).

4. Imaging appearance

a. Eccentric, lytic lesions located in the metaphysis (**Figure 16, A**)

b. Can aggressively destroy/expand the cortex and extend into the soft tissues

c. Lesion can expand to greater than the width of the epiphyseal plate (**Figure 16, B**).

d. Usually maintains a periosteal rim around the lesion

e. Can grow contiguously across adjacent spinal segments or extend through epiphyseal plate

f. No matrix mineralization

g. MRI shows fluid-fluid levels on T2-weighted images (separation of serum and blood products) (**Figure 16, C**).

h. Radiographic differential diagnosis includes UBC and telangiectatic osteosarcoma.

5. Pathology

a. Blood-filled cyst without a true endothelial lining

b. Lining contains giant cells, new (woven) bone, spindle cells (**Figure 16, D**).

c. Solid areas are common.

d. May be histologic evidence of an underlying primary lesion

e. No cellular atypia, but mitoses are common

f. Histologic differential diagnosis includes telangiectatic osteosarcoma and giant cell tumor.

6. Treatment/outcome

a. Surgical treatment is curettage and bone grafting of the lesion.

b. Local adjuvants (eg, phenol) can be used after curettage.

c. Highest local recurrence is in patients with an open physeal plate.

d. For local recurrence, repeat curettage and grafting is indicated.

e. May resect expendable bones (proximal fibula)

f. Embolization can be useful for pelvic or spinal lesions alone or in combination with surgical treatment.

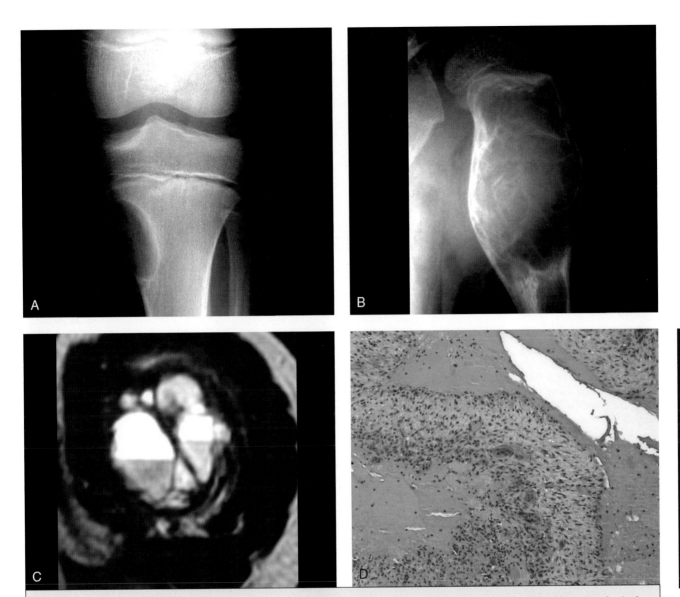

Figure 16 Aneurysmal bone cysts. **A,** AP view of a proximal tibia shows an eccentric lytic lesion located in the metaphysis that expands into the soft tissues with a periosteal rim consistent with an ABC. **B,** AP view of a proximal humerus showing a septated expansile lesion wider than the epiphyseal plate in a very young child, consistent with an ABC. **C,** An axial MRI reveals the presence of fluid-fluid levels within the lesion. **D,** Higher power magnification of an ABC shows multinucleated giant cells within the fibrohistiocystic stroma. No cellular atypia is seen. (*Part D reproduced from Schwartz HS [ed]: Orthopaedic Knowledge Update: Musculoskeletal Tumors 2. Rosemont, IL, American Academy of Orthopaedic Surgeons, 2007, p 89.*)

4: Orthopaedic Oncology and Systemic Disease

V. Miscellaneous

A. Giant cell tumor—A benign, aggressive bone tumor consisting of distinct undifferentiated mononuclear cells.

1. Demographics

   a. Most occur in patients 30 to 50 years of age (90% are older than 20 years)

   b. Affects females more than males

2. Genetics/etiology

   a. Etiology is unknown.

   b. Stromal cells have alterations in the *C-myc*, C-*fos*, and N-*myc* oncogenes.

3. Clinical presentation

   a. Pain and swelling for 2 to 3 months are main symptoms.

   b. Decreased range of motion around a joint

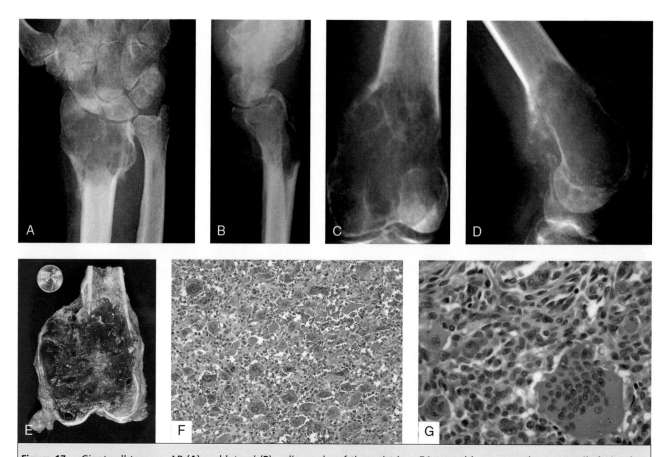

Figure 17 Giant cell tumors. AP (**A**) and lateral (**B**) radiographs of the wrist in a 54-year-old man reveal an expansile lesion located within the epiphysis of the distal radius. No matrix is produced, and there is no sclerotic rim. There has been a pathologic fracture through the lesion. AP (**C**) and lateral (**D**) radiographs of the distal femur in a 33-year-old woman demonstrate an aggressive lytic lesion expanding and destroying the medial and posterior cortices. The differential includes malignant bone tumors, but a biopsy revealed a giant cell tumor. **E**, Gross view of the resection specimen (an intralesional procedure was not deemed appropriate) from the same patient shown in **C** and **D**. **F**, Low-power photomicrograph shows abundant multinucleated giant cells amid a background of mononuclear stromal cells (hematoxylin and eosin, x100). **G**, A higher power photomicrograph shows the multinucleated giant cells with abundant nuclei. The nuclei of the stromal cells resemble those of the giant cells. No cellular atypia or matrix production is noted (hematoxylin and eoxin, x400). (*Parts F and G reproduced from Schwartz HS [ed]: Orthopaedic Knowledge Update: Musculoskeletal Tumors 2. Rosemont, IL, American Academy of Orthopaedic Surgeons, 2007, p 135.*)

c. Sometimes presents with a pathologic fracture (10%)

d. Located most commonly in distal femur, proximal tibia, distal radius, proximal humerus, proximal femur, sacrum, and pelvis

e. 1% of cases are multicentric.

4. Imaging appearance

a. Eccentric, lytic lesions located in the epiphysis/metaphysis of long bones

b. May arise in an apophysis

c. Lesions extend to the subchondral surface with no sclerotic rim (**Figure 17**, *A* and *B*).

d. Can destroy the cortex and extend into the surrounding tissues (**Figure 17**, *C* and *D*)

e. Located in the anterior vertebral body when involving the spine

f. Commonly have a secondary ABC component

g. May be associated soft-tissue calcifications

h. Bone scan shows increased uptake in the lesion.

i. MRI helpful only to define the extent of soft-tissue involvement, as plain radiographs are usually diagnostic.

5. Pathology

a. Gross: soft, red-brown, hemorrhage, necrosis (**Figure 17**, *E*)

b. Histology: uniformly scattered multinucleated giant cells within a background of mononuclear stromal cells (**Figure 17**, *F* and *G*)

c. The stromal cells represent the neoplastic cell.

d. Can have secondary changes of necrosis or fibrohistiocytic change

e. Mitoses are frequent, but there should be no cellular atypia.

f. No matrix production unless there is a pathologic fracture

g. Frequent ABC component

h. There is no histologic grading system for giant cell tumor or way to predict prognosis.

6. Treatment/outcome

a. Most lesions can be treated with thorough curettage and a high-speed burr.

b. Thorough intralesional treatment requires making a large cortical window.

c. Local adjuvants are commonly used to decrease local recurrence (phenol, cryotherapy, argon beam).

d. Can fill defect with either bone graft or methylmethacrylate (equivalent recurrence rate), with or without internal fixation, depending on the defect size

e. Can bear weight as tolerated after using methylmethacrylate; protect from weight bearing after using bone graft until consolidation

f. Local recurrence with intralesional treatment is 10% to 15%.

g. Local recurrence can be in the adjacent bone or manifest as soft-tissue masses.

h. Aggressive lesions may require resection and reconstruction.

i. Embolization should be used for large pelvic or spinal lesions alone or in combination with surgical treatment.

j. Radiation occasionally used in multiply recurrent or surgically inaccessible lesions

k. Metastasizes to the lungs in 2% of patients (benign metastasizing giant cell tumor)

    i. Treatment includes thoracotomy, radiation, chemotherapy, or observation.

    ii. 10% to 15% of patients with metastatic disease die of the disease.

l. Rare cases (~1%) of malignant giant cell tumor

Top Testing Facts

Bone

1. Osteoid osteoma has a radiolucent nidus with surrounding sclerosis.

2. The bone scan is always intensely positive in an osteoid osteoma.

3. Thin-cut CT scans most often identify the nidus and make the diagnosis of osteoid osteoma.

4. The proximal femur is the most common location for an osteoid osteoma.

5. Osteoid osteoma is the most common cause of a painful scoliosis in a young patient.

6. RFA is the current standard of care to treat osteoid osteoma.

7. An osteoid osteoma can be differentiated from an osteoblastoma by its smaller size and less aggressive behavior, although the histologic appearance is similar.

8. Osteoblastoma is a large radiolucent lesion that occurs most commonly in the posterior elements of the spine.

9. Parosteal osteoma must be differentiated from parosteal osteosarcoma.

10. A bone island is an inactive lesion most commonly found in the pelvis and proximal femur.

Cartilage

1. Enchondromas are usually asymptomatic; a painful presentation is usually due to an unrelated condition.

2. The clinical presentation and radiographic appearance are more important than the histologic appearance in differentiating enchondroma from low-grade chondrosarcoma.

3. Patients with either Ollier disease or Maffucci syndrome have an increased risk for malignant transformation of an enchondroma to a low-grade chondrosarcoma.

4. A periosteal chondroma is a surface lesion that creates a saucerized defect in the underlying cortex.

5. The medullary cavity of the underlying bone is continuous with the stalk of an osteochondroma.

6. Secondary chondrosarcomas arising from osteochondromas are low grade and occur more often in patients with multiple lesions.

7. EXT1, EXT2, and EXT3 are genetic loci commonly mutated in patients with multiple hereditary exostoses.

8. Chondroblastoma most commonly occurs in the epiphyses and apophyses of long bones.

9. Chondroblastoma rarely metastasizes to the lung.

10. Chondromyxoid fibroma is a lucent, eccentric lesion with a sclerotic, scalloped rim seen in long bones, pelvis, and hands/feet.

Top Testing Facts (cont.)

Fibrous/Histiocytic

1. Nonossifying fibromas are usually incidental findings that spontaneously regress and should be observed.

2. Nonossifying fibromas are developmental abnormalities that occur in 30% of children.

3. Nonossifying fibromas occur as scalloped lytic lesions with a sclerotic border within the metaphysis.

4. Fibrous dysplasia is a long lesion in a long bone with a ground glass appearance.

5. The histologic appearance of fibrous dysplasia is woven bone shaped like "Chinese letters" or "alphabet soup" in a cellular, fibrous stroma.

6. Polyostotic fibrous dysplasia occurs in McCune-Albright syndrome along with precocious puberty and café-au-lait spots.

7. Osteofibrous dysplasia affects children in the first decade, with a predilection for the anterior cortex of the tibia.

8. The histologic appearance of osteofibrous dysplasia is a cellular, fibrous stroma with prominent osteoblastic rimming around the woven bone, which differentiates it from fibrous dysplasia.

9. Langerhans cell histiocytosis is the great mimicker; think of it with lytic lesions in children.

10. In Langerhans cell histiocytosis, the histiocyte (not the eosinophil) is the tumor cell and stains with CD1A.

Cystic/Miscellaneous

1. UBCs are centrally located in the metaphysis and appear to move to the diaphysis.

2. UBCs present with a pathologic fracture—rare fallen leaf sign on radiographs.

3. Treat UBCs with an intralesional steroid injection.

4. ABCs are destructive, expansile, blood-filled cysts.

5. ABCs occur around the knee, pelvis, and posterior elements of the spine.

6. At least 30% of the time, ABCs are secondary to an underlying primary bone tumor.

7. Giant cell tumors are epiphyseal or apophyseal and extend into the metaphysis and subchondral bone.

8. The mononuclear stromal cell is the neoplastic cell in giant cell tumor.

9. The treatment of giant cell tumor is careful curettage with a large cortical window (low local recurrence rate of 5% to 15%).

10. Giant cell tumor metastasizes to the lung in 2% of patients.

Bibliography

Arata MA, Peterson HA, Dahlin DC: Pathological fractures through non-ossifying fibromas. Review of the Mayo Clinic experience. *J Bone Joint Surg Am* 1981;63:980-988.

Campanacci M, Capanna R, Picci P: Unicameral and aneurysmal bone cysts. *Clin Orthop Relat Res* 1986;204:25-36.

Frassica FJ, Waltrip RL, Sponseller PD, Ma LD, McCarthy EF: Clinicopathologic features and treatment of osteoid osteoma and osteoblastoma in children and adolescents. *Orthop Clin North Am* 1996;27:559-574.

Guille JT, Kumar SJ, MacEwen GD: Fibrous dysplasia of the proximal part of the femur. Long-term results of curettage and bone-grafting and mechanical realignment. *J Bone Joint Surg Am* 1998;80:648-658.

Lersundi A, Mankin HJ, Mourikis A, Hornicek FJ: Chondromyxoid fibroma: A rarely encountered and puzzling tumor. *Clin Orthop Relat Res* 2005;439:171-175.

McCarthy EF, Frassica FJ: *Pathology of Bone and Joint Disorders.* Philadelphia, PA, Saunders, 1998.

Ozaki T, Hamada M, Sugihara S, Kunisada T, Mitani S, Inoue H: Treatment outcome of osteofibrous dysplasia. *J Pediatr Orthop B* 1998;7:199-202.

Park YK, Unni KK, Beabout JW, Hodgson SF: Oncogenic osteomalacia: A clinicopathologic study of 17 bone lesions. *J Korean Med Sci* 1994;9:289-298.

Ramappa AJ, Lee FY, Tang P, Carlson JR, Gebhardt MC, Mankin HJ: Chondroblastoma of bone. *J Bone Joint Surg Am* 2000;82-A:1140-1145.

Rosenthal DI, Hornicek FJ, Torriani M, Gebhardt MC, Mankin HJ: Osteoid osteoma: Percutaneous treatment with radiofrequency energy. *Radiology* 2003;229:171-175.

Taconis WK, Schutte HE, van der Heul RO: Desmoplastic fibroma of bone: A report of 18 cases. *Skeletal Radiol* 1994;23:283-288.

Turcotte RE, Wunder JS, Isler MH, et al: Giant cell tumor of long bone: A Canadian Sarcoma Group study. *Clin Orthop Relat Res* 2002;397:248-258.

Unni KK: Cartilaginous lesions of bone. *J Orthop Sci* 2001;6:457-472.

Wuyts W, Van Hul W: Molecular basis of multiple exostoses: Mutations in the EXT1 and EXT2 genes. *Hum Mutat* 2000;15:220-227.

Yasko AW, Fanning CV, Ayala AG, Carrasco CH, Murray JA: Percutaneous techniques for the diagnosis and treatment of localized Langerhans-cell histiocytosis (eosinophilic granuloma of bone). *J Bone Joint Surg Am* 1998;80:219-228.

4: Orthopaedic Oncology and Systemic Disease

Chapter 39
Malignant Bone Tumors

Kristy Weber, MD

I. Bone Tumors

A. Osteosarcoma—Classic intramedullary osteosarcoma is a malignant bone-forming tumor.

1. Demographics

   a. Male to female ratio = 1.5:1

   b. Most common malignant bone tumor in children (1,000 to 1,500 new cases/year in United States)

   c. Bimodal age distribution

      i. Most common in second decade of life

      ii. Late peak in sixth decade of life

2. Genetics/etiology

   a. Associated with retinoblastoma gene (*RB1*), which is a tumor-suppressor gene

   b. Increased incidence in patients with p53 mutations, Paget disease, prior radiation, Rothmund-Thomson syndrome, and retinoblastoma

   c. *MDM2*, *HER2/neu*, c-*myc*, and c-*fos* are oncogenes overexpressed in osteosarcoma.

3. Clinical presentation

   a. Commonly presents with intermittent pain progressing to constant (rest, night) pain unrelieved by medications

   b. Swelling, decreased range of motion, limp, and weakness depending on location

   c. Often present after injury or sporting activity (coincident with age group, no causality known to trauma)

   d. Most commonly noted in metaphysis of distal femur, proximal tibia, proximal humerus, and pelvis

   e. 10% of patients present with a pathologic fracture.

4. Imaging

   a. Classically, osteosarcomas have a mixed appearance with bone destruction and bone formation (**Figures 1** and **2**).

   b. In skeletally immature patients, most do not extend past the epiphyseal plate.

   c. Most have cortical destruction and soft-tissue mass with adjacent Codman triangle (normal reactive bone near tumor)

   d. Classic osteosarcomas originate in medullary canal.

   e. Radiographic differential diagnosis includes osteomyelitis and Ewing sarcoma.

   f. Technetium Tc 99m bone scan can identify skip lesions.

   g. MRI delineates extent of marrow involvement, proximity of soft-tissue mass to adjacent neurovascular structures, and skip lesions (**Figures 1**, *C* and **2**, *C*).

5. Pathology

   a. The gross appearance varies from a soft, fleshy mass to a firm, fibrous or sclerotic lesion (**Figure 1**, *D*).

   b. The low-power histologic appearance is frankly sarcomatous stroma forming tumor osteoid that permeates existing trabeculae (**Figure 1**, *E*).

   c. On high power, the osteoblastic cells are malignant and form the neoplastic new bone (**Figure 1**, *F*).

   d. Osteosarcoma is defined by the presence of malignant osteoid.

   e. Extensive pleomorphism and numerous mitotic figures are present.

   f. Areas of necrosis, cartilage, or giant cells may be present within the lesion.

   g. The histologic differential diagnosis includes fibrous dysplasia.

6. Treatment/outcome

   a. The standard treatment of osteosarcoma is neoadjuvant chemotherapy followed by surgical resection (limb-sparing or amputation), followed by additional adjuvant chemotherapy.

   b. The most common chemotherapy agents in-

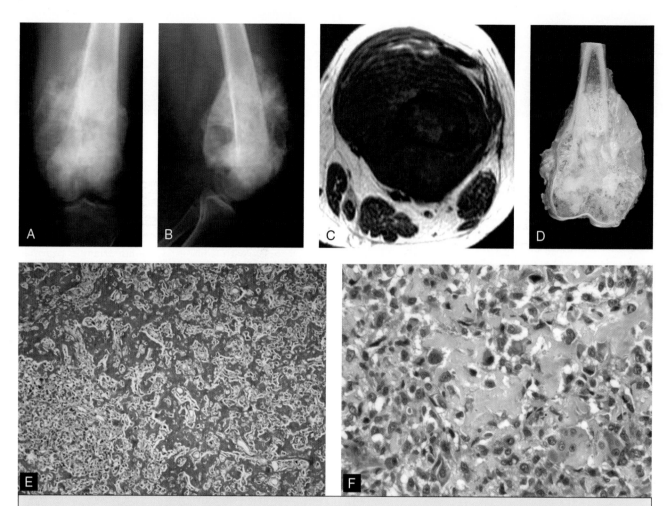

Figure 1 Osteosarcoma of the left distal femur in a 15-year-old boy. AP (**A**) and lateral (**B**) radiographs demonstrate extensive bone formation and an ossified soft-tissue mass after several cycles of chemotherapy. **C,** Axial MRI reveals an extensive circumferential soft-tissue mass abutting the neurovascular bundle posteriorly. **D,** Gross specimen after distal femoral resection showing a clear proximal margin and tumor extending into the epiphysis. **E,** Low-power histology shows the classic osteoid formed by malignant stromal cells. Note the lacelike pattern. **F,** High power reveals the pleomorphic cells producing the new bone. (*Part E reproduced from Scarborough MT (ed): 2005 Musculoskeletal Tumors and Diseases Self-Assessment Examination. Rosemont, IL, American Academy of Orthopaedic Surgeons, 2005, question 89, figure 52 C.*)

clude adriamycin (doxorubicin), cis-platinum, methotrexate, and ifosfamide (**Table 1**).

c. Radiation plays no role in the standard treatment of osteosarcoma.

d. Limb-sparing surgery can be performed in 90% of cases.

e. Patients who present with a pathologic fracture can be treated with limb-salvage surgery but have a higher risk of local recurrence if the fracture is widely displaced.

f. Local recurrence after surgical resection is approximately 5%; these patients have a dismal prognosis.

g. Good histologic response and wide surgical margins are associated with a low risk of local recurrence.

h. Reconstructive options depend on patient age and tumor location but include metal prostheses, osteoarticular/intercalary allografts, allograft-prosthetic composites, expandable prostheses, or vascularized fibular autografts.

i. Tumor stage is the most important prognostic indicator.

j. The percentage of necrosis within the tumor after neoadjuvant chemotherapy is related to overall survival (>90% necrosis is associated with significantly increased survival).

k. Elevated lactate dehydrogenase (LDH) and alkaline phosphatase have been reported to be poor prognostic factors.

l. Survival

i. The 5-year survival of patients with localized

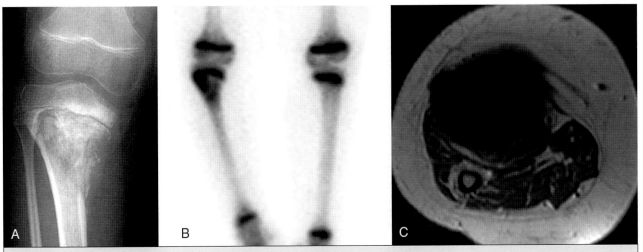

Figure 2   Osteosarcoma of the right proximal tibia in an 8-year-old boy. **A,** AP radiograph demonstrates collapse of the medial cortex with a minimally displaced fracture. There is both bone destruction and formation. **B,** A technetium Tc 99m bone scan reveals avid uptake in the area of the tumor. **C,** Axial MRI reveals a small medial soft-tissue mass.

4: Orthopaedic Oncology and Systemic Disease

osteosarcoma in an extremity is 65% to 70%.

   ii. The 5-year survival of patients with localized pelvic osteosarcoma is 25%.

   iii. The 5-year survival of patients who present with metastatic disease is 20%.

m. The most common site of metastasis is the lungs, followed by the bones.

   i. Aggressive treatment of late (>1 year) pulmonary metastasis with thoracotomy allows ~30% 5-year survival.

   ii. Patients with bone metastasis usually die of the disease.

n. Skip lesions occur in 10% of patients; prognosis is similar to those with lung metastasis.

B. Osteosarcoma subtypes

1. Parosteal osteosarcoma—Low-grade surface osteosarcoma composed of dense bone.

   a. Demographics

      i. Female to male ratio = 2:1

      ii. Accounts for 5% of all osteosarcomas

      iii. Most patients are 20 to 45 years of age.

   b. Clinical presentation

      i. Classic presentation is swelling of long duration (often years).

      ii. Pain, limited joint range of motion, limp are variable

      iii. The most common location is the posterior aspect of the distal femur (75%), followed

Table 1

Chemotherapy Drugs Used in the Treatment of Osteosarcoma

Drug	Mechanism of Action	Major Toxicities
Adriamycin/ doxorubicin	Blocks DNA/RNA synthesis Inhibits topoisomerase II	Cardiotoxicity
Cis-platinum	DNA disruption by covalent binding	Hearing loss Neuropathy Renal failure
Methotrexate	Inhibits dehydrofolate reductase (inhibits DNA synthesis)	Mucositis
Ifosfamide	DNA alkylating agent	Renal failure Encephalopathy

by the proximal tibia and the proximal humerus.

   c. Imaging

      i. Dense, lobulated lesion on the surface of the bone (**Figure 3,** *A*)

      ii. May have underlying cortical thickening

      iii. Attachment to the cortex may be broad.

      iv. Occasional minor intramedullary involvement

      v. The tumor is most dense in the center and least ossified peripherally.

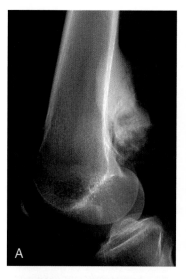

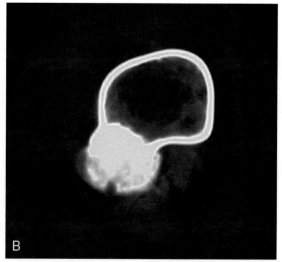

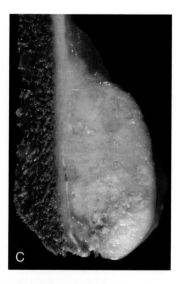

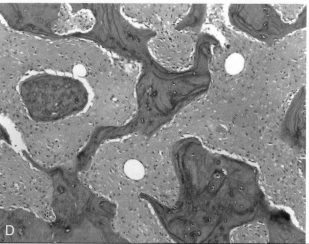

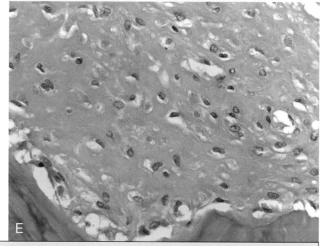

Figure 3 Parosteal osteosarcoma of the distal femur. **A,** Lateral radiograph of the knee reveals a densely ossified surface lesion on the posterior distal femur that is consistent with a parosteal osteosarcoma. **B,** CT scan demonstrates the relationship between the tumor and the femoral cortex. **C,** Gross specimen confirms that it is truly a surface osteosarcoma. **D,** Low-power histology reveals a bland appearance with regular, ordered, dense trabeculae and interspersed fibrous stroma. **E,** Higher power reveals minimal cellular atypia. (*Part A reproduced from Scarborough MT (ed): 2005 Musculoskeletal Tumors and Diseases Self-Assessment Examination. Rosemont, IL, American Academy of Orthopaedic Surgeons, 2005, question 86, figure 50 A.*)

vi. Radiographic differential diagnosis includes myositis ossificans and osteochondroma.

vii. MRI or CT scans are helpful in defining the lesional extent before surgery (**Figure 3,** *B*).

viii. Dedifferentiated parosteal osteosarcoma has ill-defined areas on the surface of the lesion and hypervascularity on angiographic studies.

d. Pathology

  i. Regular, ordered osseous trabeculae (**Figure 3,** *D* and *E*)

  ii. Bland, fibrous stroma with occasional slightly atypical cells (grade 1)

  iii. Dedifferentiated parosteal osteosarcoma contains a high-grade sarcoma juxtaposed to the underlying low-grade lesion.

e. Treatment/outcome

  i. Wide surgical resection is the treatment of choice (**Figure 4**).

  ii. High risk of local recurrence with inadequate resection

  iii. Often the knee joint can be maintained after resection of the lesion and posterior cortex of the femur.

  iv. Survival is 95% if wide resection is achieved.

  v. Dedifferentiated variants occur in 25% of patients and are more common after multiple recurrences; survival is 50%.

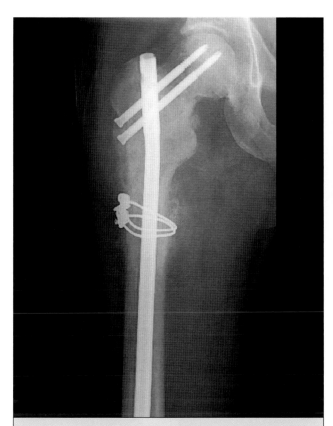

Figure 4 Radiograph of the proximal femur of a 43-year-old man who was assumed to have metastatic disease; an intramedullary rod was placed in the right femur. Note the osteoblastic appearance of the proximal femur. A later biopsy after continued pain revealed an osteosarcoma. The patient required a hindquarter amputation. This case highlights the importance of a preoperative biopsy.

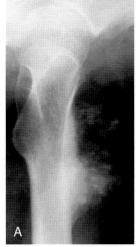
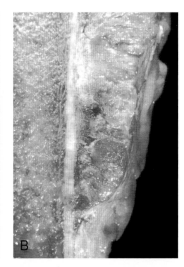
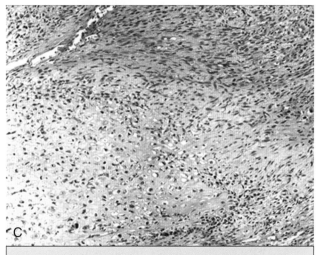

Figure 5 Periosteal osteosarcoma. **A,** Radiograph demonstrates a lesion in the proximal femur. **B,** Gross pathology. **C,** The histology reveals a lobular cartilaginous lesion with moderate cellularity. From this appearance, a malignant cartilage lesion would be suspected. One area reveals osteoid production confirming the diagnosis of periosteal osteosarcoma, which is typically chondroblastic in appearance. *(Reproduced from Hornicek FJ: Osteosarcoma of bone, in Schwartz HS (ed): Orthopaedic Knowledge Update: Musculoskeletal Tumors 2. Rosemont, IL, American Academy of Orthopaedic Surgeons, 2007, p 167.)*

2. Periosteal osteosarcoma—Rare, intermediate-grade surface osteosarcoma.

   a. Demographics

      i. Occurs in patients 15 to 25 years of age

      ii. Extremely rare

   b. Clinical presentation

      i. Pain is the most common presenting symptom.

      ii. Most commonly occurs in the femoral or tibial diaphysis

   c. Imaging

      i. Lesion has a sunburst periosteal elevation in the diaphysis of long bones (**Figure 5,** *A*).

      ii. The underlying cortex may be saucerized.

      iii. No involvement of the medullary canal

   d. Pathology

      i. Gross appearance is lobular and cartilaginous (**Figure 5,** *B*)

      ii. Histology reveals extensive areas of chondroblastic matrix, but the tumor produces osteoid (**Figure 5,** *C*).

      iii. Without any osteoid production, the lesion would be a chondrosarcoma.

      iv. Cellular appearance is grade 2 to 3.

   e. Treatment/outcome

      i. Some controversy exists whether to use che-

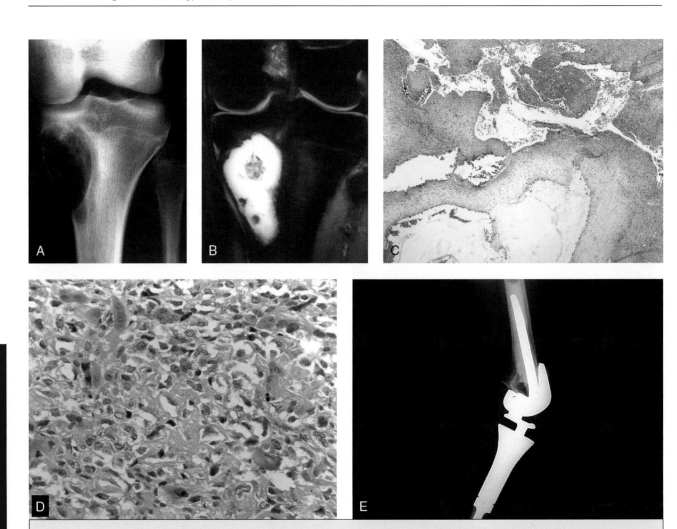

Figure 6 Telangiectatic osteosarcoma. **A,** AP radiograph of a 14-year-old girl with an osteolytic lesion in the medial aspect of the left proximal tibia. The differential diagnosis includes telangiectatic osteosarcoma or ABC. **B,** Coronal MRI reveals a lesion of high intensity on T2-weighted imaging, but no fluid levels are seen. **C,** Low-power histology reveals large blood-filled spaces with intervening fibrous septa. **D,** The high-power view is required to determine that this is a telangiectatic osteosarcoma with pleomorphic osteoblasts producing osteoid. **E,** Postoperative radiograph after wide resection of the proximal tibia and reconstruction with a modular proximal tibial endoprosthesis. (*Parts A and B reproduced from Scarborough MT (ed):* 2005 Musculoskeletal Tumors and Diseases Self-Assessment Examination. *Rosemont, IL, American Academy of Orthopaedic Surgeons, 2005, question 13, figure 10 A, B, C.*)

motherapy, but the current standard is neoadjuvant chemotherapy followed by wide surgical resection followed by additional chemotherapy.

   ii. Metastasis develops in 25% of patients.

3. High-grade surface osteosarcoma

   a. Definition—rare, high-grade variant of osteosarcoma that occurs on the bone surface

   b. Demographics, genetics, etiology, clinical presentation, and pathology are the same as for classic osteosarcoma (see I.A.).

   c. Radiographic appearance

      i. Similar to the appearance of a classic osteosarcoma except that it occurs solely on the cortical surface

   ii. No intramedullary involvement

4. Telangiectatic osteosarcoma—Rare histologic variant of osteosarcoma containing large, blood-filled spaces.

   a. Demographics, genetics/etiology, clinical presentation

      i. Similar to classic osteosarcoma

      ii. Rare (only 4% of all osteosarcomas)

      iii. 25% present with pathologic fracture.

   b. Imaging

      i. Purely lytic lesion that occasionally obliterates entire cortex

      ii. Differential diagnosis primarily includes aneurysmal bone cyst (ABC) (**Figure 6**).

iii. Osteosarcoma has more intense uptake than ABC on bone scan.

iv. MRI may show fluid-fluid levels and extensive surrounding edema.

c. Pathology

i. Grossly, the tumor is described as a "bag of blood."

ii. Histology shows large blood-filled spaces (**Figure 6,** *C*).

iii. Intervening septa contain areas of high-grade sarcoma with atypical mitoses (**Figure 6,** *D*).

iv. May produce only minimal osteoid

v. Occasionally contains benign giant cells

vi. Differential diagnosis: primarily ABC

d. Treatment/outcome—Same as classic osteosarcoma (see I.A.6).

II. Fibrous/Histiocytic Tumors

A. Malignant fibrous histiocytoma—Malignant fibrous histiocytoma (MFH) is a primary malignant bone tumor similar to osteosarcoma but with histiocytic differentiation and no osteoid (**Figures 7 and 8**).

1. Demographics

a. Occurs in patients 20 to 80 years of age (most are >40 years)

b. Slight male predominance

2. Genetics/etiology—25% of cases occur as secondary lesions in the setting of a bone infarct, Paget disease, or prior radiation.

3. Clinical presentation

a. Pain is the primary symptom, followed by swelling, limp, decreased range of motion, and pathologic fracture.

b. MFH of bone most commonly occurs in the metaphyses of long bones, primarily the distal femur, proximal tibia, and proximal humerus.

4. Imaging

a. Lytic, destructive lesion with variable periosteal reaction (**Figures 7,** *A* **and** *B*, **and 8**)

b. No bone production

c. Often has cortical destruction with a soft-tissue mass

d. Appearance is often nonspecific, and the differential diagnosis includes any malignant bone tumor or metastasis.

5. Pathology

a. MFH of bone is the same entity as "undifferentiated pleomorphic sarcoma."

b. Storiform appearance with marked pleomorphism and mitotic figures (**Figure 7,** *D*)

c. Fibrous fascicles radiate from focal hypocellular areas.

d. Multinucleated tumor cells with histiocytic nuclei (grooved)

e. Areas of chronic inflammatory cells

f. Variable collagen production

6. Treatment/outcome

a. Treat MFH of bone similarly to osteosarcoma with neoadjuvant chemotherapy, wide surgical resection, and postoperative chemotherapy.

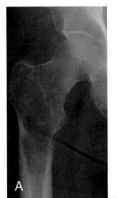 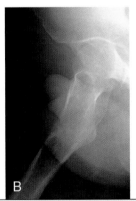 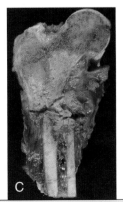 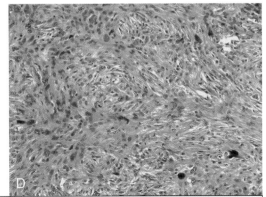

Figure 7 Malignant fibrous histiocytoma. AP (**A**) and lateral (**B**) radiographs in a 43-year-old man with a destructive lesion in the intertrochanteric region of the right femur. A needle biopsy revealed MFH of bone. He sustained a pathologic fracture during preoperative chemotherapy. **C,** Gross specimen after proximal femoral resection and reconstruction with a modular endoprosthesis. **D,** The histology reveals a storiform pattern with marked pleomorphism and a few multinucleated cells.

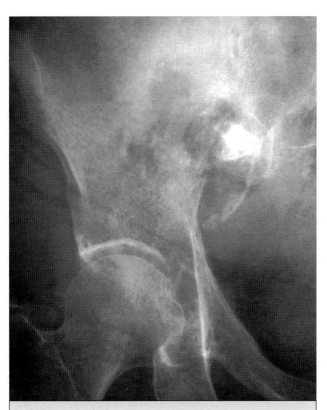

Figure 8 AP radiograph of the right hip and pelvis of a 54-year-old woman with a destructive lesion in the ilium. It is poorly defined, and cortical disruption is seen along the medial wall. A biopsy was consistent with MFH of bone.

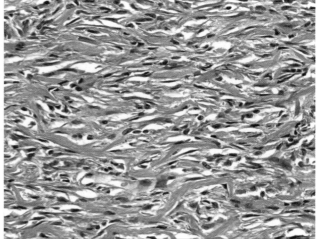

Figure 9 High-power histologic view of a fibrosarcoma of bone reveals moderately atypical spindle cells arranged in a herringbone pattern along with collagen fibers.

b. As with osteosarcoma, reconstructive options depend on patient age and tumor location but include metal prostheses, osteoarticular/intercalary allografts, allograft-prosthetic composites, expandable prostheses, or vascularized fibular autografts.

c. Survival is slightly worse than osteosarcoma, with metastasis primarily to the lung and bones.

d. Secondary MFH in a preexisting lesion has a worse prognosis.

B. Fibrosarcoma of bone—Rare malignant bone tumor characterized by spindle cells.

1. Demographics—Presents in patients from 20 to 70 years of age (most >40 years).

2. Clinical presentation

a. Pain is the predominant symptom.

b. Variable swelling, limp, decreased range of motion

c. Occurs most commonly in the femur

d. 25% present secondary to preexisting lesions such as Paget disease, prior radiation, or an infarct.

3. Imaging

a. Purely lytic lesion that occurs primarily in the metaphysis

b. Focal periosteal reaction

c. Poorly defined margins

d. May have a soft-tissue mass best defined with MRI

e. Appearance is often nonspecific; the differential diagnosis includes any malignant bone tumor or metastasis.

4. Pathology

a. Histology is spindle cells arranged in a herringbone pattern—fascicles at right angles (**Figure 9**).

b. Can occur in low- to high-grade variants

c. Differential diagnosis includes desmoplastic fibroma.

d. The number of mitotic figures correlates with the grade of the lesion.

5. Treatment/outcome

a. The standard treatment of high-grade fibrosarcoma is similar to that for osteosarcoma: neoadjuvant chemotherapy, wide surgical resection, and postoperative chemotherapy.

b. Overall survival is correlated with grade of the tumor (30% for high grade, 80% for low grade).

c. Overall survival is slightly worse than for osteosarcoma.

III. Cartilage Tumors

A. Chondrosarcoma—Classic intramedullary chondrosarcoma is a malignant cartilage-producing bone tumor that arises de novo or secondary to other lesions.

1. Demographics

   a. Occurs in adult patients (40 to 75 years)

   b. Slight male predominance

   c. Central and surface lesions occur with equal frequency.

   d. Incidence

      i. Grade 1 = 60%

      ii. Grade 2 = 25%

      iii. Grade 3 = 5%

      iv. Dedifferentiated = 10%

2. Genetics/etiology—correlation between high expression of telomerase RT and metastasis

3. Clinical presentation

   a. Pain of prolonged duration (pain can differentiate low-grade chondrosarcoma from benign enchondroma)

   b. Slow-growing firm mass

   c. Bowel/bladder symptoms may develop with large pelvic lesions.

   d. Most common locations include pelvis, proximal femur, scapula

   e. Location is important for diagnosis (scapula = malignant, hand = benign).

   f. Wide range of aggressiveness, depending on grade

   g. Secondary chondrosarcomas occur in the setting of a solitary osteochondroma (<1%), multiple hereditary osteochondromas (1% to 10%), Ollier disease (25% to 40%), or Maffucci disease (100%).

4. Imaging

   a. Radiographic appearance varies by grade of tumor.

   b. Low-grade intramedullary lesions are similar to enchondromas but they have cortical thickening/expansion, extensive endosteal erosion, and occasional soft-tissue extension (**Figure 10**).

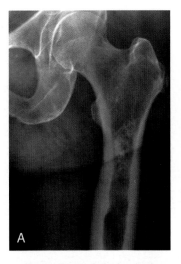
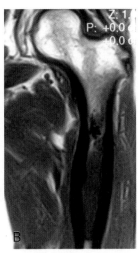
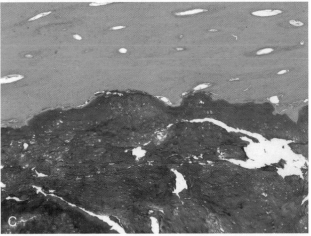
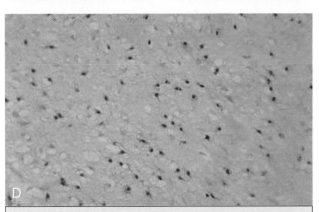

Figure 10   Low-grade chondrosarcoma. **A,** AP radiograph of the left proximal femur in a 65-year-old woman with constant thigh pain shows thickened cortices and proximal intramedullary calcification within the lesion. These findings are consistent with a low-grade chondrosarcoma. **B,** Coronal MRI reveals the intramedullary extent of the lesion. There is no soft-tissue mass. **C,** Low-power histology reveals the interface between the bone and a relatively hypocellular cartilage lesion. **D,** Higher power reveals a grade 1 chondrosarcoma with a bland cellular appearance, extensive basophilic cytoplasm, and no mitotic figures.

4: Orthopaedic Oncology and Systemic Disease

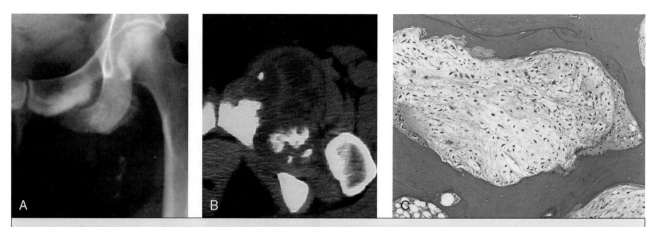

Figure 11   High-grade chondrosarcoma. **A,** AP radiograph of the left anterior pelvis in a 42-year-old woman reveals a destructive lesion of the inferior pubic ramus with a soft-tissue mass. **B,** CT scan defines the mass. There is evidence of intralesional calcium within the mass. This radiographic appearance is consistent with a chondrosarcoma. **C,** The histology reveals a hypercellular lesion with atypical cells and permeation of the trabecular spaces consistent with a high-grade lesion. *(Parts A and B reproduced from Scarborough MT (ed): 2005 Musculoskeletal Tumors and Diseases Self-Assessment Examination. Rosemont, IL, American Academy of Orthopaedic Surgeons, 2005, question 73, figure 42 A, B.)*

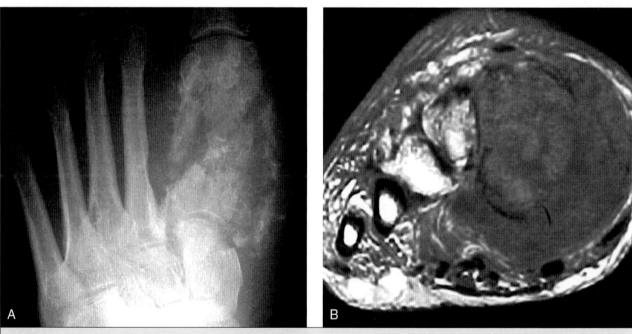

Figure 12   Grade 2 chondrosarcoma. **A,** AP radiograph of the left foot in a 68-year-old man with a destructive lesion in the metatarsal. **B,** Axial MRI reveals an extensive soft-tissue mass and the tissue diagnosis was a grade 2 chondrosarcoma. He required a below-knee amputation.

c. Low-grade lesions have rings, arcs, and stipples and are usually mineralized.

d. Low-grade chondrosarcoma is usually >8 cm in the long bones.

e. Low-grade pelvic chondrosarcoma can grow to large size (>10 cm) with extensive soft-tissue extension toward surrounding viscera.

f. Intermediate- or high-grade chondrosarcoma is less well defined, involves frank cortical de-

struction, and often has an associated soft-tissue mass (**Figures 11 through 13**).

g. Dedifferentiated chondrosarcoma is a high-grade sarcoma juxtaposed to a benign or low-grade malignant cartilage lesion, noted radiographically by a calcified intramedullary lesion with an adjacent destructive lytic lesion (**Figure 14**).

h. Secondary chondrosarcomas appear with ill-defined edges or thickened cartilage caps (>2 cm) next to an enchondroma or osteochondroma, respectively (**Figure 15**).

   i. Bone scan shows increased uptake in all variants and grades of chondrosarcoma.

   j. CT or MRI scans are helpful in defining cortical destruction and marrow involvement, respectively.

5. Pathology

   a. Low-grade tumors are grossly lobular, whereas higher grade tumors may be myxoid.

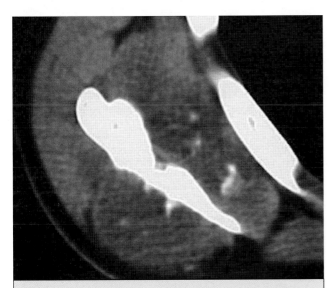

Figure 13   CT scan of the scapula reveals a large soft-tissue mass with tissue consistent with a grade 3 chondrosarcoma. There are intralesional calcifications. The scapula is a common location for this tumor.

   b. Needle biopsy is not helpful in determining the grade of a cartilage tumor.

   c. Low-grade chondrosarcomas have a bland histologic appearance, but permeation and entrapment of the existing trabeculae are present (**Figure 10, C and D**).

   d. Mitotic figures are rare.

   e. Higher grade chondrosarcomas have a hypercellular pattern with binucleate forms and occasional myxoid change (**Figure 11, C**).

   f. Dedifferentiated chondrosarcomas reveal a high-grade sarcoma (MFH, fibrosarcoma, osteosarcoma) adjacent to a low-grade or benign cartilage tumor (**Figure 14, D**).

6. Treatment/outcome

   a. Grade 1 chondrosarcomas in the extremities can be treated with careful intralesional curettage or wide resection.

   b. All pelvic chondrosarcomas should be resected with an adequate margin (may require amputation).

   c. Local recurrence rate at 10 years is ~20%.

   d. Recurrent lesions have a 10% chance of increasing in grade.

   e. Grade 2, 3, or dedifferentiated chondrosarcomas require wide surgical resection regardless of location.

   f. No current role for chemotherapy or radiation except in dedifferentiated chondrosarcoma (receive chemotherapy depending on patient age/condition)

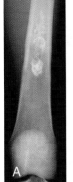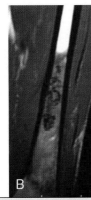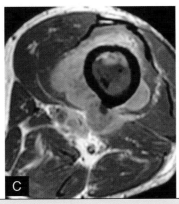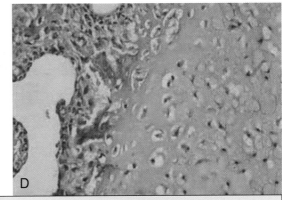

Figure 14   Dedifferentiated chondrosarcoma. **A,** AP radiograph of the femur in a 73-year-old man reveals a lesion similar to an enchondroma within the medullary canal but there is an ill-defined lucency distal to the lesion. **B,** Coronal MRI reveals the intramedullary extent of the lesion, which is much different from an enchondroma and raises the concern for a dedifferentiated chondrosarcoma. **C,** Axial MRI demonstrates a circumferential soft-tissue mass consistent with a high-grade lesion. **D,** A high-power histologic view shows low-grade cartilage juxtaposed to a high-grade sarcomatous lesion. This is a dedifferentiated chondrosarcoma. *(Parts A and B reproduced from Scarborough MT (ed): 2005 Musculoskeletal Tumors and Diseases Self-Assessment Examination. Rosemont, IL, American Academy of Orthopaedic Surgeons, 2005, question 33, figure 19 A, B.)*

4: Orthopaedic Oncology and Systemic Disease

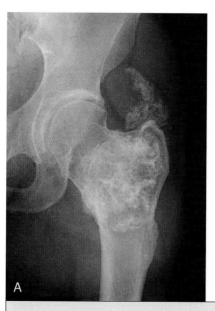
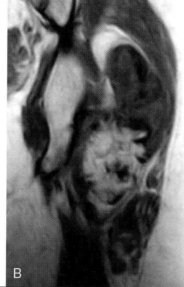
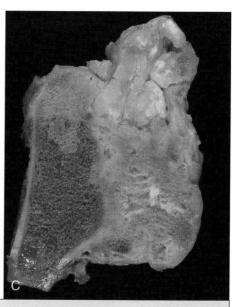

Figure 15 Chondrosarcoma. **A,** AP radiograph in a 35-year-old woman with multiple hereditary osteochondromas who has new onset of hip pain that has become constant. Note the proximal femoral osteochondroma with an ill-defined area proximal to the lesion. **B,** Coronal MRI reveals the osteochondroma to have the same appearance as the adjacent pelvic marrow, but the proximal aspect is composed of soft tissue consistent with malignant degeneration. **C,** Gross appearance of the lesion after resection of the proximal femur. The histology revealed a grade 1 chondrosarcoma.

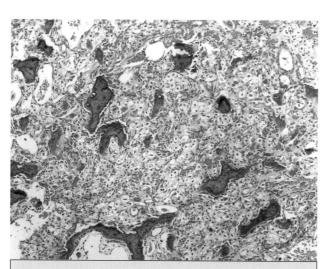

Figure 16 The low-power view of a clear cell chondrosarcoma reveals a cellular lesion with minimal matrix. The cartilage cells have clear cytoplasm, and there are additional benign giant cells within the lesion.

g. Metastasis to the lungs is treated with thoracotomy.

h. Slow progression of disease requires long-term follow-up (~20 years).

i. Overall survival depends on the grade of the tumor.

   i. Grade 1 = 90%

   ii. Grade 2 = 60% to 70%

   iii. Grade 3 = 30% to 50%

   iv. Dedifferentiated = 10%

B. Chondrosarcoma subtypes

  1. Clear cell chondrosarcoma—Rare malignant cartilage tumor with immature cartilaginous histiogenesis.

   a. Demographics, genetics/etiology, and clinical presentation are the same as for classic chondrosarcoma (see III.A.1-3).

   b. Radiographic appearance

    i. Clear cell chrondrosarcoma occurs in the epiphysis of long bones, most commonly in the proximal femur or proximal humerus.

    ii. Lytic, round, expansile well-defined lesion

    iii. No periosteal reaction

    iv. Mineralization may be evident within the lesion.

    v. Most often confused with a benign chondroblastoma

   c. Pathology

    i. Intermediate- to high-grade lesion formed of immature cartilage cells (**Figure 16**)

    ii. Lobular growth pattern

    iii. Benign giant cells throughout the tumor

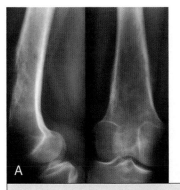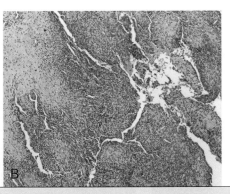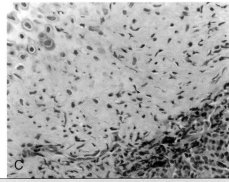

Figure 17 Chondrosarcoma. **A,** A composite lateral and AP radiograph of the distal femur in a 28-year-old woman reveals a poorly defined lytic lesion with destruction of the anterior cortex. **B,** Low-power histology reveals a biphasic appearance to the lesion with cartilage as well as small round cells consistent with a mesenchymal chondrosarcoma. **C,** Higher power of the junction between the low-grade cartilage and the sheets of small cells.

iv. Extensive clear cytoplasm with minimal matrix

d. Treatment/outcome

 i. Wide surgical resection required for cure

 ii. Chemotherapy and radiation not effective

 iii. Metastasis to bones and lungs

 iv. Good prognosis—5-year survival is 80%

2. Mesenchymal chondrosarcoma—Rare primary bone tumor composed of a biphasic pattern of cartilage and small round cell components (**Figure 17**).

a. Demographics—Occurs in younger individuals (10 to 40 years of age) than classic chondrosarcoma.

b. Clinical presentation

 i. Most common in the flat bones (ilium, ribs, skull), but can occur in the long bones

 ii. 30% of cases involve only soft tissue.

 iii. May involve multiple skeletal sites at presentation

 iv. Pain and swelling of long duration are the most common symptoms.

c. Radiographic appearance

 i. Lytic destructive lesions with stippled calcification within the lesion (**Figure 17,** *A*)

 ii. Expansion of bone with cortical thickening and poor margination

 iii. Nonspecific appearance can be included in a differential of any malignant or metastatic lesion.

d. Pathology—Biphasic histologic pattern of low-grade islands of cartilage alternating with sheets of small anaplastic round cells (**Figure 17,** *B* and *C*).

e. Treatment/outcome

 i. Treatment: chemotherapy and wide surgical resection

 ii. Survival: 30% to 60% at 5 years

 iii. Few series in the literature

IV. Round Cell Lesions

A. Ewing sarcoma/primitive neuroectodermal tumor (PNET)—Malignant bone tumor composed of small round blue cells.

1. Demographics

 a. Male to female ratio = 3:2

 b. Uncommon in African Americans and Chinese

 c. Second most common primary bone tumor in children (80% are younger than 20 years)

2. Genetics/etiology

 a. Cell of origin unknown

 b. Hypothesized to be of neuroectodermal differentiation. PNET is thought to be the differentiated neural tumor, whereas Ewing sarcoma is the undifferentiated variant.

 c. Classic 11:22 chromosomal translocation (*EWS/FLI1* is the fusion gene)

3. Clinical presentation

 a. Pain is the most common symptom.

 b. Swelling, limp, and decreased range of motion are variable.

 c. Frequent fever, occasional erythema (mistaken for infection)

4: Orthopaedic Oncology and Systemic Disease

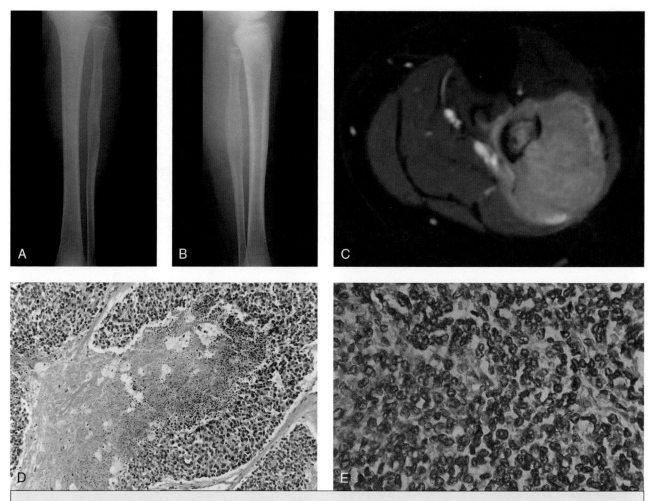

Figure 18 Ewing sarcoma/PNET. **A,** AP and **B,** lateral radiographs of the left tibia/fibula in an 11-year-old boy reveal a lesion in the fibular diaphysis. After needle biopsy, it was diagnosed as a Ewing sarcoma. The initial periosteal reaction ossified slightly after two cycles of neoadjuvant chemotherapy. **C,** Axial MRI reveals an extensive soft-tissue mass at diagnosis consistent with a small round cell lesion. **D,** Low-power histology reveals a small round blue cell lesion with large sheets of necrosis. **E,** Higher power reveals the monotonous small cells with prominent nuclei and scant cytoplasm.

d. Elevated erythrocyte sedimentation rate (ESR), LDH, white blood cell count

e. The most common locations are the pelvis, diaphysis of long bones, and scapula.

f. Staging workup includes a bone marrow biopsy in addition to the standard studies (CT chest, radiograph/MRI of primary lesion, bone scan).

4. Imaging

a. Purely lytic bone destruction

b. Periosteal reaction in multiple layers (the classic reaction, called "onion skin") or sunburst pattern (**Figure 18,** A and B).

c. Poorly marginated and permeative

d. Extensive soft-tissue mass often present despite more subtle bone destruction (**Figures 19 and 20**)

e. MRI necessary to identify soft-tissue extension and marrow involvement (**Figure 18,** C)

f. Radiographic differential diagnosis includes osteomyelitis, osteosarcoma, eosinophilic granuloma, osteoid osteoma, lymphoma.

5. Pathology

a. Gross appearance may be a liquid consistency, mimicking pus.

b. Small round blue cells with round/oval nuclei (**Figure 18,** D and E)

c. Indistinct cell outlines

d. Prominent nuclei and minimal cytoplasm

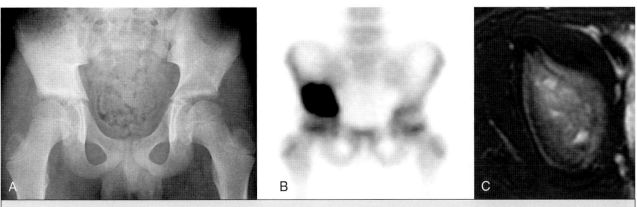

Figure 19   Ewing sarcoma of the pelvis. **A,** AP radiograph reveals an indistinct abnormality in the right supra-acetabular region. **B,** Technetium Tc 99m bone scan reveals avid uptake in this area. **C,** Axial MRI of the acetabular region reveals an elevated periosteum. A biopsy was consistent with Ewing sarcoma.

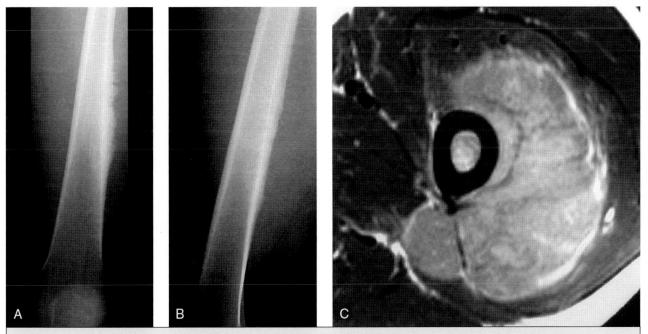

Figure 20   Ewing sarcoma in a 14-year-old boy. AP **(A)** and lateral **(B)** radiographs of the femur reveal a diaphyseal lesion with a sunburst pattern of periosteal reaction. **C,** Axial MRI reveals an extensive soft-tissue mass. A biopsy revealed Ewing sarcoma.

e. Reactive osseous or fibroblastic tissue may be present.

f. Can be broad sheets of necrosis and widely separated fibrous strands

g. Differential diagnosis includes lymphoma, osteomyelitis, neuroblastoma, rhabdomyosarcoma, eosinophilic granuloma, leukemia.

h. Immunohistochemical stains helpful—CD99 positive (013 antibody)

i. 11:22 chromosomal translocation produces *EWS/FLI1*, which can be identified by polymerase chain reaction and differentiates Ewing

sarcoma from other round cell lesions.

j. Additional features seen only in PNET include a more lobular pattern and arrangement of the cells in poorly formed rosettes around an eosinophilic material (**Figure 21**).

6. Treatment/outcome

a. Standard treatment of Ewing sarcoma is neoadjuvant chemotherapy.

b. Most common chemotherapy drugs include vincristine, adriamycin (doxorubicin), ifosfamide, etoposide, cytoxan, and actinomycin D.

4: Orthopaedic Oncology and Systemic Disease

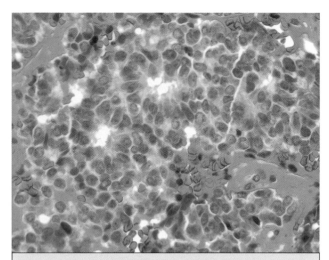

Figure 21 High-power histology of a PNET lesion. Note that the cells are arranged in a rosette pattern around a central eosinophilic substance.

c. Local control of the primary tumor can be achieved by either wide surgical resection or external beam radiation.

d. Most isolated extremity lesions are treated with surgical resection rather than radiation because of potential side effects of radiation and better local control with surgery.

e. Radiation is often used for the primary lesion when patients present with metastatic disease.

f. Local control is controversial for pelvic Ewing sarcoma: surgery or radiation or both.

g. Complications of radiation in skeletally immature patients include joint contractures, fibrosis, growth arrest, fracture, and secondary malignancy (usually 10 to 20 years later).

h. Response to chemotherapy (percent necrosis) is used as a prognostic indicator for overall survival.

i. Patients with isolated extremity Ewing sarcoma have a 5-year survival of 65% to 70%.

j. Patients who present with metastatic disease have a poor prognosis (5-year survival <20%).

k. Metastases occur primarily in the lungs but also in the bone and bone marrow.

l. Adverse prognostic factors include nonpulmonary metastasis, <90% necrosis, large tumor volume, pelvic lesions.

m. PNET is thought to have a slightly worse prognosis than Ewing sarcoma.

V. Notochordal and Miscellaneous

A. Chordoma—Slow-growing malignant bone tumor arising from notochordal rests and occurring in the spinal axis.

1. Demographics

   a. Male to female ratio = 3:1 (most apparent in sacral lesions)

   b. Occurs in adult patients (older than 40 years)

   c. Lesions at base of skull present earlier than sacral lesions

2. Genetics/etiology—Chordoma is thought to develop from residual notochordal cells that eventually undergo neoplastic change.

3. Clinical presentation

   a. Insidious onset of low back or sacral pain

   b. Frequently misdiagnosed as osteoarthritis, nerve impingement, disk herniation

   c. Infrequent distal motor/sensory loss because most lesions occur below S1

   d. Bowel/bladder symptoms are common.

   e. 50% can be identified on a careful rectal examination. (Do not perform a transrectal biopsy.)

   f. 50% occur in the sacrococcygeal region, 35% in the spheno-occipital region, and 15% in the mobile spine.

4. Imaging

   a. Chordomas occur in the midline, consistent with prior notochord location.

   b. Subtle findings on plain radiographs because of overlying bowel gas

   c. Cross-sectional imaging with CT or MRI required (**Figure 22, *A* through** C)

   d. CT reveals areas of calcification within the lesion.

   e. MRI (low intensity on T1-weighted images, high intensity on T2-weighted images) defines the extent of the frequent anterior soft-tissue mass and the bony involvement (usually involves multiple sacral levels).

   f. Radiographic differential diagnosis includes chondrosarcoma, multiple myeloma, metastatic disease, giant cell tumor, and lymphoma (**Table 2**).

5. Pathology

   a. Grossly, chordoma appears lobulated and jelly-

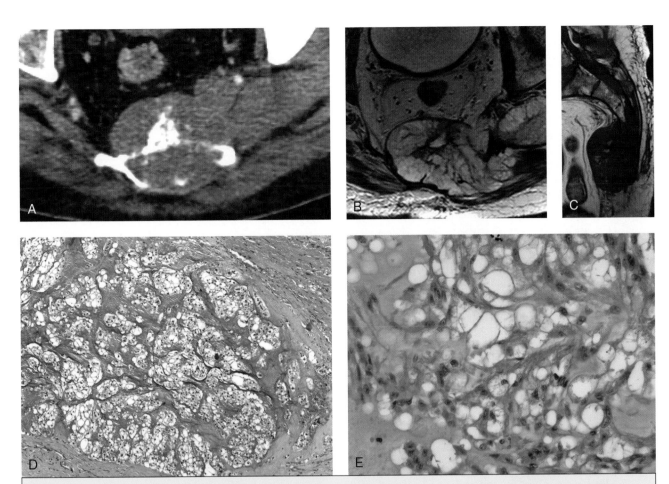

Figure 22   Chordoma. **A,** CT scan of the sacrum in a 66-year-old man reveals a destructive lesion with an anterior soft-tissue mass containing calcifications. **B,** Axial MRI further defines the soft-tissue extension anteriorly and toward the left pelvic sidewall. **C,** Sagittal T1-weighted MRI shows the lesion at S3 and below. The anterior extension abuts the rectum. **D,** Low-power histology of this lesion reveals a tumor lobule surrounded by fibrous tissue. **E,** Higher power reveals the physaliferous cells of a chordoma with a bubbly appearance to the cytoplasm.

like, with tumor tracking along the nerve roots.

b. The signature cell is the physaliferous cell, which contains intracellular vacuoles and appears bubbly (cytoplasmic mucous droplets) (**Figure 22,** *D* and *E*).

c. Lobules of the tumor are separated by fibrous septa.

d. Physaliferous cells are keratin-positive, which differentiates this tumor from chondrosarcoma.

e. Weakly S100-positive

f. Differential diagnosis includes chondrosarcoma and metastatic carcinoma.

6. Treatment/outcome

a. The main treatment is wide surgical resection.

b. Local recurrence is common (50%) and is directly related to the surgical margin achieved.

Table 2
Tumors Occurring in the Vertebrae
Anterior (Vertebral Body)
Giant cell tumor
Metastatic disease
Multiple myeloma
Ependymoma
Chordoma
Lymphoma
Primary bone tumors (chondrosarcoma, osteosarcoma)
Posterior Elements
Osteoid osteoma
Osteoblastoma
Aneurysmal bone cyst

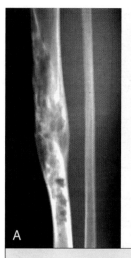
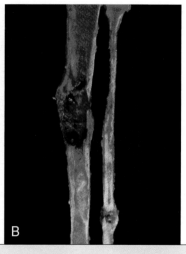
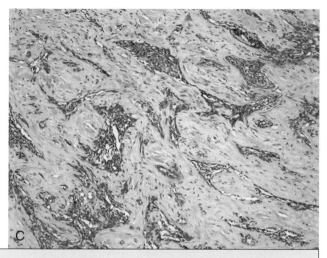

Figure 23   Adamantinoma. **A,** AP radiograph of the tibia in a 38-year-old woman reveals multiple diaphyseal lucent lesions separated by sclerotic bone. They have a bubbly appearance consistent with adamantinoma. **B,** A gross specimen from a different patient reveals lesions in both the tibia and fibula that expand the bone. **C,** The histologic appearance is nests of epithelial cells in a fibrous stroma.

c. To achieve a satisfactory wide margin, the surgeon must be willing to sacrifice involved nerve roots, viscera, etc.

d. Radiation can be used as an adjunct for locally recurrent disease, positive margins, or as primary treatment of inoperable tumors (protons or external beam).

e. Radiation alone is generally not effective for local control.

f. Chemotherapy is not effective and is currently not indicated.

g. Chordoma metastasizes late to the lungs and occasionally bone; requires long-term follow-up (20 years).

h. Long-term survival is 25% to 50%, due in part to local progression.

B. Adamantinoma—Unusual, rare, slow-growing malignant bone tumor with a predilection for the tibia (**Figure 23**)

1. Demographics

a. No gender predilection

b. Patients are generally 20 to 40 years of age.

c. Fewer than 300 cases in the literature

2. Genetics/etiology—Controversy whether adamantinoma evolves from osteofibrous dysplasia; most believe it does not.

3. Clinical presentation

a. Pain of variable duration and intensity is the major symptom.

b. Occasional tibial deformity or a mass

c. Tenderness over the subcutaneous tibial border

d. History of preceding trauma is common.

e. 90% of lesions occur in the tibial diaphysis.

4. Imaging

a. Classic radiographic appearance is multiple well-circumscribed lucent defects, usually with one dominant defect that may locally expand the bone (**Figure 23,** *A*).

b. Sclerotic bone between defects

c. "Soap bubble" appearance

d. Lesions may be intracortical or intramedullary, with occasional (10%) soft-tissue mass.

e. No periosteal reaction

5. Pathology

a. Nests of epithelial cells in a benign fibrous stroma (**Figure 23,** *C*)

b. Epithelial cells are columnar in appearance and keratin-positive.

c. Epithelial cells are bland without mitosis.

6. Treatment/outcome

a. Standard of care is wide surgical resection.

b. Chemotherapy and radiation are not indicated.

c. Local recurrence is more common when adequate margins are not achieved.

d. Given diaphyseal location, common reconstruction is intercalary allograft

e. Late metastasis to lungs, bones, lymph nodes in 15% to 20%

f. Requires long-term follow-up

g. Case series from 2000 described 87% survival at 10 years.

VI. Systemic Disease

A. Multiple myeloma—Neoplastic proliferation of plasma cells producing a monoclonal protein.

1. Demographics

   a. Considered the most common primary malignant bone tumor

   b. Affects patients >40 years of age

   c. Twice as common in blacks as whites

   d. Affects males more than females

2. Genetics/etiology

   a. Immunoglobulins (Igs) are composed of two heavy chains and two light chains.

      i. Heavy chains = IgG, IgA, IgM, IgD, and IgE (IgG and IgA common in myeloma)

      ii. Light chains = κ and λ (Bence Jones proteins)

   b. In myeloma, both heavy and light chains are produced.

   c. Major mediators of osteoclastogenesis in myeloma include receptor activator of nuclear factor κ B ligand (RANKL), interleukin-6, and macrophage inflammatory protein-1α.

   d. Osteoblastic bone formation is suppressed by tumor necrosis factor and Dickkopf-1 (Dkk-1).

3. Clinical presentation

   a. Common symptoms include bone pain, pathologic fractures, cord compression, and recurrent infections.

   b. Occurs throughout the skeleton but is common in bones that contain hematopoietic marrow, including the skull, spine, and long bones (**Figure 24**)

   c. Laboratory findings: normochromic, normocytic anemia, hypercalcemia, renal failure, amyloidosis, elevated ESR

   d. Electrophoresis (99% of patients have a spike on one or both)

      i. Serum—identifies types of proteins present.

      ii. Urine—identifies Bence Jones proteins.

   e. 24-hour urine collection—quantifies protein in urine.

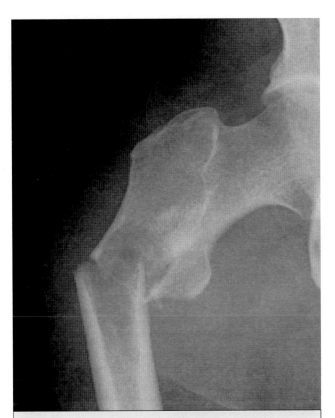

Figure 24   This 47-year-old woman presented with a pathologic fracture through a lytic lesion, and open biopsy at the time of surgery showed a plasma cell lesion consistent with multiple myeloma.

f. β2 microglobulin—tumor marker with prognostic ability (increased β2 microglobulin = poor prognosis)

g. Diagnosis—One major and one minor (or three minor) diagnostic criteria must be present.

   i. Major criteria

      (a) Plasmacytoma—tissue diagnosis on biopsy

      (b) >30% plasma cells in bone marrow

      (c) Serum IgG >3.5 g/dL, IgA >2 g/dL or urine >1 g/24 hours, or Bence Jones protein

   ii. Minor criteria

      (a) 10% to 30% plasma cells in bone marrow

      (b) Serum/urine protein levels lower than listed for major criteria

      (c) Lytic bone lesions

      (d) Lower than normal IgG levels

4: Orthopaedic Oncology and Systemic Disease

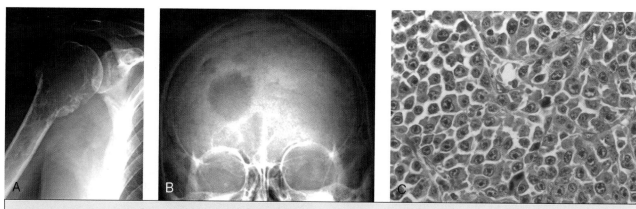

Figure 25 Multiple myeloma. **A,** AP radiograph in a 67-year-old woman with constant right shoulder pain shows a lytic lesion in the humeral head. **B,** A workup included a skeletal survey after a positive serum protein electrophoresis. A punched-out lytic lesion was noted in the skull, consistent with multiple myeloma. **C,** A high-power view of myeloma reveals numerous plasma cells with eccentric nuclei and extensive vascularity.

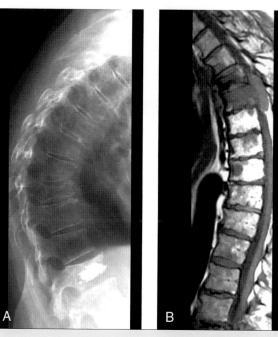

Figure 26 Multiple myeloma. **A,** A lateral thoracic spine radiograph demonstrates the severe osteopenia present in multiple myeloma contributing to compression fractures. Note the prior injection of cement to stabilize a vertebral body in the lower part of the figure. **B,** Sagittal MRI of the thoracic spine in a patient with long-standing multiple myeloma shows multiple vertebral lesions with an area of epidural extension.

   d. Diffuse osteopenia (**Figure 26,** *A*)

   e. Bone scan is usually negative because there is minimal osteoblastic response in myeloma.

   f. Skeletal survey is the screening tool of choice.

   g. MRI is not necessary for screening but is helpful in defining vertebral lesions (**Figure 26,** *B*).

5. Pathology

   a. Lesion consists of sheets of plasma cells with eccentric nuclei; little intercellular material (**Figure 25,** *C*).

   b. Nuclear chromatin arranged in a "clock face" pattern

   c. Abundant eosinophilic cytoplasm

   d. Rare mitotic figures

   e. Extremely vascular, with extensive capillary system

   f. Immunohistochemistry stains—CD38+

6. Treatment/outcome

   a. Primary treatment is cytotoxic chemotherapy (often in combination with prednisone or dexamethasone).

   b. Chemotherapy agents include melphalan, cyclophosphamide, doxorubicin, thalidomide (second line).

   c. Bisphosphonates help to decrease number of lesions, bone pain, and serum calcium.

   d. Autologous stem cell transplant improves survival.

   e. Radiation effective to decrease pain, avoid surgery

4. Imaging

   a. Classic appearance is multiple "punched-out" lytic lesions throughout the skeleton (**Figures 25,** *A* and *B*, **and 26,** *A*)

   b. No surrounding sclerosis

   c. Skull lesions and vertebral compression fractures are common (**Figures 25,** *B* and **26,** *A*).

f. Surgical stabilization of pathologic fractures or impending fractures (similar principles as used in metastatic disease)

g. Kyphoplasty/vertebroplasty common to treat vertebral compression fractures

h. Survival worse with renal failure

i. 10-year survival is 10%.

j. Median survival is 3 years.

B. Plasmacytoma

1. Plasma cell tumor in a single skeletal site

2. Represents 5% of patients with plasma cell lesions

3. Negative serum/urine protein electrophoresis

4. Bone marrow biopsy/aspirate negative

5. Treated with radiation alone (4,500 to 5,000 cGy)

6. Progresses to myeloma in ~55% of patients

C. Osteosclerotic myeloma

1. Accounts for 3% of cases

2. POEMS syndrome = *p*olyneuropathy, *o*rganomegaly, *e*ndocrinopathy, *M*-spike, *s*kin changes

D. B-cell lymphoma—Clonal proliferation of B-cells commonly presenting as nodal disease and occasionally affecting the skeleton.

1. Demographics

a. Can occur at any age but most commonly in patients aged 35 to 55 years

b. Affects males more than females

c. Non-Hodgkin lymphoma most commonly affects the bone (B-cell much more common than T-cell variants).

d. 10% to 35% of patients with non-Hodgkin lymphoma have extranodal disease.

e. Primary lymphoma of bone can occur but is quite rare.

2. Genetics/etiology—Risk factors for B-cell lymphoma include immunodeficiency (human immunodeficiency virus, hepatitis) and viral/bacterial infection.

3. Clinical presentation

a. Constant pain unrelieved by rest

b. A large soft-tissue mass that is tender or warm is common.

c. Lymphoma affects bones with persistent red marrow (femur, spine, pelvis).

d. Neurologic symptoms from spinal lesions

e. 25% present with pathologic fracture.

f. B-symptoms = fever, weight loss, and night sweats

g. Primary lymphoma of bone is rare and occurs when there are no extraskeletal sites of disease (other than a single node) for 6 months after diagnosis.

4. Imaging appearance

a. Lytic, permeative lesions that can show subtle bone destruction (**Figure 27, *A***)

b. Generally involves the diaphysis in long bones

c. Can involve multiple sites in the skeleton

d. Intensely positive on bone scan

e. Extensive marrow involvement noted on MRI

f. Often large soft-tissue mass (**Figure 27, *B* and *C***)

g. PET helpful in staging and follow-up of disease

h. Radiographic differential diagnosis includes metastatic disease, myeloma. and osteomyelitis.

5. Pathology

a. Difficult to diagnose on needle biopsy because the tissue is often crushed

b. Diffuse infiltrative rather than nodular pattern

c. Lesion comprised of small round blue cells (2× size of lymphocytes and can be variable) (**Figure 27, *D***)

d. Immunohistochemistry stains—CD20+, CD45+

e. Primary lymphoma of bone; increased percentage of cleaved cells improves prognosis.

6. Treatment/outcome

a. Bone marrow biopsy and CT of the chest, abdomen, and pelvis are required as part of staging/workup.

b. Chemotherapy is the primary treatment. Chemotherapeutic agents include cyclophosphamide, doxorubicin, prednisone, and vincristine.

c. Radiation of the primary site is used in some individuals for persistent disease.

d. Surgical treatment is necessary only for pathologic fractures because chemotherapy alone is effective for most lesions.

e. 5-year survival is as high as 70% in series where chemotherapy and radiation were used for disseminated disease.

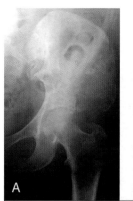
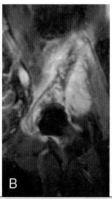
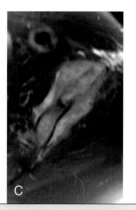
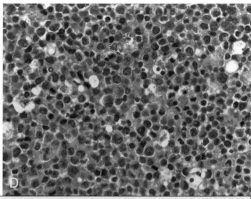

Figure 27   Lymphoma. **A,** AP radiograph of the left pelvis in a 72-year-old woman with lateral hip pain reveals an extensive lytic lesion of the ilium causing a pathologic fracture. Coronal (**B**) and axial (**C**) MRI scans reveal the extent of the surrounding soft-tissue mass. **D,** A high-power histologic view reveals a small round blue cell lesion (larger than lymphocytes). A CD20 stain was positive for a B-cell lymphoma.

f. Secondary involvement of bone in lymphoma has a worse prognosis than primary lymphoma of bone.

VII. Secondary Lesions

A. Overview

1. Secondary lesions can be benign (secondary ABC), but most commonly they are malignant (postradiation sarcoma, Paget sarcoma, sarcomas emanating from infarct or fibrous dysplasia, squamous carcinomas from osteomyelitis/ draining sinus) (**Table 3 and Figures 28 and 29**).

2. These lesions develop from a preexisting tumor, process, or treatment.

B. Postradiation sarcoma—A postradiation sarcoma develops with a latent period after radiation has been used to treat a benign or malignant bone, soft-tissue, or visceral tumor.

1. Demographics

a. These lesions can occur at any age after radiation of a prior tumor (Ewing sarcoma, cervical/breast/prostate cancer, giant cell tumor, soft-tissue sarcoma, retinoblastoma).

b. More common in children exposed to radiation than in adults

c. Latent period is variable (4 to 40 years; median ~10 years)

d. Literature suggests children with Ewing sarcoma treated with radiation have a 5%-10% risk of postradiation malignancy at 20 years (7% for a postradiation sarcoma).

2. Genetics/etiology

a. Ionizing radiation causes DNA damage and creates free radicals.

Table 3

Secondary Lesions

Type	Histology
Benign	Aneurysmal bone cyst
Postradiation (for Ewing sarcoma, carcinoma, giant cell tumor)	Osteosarcoma Malignant fibrous histiocytoma Fibrosarcoma Chondrosarcoma
Paget sarcoma	Osteosarcoma Malignant fibrous histiocytoma Fibrosarcoma
Secondary to infarct	Malignant fibrous histiocytoma
Secondary to fibrous dysplasia	Osteosarcoma Malignant fibrous histiocytoma Fibrosarcoma
Secondary to benign cartilage lesion (enchondroma/osteosarcoma)	Chondrosarcoma
Secondary to chronic osteomyelitis/draining sinus	Squamous cell carcinoma

b. Incidence dependent on dose, type, and rate of radiation treatment

c. May be affected by the use of chemotherapy (especially alkylating agents)

3. Clinical presentation

a. Gradual onset of intermittent, then constant, pain in a previously radiated site

b. Can affect any skeletal site

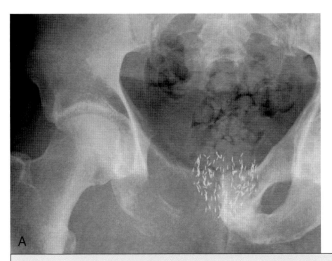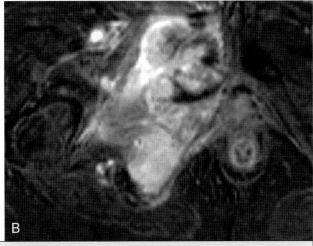

Figure 28 Secondary sarcoma. **A,** AP radiograph of the right anterior pelvis in a 68-year-old man with a history of prostate cancer (note radiation seeds) shows a destructive lesion in the right pubic rami. **B,** Axial MRI shows the extent of the surrounding soft-tissue mass. The biopsy revealed a high-grade sarcoma that was presumably radiation-induced.

4. Imaging appearance

    a. Lytic, aggressive, destructive bone lesion (**Figure 28,** *A*)

    b. Possible soft-tissue mass (**Figure 28,** *B*)

    c. MRI used to define the extent of the lesion

5. Pathology

    a. Histology shows the high-grade sarcoma (osteosarcoma, MFH, fibrosarcoma).

    b. May be histologic evidence of prior irradiation in the surrounding tissues

6. Treatment/outcome

    a. Treatment is chemotherapy and surgical resection.

    b. Poor prognosis, with 25% to 50% 5-year survival (worse in sites not amenable to surgical resection)

    c. Metastasis primarily to the lung

C. Paget sarcoma—Arises from a skeletal area affected by Paget disease.

    1. Demographics

        a. Occurs in older patients (>50 years of age)

        b. Occurs in ~1% of patients with Paget disease

    2. Clinical presentation

        a. New onset of pain in an area affected by Paget disease

        b. Possible swelling or pathologic fracture

        c. Commonly affects pelvis, proximal femur

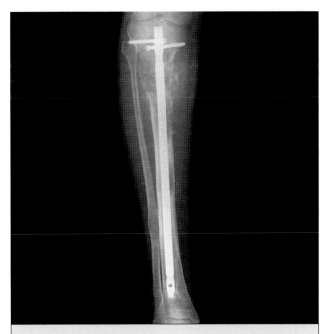

Figure 29 Radiograph of the right lower extremity of a 64-year-old man with a diagnosis of polyostotic fibrous dysplasia. He sustained a pathologic fracture of the right proximal tibia through a lytic lesion, and an intramedullary device was placed without a preoperative biopsy. The eventual biopsy revealed a high-grade osteosarcoma developing from an area of fibrous dysplasia. The patient required an above-knee amputation.

3. Imaging appearance

    a. Marked bone destruction and possible soft-tissue mass in a skeletal site affected by Paget disease

4: Orthopaedic Oncology and Systemic Disease

b. Helpful to have prior documentation of the radiographic appearance

c. MRI helpful to define the extent of the sarcoma within the abnormal bone

4. Pathology—Histology shows a high-grade sarcoma (osteosarcoma, MFH, fibrosarcoma, chondrosarcoma) within an area of pagetoid bone.

5. Treatment/outcome

a. Poor prognosis, with <10% 5-year survival rate

b. Treat as a primary bone sarcoma with chemotherapy and surgical resection

c. Radiation is palliative only.

d. High rate of metastasis to the lung

Top Testing Facts

Osteosarcoma and Malignant Fibrous Histiocytoma

1. Osteosarcoma is the most common malignant bone tumor in children.

2. Osteosarcoma classically occurs in the metaphysis of long bones and presents with progressive pain.

3. Osteosarcoma has a radiographic appearance of bone destruction and bone formation starting in the medullary canal.

4. The osteoblastic stromal cells are malignant in osteosarcoma.

5. The 5-year survival of patients with osteosarcoma is 65% to 70%.

6. Parosteal and periosteal osteosarcomas occur on the surface of the bone.

7. Parosteal osteosarcoma is a low-grade lesion that appears fibrous histologically and is treated with wide surgical resection alone.

8. Periosteal osteosarcoma is an intermediate-grade lesion that appears cartilaginous and is treated with chemotherapy and surgical resection.

9. Telangiectatic osteosarcoma can be confused with an aneurysmal bone cyst.

10. Malignant fibrous histiocytoma of bone presents and is treated like osteosarcoma but no osteoid is noted histologically.

Chondrosarcoma

1. Chondrosarcoma occurs de novo or secondary to an enchondroma or osteochondroma.

2. Chondrosarcoma occurs in adults, whereas osteosarcoma and Ewing sarcoma occur primarily in children.

3. The pelvis is the most common location for chondrosarcoma.

4. Pelvic chondrosarcomas require wide resection regardless of grade.

5. Chemotherapy is used only in the dedifferentiated and mesenchymal chondrosarcoma variants.

6. Tumor grade is a major prognostic factor for chondrosarcoma.

7. Grade 1 chondrosarcomas rarely metastasize and have a >90% survival.

8. The survival for patients with dedifferentiated chondrosarcoma is the lowest of all bone sarcomas (10%).

9. Clear cell chondrosarcoma has a radiographic appearance similar to chondroblastoma.

10. Radiation is not used in the treatment of chondrosarcoma.

Top Testing Facts (cont.)

Ewing Sarcoma/PNET

1. Ewing sarcoma is one of a group of small round blue cell tumors not distinguishable based on histology alone.
2. Ewing sarcoma is the second most common malignant bone tumor in children.
3. Ewing sarcoma is found most commonly in the diaphysis of long bones as well as in the pelvis.
4. No matrix is produced by the tumor cells, so the radiographs are purely lytic.
5. There may be extensive periosteal reaction and a large soft-tissue mass.
6. Ewing sarcoma is CD99-positive and has the 11:22 chromosomal translocation.
7. Ewing sarcoma is radiation-sensitive, but surgery is used more commonly for local control unless the patient has metastatic disease.
8. Ewing sarcoma requires multiagent chemotherapy
9. Ewing sarcoma can metastasize to the lungs, bone, and bone marrow.
10. The 5-year survival rate of patients with isolated extremity Ewing sarcoma is 65% to 70%.

Chordoma and Adamantinoma

1. Chordoma occurs exclusively in the spinal axis, although many lesions should be considered in the differential of a destructive sacral lesion.
2. Chordoma occurs in adults and has a prolonged course; misdiagnosis is common.
3. Plain radiographs often do not identify sacral destruction from chordoma—cross-sectional imaging is required.
4. CT scan of a chordoma shows calcified areas within the tumor.
5. Chordoma consists of physaliferous cells on histologic examination.
6. Surgical cure of chordoma requires a wide resection—possibly removing nerve roots, bowel, bladder, etc.
7. Radiation can be used in an adjunct fashion for chordoma, but chemotherapy has no role.
8. Adamantinoma occurs primarily in the tibial diaphysis and has a soap bubble radiographic appearance.
9. Adamantinoma consists of nests of epithelial cells in a fibrous stroma and is keratin-positive.
10. Adamantinoma requires a wide surgical resection for cure.

Multiple Myeloma and Lymphoma

1. Multiple myeloma is the most common primary malignant bone tumor.
2. Myeloma often presents with normochromic, normocytic anemia.
3. Myeloma presents radiographically with multiple punched-out lytic lesions.
4. Myeloma is typically "cold" on bone scan.
5. Myeloma is composed of sheets of plasma cells.
6. Myeloma is treated with chemotherapy, bisphosphonates, and possibly autologous stem cell transplant.
7. Lymphoma affecting bone is usually non-Hodgkin B-cell subtype.
8. Subtle radiographic bone destruction with extensive marrow and soft-tissue involvement is typical.
9. Lymphoma cells are CD20+ on immunohistochemistry staining.
10. B-cell lymphoma is treated with chemotherapy and radiation and rarely requires surgery.

Secondary Lesions

1. Secondary lesions can be benign (secondary ABC or giant cell tumor) but are most commonly sarcomas.
2. Secondary sarcomas arise in areas of Paget disease, prior radiation, or previous lesions (bone infarcts, fibrous dysplasia).
3. New onset pain in the site of a previous lesion or site of radiation is suspicious for a secondary lesion.
4. Radiographic appearance of a secondary sarcoma is an aggressive, destructive bone tumor.
5. Histologic appearance is of a high-grade sarcoma (osteosarcoma, MFH, fibrosarcoma, chondrosarcoma).
6. Secondary sarcomas have a uniformly poor prognosis; treatment is with chemotherapy and surgery.
7. MFH of bone can arise in a prior infarct and has a poor prognosis.
8. Fewer than 1% of fibrous dysplasia lesions undergo malignant change to MFH or osteosarcoma.
9. Secondary squamous cell carcinoma can arise in long-standing osteomyelitis with a draining sinus tract.
10. Secondary chondrosarcomas can occur in prior enchondromas or osteochondromas (more commonly in patients with Ollier, Maffucci, or multiple hereditary osteochondromas).

4: Orthopaedic Oncology and Systemic Disease

Bibliography

Bacci G, Longhi A, Versari M, Mercuri M, Briccoli A, Picci P: Prognostic factors for osteosarcoma of the extremity treated with neoadjuvant chemotherapy: 15-year experience in 789 patients treated at a single institution. *Cancer* 2006;106: 1154-1161.

Bacci G, Picci P, Mercuri M, Bertoni F, Ferrari S: Neoadjuvant chemotherapy for high grade malignant fibrous histiocytoma of bone. *Clin Orthop Relat Res* 1998;346:178-189.

Bjornsson J, McLeod RA, Unni KK, Ilstrup DM, Pritchard DJ: Primary chondrosarcoma of long bones and limb girdles. *Cancer* 1998;83:2105-2119.

Bullough PG: *Atlas of Orthopaedic Pathology with Clinical and Radiologic Correlations*, ed 2. New York, NY, Gower Medical Publishing, 1992, pp 16.5-17.21.

Carvajal R, Meyers P: Ewing's sarcoma and primitive neuroectodermal family of tumors. *Hematol Oncol Clin North Am* 2005;19:501-525.

Durie BGM, Salmon SE: A clinical staging system for multiple myeloma: Correlation of measured myeloma cell mass with presenting clinical features, response to treatment and survival. *Cancer* 1975;36:842-852.

Fuchs B, Dickey ID, Yaszemski MJ, Inwards CY, Sim FH: Operative management of sacral chordoma. *J Bone Joint Surg Am* 2005;87:2211-2216.

Gibbs CP, Weber K, Scarborough MT: Malignant bone tumors. *Instr Course Lect* 2002;51:413-428.

Hornicek FJ: Osteosarcoma of bone, in Schwartz HS (ed): *Orthopaedic Knowledge Update: Musculoskeletal Tumors 2*. Rosemont, IL, American Academy of Orthopaedic Surgeons, 2007, pp 163-174.

Keeney GL, Unni KK, Beabout JW, Pritchard DJ: Adamantinoma of long bones: A clinicopathologic study of 85 cases. *Cancer* 1989;64:730-737.

Kuttesch JF Jr, Wexler LH, Marcus RB, et al: Second malignancies after Ewing's sarcoma: Radiation dose-dependency of secondary sarcomas. *J Clin Oncol* 1996;14:2818-2825.

McCarthy EF, Frassica FJ: *Pathology of Bone and Joint Disorders*. Philadelphia, PA, WB Saunders, 1998, pp 185-269.

Ostrowski ML, Unni KK, Banks PM, Shives TC, Evans RG, O'Connell MJ: Malignant lymphoma of bone. *Cancer* 1986; 58:2646-2655.

Patterson FR, Basra SK: Ewing's sarcoma, in Schwartz HS (ed): *Orthopaedic Knowledge Update: Musculoskeletal Tumors 2*. Rosemont, IL, American Academy of Orthopaedic Surgeons, 2007, pp 175-183.

Qureshi AA, Shott S, Mallin BA, Gitelis S: Current trends in the management of adamantinoma of long bones: An international study. *J Bone Joint Surg Am* 2000;82:1122-1131.

Seo SW, Remotti F, Lee FY: Chondrosarcoma of bone, in Schwartz HS (ed): *Orthopaedic Knowledge Update: Musculoskeletal Tumors 2*. Rosemont, IL, American Academy of Orthopaedic Surgeons, 2007, pp 185-195.

Unni KK: *Dahlin's Bone Tumors: General Aspects and Data on 11,087 Cases*, ed 5. Philadelphia, PA, Lippincott-Raven, 1996, pp 71-342.

Wold LE, Adler CP, Sim FH, Unni KK: *Atlas of Orthopedic Pathology*, ed 2. Philadelphia, PA, WB Saunders, 1990, pp 179-396.

Chapter 40

Benign Soft-Tissue Tumors and Reactive Lesions

Kristy Weber, MD

I. Lipoma

A. Definition and demographics

1. Lipoma is a benign tumor of adipose tissue.

2. Slightly more common in men than in women

3. Occurs primarily in patients 40 to 60 years of age

4. Superficial/subcutaneous lesions are common; deep lesions are uncommon.

5. Hibernomas are tumors of brown fat; they occur in slightly younger patients (20 to 40 years of age).

B. Genetics/etiology

1. White (common) versus brown fat (usually in hibernating animals or human infants)

2. Lipomas occur when white fat accumulates in inactive people.

3. Chromosomal abnormalities have been described.

C. Clinical presentation

1. Soft, painless, mobile mass characterizes the common superficial variety.

2. 5% to 8% of patients with superficial lipomas have multiple lesions.

3. Superficial lipomas are common in the upper back, the shoulders, the arms, the buttocks, and the proximal thighs.

4. Deep lipomas are usually intramuscular, fixed, and painless and can be large.

5. Deep lesions are found frequently in the thigh, shoulder, and calf.

6. Most are stable after an initial period of growth.

D. Imaging appearance

1. Plain radiographs are not helpful; may see a radiolucency in deep lipomas

2. CT scan: appearance of subcutaneous fat

3. Magnetic resonance imaging

a. Bright on T1-weighted images, moderate on T2-weighted images (**Figure 1, A** and **B**)

b. Lipomas will image exactly as fat on all sequences (suppress with fat-suppressed images).

c. They have a homogenous appearance, although minor linear streaking may occur.

d. Hibernomas have increased signal on T1-weighted images, but not always the same appearance as fat.

4. Occasionally, lipomas contain calcific deposits, bone.

5. Usually classic in MRI appearance and do not require a biopsy

E. Pathology

1. Gross appearance of lipoma is soft, lobular, white or yellow, with a capsule; hibernoma is red-brown in color because of profusion of mitochondria and more extensive vascularity than lipoma.

2. Histology reveals mature fat cells with moderate vascularity (**Figure 1, C**).

3. Occasionally note focal calcium deposits, cartilage, bone

4. Histologic variants include spindle cell lipoma, pleomorphic lipoma, angiolipoma—all benign but can be confused histologically with malignant lesions.

F. Treatment/outcome

1. Observation or local excision (can do excisional biopsy with marginal margin if imaging studies clearly document a lipoma).

2. Local recurrence is <5% if removed.

3. Malignant transformation is not clinically relevant; few cases reported.

G. Atypical lipoma

1. Usually very large, deep tumors

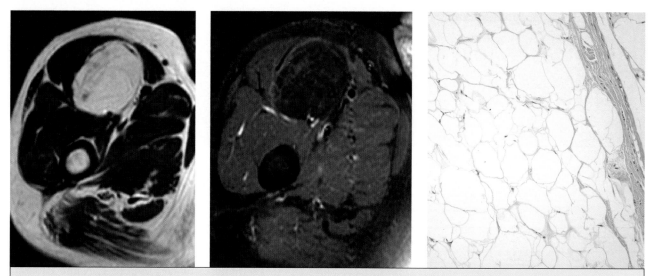

Figure 1   Intramuscular lipoma. Axial T1 fat-suppressed (**A**) and T2 fat-suppressed (**B**) MRIs of the right thigh reveal a well-circumscribed lesion with the same signal as the subcutaneous fat. Note that the lesion suppresses on the fat-suppressed images. This is classic for an intramuscular lipoma. **C,** The histologic appearance is of mature fat cells without atypia. A loose fibrous capsule is visible.

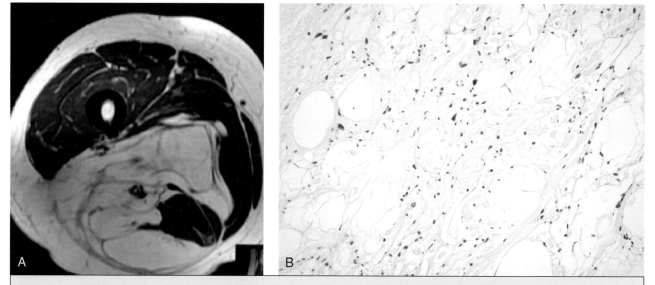

Figure 2   Atypical lipoma. **A,** Axial MRI reveals an extensive intramuscular lipomatous lesion infiltrating the posterior thigh musculature. Note the extensive stranding within the lesion. From this appearance, an intramuscular lipoma cannot be differentiated from an atypical lipoma. **B,** The histologic appearance of this atypical lipoma is more cellular than a classic lipoma.

2. May look identical to classic lipomas or may have increased stranding on MRI (**Figure 2,** *A* and *B*)

3. Histology shows greater cellularity than classic lipoma (**Figure 2,** *C*).

4. Often called atypical lipoma in extremities and well-differentiated liposarcoma in the retroperitoneum

5. Treatment is marginal excision; often not differentiated from classic lipoma until after excision (based on histology).

6. Higher chance of local recurrence (50% at 10 years) compared with lipoma, but does not metastasize

II. Intramuscular Hemangioma

A. Definition and demographics

1. Intramuscular hemangioma is a benign vascular neoplasm occurring in the deep tissues.

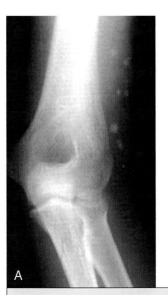
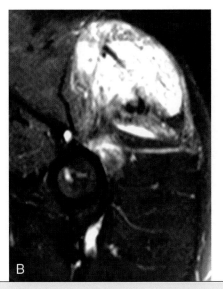
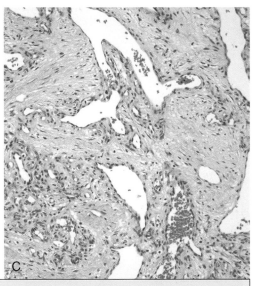

Figure 3 Intramuscular hemangiomas. **A,** Phleboliths seen in the lateral arm on this plain radiograph suggest a hemangioma. **B,** Axial T2-weighted MRI of the thigh reveals a poorly circumscribed soft-tissue lesion with both fatty and vascular features within the muscle, consistent with a hemangioma. **C,** Histologic view of this capillary hemangioma shows large blood-filled spaces but no cellular atypia.

2. Accounts for <1% of all benign vascular tumors

3. Males and females affected equally

4. Usually seen in patients <30 years of age

5. Often confused with other vascular malformations (arteriovenous malformations, cavernous hemangioma, angiomatosis, vascular ectasias, etc)

B. Genetics/etiology

1. Vascular malformations are caused by errors in morphogenesis affecting any segment of the vascular system.

2. Possible hormonal modulation

3. 20% associated with a history of trauma (no causal relationship)

C. Clinical presentation

1. Lesions are usually deep in the lower extremities but can involve any muscle.

2. Variable growth; often fluctuates with activity

3. Pain is variable and can increase with activity.

4. Usually no overlying skin lesions or bruits

5. Usually isolated lesions, but a rare form called diffuse hemangioma manifests in childhood and involves a limb extensively

D. Imaging appearance

1. Plain radiographs may reveal phleboliths or calcifications within the lesion (**Figure 3,** *A*).

2. May erode the adjacent bone

3. MRI reveals increased signal on T1- and T2-weighted images (**Figure 3,** *B*).

4. Focal low-signal areas are due to blood flow or calcifications.

5. Often ill-defined or described as a bag of worms; can appear infiltrative within the muscle

6. Frequently mistaken for a malignant soft-tissue tumor

E. Pathology

1. Gross appearance varies depending on whether the lesion is the capillary type or the cavernous type (capillary more common).

2. Color varies from red to tan to yellow.

3. Histology shows capillary-sized vessels with large nuclei (**Figure 3,** *C*).

4. Well-developed vascular lumens, infiltration of muscle fibers

5. No significant cellular pleomorphism

6. Cavernous type composed of large vessels with a large degree of adipose tissue

7. Differential diagnosis includes angiosarcoma.

F. Treatment/outcome

1. Most should be treated with observation, anti-inflammatory medications, compressive sleeves.

2. Many are amenable to interventional radiology techniques of embolization or sclerotherapy to decrease size of lesion or symptoms.

4: Orthopaedic Oncology and Systemic Disease

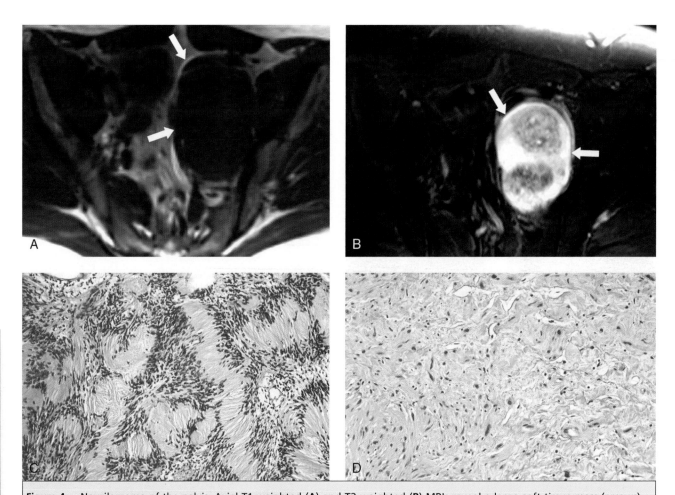

Figure 4   Neurilemoma of the pelvis. Axial T1-weighted (**A**) and T2-weighted (**B**) MRIs reveal a large soft-tissue mass (arrows) that has low signal intensity on T1 sequences and high signal intensity on T2 sequences. It would enhance after gadolinium administration. **C,** Low-power histologic view reveals the compact spindle cell areas (Antoni A) of a neurilemoma. Note the palisading nuclei and verocay bodies. **D,** Within the same tumor, there are areas of loosely arranged cells within a haphazard collagenous stroma (Antoni B). Antoni B areas contain numerous blood vessels.

3. Surgical excision carries a high risk of local recurrence.

4. No incidence of malignant transformation

III. Neurilemoma (Schwannoma)

A. Definition and demographics

1. Neurilemoma (schwannoma) is an encapsulated benign soft-tissue tumor composed of Schwann cells.

2. Commonly discovered in patients 20 to 50 years of age (may also occur in older patients)

3. Affects males and females equally

4. Can affect any motor or sensory nerve

5. More common than neurofibroma

B. Genetics/etiology—Often associated with mutations affecting the *NF2* gene.

C. Clinical presentation

1. Usually asymptomatic; sometimes causes pain with stretch or activity

2. Occurs frequently on the flexor surfaces of the extremities as well as the head/neck

3. Pelvic lesions can become quite large.

4. May change in size given frequent occurrence of cystic degeneration

5. Multiple lesions occur rarely.

6. Positive Tinel sign may be present.

D. Imaging appearance

1. Low signal intensity on T1-weighted MRI, high signal intensity on T2-weighted MRI (**Figure 4,** *A* and *B*)

2. Diffusely enhanced signal with gadolinium administration

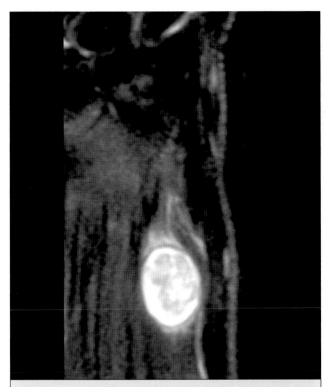

Figure 5 Coronal T2-weighted MRI of the wrist reveals a small, oval soft-tissue mass in continuity with a nerve, consistent with a neurilemoma.

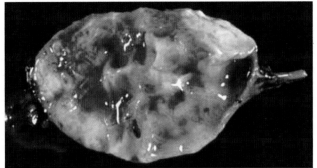

Figure 6 Gross appearance of a bisected neurilemoma (schwannoma) reveals cystic degeneration of the well-encapsulated lesion.

3. In sagittal or coronal images, may see in continuity with affected nerve (**Figure 5**)

4. Difficult to differentiate neurilemoma and neurofibroma

E. Pathology

1. Gross appearance is a well-encapsulated lesion, gray-tan in color (**Figure 6**).

2. Grows eccentrically from the nerve

3. Histology shows alternating areas of compact spindle cells (Antoni A) (**Figure 4,** C) and loosely arranged cells with large vessels (Antoni B) (**Figure 4,** D).

4. Verocay bodies are composed of two rows of aligned nuclei in a palisading formation, and their appearance is pathognomonic.

5. Strongly uniform positive staining for S100 antibody

F. Treatment/outcome

1. Observation or marginal/intralesional excision with nerve fiber preservation as symptoms dictate

2. Small risk of sensory deficits or long-standing palsies after dissection

3. Extremely rare risk of malignant degeneration

IV. Neurofibroma

A. Definition and demographics

1. Neurofibroma is a benign neural tumor involving multiple cell types.

2. Occurs in patients 20 to 40 years of age (younger when associated with neurofibromatosis)

3. Males and females are affected equally.

B. Genetics/etiology

1. Most neurofibromas arise sporadically.

2. Neurofibromatosis type 1 is an autosomal dominant syndrome characterized by multiple neurofibromas.

3. NF1—abnormal chromosome 17 (1 in 4,000 births)

4. NF2—abnormal chromosome 22 (1 in 40,000 births)

C. Clinical presentation

1. Can affect any nerve; may be cutaneous or plexiform (infiltrative)

2. Most are asymptomatic, but sometimes neurologic symptoms are present.

3. Tumors are slow-growing.

4. May have positive Tinel sign

5. National Institutes of Health criteria for neurofibromatosis:

- More than 6 café-au-lait spots
- Lisch nodule (melanocyte hamartoma affecting the iris)
- Axillary freckling
- Two neurofibromas or one plexiform neurofibroma
- Optic glioma
- Bone scalloping
- Relative with NF1 disease

4: Orthopaedic Oncology and Systemic Disease

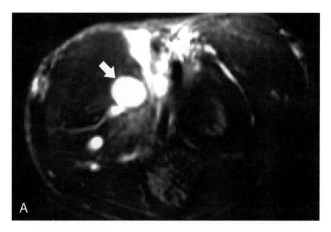

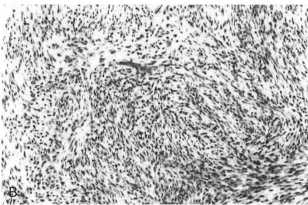

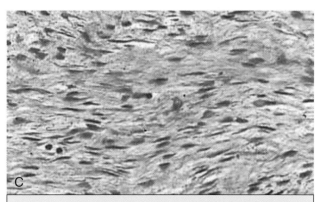

Figure 7   Neurofibroma of the elbow. **A,** Axial T2-weighted MRI of the elbow in a 26-year-old man with neurofibromatosis reveals an area of high signal intensity (arrow) consistent with a neurofibroma within the volar forearm muscles. The same lesion would be dark on T1-weighted sequences. **B,** Low-power histology reveals a cellular lesion with a wavy or storiform appearance. **C,** Higher power reveals elongated cells with dark nuclei and no atypia.

6. Rapid enlargement of a neurofibroma suggests malignant transformation.

D. Imaging appearance

   1. Varies in size; usually a fusiform expansion of the nerve

2. MRI—Low signal intensity on T1-weighted sequences, high on T2-weighted sequences (**Figure 7, A**).

3. Dumbbell-shaped lesion that can expand a neural foramen

4. More common than neurilemoma to have target sign (peripheral T2-hyperintensity and low signal center)

5. Bone changes include penciling of the ribs, sharp vertebral end plates, tibial pseudarthrosis, nonossifying fibromas, or scoliosis.

6. Plexiform neurofibroma has extensive signal on MRI scan; infiltrative

E. Pathology

   1. Gross appearance is fusiform expansion of the nerve, usually unencapsulated.

   2. Histology contains interlacing bundles of elongated cells with wavy, dark nuclei (**Figure 7, B** and **C**).

   3. Cells are associated with wirelike collagen fibrils.

   4. Sometimes the cells are arranged in fascicles or a storiform pattern.

   5. Mixed cell population of Schwann cells, mast cells, lymphocytes

   6. Stroma may have a myxoid appearance.

   7. S100 staining is variable.

F. Treatment/outcome

   1. Observe if asymptomatic

   2. Surgical excision can leave significant nerve deficit and may require grafting.

   3. 5% of patients with neurofibromatosis develop malignant transformation of a lesion (often a plexiform neurofibroma).

   4. Malignant transformation of a solitary lesion is rare.

V. Nodular Fasciitis

A. Definition and demographics

   1. Nodular fasciitis is a self-limited reactive process often mistaken for a fibrous neoplasm.

   2. Most common in adults 20 to 40 years of age

   3. Males and females affected equally

   4. Most common fibrous soft-tissue lesion

B. Genetics/etiology—Reactive rather than neoplastic process.

C. Clinical presentation

   1. Rapid growth of a nodule over 1 to 2 weeks

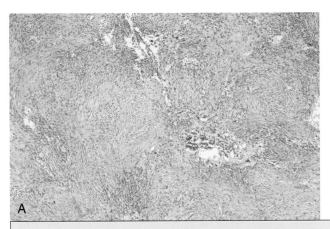
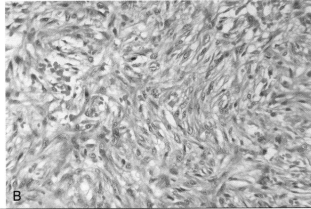

Figure 8   Nodular fasciitis. **A**, Low-power histology reveals a highly cellular lesion with a nodular pattern. **B**, Higher power shows regular plump fibroblasts with vessels, erythrocytes, and lipid macrophages consistent with nodular fasciitis.

2. 50% of patients have pain and/or tenderness.

3. Lesion is usually 1 to 2 cm in size.

4. Commonly occurs on volar forearm, back, chest wall, head/neck

5. Occurs as a solitary lesion

D. Imaging appearance

1. MRI shows nodularity, extension along fascial planes, and avid enhancement with gadolinium.

2. Usually small in size

3. Occurs superficially (most common), intramuscularly, or along the superficial fascial planes

E. Pathology

1. Grossly nodular without a surrounding capsule

2. Histology is cellular with numerous mitotic figures (**Figure 8, A**).

3. Cells are plump, regular fibroblasts arranged in short bundles or fascicles (**Figure 8, B**).

4. Additional cells include lymphoid cells, erythrocytes, giant cells, and lipid macrophages.

F. Treatment/outcome

1. Local resection with marginal or intralesional margin has a low risk of local recurrence.

2. No risk of malignant transformation

3. Reports of resolution of lesion after needle biopsy

VI. Intramuscular Myxoma

A. Definition and demographics

1. Intramuscular myxoma is a benign, nonaggressive myxomatous soft-tissue tumor.

2. Occurs in adults 40 to 70 years of age

3. Male to female ratio = 1:2

B. Clinical presentation

1. Usually presents as a painless mass

2. Pain/tenderness in ~20% of patients

3. Possible numbness or paresthesias in patients with large lesions

4. Usually solitary

5. Most commonly located in the thigh, buttocks, shoulder, and upper arm

6. Multiple intramuscular myxomas associated with fibrous dysplasia (Mazabraud syndrome)

C. Imaging appearance

1. MRI appearance is homogenous.

2. Low signal intensity (lower than muscle) on T1-weighted sequences, high on T2-weighted sequences (**Figure 9, A and B**)

3. Located within the muscle groups; usually 5 to 10 cm in size

4. In Mazabraud syndrome, fibrous dysplasia develops at a young age and the myxomas occur later in the same general anatomic area.

D. Pathology

1. Grossly lobular and gelatinous with cyst-like spaces (**Figure 9, C**)

2. Histology shows minimal cellularity with cells suspended in abundant mucoid material (**Figure 9, D**).

3. Loose network of reticulin fibers

4. No atypia and only sparse vascularity

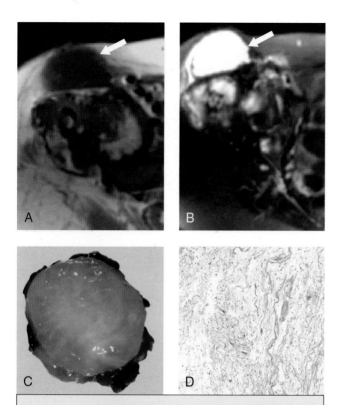

Figure 9 Intramuscular myxoma. Axial T1-weighted (**A**) and T2-weighted (**B**) MRIs in a 52-year-old woman with Mazabraud syndrome show a large soft-tissue lesion (arrows) along the anterior aspect of the right hip consistent with an intramuscular myxoma. It has lower signal intensity than muscle on T1-weighted images and is bright on T2-weighted images. **C**, Gross appearance of a bisected intramuscular myxoma reveals a white, gelatinous surface. **D**, The histologic appearance reveals a paucicellular lesion with extensive reticulin fibers and a mucoid stroma.

5. "Cellular myxoma" has increased cellularity and can be mistaken for a malignant myxoid neoplasm.

E. Treatment/outcome

1. Marginal excision is the preferred treatment.

2. Very rarely recurs locally and does not metastasize

VII. Desmoid Tumor (Extra-abdominal Fibromatosis)

A. Definition and demographics

1. Desmoid tumor is a benign, locally aggressive fibrous neoplasm with a high risk of local recurrence.

2. Common tumor; approximately 900 cases/year in United States

3. Occurs in young individuals (15 to 40 years of age)

4. Slight female predominance

5. Desmoid tumors occur within a family of fibromatoses that also includes superficial lesions in the palmar and plantar fascia (Dupuytren contracture, Ledderhose disease).

B. Genetics/etiology

1. Can have mutations in the adenomatous polyposis coli gene (more common in patients with familial polyposis)

2. Cytogenetic abnormalities include trisomy of chromosomes 8 or 20.

C. Clinical presentation

1. Usually present with painless mass

2. Rock hard, fixed, and deep on examination

3. Most commonly occurs in the shoulder, chest wall/back, thigh

4. >50% are extra-abdominal; 50% are intra-abdominal (pelvis, mesentery).

5. Occasionally multicentric; usually the subsequent lesion is more proximal in the same limb.

D. Imaging appearance

1. Typical MRI appearance: low signal intensity on T1-weighted sequences, low to medium signal intensity on T2-weighted sequences (**Figure 10**, *A* and *B*)

2. Gadolinium administration enhances appearance.

3. Infiltrative within the muscles; usually 5 to 10 cm in size

4. May have adjacent osseous changes (erosion)

E. Pathology

1. Gross characteristics: gritty, white, poorly encapsulated

2. Histology: bland fibroblasts with abundant collagen (**Figure 10**, *C* and *D*)

3. Uniform spindle cells with elongated nuclei and only occasional mitoses

4. Moderate vascularity

5. Sweeping bundles of collagen less defined than fibrosarcoma

6. Often infiltrates into adjacent tissues

F. Treatment/outcome

1. Treat similar to sarcoma, with wide resection

2. High risk of local recurrence given infiltrative pattern

3. Difficult to differentiate recurrent tumor from scar tissue

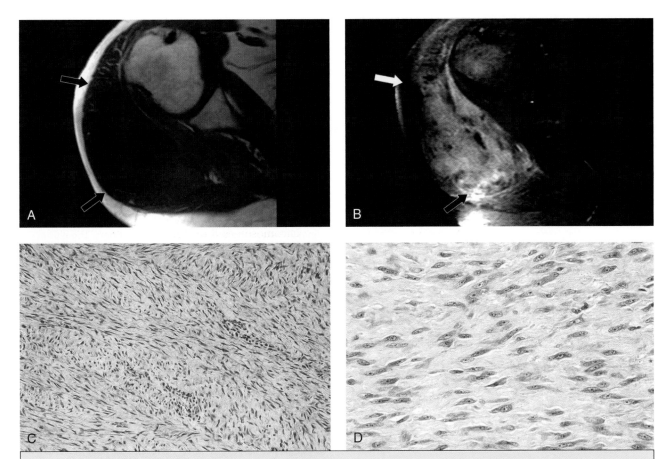

Figure 10 Desmoid tumors. Axial T1-weighted (**A**) and short tau inversion recovery (STIR) (**B**) MRIs of the right shoulder of a 58-year-old woman reveal a desmoid tumor (arrows). The STIR sequence is fluid-sensitive and reveals findings similar to those found on a fat-sensitive T2 image. There is low signal noted on both images. **C,** Low-power histologic view reveals sweeping bundles of collagen. **D,** Higher power demonstrates bland, elongated, fibrous cells without atypia.

4. External beam radiation (up to 60 Gy) is often used for recurrent lesions.

5. Low-dose chemotherapy ± radiation is used for inoperable lesions.

6. Unusual natural history: hard-to-predict behavior, occasional spontaneous regression

7. Treatment should not be worse than the disease; avoid amputation.

8. No risk of metastasis or malignant transformation unless related to radiation

VIII. Elastofibroma

A. Definition and demographics

1. Elastofibroma is an unusual, tumorlike reactive process that frequently occurs between the scapula and chest wall.

2. Occurs in patients 60 to 80 years of age

3. More common in females than males

B. Genetics/etiology

1. High familial incidence

2. Often occurs after repeated trauma

C. Clinical presentation

1. Usually asymptomatic; found in ~17% of elderly people at autopsy

2. Snapping scapula on examination

3. Firm, deep lesion

4. Occurs almost exclusively in the soft tissues between the tip of the scapula and the chest wall (rare in deltoid, greater trochanter)

5. Bilateral in 10% of cases (often noted on chest CT scans)

D. Imaging appearance

1. Ill-defined lesion with appearance of muscle on CT scan

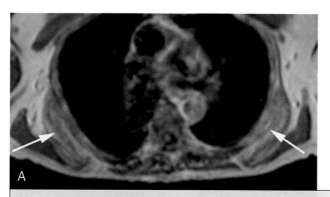
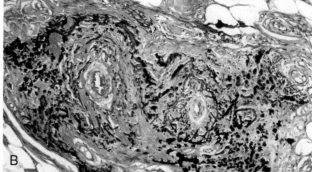

Figure 11 Elastofibroma. **A**, Axial MRI of the chest in a 73-year-old woman reveals bilateral soft-tissue masses between the inferior tip of the scapula and the underlying chest wall consistent with elastofibromas (arrows). **B**, High-power histology reveals the beaded appearance of the elastic fibers admixed with the extensive collagen fibers. The elastin stain highlights the elastic fibers throughout the lesion. Note the extensive vascularity.

2. MRI: mixed low and high signal intensity on both T1- and T2-weighted sequences (**Figure 11, A**)

E. Pathology

1. Gross appearance is gray with cystic degeneration, 5 to 10 cm in length.

2. Histology shows elastic fibers having a beaded appearance with characteristic staining for elastin (**Figure 11, B**).

3. Equal proportion of intertwined collagen fibers

F. Treatment/outcome

1. Observation if asymptomatic

2. Simple excision is curative.

3. No risk of malignant transformation

Figure 12 Low-power histology of a glomus tumor reveals small, rounded cells with dark nuclei in well-defined clumps. On higher power, the glomus cells and the admixed capillaries would be present within a myxoid stroma.

IX. Glomus Tumor

A. Definition and demographics

1. Glomus tumor is a rare, benign tumor of the normal glomus body usually occurring in the subungual region.

2. Extremely rare

3. Occurs in patients 20 to 40 years of age

4. Males and females are affected equally (except with subungual tumors, in which the male to female ratio = 1:3)

B. Clinical presentation

1. Small (<1 cm) red-blue nodule in the subungual region or other deep dermal layers in the extremities

2. More difficult to see color in subungual region; may have ridging of the nail or discoloration of the nail bed

3. Characteristic triad of symptoms includes paroxysmal pain, cold insensitivity, and localized tenderness.

4. Frequent delay in diagnosis

5. Less common locations include the palm, wrist, forearm, and foot.

6. Multiple in 10% of cases

C. Imaging appearance

1. MRI is the best imaging modality to identify glomus tumors.

2. MRI sensitivity 90% to 100%, specificity 50%

3. Low signal intensity on T1-weighted sequences, high on T2-weighted sequences

4. Plain radiographs not very helpful in diagnosis, but can show a scalloped osteolytic defect with a sclerotic border in the distal phalanx

D. Pathology

1. Gross: small, red-blue nodule

2. Histology shows a well-defined lesion of small vessels surrounded by glomus cells in a hyaline or myxoid stroma (**Figure 12**).

3. A glomus cell is a uniform, round cell with a prominent nucleus and eosinophilic cytoplasm.

4. Periodic acid-Schiff stain gives a chicken-wire appearance to the matrix between cells.

E. Treatment/outcome

1. Marginal excision is curative

2. Extremely rare reports of malignant glomus tumors

X. Synovial Chondromatosis

A. Definition and demographics

1. Synovial chondromatosis is a metaplastic proliferation of hyaline cartilage nodules in the synovial membrane.

2. Occurs in patients 30 to 50 years of age

3. Male to female ratio = 2:1

B. Genetics/etiology

1. Generally thought to be a metaplastic condition

2. Occasional chromosome 6 abnormalities have been identified.

C. Clinical presentation

1. Symptoms include joint pain, clicking, and limited range of motion.

2. Pain worse with activity

3. May have warmth, erythema, or tenderness, depending on location

4. Slow progression of symptoms over years

5. Most common in the hip and knee, followed by shoulder and elbow

6. Occasionally occurs in the bursa overlying an osteochondroma

D. Imaging appearance

1. Plain radiographs show variable appearance depending on early or late disease.

2. Initially the cartilage nodules are not visible, except on MRI.

3. Over time, the nodules calcify, then undergo endochondral ossification (**Figure 13**, *A* and *B*).

4. The densities are smooth, well-defined, and remain in the confines of the synovial membrane.

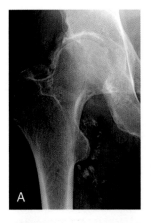
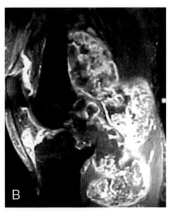
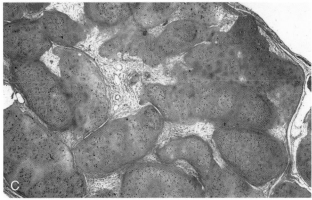
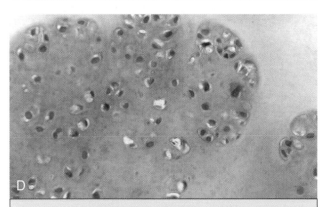

Figure 13   Synovial chondromatoses. **A**, AP radiograph of the right hip in a 46-year-old male with synovial chondromatosis demonstrates discrete calcifications superior and inferior to the femoral head, both within and external to the hip capsule. **B**, Sagittal MRI of the knee in a 33-year-old man with extensive synovial osteochondromatosis. The patient had multiple ossified nodules within the joint and required open synovectomies of the anterior and posterior compartments of the knee. **C**, Low-power histology of synovial osteochondromatosis reveals discrete hyaline cartilage nodules. **D**, Higher power reveals increased cellularity with occasional binucleate cells.

5. Process may erode cartilage and underlying bone.

6. CT scan can define the intra-articular loose bodies.

7. MRI shows lobular appearance with signal dropout consistent with calcification.

E. Pathology

1. Gross: may be hundreds of osteocartilaginous loose bodies within an affected joint

2. Histology shows discrete hyaline cartilage nodules in various phases of calcification or ossification (**Figure 13**, *C*).

3. Ossification starts on the periphery of the nodules.

4. Cellular appearance of chondrocytes includes mild atypia, binucleate cells, and occasional mitoses (more cellular atypia than allowed in an intramedullary benign cartilage tumor) (**Figure 13**, *D*).

F. Treatment/outcome

1. Open or arthroscopic synovectomy

2. Less than adequate removal of nodules increases risk for local recurrence.

3. Natural history is self-limited, but the process can damage the joint.

XI. Pigmented Villonodular Synovitis

A. Definition and demographics

1. Pigmented villonodular synovitis (PVNS) is a proliferative synovial process characterized by mononuclear stromal cells, hemorrhage, histiocytes, and giant cells.

2. Most commonly affects patients 30 to 50 years of age, occasionally teenagers

3. Males and females affected equally

4. Occurs in focal or diffuse forms

5. Can be intra-articular or extra-articular (giant cell tumor of tendon sheath)

B. Genetics/etiology

1. 50% of patients report an earlier traumatic incident

2. Reactive rather than neoplastic

C. Clinical presentation

1. Pain, swelling, effusion, erythema, and decreased joint range of motion with diffuse joint involvement

2. Mechanical joint symptoms with focal involvement

3. Most commonly affects the knee (80%), followed by hip, shoulder, ankle

4. Extra-articular form (giant cell tumor of tendon sheath) usually affects the hand/wrist with a small, painless, superficial soft-tissue nodule.

D. Imaging appearance

1. Well-defined erosions on both sides of a joint noted on plain radiographs signify advanced, diffuse disease (**Figure 14**, *A*).

2. MRI reveals either a focal low-signal nodule within a joint or a diffuse process with low signal intensity (due to hemosiderin deposits) on T1- and T2-weighted images (**Figure 14**, *B* and *C*).

3. MRI shows presence of fat signal within the lesion.

4. MRI may reveal extra-articular extension of the process.

5. Differential diagnosis includes reactive or inflammatory synovitis, hemophilia, or synovial chondromatosis.

E. Pathology

1. Gross appearance: reddish-brown stained synovium with extensive papillary projections (**Figure 14**, *D*).

2. Histology: diagnostic mononuclear stromal cell infiltrate within the synovium (**Figure 14**, *E*)

3. Cells are round with a large nucleus and eosinophilic cytoplasm.

4. Hemosiderin-laden macrophages, multinucleated giant cells, and foam cells present; not required for diagnosis

5. Mitotic figures relatively common

F. Treatment/outcome

1. Treatment is arthroscopic or open removal of a focal PVNS lesion (arthroscopic preferred).

2. Diffuse form requires aggressive total synovectomy using arthroscopic, open, or combined arthroscopic and open techniques.

3. Often an anterior arthroscopic synovectomy is combined with open posterior removal of any extra-articular disease.

4. High local recurrence rate suggests frequent incomplete synovectomy.

5. Total joint arthroplasty is indicated for advanced disease with secondary degenerative changes.

6. Occasionally, external beam radiation is used following multiple local recurrences.

7. Giant cell tumor of tendon sheath is treated with marginal excision.

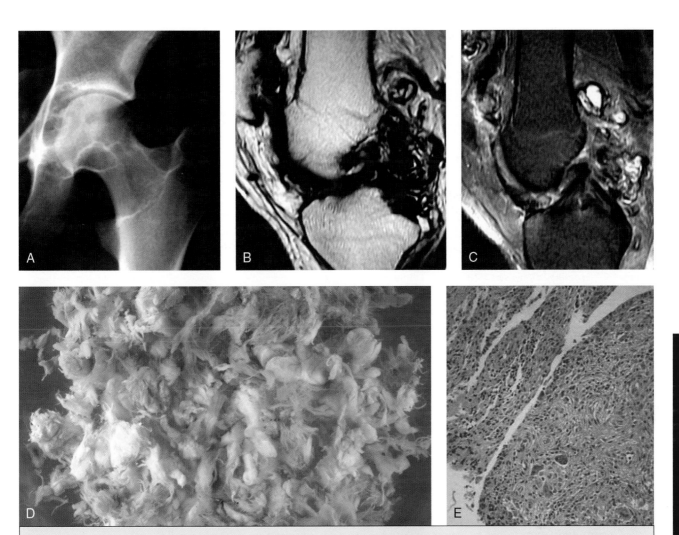

Figure 14 Examples of pigmented villonodular synovitis. **A**, AP radiograph of the left hip in a patient with PVNS reveals osteolytic lesions with sclerotic rims on both sides of the joint. Sagittal T1-weighted (**B**) and T2-weighted (**C**) images of a knee show extensive disease in the posterior aspect of the knee. The lesion is both intra-articular and extra-articular. There is dark signal on both of the images as a result of the hemosiderin deposits within the synovium. **D**, Gross appearance of the reddish-brown synovial fronds seen in PVNS. **E**, Histologic examination reveals a cellular infiltrate within the synovium with multinucleated giant cells and faint hemosiderin. The round, mononuclear stromal cells are the key to the diagnosis.

XII. Myositis Ossificans

A. Definition and demographics

1. Myositis ossificans is a reactive process characterized by a well-circumscribed proliferation of fibroblasts, cartilage, and bone within a muscle (or, rarely, within a nerve, tendon, or fat).

2. Occurs in young, active individuals (most common in individuals 15 to 35 years of age)

3. Occurs in males more than females

B. Genetics/etiology—Almost always a posttraumatic condition.

C. Clinical presentation

1. Pain, tenderness, swelling, decreased range of motion usually within days of an injury

2. Mass increases in size over several months (usually 3 to 6 cm)

3. Growth stops and mass becomes firm

4. Commonly occurs in the quadriceps, brachialis, gluteal muscles

D. Imaging appearance

1. Mineralization begins 3 weeks after injury.

2. Initially, irregular, fluffy densities in the soft tissues are noted on plain radiographs (**Figure 15**, *A*).

3. There may be adjacent periosteal reaction in the bone.

4. Rim enhancement is seen on MRI with gadolinium within the first 3 weeks.

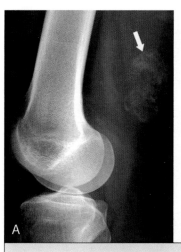
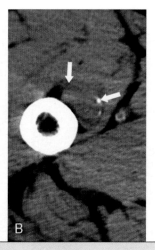
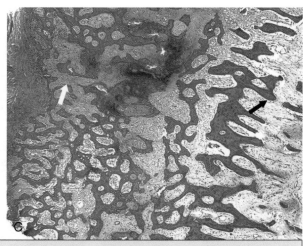

Figure 15   Examples of myositis ossificans. **A**, Lateral radiograph of the knee obtained 4 weeks after a football injury to the posterior thigh in a 19-year-old man reveals fluffy calcifications (arrow) in the posterior thigh musculature consistent with early myositis ossificans. **B**, CT scan of the thigh in a patient with traumatic myositis ossificans reveals the calcified outline of the lesion (arrows) with more mature tissue on the periphery. **C**, Histologic view of a myositis ossificans lesion reveals a zonal pattern, with more mature bone toward the periphery (white arrow) and looser fibrous tissue toward the center (black arrow).

5. With time and maturation, a zoning pattern occurs, with increased peripheral mineralization and a radiolucent center.

6. CT scan defines the ossified lesion (looks like an eggshell) (**Figure 15, B**).

7. Differential diagnosis includes extraskeletal or parosteal osteosarcoma (more ossified in the center with peripheral lucencies).

E. Pathology

1. Grossly immature tissue in center of lesion with mature bone around outer edge

2. Histology reveals a zonal pattern (**Figure 15, C**).

   a. Periphery—mature lamellar bone

   b. Intermediate—poorly defined trabeculae with osteoblasts, fibroblasts, and large ectatic blood vessels

   c. Center—immature, loose, fibrous tissue with moderate pleomorphism and mitoses

3. Skeletal muscle can be entrapped in the periphery of the lesion.

4. No cytologic atypia

5. Differential diagnosis includes extraskeletal osteosarcoma (periphery is least ossified and cells show extreme pleomorphism).

F. Treatment/outcome

1. Myositis ossificans is a self-limited process, so observation and physical therapy to maintain motion are indicated.

2. Repeat radiographs to confirm maturation and stability of the lesion

3. Excision only when lesion is mature (~6 to 12 months) and if symptomatic; excision at initial stages predisposes to local recurrence

4. Often, the size of the mass decreases after 1 year.

Bibliography

Blei F: Basic science and clinical aspects of vascular anomalies. *Curr Opin Pediatr* 2005;17:501-509.

Enzinger FM, Weiss SW: *Soft Tissue Tumors*, ed 3. St. Louis, MO, Mosby, 1995, pp 165-230, 381-430, 579-628, 735-756, 821-888.

Fayad LM, Hazirolan T, Bluemke D, Mitchell S: Vascular malformations in the extremities: Emphasis on MR imaging features that guide treatment options. *Skeletal Radiol* 2006; 35:127-137.

Furlong MA, Fanburg-Smith JC, Miettinen M: The morphologic spectrum of hibernoma: A clinicopathologic study of 170 cases. *Am J Surg Pathol* 2001;25:809-814.

Giebel BD, Bierhoff E, Vogel J: Elastofibroma and preelastofibroma: A biopsy and autopsy study. *Eur J Surg Oncol* 1996; 22:93-96.

Gonzalez Della Valle AG, Piccaluga F, Potter H, Salvati EA, Pusso R: Pigmented villonodular synovitis of the hip: 2- to 33-year follow-up study. *Clin Orthop Relat Res* 2001;388: 187-199.

Jee W-H, Oh S-N, McCauley T, et al: Extraaxial neurofibromas versus neurilemomas: Discrimination with MRI. *AJR Am J Roentgenol* 2004;183:629-633.

Kransdorf MJ, Meis JM, Jelinek JS: Myositis ossificans: MR appearance with radiologic-pathologic correlation. *AJR Am J Roentgenol* 1991;157:1243-1248.

Lim ST, Chung HW, Choi YL, Moon YW, Seo JG, Park YS: Operative treatment of primary synovial osteochondromatosis of the hip. *J Bone Joint Surg Am* 2006;88:2456-2464.

Masih S, Antebi A: Imaging of pigmented villonodular synovities. *Semin Musculoskelet Radiol* 2003;7:205-216.

Murphey MD, Vidal JA, Fanburg-Smith JC, Gajewski DA: Imaging of synovial chondromatosis with radiologic-pathologic correlation. *Radiographics* 2007;27:1465-1488.

Okuno S: The enigma of desmoid tumors. *Curr Treat Options Oncol* 2006;7:438-443.

Schwartz HS: *Orthopaedic Knowledge Update: Musculoskeletal Tumors 2.* Rosemont, IL, American Academy of Orthopaedic Surgeons, 2007, pp 225-269.

Top Testing Facts

1. Lipomas should image the same as fat on all MRI sequences.

2. Intramuscular hemangiomas or other vascular malformations are best treated nonsurgically.

3. NF1 involves an abnormal chromosome 17, and 5% of patients will develop malignant transformation of a lesion.

4. Neurilemomas have Antoni A (cellular) and Antoni B (myxoid) areas on histology.

5. Desmoid tumors are one of the few benign soft-tissue lesions to require a wide resection.

6. Radiation is often part of the treatment regimen for recurrent desmoid tumors.

7. Elastofibromas commonly occur between the scapula and chest wall; they stain with elastin.

8. Glomus tumors usually occur in a subungual location.

9. Synovial chondromatosis and PVNS require a complete synovectomy to achieve local control.

10. The imaging and histologic appearance of myositis ossificans shows a zonal pattern with increased peripheral mineralization and immature tissue in the center.

4: Orthopaedic Oncology and Systemic Disease

Chapter 41

Malignant Soft-Tissue Tumors

Kristy Weber, MD

I. Soft-Tissue Sarcoma Treatment

A. Overview

1. Ratio of benign to malignant soft-tissue masses = 100:1 (sarcomas rare)

2. Males affected more than females

3. Extremities (upper and lower)—60% of sarcomas

4. 85% occur in individuals older than 15 years.

5. Appearance of most sarcomas on MRI is indeterminate; a biopsy is required.

6. Staging—The most common system is the AJCC system, which relies on histologic grade, tumor size, nodal status, and whether distant metastases are present.

B. Surgery

1. Goal is to achieve an acceptable margin to minimize local recurrence and maintain reasonable function; limb salvage procedures performed in ~90% of patients.

2. Sarcomas have a centripetal growth pattern.

3. Reactive zone around tumor includes edema, fibrous tissue (capsule), inflammatory cells, and tumor cells

4. "Shelling out" a sarcoma usually means excising it through the reactive zone, which leaves tumor cells behind in most cases.

5. Definition of surgical margins (Enneking)

   a. Intralesional: resection through the tumor mass for gross total resection

   b. Marginal: resection through the reactive zone

   c. Wide: resection with a cuff of normal tissue

   d. Radical: resection of the entire compartment (eg, quadriceps)

6. Amputation is indicated if necessary to resect the entire tumor, if major nerves cannot be saved, or if the patient has significant comorbidities that preclude a limb-sparing surgery.

7. Standard oncologic techniques are used to resect soft-tissue sarcomas.

   a. Tourniquet without exsanguination

   b. Excise biopsy tract

   c. Drains distal, close, and in line with incision

8. Surgical resection alone of large, deep, high-grade tumors has unacceptably high rate of local recurrence—requires adjuvant treatment (radiation with or without chemotherapy).

9. Soft-tissue reconstruction by free or rotational tissue transfer frequently is necessary and minimizes wound complications after major resection (Figure 1).

C. Radiation

1. Used routinely in the treatment of soft-tissue sarcoma (noted exceptions being when an amputation is performed or when the sarcoma is small, superficial, low grade, and amenable to a wide surgical resection)

2. Radiation can be administered by external beam techniques, brachytherapy (percutaneous flexible catheters placed directly on tumor bed and loaded with radiation sources [beads or wires] over 48 to 96 hours) (Figure 2), or intraoperatively.

3. Early radiation effects: desquamation, delayed wound healing, infection. Late effects: fibrosis, fractures, joint stiffness, secondary sarcoma (depending on treatment dose, volume, and length of follow-up).

4. Preoperative radiation requires a lower dose (~50 Gy) than postoperative radiation (~66 Gy), decreases the surrounding edema, and helps form a thick fibrous capsule around the tumor. Surgery is delayed 3 to 4 weeks after completion of radiation.

5. Preoperative radiation incurs a higher wound complication rate (35%) than postoperative radiation (17%) (Figure 3).

6. No difference in overall survival or functional outcomes related to timing of radiation has been reported.

7. External beam radiation combined with extensive periosteal stripping during tumor resection increases the risk of postradiation fracture. In these cases, consider prophylactic intramedullary or plate stabilization.

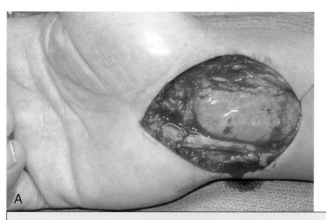

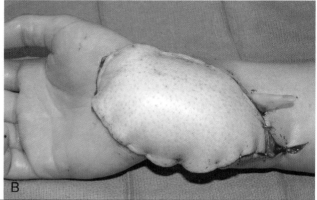

Figure 1 Clinical photographs after soft-tissue sarcoma resection. **A,** Soft-tissue defect after wide resection of a clear cell sarcoma of the volar wrist. **B,** Soft-tissue reconstruction using free tissue transfer is commonly performed to minimize wound breakdown and infection, especially when the patient has had preoperative radiation.

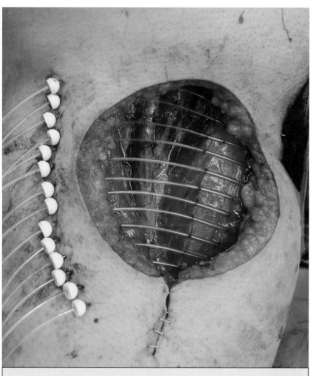

Figure 2 Brachytherapy catheters are shown overlying a tumor bed after resection. A free flap was used to cover the defect.

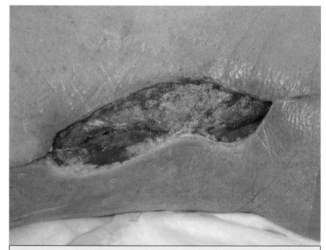

Figure 3 Wound breakdown after preoperative radiation and surgical resection of a high-grade liposarcoma of the medial thigh.

D. Chemotherapy

1. Controversial for soft-tissue sarcoma in general. (May delay local or systemic recurrent disease, but no statistically significant survival benefit at 10 years.)

2. Key component of treatment for rhabdomyosarcoma and soft-tissue Ewing sarcoma/primitive neuroectodermal tumor. Studies show possible benefit for synovial sarcoma.

3. Common agents include ifosfamide and doxorubicin (adriamycin), which have considerable toxicity in high doses.

4. Patients with soft-tissue sarcoma commonly are older, with more comorbidities, and cannot tolerate high-dose systemic treatment.

E. Outcomes

1. The use of radiation and surgery minimizes the risk of local recurrence to <10%.

2. Stage is the most important factor in determining overall prognosis/outcome.

3. Other prognostic factors include presence of metastasis, grade, size, and depth of tumor.

4. Tumor grade is related to risk of metastasis (low grade, <10%; intermediate grade, 10% to 25%; high grade, >50%).

5. Most common site of metastasis is to the lungs.

6. Lymph node metastasis (~5%) occurs most frequently in rhabdomyosarcoma, synovial sarcoma, epithelioid sarcoma, and clear cell sarcoma.

7. The outcome of individual soft-tissue sarcoma subtypes is rarely reported; ~50% of patients with high-grade soft-tissue sarcomas die of the disease.

8. Resection of pulmonary metastasis can cure up to 25% of patients.

9. Patients require follow-up of primary site of resection (MRI with contrast, or ultrasound) and chest (radiograph or CT scan) every 3 to 4 months for 2 years, every 6 months for 3 years, and then yearly with chest studies.

II. Malignant Fibrous Histiocytoma

A. Definition and demographics

1. Pleomorphic in histologic appearance (recently reclassified as "undifferentiated high-grade pleomorphic sarcoma")

2. Most common soft-tissue sarcoma in adults 55 to 80 years of age

3. Male to female ratio = 2:1

4. More common in Caucasian than in African-American or Asian populations

B. Genetics/etiology—No data yet.

C. Clinical presentation

1. Usually a deep, slow-growing, painless mass

2. More common in the extremities (lower more common than upper) than retroperitoneum

3. Patients occasionally present with fever, elevated white blood cell count, and hypoglycemia.

D. Imaging appearance (indeterminate)—Low intensity on T1-weighted MRI; high intensity on T2-weighted MRI (**Figure 4,** *A* and *B*).

E. Pathology

1. Grossly, a gray-white multinodular mass

2. Histologic subtypes include pleomorphic (80% to 85%), giant cell (10%), and inflammatory (<10%).

3. Low-power histology shows storiform or cartwheel growth pattern (**Figure 4,** *C*).

4. Cells are plump, spindled, and arranged around narrow vessels.

5. Haphazard histiocytic cells

6. Multinucleated eosinophilic giant cells (**Figure 4,** *D*)

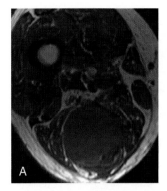
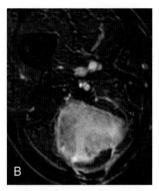
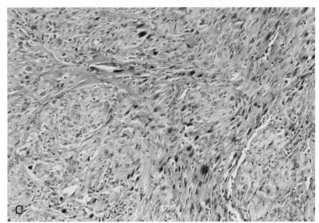
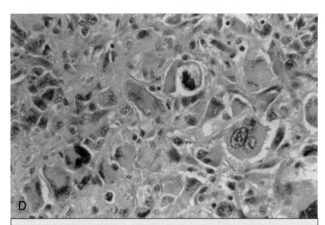

Figure 4 Malignant fibrous histiocytoma in a 68-year-old man who presented with a painless soft-tissue mass in the right posterior thigh. Axial T1-weighted (**A**) and T2-weighted (postcontrast) (**B**) MRI scans are indeterminate in appearance; a biopsy is required. **C,** Low-power histology reveals a storiform pattern with bizarre pleomorphic tumor cells and hyalinized collagen bundles consistent with malignant fibrous histiocytoma (undifferentiated high-grade pleomorphic sarcoma). **D,** Higher power reveals anaplastic tumor cells, multinucleated cells, and mitotic figures.

7. Marked atypia, mitotic activity, and pleomorphism

F. Treatment/outcome

1. Radiation and wide surgical resection

2. Chemotherapy in selected cases

3. Overall 5-year survival of 50% to 60% (depending on size, grade, depth, presence of metastasis)

III. Liposarcoma

A. Definition and demographics

1. Composed of a variety of histologic forms related to the developmental stages of lipoblasts

2. Second most common soft-tissue sarcoma in adults

3. Occurs most commonly in patients 50 to 80 years of age

4. Affects males more than females

B. Genetics/etiology

1. Origin of liposarcoma is from primitive mesenchymal cells; diagnosis does not require adipose cells.

2. Lipomas do not predispose a patient to liposarcomas.

3. Histologic types include well-differentiated, myxoid (most common—50%), round cell, pleomorphic, and dedifferentiated.

4. Well-differentiated variants have giant marker and ring chromosomes.

5. Myxoid liposarcoma is associated with a translocation between chromosomes 12 and 16.

C. Clinical presentation

1. Wide spectrum of disease depending on histologic type

2. Slow-growing; may become extremely large (10 to 20 cm), painless masses

3. Pain may occur in larger lesions.

4. Occur in extremities (lower [thigh] more common than upper) and retroperitoneum (15% to 20%) (present at later age)

5. Well-differentiated liposarcoma is essentially the same entity as atypical lipoma/atypical lipomatous tumor (some use the former term for retroperitoneal lesions and the latter term for extremity lesions).

6. Well-differentiated liposarcomas can rarely dedifferentiate. Watch for rapid growth of a long-standing (usually >5 years) painless mass.

D. Imaging appearance

1. Plain radiographs occasionally show foci of calcification or ossification in well-differentiated variants.

2. MRI appearance of well-differentiated variant is the same as a lipoma. Watch for rare areas of dedifferentiation (**Figure 5,** *A* and *B*).

3. MRI appearance of high-grade liposarcoma is indeterminate and similar to all sarcomas (low intensity on T1-weighted images; high intensity on T2-weighted images) (**Figure 6,** *A* and *B*).

4. Myxoid liposarcomas can metastasize to sites other than the lungs (eg, abdomen), so staging for this tumor should include a CT scan of the abdomen and pelvis as well as a chest CT scan.

E. Pathology

1. Grossly, liposarcomas are large, well-circumscribed, and lobular.

2. Well-differentiated liposarcoma—Low-grade tumor with lobulated appearance of mature adipose tissue (**Figure 5,** *C*).

3. Myxoid liposarcoma

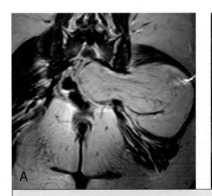
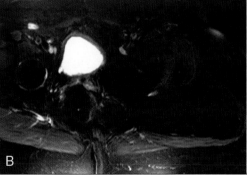
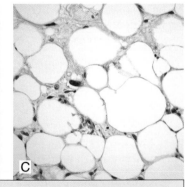

Figure 5   Well-differentiated liposarcoma. **A,** Coronal T1-weighted image reveals a large left retroperitoneal lipomatous lesion extending through the sciatic notch into the gluteal muscles. **B,** Axial T2-weighted fat-suppressed MRI scan reveals that the lesion completely suppresses with no concern for high-grade areas. **C,** Histology of the resected specimen reveals slight variation in the size and shape of the fat cells with hyperchromatic nuclei, consistent with a well-differentiated liposarcoma.

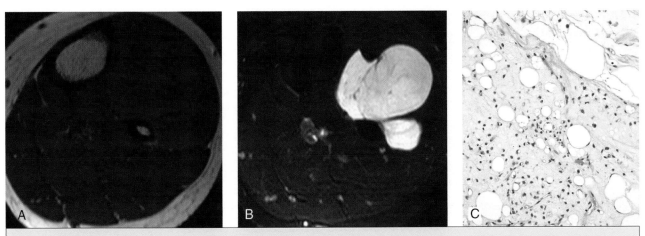

Figure 6 Myxoid liposarcoma in the left calf of a 27-year-old woman. Axial T1-weighted (**A**) and T2-weighted short tau inversion recovery (STIR) (**B**) MRI sequences reveal an indeterminate lesion that is low intensity on T1-weighted images and high intensity on T2-weighted images. There is no bony involvement, but the mass is adjacent to the proximal fibula. **C,** The histology reveals lipoblasts (some with signet-ring appearance), numerous capillaries, and a myxoid stroma between the tumor cells. No significant round cell component is noted.

a. Low- to intermediate-grade tumor with lobulated appearance

b. Composed of proliferating lipoblasts, a plexiform capillary network, and a myxoid matrix (**Figure 6, C**)

c. Signet ring (univacuolar) lipoblasts occur at the edge of the tumor lobules.

d. Few mitotic figures

4. Round cell liposarcoma

a. Also considered a poorly differentiated myxoid liposarcoma

b. Characteristic small round blue cells

c. Rare intracellular lipid formation and minimal myxoid matrix

5. Pleomorphic liposarcoma

a. High-grade tumor with marked pleomorphic appearance

b. Giant lipoblasts with hyperchromatic bizarre nuclei

c. Deeply eosinophilic giant cells

6. Dedifferentiated liposarcoma—high-grade sarcoma (malignant fibrous histiocytoma, fibrosarcoma, leiomyosarcoma) juxtaposed to well-differentiated lipomatous lesion.

F. Treatment/outcome

1. Well-differentiated liposarcoma

a. Marginal resection without radiation or chemotherapy

b. Metastasis extremely rare

c. Risk of local recurrence is 25% to 50% at 10 years.

d. Dedifferentiation risk is 2% for extremity lesions and 20% for retroperitoneal lesions.

2. Intermediate- and high-grade variants

a. Radiation and wide surgical resection

b. Chemotherapy in selected patients

c. Incidence of pulmonary metastasis increases with grade.

d. Myxoid liposarcomas with >10% round cells have higher likelihood of metastasis.

e. Local recurrence is higher in retroperitoneal lesions.

IV. Fibrosarcoma

A. Definition and demographics

1. Rare soft-tissue sarcoma of fibroblastic origin that shows no tendency toward other cellular differentiation

2. Occurs in adults 30 to 55 years of age

3. Affects males more than females

B. Genetics/etiology—No data yet.

C. Clinical presentation

1. Slow-growing, painless mass (4 to 8 cm) most commonly noted around the thigh or knee

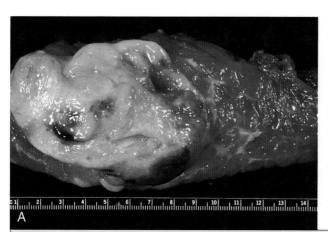 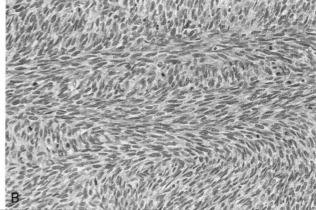

Figure 7 Fibrosarcomas. **A,** Gross appearance of a fibrosarcoma within the muscles of the anterior thigh. There are areas of hemorrhage and cyst formation. **B,** High-power view of a fibrosarcoma reveals the distinct fascicular appearance of cells with little variation in size or shape. When the cells are cut in cross section, they appear round. The overall appearance is a herringbone pattern of spindle cells.

2. Ulceration of the skin in superficial lesions

D. Imaging appearance (indeterminate)—Low intensity on T1-weighted MRI; high intensity on T2-weighted MRI.

E. Pathology

 1. Gross appearance (**Figure 7, *A***)

 2. Histology

  a. Uniform fasciculated growth pattern (herringbone) (**Figure 7, *B***)

  b. Spindle cells with minimal cytoplasm

  c. Collagen fibers commonly aligned in parallel throughout tumor

  d. Mitotic activity varies

F. Treatment/outcome

 1. Wide surgical resection and radiation

 2. Chemotherapy for selected patients

 3. Metastasis in ~50% of high-grade lesions

V. Synovial Sarcoma

A. Definition and demographics

 1. Distinct lesion occurring in para-articular regions

 2. Most common soft-tissue sarcoma in young adults

 3. Occurs most commonly in patients 15 to 40 years of age

 4. Affects males more than females

B. Genetics/etiology

 1. Characteristic translocation (X;18)

 2. Represents the fusion of *SYT* with either *SSX1* or *SSX2*

C. Clinical presentation

 1. Slow-growing soft-tissue mass (3 to 5 cm)

 2. Sometimes 2 to 4 years before a correct diagnosis

 3. Pain in 50% of patients; some have history of trauma

 4. Most commonly occur in para-articular regions around the knee, shoulder, arm, elbow, and foot (lower extremity in 60%)

 5. Can arise from tendon sheaths, bursa, fascia, and joint capsule, but only rarely involves a joint (**Figure 8, *A* and *B***)

D. Imaging appearance

 1. Calcification noted on plain radiographs in 15% to 20% of synovial sarcomas

 2. MRI appearance indeterminate: low intensity on T1-weighted images; high intensity on T2-weighted images (**Figure 8, *A* and *B***)

E. Pathology

 1. Classically occurs as biphasic type, with epithelial cells forming glandlike structures alternating with elongated spindle cells (**Figure 8, *C***)

 2. Epithelial cells are large and round with distinct cell borders and pale cytoplasm.

 3. Epithelial cells are arranged in nests or chords and stain positive with keratin.

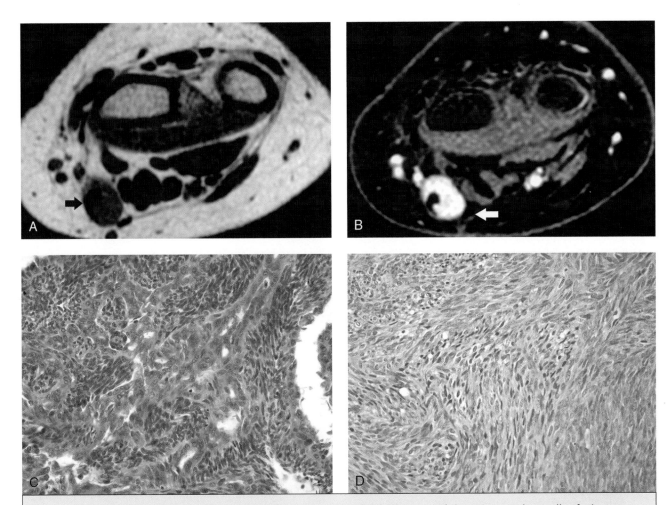

Figure 8 Synovial sarcomas. Axial T1-weighted (**A**) and T2-weighted (**B**) MRI scans of the wrist reveal a small soft-tissue mass associated with the flexor carpi radialis tendon sheath (arrow). It is indeterminate in appearance, and a biopsy revealed a synovial sarcoma. **C,** Histology of a biphasic synovial sarcoma showing the typical pattern of epithelial cells and fibrosarcoma-like spindle cells. **D,** Monophasic synovial sarcoma variant showing only spindle cells (would be keratin positive).

4. Fibrous component involves plump, malignant spindle cells with minimal cytoplasm and dark nuclei; mast cells are common in fibrous sections.

5. Calcification more common at periphery

6. Variable vascularity

7. Less commonly, a monophasic histology is seen (either fibrous or epithelial) (**Figure 8, *D***).

F. Treatment/outcome

1. Wide resection and radiation

2. Chemotherapy used more commonly; younger patients tolerate it better.

3. Lymph node metastasis occurs in 20% of patients; can stage with sentinel node biopsy.

4. 5-year survival = 50%, 10-year survival = 25% (better in heavily calcified lesions)

VI. Epithelioid Sarcoma

A. Definition and demographics

1. Distinct soft-tissue sarcoma occurring in young adults that is often mistaken for a benign granulomatous process

2. Occurs in adolescents and young adults (10 to 35 years)

3. Male to female ratio = 2:1

B. Genetics/etiology—No data yet.

C. Clinical presentation

1. Small, slow-growing soft-tissue tumor that can be superficial or deep

2. Frequently involves hand, forearm, fingers; 3 to 6 cm in size (**Figure 9, *A***)

4: Orthopaedic Oncology and Systemic Disease

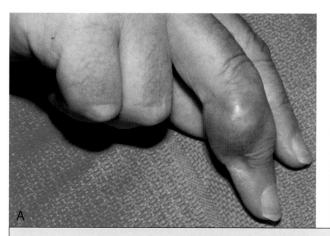
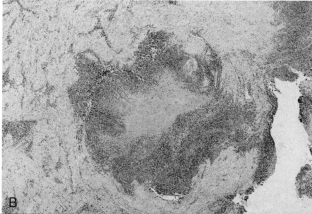

Figure 9 Epithelioid sarcoma. **A,** Clinical photograph of an epithelioid sarcoma in the dorsal aspect of the distal long finger. Note the nodule in the superficial tissues. **B,** Low-power histology reveals a nodule with central necrosis consistent with an epithelioid sarcoma but often mistaken for a benign granulomatous process. *(Reproduced from Scarborough MT (ed): 2008 Musculoskeletal Tumors and Diseases Self-Assessment Examination. Rosemont, IL, American Academy of Orthopaedic Surgeons, 2008, question 21, figures 18A and 18B.)*

3. Most common soft-tissue sarcoma in the hand/wrist

4. Occurs as firm, painless nodule(s); may ulcerate when superficial

5. When deep, attached to tendons, tendon sheaths, or fascia

6. Confused with granuloma, rheumatoid nodule, or skin cancer, often resulting in delay in diagnosis or inappropriate treatment

D. Imaging appearance

1. Occasional calcification within lesion

2. Can erode adjacent bone

3. MRI reveals nodule along tendon sheaths of upper or lower extremity.

   a. Low intensity on T1-weighted images; high intensity on T2-weighted images

   b. Indeterminate in appearance; requires biopsy

E. Pathology

1. Low-power histology reveals a nodular pattern with central necrosis within granulomatous areas (**Figure 9**, *B*).

2. Higher power reveals an epithelial appearance with eosinophilic cytoplasm.

3. Minimal cellular pleomorphism

4. Intercellular deposition of dense hyalinized collagen

5. Calcification/ossification in 10% to 20% of patients

6. Cells are keratin positive

F. Treatment/outcome

1. Wide surgical resection with adjuvant radiation if necessary

2. Regional lymph node metastasis is common. Sentinel node biopsy may be indicated.

3. Often mistaken for a benign lesion and inadequately excised, leading to high rate of multiple recurrences

4. Amputation is frequently necessary to halt spread of disease.

5. Late regional or systemic metastasis to lungs is common.

6. Overall, extremely poor prognosis

VII. Clear Cell Sarcoma

A. Definition and demographics

1. Rare soft-tissue sarcoma that has the ability to produce melanin

2. Occurs in young adults (age 20 to 40 years)

3. Affects females more than males

4. Often called "malignant melanoma of soft parts"

B. Genetics/etiology

1. Frequent translocation of chromosomes 12 and 22 (not seen in malignant melanoma)

2. Etiology thought to be neuroectodermal

C. Clinical presentation

1. Occurs in deep tissues associated with tendons, aponeuroses

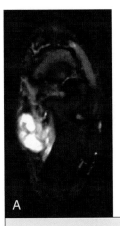
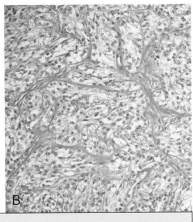

Figure 10 Clear cell sarcoma. **A,** STIR sequence of the left foot reveals a soft-tissue lesion abutting the medial calcaneous. Additional views revealed involvement of the neurovascular bundle. **B,** Histology shows fibrous septa separating the tumor into well-defined fascicles of cells with clear cytoplasm consistent with a clear cell sarcoma.

2. Most common soft-tissue sarcoma of the foot; also occurs in ankle, knee, and hand

3. 2 to 6 cm in size

4. Slow-growing mass; pain in 50% of patients and present for many years prior to diagnosis

5. Often mistaken for a benign lesion and inadequately excised

D. Imaging appearance

1. Nonspecific appearance; may be nodular in foot

2. MRI: indeterminate; requires a biopsy. Low intensity on T1-weighted images; high intensity on T2-weighted images (**Figure 10,** *A*)

E. Pathology

1. Grossly, no connection to overlying skin, but may be attached to tendons

2. Histology shows nests of round cells with clear cytoplasm (**Figure 10,** *B*)

3. Uniform pattern of cells with a defined fibrous border that might be continuous with surrounding tendons or aponeuroses

4. Occasional multinucleated giant cells but rare mitotic figures

5. Intracellular melanin noted in 50% of patients with appropriate staining

F. Treatment/outcome

1. Wide surgical resection with adjuvant radiation

2. Local recurrence is common.

3. Frequent regional lymph node metastasis; consider sentinel lymph node biopsy

4. High rate of pulmonary metastasis with extremely poor prognosis

5. No effective chemotherapy

VIII. Rhabdomyosarcoma

A. Definition, demographics, and genetics

1. Soft-tissue sarcoma of primitive mesenchyme, occurring primarily in children

2. Most common soft-tissue sarcoma in children/adolescents (embryonal and alveolar types)

3. Embryonal type occurs in infants/children, alveolar in adolescents/young adults.

4. Affects males more than females

5. Histologic subtypes include embryonal (most common), alveolar, botryoid, and pleomorphic (affects adults 40 to 70 years of age)

6. In alveolar rhabdomyosarcoma, translocation between chromosome 2 and 13 is common.

B. Clinical presentation

1. Most lesions occur in head/neck, genitourinary, and retroperitoneal locations.

2. 15% occur in extremities (incidence equal in upper and lower)—forearm, thigh, foot, hand.

3. Often rapidly enlarging, deep, painless soft-tissue masses

4. Staging should include bone marrow biopsy.

C. Imaging appearance (indeterminate): low intensity on T1-weighted MRI; high intensity on T2-weighted MRI

D. Pathology

1. Immunohistochemical markers for rhabdomyosarcoma: desmin, myoglobin, *MyoD1*

2. Embryonal—Composed of small round cells that resemble normal skeletal muscle in various stages of development, with cross striations visible in 50% of patients.

   a. Alternating dense hypercellular areas with loose myxoid areas (**Figure 11,** *A*)

   b. Mixture of undifferentiated, hyperchromatic cells and differentiated cells with eosinophilic cytoplasm

   c. Matrix with minimal collagen and more prominent myxoid material

3. Alveolar—Aggregates of poorly differentiated round tumor cells and irregular alveolar spaces.

4. Orthopaedic Oncology and Systemic Disease

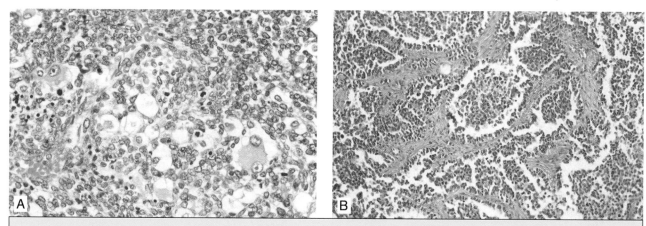

Figure 11   Rhabdomyosarcomas. **A,** Histology of embryonal rhabdomyosarcoma shows undifferentiated small round cells in addition to rhabdomyoblasts in various stages of differentiation. **B,** Histology of alveolar rhabdomyosarcoma shows aggregates of small round tumor cells separated by fibrous septa.

a. Cellular aggregates surrounded by dense, hyalinized fibrous septa arranged around dilated vascular spaces (**Figure 11,** *B*)

b. Multinucleated giant cells prominent

4. Pleomorphic—Loosely arranged polygonal tumor cells with eosinophilic cytoplasm.

   a. Difficult to differentiate from other pleomorphic sarcomas

   b. Requires either cells with cross striations or positive staining for desmin and myoglobin

E. Treatment/outcome

1. Treatment is wide surgical resection and chemotherapy.

2. For unresectable lesions or tumors with positive margins after surgery, radiation is indicated.

3. Common chemotherapy agents include vincristine, dactinomycin, cyclophosphamide.

4. Regional lymph node metastasis is common. May consider sentinel lymph node biopsy.

5. Tendency to metastasize to the bone marrow

6. 5-year survival of embryonal form is 80%, alveolar 60%

7. For pleomorphic variant in adults, treatment is wide resection and radiation. Chemotherapy is not effective—5-year survival of 25%.

IX. Malignant Peripheral Nerve Sheath Tumor

A. Definition and demographics

1. Malignant peripheral nerve sheath tumor (MPNST), or neurofibrosarcoma, is a sarcoma arising from a peripheral nerve or neurofibroma.

2. MPNSTs that arise from solitary neurofibromas occur in patients 30 to 55 years of age.

3. MPNSTs that arise in setting of neurofibromatosis type 1 (NF1) occur in patients 20 to 40 years of age

4. Affects males more than females in NF1 patients; male to female ratio = 1 in sporadic cases

B. Genetics/etiology

1. Most cases (50%) associated with NF1

2. Patients with NF1 have ~5% risk of malignant transformation (latent period of 10 to 20 years).

C. Clinical presentation

1. Slow or rapid enlargement of a long-standing benign soft-tissue mass

2. Pain is variable but more common in patients with NF1.

3. Most arise from large nerves (sciatic, sacral roots, brachial plexus) (5 to 8 cm in size).

D. Imaging appearance

1. Indeterminate MRI appearance: low intensity on T1-weighted images; high intensity on T2-weighted images (**Figure 12,** *A* and *B*)

2. Fusiform appearance; eccentrically located within a major nerve

3. Serial MRI scans documenting enlargement of a previously documented benign nerve sheath tumor suggest malignant degeneration.

E. Pathology

1. Spindle cells closely resemble fibrosarcoma; pattern is sweeping fascicles (**Figure 12,** *C*).

2. Histology reflects Schwann cell differentiation; cells arranged asymmetrically

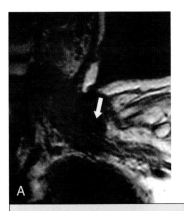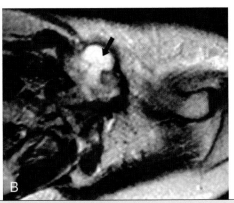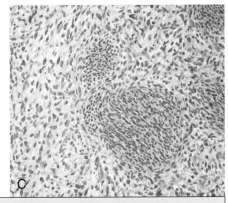

Figure 12 Malignant peripheral nerve sheath tumor arising from a solitary neurofibroma. Coronal T1-weighted (**A**) and axial T2-weighted (**B**) images of the left neck area. The tumor (arrows) is indeterminate in appearance but involves the brachial plexus, causing decreased motor function of the left arm. **C,** Histology is similar to a fibrosarcoma, with spindle cells arranged in long fascicles. The nuclei, however, are wavy or comma-shaped in appearance, which is unique to MPNSTs.

3. Spindle cells have wavy nuclei.

4. Dense cellular areas alternate with myxoid areas.

5. Mature islands of cartilage, bone, or muscle present in 10% to 15% of lesions.

6. Staining for S100 is positive in most tumors but usually focal.

7. Keratin staining is negative.

F. Treatment/outcome

1. Wide surgical resection (requires nerve resection)

2. Adjuvant radiation preoperatively (or postoperatively, especially if margins are close)

3. Chemotherapy has not been effective.

4. 5-year survival for MPNST in a solitary lesion is 75%; 5-year survival in a patient with NF1 is 30%.

Top Testing Facts

1. Soft-tissue sarcomas are usually categorized as indeterminate lesions on MRI (low intensity on T1-weighted images and high intensity on T2-weighted images) and require a biopsy for definitive diagnosis.

2. Liposarcomas (other than low-grade well-differentiated subtypes) do not have any resemblance to fat on MRI studies.

3. Myxoid liposarcoma has a classic 12;16 chromosomal translocation.

4. Synovial sarcoma has a classic X;18 chromosomal translocation.

5. Epithelioid sarcoma is the most common soft-tissue sarcoma found in the hand/wrist.

6. Common sarcomas that metastasize to regional lymph nodes include rhabdomyosarcoma, synovial sarcoma, clear cell sarcoma, and epithelioid sarcoma.

7. Chemotherapy has not been shown to have a proven benefit in the treatment of most soft-tissue sarcomas (exceptions from this chapter include rhabdomyosarcoma and synovial sarcoma).

8. Patients with a history of NF1 have a 5% chance of malignant degeneration of a neurofibroma to an MPNST.

9. Most high-grade soft-tissue sarcomas are treated with radiation and wide surgical resection.

10. Compared with postoperative radiation, preoperative radiation allows a lower dose, but wound complications are increased.

Bibliography

Cohen RJ, Curtis RE, Inskip PD, Fraumeni JF Jr: The risk of developing second cancers among survivors of childhood soft tissue sarcoma. *Cancer* 2005;103:2391-2396.

Cormier JN, Huang X, Xing Y, et al: Cohort analysis of patients with localized, high risk extremity soft tissue sarcoma treated at two cancer centers: Chemotherapy-associated outcomes. *J Clin Oncol* 2004;22:4567-4574.

Crew AJ, Clark J, Fisher C, et al: Fusion of SYT to two genes, SSX1 and SSX2, encoding proteins with homology to the Kruppel-associated box in human synovial sarcoma. *EMBO J* 1995;14:2333-2340.

Crozat A, Aman P, Mandahl N, Ron D: Fusion of CHOP to a novel RNA-binding protein in human myxoid liposarcoma. *Nature* 1993;363:640-644.

Enzinger FM, Weiss SW (eds): *Soft Tissue Tumors*, ed 3. St. Louis, MO, Mosby, 1995, pp 165-230, 381-430, 579-628, 735-756, 821-888.

Fletcher CM, Unni KK, Mertens F (eds): *World Health Organization Classification of Tumours: Pathology and Genetics of Tumours, Tumours of Soft Tissue and Bone*. Lyon, France, IARC Press, 2002.

Frustaci S, Gherlinzoni F, De Paoli A, et al: Adjuvant chemotherapy for adult soft tissue sarcomas of the extremities and girdles: Results of the Italian randomized cooperative trial. *J Clin Oncol* 2001;19:1238-1247.

Holt GE, Griffin AM, Pintilie M, et al: Fractures following radiotherapy and limb-salvage surgery for lower extremity soft-tissue sarcomas: A comparison of high-dose and low-dose radiotherapy. *J Bone Joint Surg Am* 2005;87:315-319.

Massi D, Beltrami G, Capanna R, Franchi A: Histopathological re-classification of extremity pleomorphic soft tissue sarcoma has clinical relevance. *Eur J Surg Oncol* 2004;30:1131-1136.

O'Sullivan B, Davis AM, Turcotte R, et al: Preoperative versus postoperative radiotherapy in soft-tissue sarcoma of the limbs: A randomized trial. *Lancet* 2002;359:2235-2241.

Pappo AS, Shapiro DN, Crist WM, Maurer HM: Biology and therapy of pediatric rhabdomyosarcoma. *J Clin Oncol* 1995; 13:2123-2139.

Pisters PW, Harrison LB, Leung DH, Woodruff JM, Casper ES, Brennan MF: Long-term results of a prospective randomized trial of adjuvant brachytherapy in soft tissue sarcoma. *J Clin Oncol* 1996;14:859-868.

Schwartz HS (ed): *Orthopaedic Knowledge Update: Musculoskeletal Tumors 2*. Rosemont, IL, American Academy of Orthopaedic Surgeons, 2007, pp 225-269.

Zagars GK, Ballo MT, Pisters PW, Pollack RE, Patel SR, Benjamin RS: Surgical margins and re-resection in the management of patients with soft tissue sarcoma using conservative surgery and radiation therapy. *Cancer* 2003;97:2544-2553.

4: Orthopaedic Oncology and Systemic Disease

I. Melorheostosis

A. Definition and demographics

   1. Melorheostosis is a rare, painful disorder of the extremities characterized by large amounts of periosteal new bone formation occurring on the surface of multiple bones.

   2. No sex predilection

   3. Usually discovered by age 40 years

B. Genetics/etiology

   1. Nonhereditary

   2. Often follows sclerotomal pattern

C. Clinical presentation

*Frank J. Frassica, MD, is a consultant or employee for SLACK Inc.

   1. Pain, reduced range of motion, contractures

   2. Soft tissues—tense, erythematous skin, induration and fibrosis of subcutaneous tissue

D. Radiographic appearance (**Figure 1**)

   1. More common in the lower extremity and usually involves one extremity

   2. Cortical hyperostosis ("dripping candle wax")

   3. Wavy appearance that flows across and involves joints

E. Pathology

   1. Enlarged bony trabeculae

   2. Normal haversian systems

F. Treatment

   1. Symptomatic treatment of pain

   2. Occasionally, correction of contractures by excision of hyperostotic and fibrotic areas

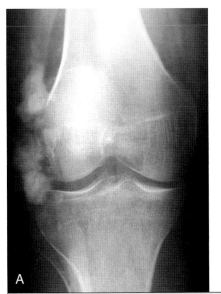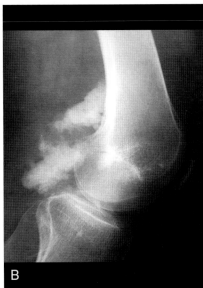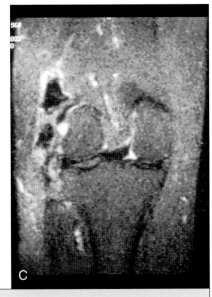

Figure 1   Melorheostasis. **A**, AP view of the knee showing periosteal new bone formation on the lateral aspect of the joint. Note the nodular appearance of the heavily ossified bone formation. **B**, Lateral view of the knee showing the large amount of nodular bone formation arising from the posterior aspect of the distal femur. **C**, T2-weighted coronal image of the knee showing very low signal nodular masses (corresponding to bone formation) and high signal changes (corresponding to edema) around the nodules.

4: Orthopaedic Oncology and Systemic Disease

II. Massive Osteolysis

A. Definition and demographics

  1. Massive osteolysis, also called Gorham disease or vanishing bone disease, is a very rare condition that is characterized by massive resorption of entire segments of bone.

  2. Affects both sexes

  3. Most common in patients younger than 40 years

B. Etiology/clinical presentation

  1. May be related to trauma

  2. Abrupt or insidious onset

C. Radiographic appearance

  1. Massive osteolysis

  2. Progressive lytic bone loss

  3. End of the remaining bone is often tapered

  4. Often spreads to adjacent bones (crosses joints)

D. Pathology/treatment

  1. Begins with numerous vascular channels and ends with fibrosis

  2. No effective treatment

III. Gaucher Disease

A. Definition and demographics

  1. Gaucher disease is an enzyme deficiency that causes accumulation of glucocerebrosides in the marrow, leading to bone deformities and osteonecrosis.

  2. Most common in Ashkenazi Jews

B. Genetics/etiology

  1. Autosomal recessive

  2. Caused by deficiency of glucocerebrosidase (acid β-glucosidase, lysosomal enzyme)

C. Clinical presentation

  1. Types

    a. Type I: adult nonneuropathic

    b. Type II: acute neuropathic (infants)—lethal form

    c. Type III: juvenile subacute neuropathic (children)—death by second decade of life

  2. Hematologic problems—pancytopenia, thrombocytopenia

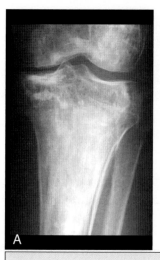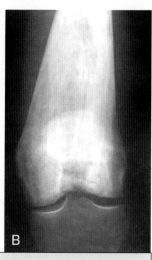

Figure 2   Gaucher disease. **A**, AP view of the tibia showing sclerosis in the medullary cavity. **B**, AP view of the distal femur showing the Erlenmeyer flask deformity, typical of Gaucher disease. Note the widened metaphyses.

  3. Easy bruisability, fatigue

  4. Bone problems

    a. Osteonecrosis

    b. Fractures

D. Radiographic appearance (**Figure 2**)

  1. Abnormal bone remodeling—Erlenmeyer flask deformity

  2. Lucent expansile lesions

  3. Subchondral collapse

  4. Vertebral collapse

E. Pathology/treatment

  1. Macrophages are enlarged and filled with abnormal material (crumpled cytoplasm).

  2. Periodic acid–Schiff (PAS)-positive, acid phosphatase-positive

  3. Treatment is enzyme replacement.

IV. Stress Fractures

A. Definition and demographics

  1. Stress fractures are overuse injuries in which normal bone is subjected to abnormal stresses, resulting in microfractures.

  2. Stress fractures occur following repetitive stress in either normal or abnormal bone.

    a. Fatigue fracture—Occurs in normal bone, such as in military recruits following marching

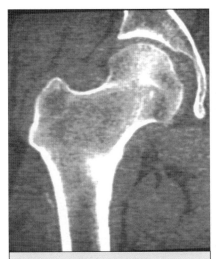

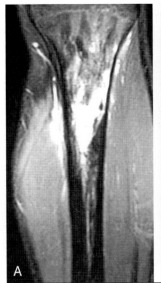

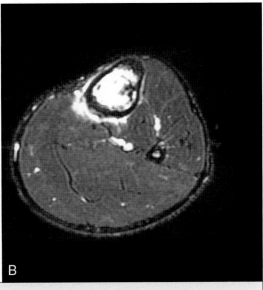

Figure 3 Coronal CT reconstruction of the proximal femur in a patient with a stress fracture. Note the focal endosteal new bone formation and the periosteal new bone formation on the medial femoral cortex.

Figure 4 Stress fracture. **A**, Coronal T2-weighted MRI showing high signal in the medullary cavity and on the periosteal surface. **B**, Axial T2-weighted MRI showing high signal in the medullary cavity and over the posteromedial cortical surface of the tibia.

(therefore sometimes called a march fracture).

b. Insufficiency fracture—Occurs in abnormal bone, such as in pagetic patients with femoral shaft bowing.

3. Common in young, athletic patients

B. Etiology/clinical presentation

1. Linear microfractures in trabecular bone from repetitive loading

2. Pain during activity located directly over the involved bone

C. Imaging appearance

1. Radiographs/CT

a. Diaphysis

i. Linear cortical radiolucency

ii. Endosteal thickening

iii. Periosteal reaction and cortical thickening

b. Metaphysis: focal linear increased mineralization (condensation of the trabecular bone)

c. Endosteal and periosteal new bone formation (**Figure 3**)

2. Technetium Tc 99m bone scan—Area of focal uptake in cortical and/or trabecular region.

3. MRI (**Figure 4**)

a. Periosteal high signal on T2-weighted images (earliest finding)

b. Linear zone of low signal on T1-weighted images

c. Broad area of increased signal on T2-weighted images

d. When a stress fracture is advanced in clinical course, linear low signal lines representing the fracture may be seen.

D. Pathology

1. Callus formation

2. Woven new bone

3. Enchondral bone formation

E. Treatment

1. Rest

2. Protected weight bearing until the fracture heals

3. Prophylactic fixation in selected cases

a. Tension-side femoral neck fractures in athletes

b. Patients with low bone mass, especially patients older than 60 years

V. Neuropathic Arthropathy

A. Definition and demographics

1. Neuropathic arthropathy is the destruction of a joint following loss of protective sensation.

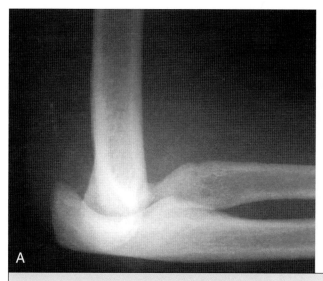
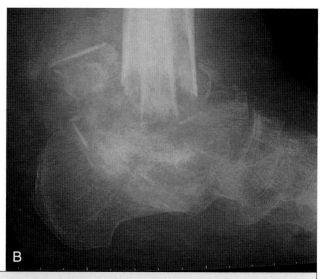

Figure 5 Neuropathic arthropathy. **A**, Lateral radiograph of the elbow in a patient with syringomyelia. There are very prominent neuropathic changes with complete destruction of the articular surfaces. **B**, Lateral radiograph of the ankle in a patient with diabetes mellitus. Note the complete destruction of the articular surfaces with dissolution and fragmentation.

   2. Common locations include the foot, ankle, elbow, and shoulder.

B. Etiology—Disease processes that damage sensory nerves.

   1. Diabetes mellitus: affects the foot and ankle

   2. Syringomyelia: affects the shoulder and elbow

   3. Syphilis: affects the knee

   4. Spinal cord tumors: affect the lower extremity joints

C. Clinical presentation

   1. Swollen, warm, and erythematous joint with little or no pain

   2. Often mimics infection, especially in patients with diabetes

D. Radiographic appearance (**Figure 5**)

   1. Characteristic features: destruction of the joint

   2. Initial changes may simulate osteoarthritis

   3. Late changes

      a. Fragmentation of the joint

      b. Subluxation/dislocation

      c. Fracture

      d. Collapse

E. Pathology

   1. Productive/hypertrophic changes secondary to the following spinal cord lesions (generally do not involve the sympathetic nervous system)

      a. Spinal cord traumatic injury

      b. Neoplasms

      c. Spinal cord malformations

      d. Syphilis

      e. Syringomyelia

   2. Destructive/atrophic changes usually secondary to peripheral nerve damage. Conditions that cause atrophic changes:

      a. Diabetes

      b. Alcoholism

   3. Histologic changes

      a. Synovial hypertrophy

      b. Fragments of bone and cartilage in the synovium (detritic synovitis)

F. Treatment

   1. Rest, elevation, protected weight bearing

   2. Total contact casting when ulcers are present in the foot and ankle

VI. Hemophilic Arthropathy

A. Definition and demographics

   1. Hemophilic arthropathy is the destruction of a joint secondary to repetitive bleeding into the synovial cavity.

   2. Classic hemophilia (hemophilia A) is caused by a

deficiency of factor VIII; Christmas disease (hemophilia B) is caused by a deficiency of factor IX.

3. Locations: knee, ankle, elbow

B. Genetics/etiology—X-linked recessive.

C. Clinical presentation

1. Hemarthrosis—Often in young males, 3 to 15 years of age.

2. Temporal changes

a. Acute hemarthrosis: tense, painful effusion

b. Subacute hemarthrosis: occurs after two previous bleeds

c. Chronic hemarthrosis: arthritis, contractures

D. Radiographic appearance

1. Arnold/Hilgartner stages

a. Stage I: soft-tissue swelling

b. Stage II: osteoporosis

c. Stage III: bone changes (subchondral cysts) with intact joint

d. Stage IV: cartilage loss

e. Stage V: severe arthritic changes

2. Radiographic changes

a. Knee

i. Overgrowth of distal femur and proximal tibia

ii. Distal condylar surface appears flattened

iii. Squaring of the inferior portion of the patella

b. Ankle: arthritic changes of the tibiotalar joint

c. Elbow: arthritic changes and contractures

E. Pathology/treatment

1. Synovial hypertrophy and hyperplasia

2. Synovium covers and destroys the cartilage.

3. Treatment is prophylaxis against recurrent hemarthroses.

Top Testing Facts

1. Melorheostosis is characterized by nodular, heavily mineralized bone on the surface of bones and in the soft tissues, which gives a "dripping candle wax" appearance on radiographs.

2. Massive osteolysis is purely lytic resorption of large segments of bone.

3. Radiographic findings for Gaucher disease include Erlenmeyer flask deformity (widened metaphyses).

4. Gaucher disease is caused by a deficiency of the enzyme glucocerebrosidase (acid β-glucosidase, lysosomal enzyme); treatment consists of enzyme replacement.

5. Imaging findings for stress fractures—radiographs: periosteal new bone formation; T1-weighted MRI: normal marrow except for low signal linear areas;

T2-weighted MRI: high signal in the medullary cavity and on the periosteal surface.

6. Neuropathic arthropathy—remember the common locations by disease state: syringomyelia—shoulder and elbow; syphilis—knee; and diabetes—foot and ankle.

7. Radiographic findings for neuropathic arthropathy include fragmentation, subluxation, and dissolution of the joint.

8. Hemophilic arthropathy—remember the factor deficiencies (hemophilia A—factor VIII, hemophilia B—factor IX), and remember the key radiographic findings (knee—squaring of the inferior patellar pole and femoral condyles).

Bibliography

McCarthy EF, Frassica FJ: Genetic diseases of bones and joints, in *Pathology of Bone and Joint Disorders*. Philadelphia, PA, Saunders, 1998, pp 54-55.

Resnick D: Neuropathic osteoarthropathy, in *Diagnosis of Bone and Joint Disorders*, ed 3. Philadelphia, PA, Saunders, 1995, pp 3413-3442.

Resnick D, Niwayama G: Enostosis, hyperostosis, and periostitis, in *Diagnosis of Bone and Joint Disorders*, ed 3. Philadelphia, PA, Saunders, 1995, pp 4410-4416.

Resnick D, Niwayama G: Osteolysis and chondrolysis, in *Diagnosis of Bone and Joint Disorders*, ed 3. Philadelphia, PA, Saunders, 1995, pp 4475-4476.

Siris ES, Roodman GD: Paget's disease of bone, in *Primer on the Metabolic Bone Diseases and Disorders of Mineral Metabolism*, ed 6. Washington, DC, American Society for Bone and Mineral Metabolism, 2006, pp 320-329.

Vigorita VJ: Osteonecrosis, Gaucher's disease, in *Orthopaedic Pathology*. Philadelphia, PA, Lippincott Williams & Wilkins, 1999, pp 503-505.

Chapter 43

Metastatic Bone Disease
Kristy Weber, MD

I. Evaluation/Diagnosis

A. Overview

1. Demographics

   a. Metastatic bone disease occurs in patients older than 40 years.

   b. Most common reason for destructive bone lesion in adults

   c. More than 1.4 million cases of cancer per year in the United States; bone metastasis develops in about 50% of patients

   d. Bone is the third most common site of metastasis (after lung and liver).

   e. Most common primary cancer sites that metastasize to bone are breast, prostate, lung, kidney, and thyroid.

2. Genetics/etiology

   a. Two main hypotheses

   i. 1889: Paget's "seed and soil" hypothesis (ability of tumor cells to survive and grow in addition to the compatible end-organ environment)

   ii. 1928: Ewing's circulation theory

      (a) Tumors colonize particular organs because of the routes of blood flow from the primary site.

      (b) Organs are passive receptacles.

      (c) Batson plexus—Valveless plexus of veins around the spine allows tumor cells to travel to the vertebral bodies, pelvis, ribs, skull, and proximal limb girdle (eg, prostate metastases).

   b. Mediators of bone destruction include tumor necrosis factors; transforming growth factors (TGFs); 1,25 dihydroxyvitamin D3; and parathyroid hormone-related protein (PTHrP).

B. Clinical presentation (Table 1)

1. History

   a. Progressive pain that occurs at rest and with weight bearing

   b. Constitutional symptoms (weight loss, fatigue, loss of appetite)

   c. Personal or family history of cancer

   d. History of symptoms related to possible primary sites (hematuria, shortness of breath, hot/cold intolerance)

   e. Primary tumors may metastasize quickly or take 10 to 15 years or longer (breast, renal, prostate).

2. Physical examination findings

   a. Occasional swelling, limp, decreased joint range of motion, neurologic deficits (10% to 20%) at metastatic bone sites

   b. Possible breast, prostate, thyroid, or abdominal mass

   c. Stool guaiac

   d. Regional adenopathy

3. Laboratory studies

   a. Complete blood cell count (anemia suggests myeloma)

Table 1

Workup of Patients Older Than 40 Years With a Destructive Bone Lesion*

Thorough history (history of cancer, weight loss, malaise, gastrointestinal bleeding, pain, etc)
Physical examination (focus on breast, lung, prostate, thyroid, lymph nodes)
Laboratory studies (electrolyte panel [calcium], alkaline phosphatase, complete blood cell count, prostate-specific antigen, serum protein electrophoresis/urine protein electrophoresis)
Plain radiographs of the bone lesion (two planes, include entire bone)
CT scan of chest, abdomen, pelvis
Total body bone scan

*Identifies primary site in 85% of patients

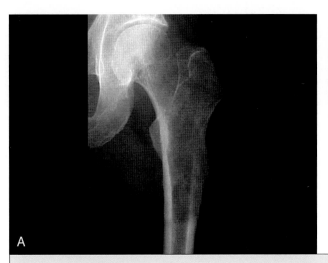 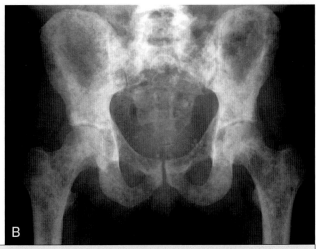

Figure 1   Osteolytic and osteoblastic metastases. **A,** Lung cancer metastases are generally purely osteolytic, as demonstrated in this radiograph. Note the lesion in the left proximal femur that is destroying the lateral cortex. **B,** Prostate cancer metastases are osteoblastic as noted throughout the pelvis, spine, and proximal femurs in this radiograph.

b. Serum protein electrophoresis/urine protein electrophoresis (abnormal in myeloma)

c. Thyroid function tests (may be abnormal in thyroid cancer)

d. Urinalysis (microscopic hematuria in renal cancer)

e. Basic chemistry panel: calcium, phosphorus, alkaline phosphatase, lactate dehydrogenase (LDH)

f. Specific tumor markers: prostate-specific antigen (PSA) (prostate); carcinoembryonic antigen (CEA) (colon, pancreas); cancer antigen 125 (CA 125) (ovarian)

4. Common scenarios

a. Known cancer patient with multiple bone lesions—Does not necessarily require confirmatory biopsy.

b. Known cancer patient with bone pain and normal radiographs—May be symptomatic from chemotherapy/bisphosphonates or may require bone scan or MRI to define an early destructive lesion.

c. Patient without history of cancer with a destructive bone lesion—Must differentiate between metastatic disease and primary malignant bone tumor.

C. Radiographic appearance/workup

1. Appearance

a. Osteolytic (most occurrences): lung, thyroid, kidney, gastrointestinal (**Figure 1,** *A*)

b. Osteoblastic: prostate, bladder (**Figure 1,** *B*)

c. Mixed osteolytic/osteoblastic: breast

d. Most common locations include spine (40%), pelvis, proximal long bones, and ribs.

e. The thoracic spine is the most common vertebral location of metastasis.

f. Metastatic carcinoma to the spine spares the intervertebral disk.

g. Lesions distal to the elbow/knee are most commonly from the lung as a primary site.

h. Pathologic fracture is a common presentation (25%).

i. An avulsion of the lesser trochanter implies a pathologic process in the femoral neck with impending fracture.

2. Workup (**Table 1**)

a. Plain radiographs—Images in two planes and of the entire bone should be obtained (consider referred pain).

b. Differential diagnosis of lytic bone lesion in patient older than 40 years includes metastatic disease, multiple myeloma, lymphoma, and, less likely, primary bone tumors, Paget sarcoma, and hyperparathyroidism (**Table 2**).

c. Bone scan

i. Detects osteoblastic activity (may be negative in myeloma, metastatic renal cancer)

ii. Identifies multiple lesions, which are common in metastatic disease (**Figure 2,** *A*)

d. CT scan of chest, abdomen, pelvis to identify primary lesion

e. Staging evaluation of lytic bone lesion will identify primary site in 85% of patients (**Table 1**).

Table 2

Differential Diagnosis of Destructive Bone Lesion in Patient Older Than 40 Years*

Metastatic bone disease
Multiple myeloma
Lymphoma
Primary bone tumors (chondrosarcoma, osteosarcoma, malignant fibrous histiocytoma, chordoma)
Sacral insufficiency fractures
Postradiation/Paget sarcoma
Giant cell tumor
Hyperparathyroidism

*From most likely (metastatic bone disease) to least likely (hyperparathyroidism)

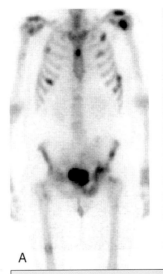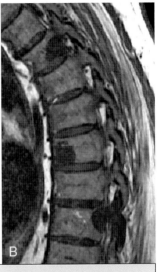

Figure 2 Metastases seen on a total body bone scan and MRI. **A,** This total body bone scan shows increased uptake in the sacroiliac region but also identifies metastases in the anterior pelvis, ribs, and shoulder girdle. **B,** MRI is not used routinely to evaluate extremity bone metastases, but it is helpful in defining vertebral lesions, as in this thoracic spine.

f. Bone marrow biopsy when considering myeloma as a diagnosis

g. MRI scan of the primary lesion is generally not necessary unless defining disease in the spine (**Figure 2,** *B*).

h. Difficult to differentiate osteoporosis from metastatic disease with a single vertebral compression fracture; tumor is suggested by soft-tissue mass and pedicle destruction.

D. Biopsy/pathology

1. A biopsy of a destructive bone lesion must be performed unless the diagnosis is certain.

2. Placing an intramedullary device in a 65-year-old patient with lytic lesions in the femur without appropriate workup is dangerous (could be a dedifferentiated chondrosarcoma).

3. An open incisional biopsy or closed needle biopsy (fine needle aspiration/core) can be performed for diagnosis.

4. Histologic appearance is islands of epithelial cells with glandular or squamous differentiation (**Figure 3,** *A* and *B*).

5. The carcinoma cells have tight junctions and reside within a fibrous stroma.

6. Thyroid (follicular): follicles filled with colloid material (**Figure 3,** *C*)

7. Renal cancer often has a clear appearance to the cytoplasm within the epithelial cells (**Figure 3,** *D*); in some cases, it may be poorly differentiated and may have a sarcomatoid pattern.

8. Epithelial cells are keratin-positive.

9. Special immunohistochemistry stains can sometimes determine the primary site of disease.

a. Thyroid transcription factor-1: lung, thyroid

b. Estrogen receptor/progesterone receptor: breast

c. PSA: prostate

II. Pathophysiology/Molecular Mechanisms

A. Metastatic cascade

1. Primary tumor cells proliferate and stimulate angiogenesis.

2. Tumor cells cross the basement membrane into capillaries and must avoid host defenses.

3. Tumor cells disseminate to distant sites.

4. Cells arrest in distant capillary bed, adhere to vascular endothelium, and extravasate into end-organ environment (integrins, cadherins, matrix metalloproteinases).

5. Tumor cells interact with local host cells and growth factors (TGF-β, insulin-like growth factor, fibroblast growth factor, bone morphogenetic protein).

6. Tumor cells proliferate to become a site of metastasis.

B. RANKL/osteoprotegerin

1. Tumor cells do not destroy bone; cytokines from the tumor stimulate osteoclasts or osteoblasts to destroy or generate new bone, respectively.

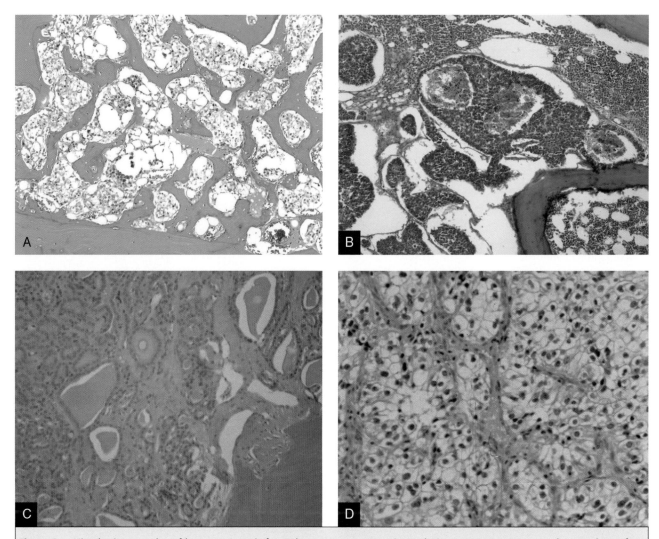

Figure 3   Histologic examples of bone metastasis from the most common primary lesions. **A,** Prostate—note the new bone formation by the osteoblasts that are stimulated by factors secreted by the tumor cells. **B,** Lung—note the clumps of epithelial cells characterized by tight cell-cell junctions. **C,** Thyroid (follicular)—the epithelial cells are forming follicles surrounding a central colloid substance. **D,** Renal—the epithelial tumor cells are characterized by clear cytoplasm.

2. Osteoblasts/stromal cells secrete receptor activator of nuclear factor κ B ligand (RANKL).

3. Osteoclasts have receptors for RANKL (RANK).

4. Increased secretion of RANKL by osteoblasts causes an increase in osteoclast precursors, which eventually results in increased bone destruction.

5. Osteoprotegerin (OPG) is a decoy receptor that binds to RANKL and inhibits an increase in osteoclasts.

C. Vicious cycle in breast cancer

1. TGF-β is stored in the bone and released during normal bone turnover.

2. TGF-β stimulates metastatic breast cancer cells to secrete PTHrP.

3. PTHrP from cancer cells stimulates osteoblasts to secrete RANKL.

4. RANKL from osteoblasts stimulates osteoclast precursors and increases osteoclasts.

5. Osteoclasts destroy bone and release TGF-β, so the cycle of destruction repeats.

D. Other disease-specific factors

1. Breast cancer cells also secrete osteoclastic stimulants (interleukin [IL]-6, IL-8).

2. Prostate cancer—Endothelin-1 stimulates osteoblasts to produce bone.

3. Overexpression of epidermal growth factor receptor is common in renal cell carcinoma.

E. Fracture healing in pathologic bone

1. Likelihood of pathologic fracture healing: multiple myeloma > renal carcinoma > breast carcinoma > lung carcinoma (ie, pathologic fracture healing is most likely in patients with myeloma and least likely in patients with metastatic lung cancer)

2. Most important factor in determining healing potential is the length of patient survival.

F. Other physiologic disruptions

1. Calcium metabolism—Hypercalcemia is present in 10% to 15% of cases.

   a. Common with lung, breast cancer metastasis

   b. Does not correlate with number of bone metastases

   c. Early symptoms: polyuria/polydipsia, anorexia, weakness, easy fatigability

   d. Late symptoms: irritability, depression, coma, profound weakness, nausea/vomiting, pruritus, vision abnormalities

   e. Treatment requires hydration and possibly intravenous bisphosphonate therapy.

2. Hematopoiesis—Normocytic/normochromic anemia is common with breast, prostate, lung, and thyroid cancer metastasis.

3. Thromboembolic disease

   a. Patients with malignancy have increased thrombotic risk.

   b. Require prophylaxis, especially after lower extremity/pelvic surgery

4. Pain control/bowel abnormalities

   a. Use narcotics for pain control.

   b. Requires laxatives/stool softener to avoid severe constipation

III. Biomechanics

A. Stress riser in bone occurs whenever there is cortical destruction.

B. Defects

1. Open section defect—When the length of a longitudinal defect in a bone exceeds 75% of diameter, there is a 90% reduction in torsional strength.

2. 50% cortical defect (centered) = 60% bending strength reduction.

3. 50% cortical defect (eccentric) = >90% bending strength reduction.

IV. Impending Fractures/Prophylactic Fixation

A. Indications for fixation

1. Snell/Beals criteria

   a. 2.5-cm lytic bone lesion

   b. 50% cortical involvement

   c. Pain persisting after radiation

   d. Peritrochanteric lesion

2. Mirels scoring system (Table 3)

   a. Four factors are scored: radiographic appearance, size (proportion of bone diameter occupied by the lesion), site, and pain.

   b. Prophylactic fixation is recommended for a score ≥9 (33% fracture risk).

3. Spinal lesions—impending fracture/collapse

   a. Thoracic

      i. Risk of fracture/collapse exists when 50% to 60% of the vertebral body is involved (without other abnormalities).

      ii. Risk of fracture/collapse exists when only 20% to 30% of the vertebral body is involved if there is also costovertebral joint involvement.

   b. Lumbar

      i. Risk of fracture/collapse exists when 35% to 40% of the vertebral body is involved (without other abnormalities).

Table 3

Mirels Scoring System for Prediction of Pathologic Fracture in Patients With Metastatic Bone Lesions

	Points		
	1	2	3
Radiographic appearance	Blastic	Mixed	Lytic
Size (as a proportion of shaft diameter)	<1/3	1/3 to 2/3	>2/3
Site	UE	LE	Peritrochanteric
Pain	Mild	Moderate	Mechanical

UE = upper extremity, LE = lower extremity. (Adapted with permission from Mirels H: Metastatic disease in long bones: A proposed scoring system for diagnosing impending pathologic fractures. Clin Orthop 1989;249:256-265.)

4: Orthopaedic Oncology and Systemic Disease

ii. Risk of fracture/collapse exists when 25% of vertebral body is involved if there is also pedicle/posterior element involvement.

B. Other factors to consider

1. Scoring systems are not exact and cannot predict all human factors.

2. Histology of primary lesion

3. Expected lifespan, comorbid conditions, and activity level

4. Most surgical decisions can be based on plain radiographs.

5. Prophylactic fixation compared with fixation of actual pathologic fracture

   a. Decreased perioperative morbidity/pain

   b. Shorter operating room time

   c. Faster recovery/shorter hospital stay

   d. Ability to coordinate care with medical oncology

V. Nonsurgical Treatment

A. Indications

1. Nondisplaced fractures

2. Non–weight-bearing bones (Figure 4)

3. Poor medical health/shortened lifespan

B. Observation/pain management/bracing

1. Observation or activity modifications are used for patients with very small lesions or advanced disease.

2. Functional bracing can be used in the upper and lower extremities and spine.

3. Pain management is important in all symptomatic patients.

   a. Opioids: fentanyl, oxycodone, hydrocodone

   b. Nonopioids: nonsteroidal anti-inflammatory drugs, trycyclic antidepressants, muscle relaxants, steroids

   c. A bowel program is necessary to prevent severe constipation.

C. Medical

1. Chemotherapy/hormonal treatment (prostate, breast metastasis)

2. Bisphosphonates

   a. Inhibit osteoclast activity by inducing apoptosis

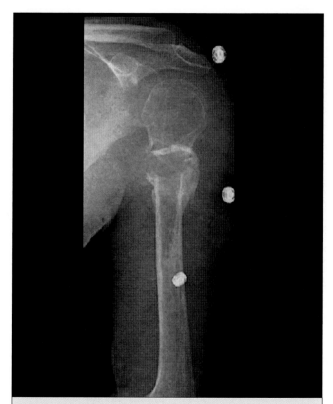

Figure 4 Radiograph of the left humerus of a 59-year-old woman with metastatic thyroid cancer that caused a pathologic fracture. She was not a safe surgical candidate and was therefore treated nonsurgically. Note the callus formation about the fracture site.

   b. Inhibit protein prenylation and act on the mevalonate pathway

   c. Significant decrease in skeletal events (breast, prostate, lung)

   d. Reduced pain

   e. Used in virtually all cases of metastatic bone disease: 4 mg zoledronic acid administered intravenously every month

   f. Complication: small incidence of osteonecrosis of the jaw

D. Radiation

1. External beam radiation

   a. Indications: pain, impending fracture, neurologic symptoms

   b. Dose: usually 30 Gy in 10 fractions to bone lesion

   c. Pain relief in 70% of patients

   d. Postoperatively, the entire implant should be irradiated after 2 weeks to decrease fixation failure and improve local control.

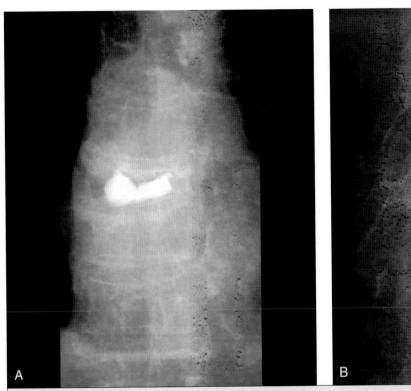
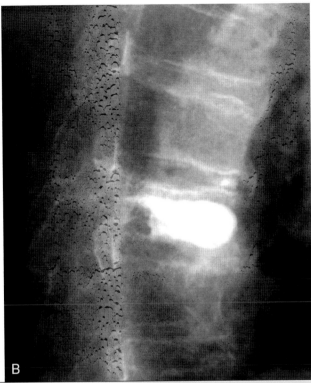

Figure 5   AP (**A**) and lateral (**B**) radiographs of the spine of a woman with metastatic lung cancer to the thoracic vertebra, causing painful collapse. The patient was treated with vertebroplasty, with marked pain relief.

4: Orthopaedic Oncology and Systemic Disease

e. Should be used for patients with radiosensitive tumors of the spine who have pain or tumor progression without instability or myelopathy

2. Radiopharmaceuticals

  a. Samarium Sm-153 or strontium chloride 89

  b. Delivery of radiation to the entire skeleton (bone scan concept)

  c. Palliation of pain—may delay progression of lesions

  d. Use requires normal renal function and blood counts.

  e. Iodine-131 is used to treat metastatic thyroid cancer.

E. Minimally invasive techniques

1. Radiofrequency ablation—Used for palliative pain control (commonly used in pelvis/acetabulum).

2. Kyphoplasty/vertebroplasty (**Figure 5**)

  a. Pain relief in patients with vertebral compression fractures from metastasis

  b. The risk of cement leakage in vertebroplasty (35% to 65%) is usually not clinically relevant.

VI. Surgical Treatment/Outcome

A. Overview

1. Goals of surgical treatment

  a. Relieve pain

  b. Improve function

  c. Restore skeletal stability

2. Considerations prior to surgery

  a. Patient selection (functional status, activity level, comorbidities)

  b. Stability/durability of planned construct (withstand force of 6× body weight around hip)

  c. Addressing all areas of weakened bone

  d. Preoperative embolization for highly vascular lesions (renal, thyroid metastasis)

  e. Extensive use of methylmethacrylate (cement) to improve stability of construct

  f. Standard of care in patients with bone metastasis is cemented joint prostheses, not uncemented prostheses

B. Upper extremity

1. Overview

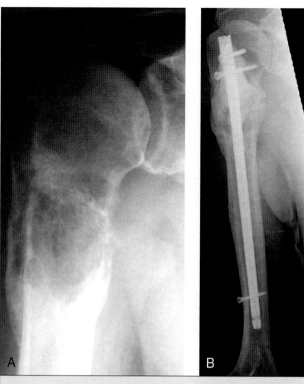
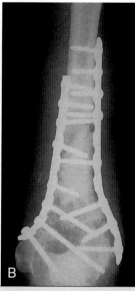

Figure 6 Radiographs of the upper extremity of a 67-year-old right-handed man with metastatic renal carcinoma that caused pain at rest and with activity. **A,** AP radiograph shows the osteolytic lesion in the right proximal humerus. **B,** Postoperative radiograph after placement of a locked right humeral intramedullary rod. This lesion was curetted and cemented during the surgery and received radiation after 2 weeks.

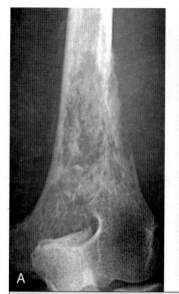

Figure 7 Radiographs of the distal humerus of a 56-year-old woman with metastatic endometrial cancer. **A,** AP view demonstrates the permeative appearance of the lesion. The patient had persistent pain after radiation of the metastasis. **B,** Postoperative radiograph after curettage, cementation, and double plating of the lesion.

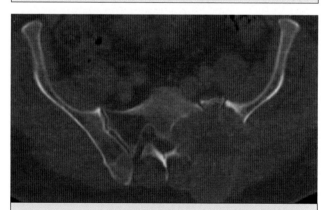

Figure 8 CT scan of the pelvis of a 47-year-old man with metastatic thyroid cancer defines a large, destructive lesion in the left sacroiliac region.

    a. Upper extremity metastases affect activities of daily living, use of external aids, bed-to-chair transfers.

    b. Much less common (20%) than lower extremity metastases

  2. Scapula/clavicle—usually nonsurgical treatment/radiation

  3. Proximal humerus

    a. Resection and proximal humeral replacement (megaprosthesis); excellent pain relief but poor shoulder function

    b. Intramedullary locked device (closed versus open with curettage/cement) (**Figure 6**)

  4. Humeral diaphysis

    a. Intramedullary fixation: closed versus open with curettage/cement

    b. Intercalary metal spacer: selected indications for extensive diaphyseal destruction or failed prior device

  5. Distal humerus

    a. Flexible nails should be supplemented with cement and extend the entire length of bone (insert at elbow).

    b. Orthogonal plating—Combine with curettage/cement (**Figure 7**).

    c. Resection and modular distal humeral prosthetic reconstruction

  6. Distal to elbow—Individualize treatment with plates or intramedullary devices.

C. Lower extremity

  1. Overview

    a. Common location for bone metastasis

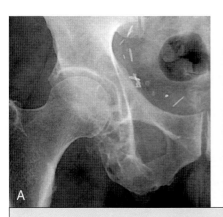
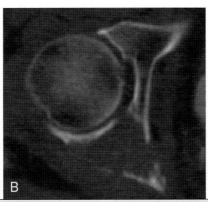
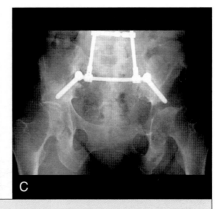

Figure 9 Imaging studies in patients with metastatic disease to the acetabulum. **A,** AP radiograph of the right pelvis in a 71-year-old man with metastatic renal cell carcinoma to the right acetabulum and ischium. The acetabular disease is not well defined on plain radiographs. **B,** CT scan of the right acetabulum defines the destruction of the posterior acetabulum, placing the patient at risk for a displaced fracture. Acetabular reconstruction would require a reinforced ring or cage device to prevent protrusion with disease progression. **C,** AP view of the pelvis in a 59-year-old woman with widely metastatic thyroid cancer and with multiple comorbidities shows destruction of the left acetabulum. Nonsurgical treatment with immobilization in a wheelchair or a Girdlestone procedure for pain relief would be reasonable options.

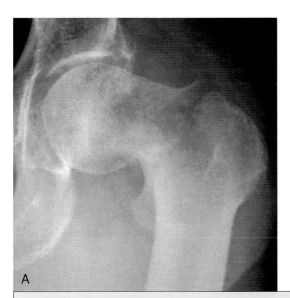
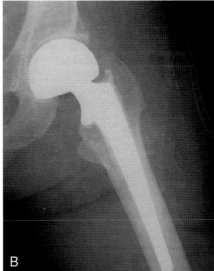
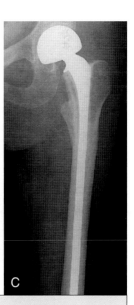

Figure 10 Metastases to the femoral neck. **A,** AP radiograph of the left hip in a 70-year-old woman with metastatic breast cancer reveals a pathologic femoral neck fracture. No other lesions were noted throughout the femur. **B,** Radiograph obtained after a cemented bipolar hip reconstruction. Most patients with femoral neck disease do not require acetabular components. Internal fixation of a pathologic hip fracture is not indicated. **C,** Radiograph of a hip after implantation of a long-stemmed femoral component, which can be used to prevent pathologic fractures in the femoral diaphysis. Patients with long-stemmed prostheses have a higher risk of cardiopulmonary complications due to intraoperative/postoperative thromboembolic events.

   b. Surgical treatment if patient has ≥3 months to live

2. Pelvis (**Figure 8**)

   a. Treat non–weight-bearing areas with radiation or minimally invasive techniques.

   b. Resection or curettage in selected cases

3. Acetabulum (**Figure 9,** *A* and *B*)

   a. Surgical treatment requires extensive preopera-

tive planning (cross-sectional imaging, embolization for vascular lesions).

   b. Extent of bone destruction delineates treatment options (standard total hip arthroplasty, acetabular mesh/cage, rebar reconstruction to transmit stresses from acetabulum to unaffected ilium/sacrum).

   c. Girdlestone procedure is appropriate in patients with end-stage disease and severe pain (**Figure 9,** *C*).

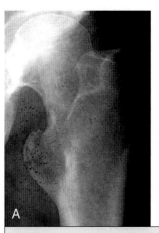
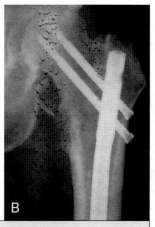

Figure 11   Intertrochanteric lesions. **A,** Radiograph of the hip of a patient with metastatic thyroid cancer. A lesser trochanter avulsion or osteolytic lesion indicates a pathologic process in the older patient. **B,** The patient was treated prophylactically with a locked femoral reconstruction nail.

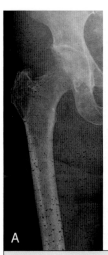
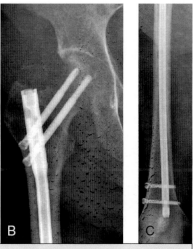
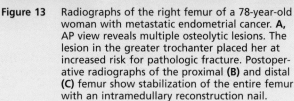

Figure 13   Radiographs of the right femur of a 78-year-old woman with metastatic endometrial cancer. **A,** AP view reveals multiple osteolytic lesions. The lesion in the greater trochanter placed her at increased risk for pathologic fracture. Postoperative radiographs of the proximal **(B)** and distal **(C)** femur show stabilization of the entire femur with an intramedullary reconstruction nail.

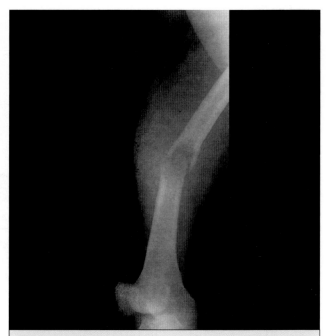

Figure 12   Radiograph of the right femur of a 60-year-old woman demonstrates a pathologic fracture. A staging workup did not reveal a primary site of disease, but a biopsy of the femoral lesion showed carcinoma. The patient should be treated with a femoral reconstruction nail.

5. Intertrochanteric (**Figure 11**)

   a. The intramedullary reconstruction nail (open versus closed) protects the entire femur.

   b. Calcar-replacement prosthesis for lesions with extensive bone destruction

   c. Rare utilization of dynamic hip screw plate/screws/cement in patients with extremely short lifespan

6. Subtrochanteric

   a. Intramedullary locked reconstruction nail

   b. Resection and prosthetic replacement (megaprosthesis)

      i. Patients with periarticular bone destruction that does not allow rigid fixation

      ii. Displaced pathologic fracture through osteolytic lesion

      iii. Radio-resistant lesion (large renal cell metastasis)

      iv. Solitary lesion (some series indicate improved survival for resection of solitary metastasis from renal carcinoma)

      v. Salvage of failed fixation devices (**Figure 12**)

7. Femoral diaphysis: intramedullary locked reconstruction nail (**Figures 13** and **14**)

4. Femoral neck (**Figure 10**)

   a. Pathologic fractures or impending fractures require prosthetic reconstruction.

   b. Internal fixation with cement has an unacceptably high failure rate because of the likelihood of disease progression.

   c. Usually a bipolar cup is satisfactory; a total hip arthroplasty should be performed only if the acetabulum is involved with metastatic disease or the patient has extensive degenerative joint disease.

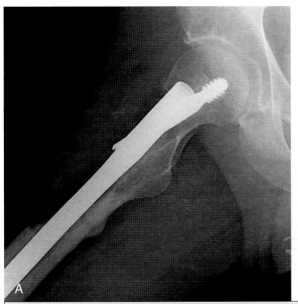
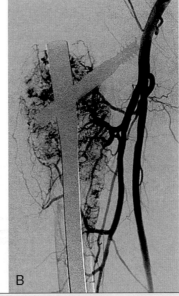
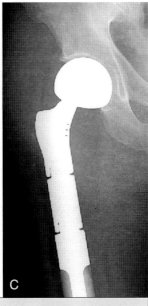

Figure 14 Imaging of a 49-year-old man with metastatic renal cell carcinoma and painful progression of disease after placement of an intramedullary reconstruction nail in the right femur. **A,** Lateral radiograph demonstrates the loss of anterior cortex proximally. **B,** Prior to salvage of the impending hardware failure, embolization of the feeding vessels is performed. This should be done routinely for patients with metastatic renal carcinoma unless a tourniquet can be used for surgery. **C,** Radiograph obtained after the proximal femur was resected and the defect reconstructed with a cemented megaprosthesis using a bipolar acetabular component.

8. Distal femur

    a. Locking plate/screws/cement

    b. Retrograde intramedullary device

    c. Resection and distal femoral replacement

9. Distal to knee

    a. Individualize treatment with prostheses, intramedullary devices, plates/screws/cement. (Figure 15)

    b. Avoid amputation if possible.

D. Spine

    1. Risk factors for progressive neurologic deficit

        a. Osteolytic lesions

        b. Pedicle involvement

        c. Posterior wall involvement

    2. Indications for surgical treatment

        a. Significant or progressive neurologic deficit

        b. Intractable pain

        c. Progression of deformity

    3. Surgical options

        a. Anterior vertebrectomy

        b. Posterior decompression/instrumentation

        c. Anterior/posterior combination approach (Figure 16)

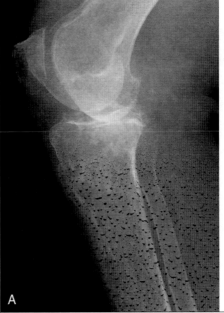
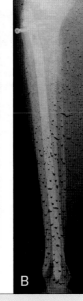

Figure 15 Radiographs of the right knee of a 67-year-old woman with metastatic breast cancer to the tibia. **A,** Lateral radiograph demonstrates the destruction of the tibia with concomitant severe osteopenia. This extends throughout the length of the bone. **B,** Lateral radiograph obtained after 18 months reveals a locked intramedullary tibial rod in good position. With postoperative radiation, bisphosphonates, and hormonal treatment, the bone quality greatly improved.

4: Orthopaedic Oncology and Systemic Disease

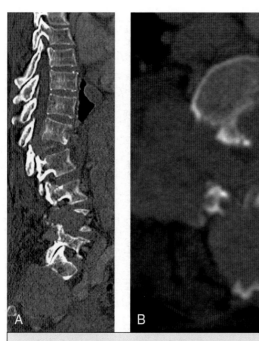 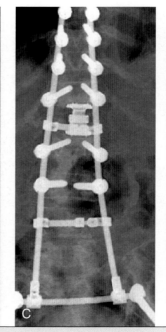 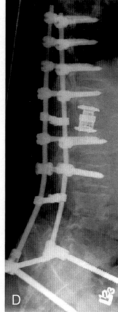

Figure 16   Images of the spine of a 57-year-old woman with metastatic thyroid cancer. **A,** A CT sagittal reconstruction of the thoracolumbar spine demonstrates complete destruction and collapse of L1, with severe central canal obstruction at this level. Note also the extensive disease at L4 and S2. **B,** Axial CT image at L4 demonstrates the canal compromise at this level and the extent of the soft-tissue mass. AP **(C)** and lateral **(D)** radiographs obtained after L1 corpectomy, partial L4 corpectomy, and posterior thoracic-lumbar-pelvic fixation with pedicle screws, rods, and a transiliac bar. A distractible cage is shown at L1.

Top Testing Facts

1. The most common primary sites that metastasize to bone are breast, prostate, lung, renal, and thyroid.

2. Careful history, physical examination, and radiographic staging will identify 85% of primary lesions; biopsy is needed when the primary lesion has not been identified.

3. The most common diagnosis of a lytic, destructive lesion in a patient older than age 40 years is bone metastasis.

4. The histology of metastatic bone disease is epithelial cells in a fibrous stroma.

5. Breast carcinoma cells secrete PTHrP, which signals osteoblasts to release RANKL, which causes osteoclast activation and bone resorption.

6. Osteolytic lesions have a greater likelihood of pathologic fracture than osteoblastic lesions.

7. Bisphosphonates cause osteoclast apoptosis by inhibiting protein prenylation and act via the mevalonate pathway.

8. External beam radiation is helpful for pain control and important in maintaining local control postoperatively.

9. Pathologic femoral neck lesions require prosthetic replacement, not for situ fixation.

10. Locked intramedullary fixation is used for diaphyseal impending or actual fractures (femoral rods must extend into the femoral neck).

Bibliography

Barragan-Campos HM, Vallee JN, Lo D, et al: Percutaneous vertebroplasty for spinal metastases: Complications. *Radiology* 2006;238:354-362.

Berenson JR: Recommendations for zoledronic acid treatment of patients with bone metastases. *Oncologist* 2005;10:52-62.

Damron TA, Morgan H, Prakash D, Grant W, Aronowitz J, Heiner J: Critical evaluation of Mirels' rating system for impending pathologic fractures. *Clin Orthop Relat Res* 2003; 415:S201-S207.

Frassica DA: General principles of external beam radiation therapy for skeletal metastases. *Clin Orthop Relat Res* 2003; 415:S158-S164.

Goetz MP, Callstrom MR, Charboneau JW, et al: Percutaneous image-guided radiofrequency ablation of painful metastases involving bone: A multicenter study. *J Clin Oncol* 2004;22:300-306.

Harrington KD: The management of acetabular deficiency secondary to metastatic malignant disease. *J Bone Joint Surg Am* 1981;63:653-664.

Lipton A: Management of bone metastases in breast cancer. *Curr Treat Options Oncol* 2005;6:161-171.

Mundy GR: Metastasis to bone: Causes, consequences and therapeutic opportunities. *Nat Rev Cancer* 2002;2:584-593.

Patchell RA, Tibbs PA, Regine WF, et al: Direct decompressive surgical resection in the treatment of spinal cord compression caused by metastatic cancer: A randomized trial. *Lancet* 2005;366:643-648.

Roodman GD: Mechanisms of bone metastasis. *N Engl J Med* 2004;350:1655-1664.

Rougraff BT: Evaluation of the patient with carcinoma of unknown primary origin metastatic to bone. *Clin Orthop Relat Res* 2003;415:S105-S109.

Silberstein EB: Teletherapy and radiopharmaceutical therapy of painful bone metastases. *Semin Nucl Med* 2005;35:152-158.

Thai DM, Kitagawa Y, Choong PF: Outcome of surgical management of bony metastases to the humerus and shoulder girdle: A retrospective analysis of 93 patients. *Int Semin Surg Oncol* 2006;3:5.

Ward WG, Holsenbeck BA, Dorey FJ, Spang J, Howe D: Metastatic disease of the femur: Surgical treatment. *Clin Orthop Relat Res* 2003;415:S230-S244.

Weber KL, Lewis VO, Randall RL, Lee AK, Springfield D: An approach to the management of the patient with metastatic bone disease. *Instr Course Lect* 2004;53:663-676.

4: Orthopaedic Oncology and Systemic Disease

Chapter 44

Metabolic Bone and Inflammatory Joint Disease
*Frank J. Frassica, MD

4: Orthopaedic Oncology and Systemic Disease

I. Osteopetrosis (Albers-Schönberg Disease)

A. Definition and demographics

1. Osteopetrosis is a rare disorder characterized by a failure of osteoclastic resorption with resultant dense bone with no medullary cavity (prone to fracture).

2. Autosomal recessive forms are discovered in children; the delayed type often is not discovered until adulthood.

B. Genetics/etiology

1. Lethal form is autosomal recessive (malignant).

2. Delayed type is autosomal dominant.

3. When osteopetrosis occurs with renal tubular acidosis and cerebral calcification, there is an associated carbonic anhydrase II deficiency.

4. Deactivating mutations in three genes have been found (inability to cause acidification in the clear zone). The sites of the defects are as follows:

   a. Carbonic anhydrase II (CA II)

   b. Alpha 3 subunit of vacuolar proton pump

   c. Chloride channel 7

C. Clinical presentation—Often discovered following:

1. Fracture

2. Complications following tooth extraction

3. Anemia

4. Cranial nerve palsy (hearing loss)

D. Radiographic appearance (**Figure 1**)

1. Symmetric increase in bone mass

2. Thickened cortical and trabecular bone

3. Often alternating sclerotic and lucent bands

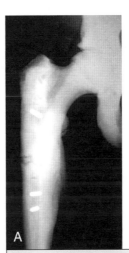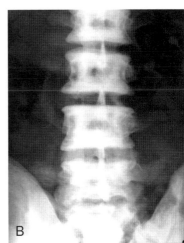

Figure 1   Osteopetrosis. **A**, AP radiograph of the hip in a patient with osteopetrosis. The medullary cavity is intensely sclerotic. There is no medullary cavity in the periacetabular region. **B**, AP view of the spine of a patient with osteopetrosis demonstrates the dense sclerosis at the superior and inferior end plates of the vertebral bodies.

4. Widened metaphyses (Erlenmeyer flask deformity)

E. Pathology

1. Islands or bars of calcified cartilage within mature trabeculae

2. Osteoclasts without ruffled borders

F. Treatment

1. Bone marrow transplantation for infantile form

2. Interferon gamma-1β for delayed type

II. Oncologic Osteomalacia (Tumor-Induced Osteomalacia)

A. Definition and demographics

1. Paraneoplastic syndrome of renal phosphate wasting caused by a bone tumor or soft-tissue tumor that secretes a substance that leads to osteomalacia

*Frank J. Frassica, MD, is a consultant or employee for SLACK Inc.

2. Putative factor is "phosphatonin"; possible gene is fibroblast growth factor-23.

3. Often a long delay in detecting the tumor

B. Genetics/etiology—Four types of tumors cause oncologic osteomalacia.

1. Phosphaturic mesenchymal tumor, mixed connective tissue type

2. Osteoblastoma-like tumors

3. Ossifying fibrous tumors

4. Nonossifying fibrous tumors

C. Clinical presentation

1. Progressive bone and muscle pain

2. Weakness and fatigue

3. Fractures of the long bones, ribs, and vertebrae

D. Imaging appearance

1. Diffuse osteopenia, pseudofractures on radiographs

2. Tumors detected on octreotide scan (indium-111–pentetreotide scintigraphy, radiolabeled somatostatin analog)

E. Laboratory features

1. Hypophosphatemia

2. Phosphaturia due to low proximal tubular reabsorption

3. Low serum 1,25-dihydroxyvitamin D

F. Treatment

1. Removal of the tumor

2. Phosphate supplementation with 1,25-dihydroxyvitamin D

III. Hypercalcemia and Malignancy

A. Definition and demographics

1. Hypercalcemia may develop in patients with cancer.

2. Two types: with diffuse lytic metastases (20%) and without (80%)

   a. Hypercalcemia with diffuse lytic metastases is commonly associated with the following types of cancers:

   i. Breast cancer

   ii. Hematologic malignancies: multiple myeloma, lymphoma, leukemia

b. Hypercalcemia without diffuse lytic metastases is commonly associated with the following types of cancers:

   i. Squamous cell carcinoma

   ii. Renal or bladder carcinoma

   iii. Ovarian or endometrial cancer

   iv. Breast cancer

B. Genetics/etiology—Local or circulating factor that causes bone resorption and release of calcium ions.

C. Clinical presentation

1. Neurologic: difficulty concentrating, sleepiness, depression, confusion, coma

2. Gastrointestinal: constipation, anorexia, nausea, vomiting

3. Genitourinary: polyuria, dehydration

4. Cardiac: shortening of QT interval, bradycardia, first-degree block

D. Radiographic appearance—Diffuse lytic metastases may or may not be present.

E. Laboratory features

1. Hypercalcemia

2. Normal or high serum phosphorus level

3. Low parathyroid hormone level

F. Pathology—Osteoclastic bone resorption.

G. Treatment

1. Bisphosphonate therapy to halt osteoclastic bone resorption

2. Combination therapy (chemotherapy and radiation) to kill the cancer cells

IV. Paget Disease

A. Definition and demographics

1. Remodeling disease characterized initially by osteoclast-mediated bone resorption and then disordered bone formation

2. Common in patients older than 50 years

B. Genetics/etiology

1. Possibly caused by a slow virus infection (paramyxovirus, respiratory syncytial virus)

2. Most common in Caucasians of Anglo-Saxon descent

3. Strong genetic tendency (autosomal dominant)

   a. Candidate genes

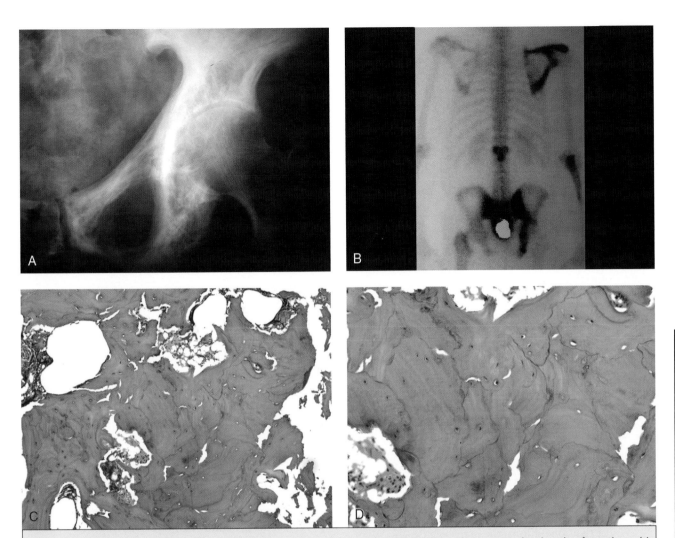

Figure 2   Paget disease. **A**, AP view of the pelvis in a patient with Paget disease. Note the coarsened trabeculae from the pubis to the supra-acetabular area and marked thickening of the iliopectineal line. **B**, Technetium Tc 99m bone scan in a patient with Paget disease. Note the intense uptake in the scapula, lumbar vertebral body, right ilium, and right ulna. **C** and **D**, Hematoxylin and eosin stain of pagetic bone. Note the disordered appearance of the bone and the multiple cement lines (curved blue lines).

b. 5q35-QTER (ubiquitin binding protein sequestosome-1)

C. Clinical presentation

1. No sex predilection

2. Generally found in patients older than 50 years

3. May be monostotic or polyostotic; the number of sites remains constant.

4. Common sites: femur, pelvis, tibia, skull, spine (**Figure 2**)

5. Often asymptomatic and found incidentally on a bone scan, chest radiograph, or in patients with elevated alkaline phosphatase levels

6. Progresses through three phases

a. Lytic phase

i. Profound resorption of the bone

ii. Purely lucent on radiographs, with expansion and thinned but intact cortices

b. Mixed phase: combination of lysis and bone formation with coarsened trabeculae

c. Sclerotic phase: enlargement of the bone with thickened cortices and with sclerotic and lucent areas

7. Bone pain may also be present, which may be caused by increased vascularity and warmth or by stress fractures.

8. Bowing of the femur or tibia

9. Fractures, most commonly femoral neck

10. Arthritis of the hip and knee

11. Lumbar spinal stenosis

12. Malignant degeneration

a. Occurs in 1% of patients

b. Most common locations: pelvis, femur, humerus

c. Patients often note a marked increase in pain, and the pain is usually constant.

D. Laboratory features

1. Increased alkaline phosphatase level

2. Increased urinary markers of bone turnover

a. Collagen cross-links

b. N-telopeptide, hydroxylproline, deoxypyridinoline

3. Normal calcium level

E. Radiographic appearance

1. Plain radiographs (**Figure 2**, *A*)

a. Coarsened trabeculae

b. Cortical thickening

c. Lucent advancing edge ("blade of grass" or "flame-shaped") in active disease

d. Loss of distinction between the cortices and medullary cavity

e. Enlargement of the bone

2. Technetium Tc 99m bone scans—Increased uptake accurately marks sites of disease (**Figure 2**, *B*).

a. Intense activity, which often outlines the shape of the bone during the active phase

b. Mild to moderate activity in the sclerotic phases

3. CT scans

a. Cortical thickening

b. Coarsened trabeculae

F. Pathology

1. Profound osteoclastic bone resorption

2. Abnormal bone formation—mosaic pattern

a. Woven bone and irregular sections of thickened trabecular bone

b. Numerous cement lines

G. Treatment

1. Therapy is aimed to stop the osteoclasts from resorbing bone and halt the pagetic bone changes.

2. Bisphosphonates

a. Oral agents: alendronate and risedronate

b. Intravenous agents: pamidronate and zoledronic acid

3. Calcitonin—Salmon calcitonin is administered subcutaneously or intramuscularly.

V. Osteonecrosis

A. Definition—Death of bone cells and bone marrow secondary to a loss of blood supply.

B. Genetics/etiology

1. Four mechanisms have been proposed.

a. Mechanical disruption of the blood vessels (trauma, such as a hip dislocation)

b. Arterial vessel occlusion

i. Nitrogen bubbles (bends), sickle cell disease

ii. Fat emboli

c. Injury or pressure on the blood vessel wall

i. Marrow diseases (such as Gaucher)

ii. Vasculitis, radiation injury

d. Venous outflow obstruction

2. Hypercoagulable states

a. Decreased anticoagulants—proteins C, S

b. Increased procoagulants

C. Clinical presentation—The patient may present with a dull pain in the joint, severe arthritic pain with collapse of the joint, or may be asymptomatic.

D. Imaging appearance

1. Initially normal radiographs

2. Sclerosis and cyst formation

3. Subchondral fracture (crescent sign), subchondral collapse

4. Arthritic changes: osteophytes, loss of joint space

5. MRI: characteristic marrow changes in the metaphyseal marrow and subchondral locations (**Figure 3**)

E. Pathology

1. Osteocyte death (no cells in the bone lacunae)

2. Marrow necrosis

3. Loss of the vascular supply

F. Treatment

1. Core decompression if the joint surfaces remain intact (no collapse)

2. Arthroplasty for joint collapse

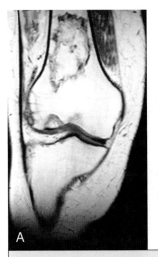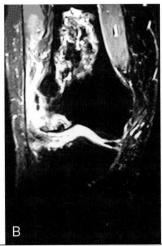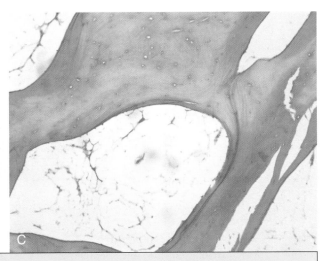

Figure 3 Osteonecrosis. **A,** T1-weighted coronal MRI in a patient with osteonecrosis showing a large metaphyseal lesion and a wedge-shaped area of necrosis at the subchondral region of the lateral femoral condyle. **B,** T2-weighted coronal MRI in a patient with osteonecrosis demonstrates a large metaphyseal lesion with a large subchondral wedge-shaped lesion in the lateral femur. **C,** Hematoxylin and eosin stain demonstrates the complete loss of the bone marrow and an absence of osteocytes in the trabecular lacunae.

VI. Rheumatoid Arthritis

A. Definition and demographics

1. Systemic inflammatory disease of the synovium

2. Twice as common in females compared with males

3. According to the American College of Rheumatology revised criteria, the patient must have four of the seven symptoms and have had symptoms 1 through 4 for at least 6 weeks (**Table 1**).

B. Genetics/etiology

1. Genetic marker human leukocyte antigen (HLA)-DR4 (patients of northern European descent)

2. Monozygotic twins have a concordance rate of 12% to 15%.

C. Clinical presentation

1. Morning stiffness, pain

2. Joint swelling (most prominent in small joints of the hands and feet)

   a. Effusions

   b. Synovial proliferation

3. Hand deformities: subluxation, ulnar drift, swan-neck deformity

D. Imaging appearance (**Figure 4**)

1. Periarticular osteopenia

2. Juxta-articular erosions

3. Joint space narrowing

Table 1

American College of Rheumatology Revised Criteria for Rheumatoid Arthritis

1. Morning stiffness
2. Arthritis of three or more joints
3. Hand arthritis
4. Symmetric arthritis
5. Rheumatoid nodules (extensor surfaces)
6. Positive serum rheumatoid factor
7. Radiographic changes

E. Laboratory features

1. Approximately 90% of patients are positive for rheumatoid factor.

2. Acute-phase reactants: erythrocyte sedimentation rate (ESR), C-reactive protein (CRP) elevated level

F. Pathology—Inflammatory agents destroy cartilage, ligaments, and bone.

G. Treatment

1. Nonsteroidal anti-inflammatory drugs

2. Aspirin

3. Disease-modifying antirheumatic drugs

   a. Methotrexate (current treatment of choice)

   b. Others (D-penicillamine, sulfasalazine, gold, antimalarials)

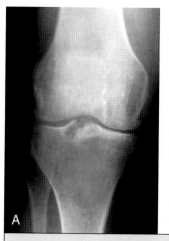
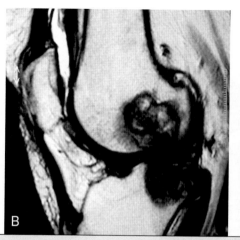
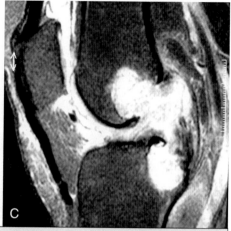

Figure 4   Rheumatoid arthritis. **A**, AP radiograph of the knee showing a subchondral cyst in the proximal tibia with narrowing of the medial compartment of the knee. **B**, T1-weighted sagittal MRI of the knee shows a large subchondral lesion in the distal femur and proximal tibia and an erosion on the tibial condylar surface. **C**, T2-weighted sagittal MRI of the knee demonstrates a large erosion on the distal femur and proximal tibia, an effusion, and diffuse synovial thickening.

4. Cytokine-neutralizing

    a. Etanercept (soluble p75 tumor necrosis factor [TNF] receptor immunoglobulin G fusion protein)

    b. Infliximab (chimeric monoclonal antibody to TNF-α)

    c. Rituximab (monoclonal antibody to CD20 antigen; inhibits B-cells)

5. Physical therapy

VII. Ankylosing Spondylitis (Marie-Strumpell Disease)

A. Definition and demographics

  1. Inflammatory disorder that affects the spine and sacroiliac joints and large joints such as the hip in young adults

  2. Male to female ratio = 3:1

B. Genetics/etiology

  1. 90% of patients with ankylosing spondylitis have HLA-B27 antigen.

  2. Autoimmune disorder

    a. High levels of TNF

    b. CD4+, CD8+ T-cells

C. Clinical presentation

  1. Young adults

  2. Low back and pelvic pain

3. Morning stiffness

4. Hip arthritis in approximately one third of patients

5. Uveitis: pain, light sensitivity

6. Heart involvement

    a. Aortic valve insufficiency

    b. Third-degree heart block

D. Radiographic appearance

  1. Sacroiliac joint inflammation

    a. Blurring of subchondral margins

    b. Erosions

    c. Bony bridging

  2. Lumbar spine involvement (**Figure 5**)

    a. Loss of lumbar lordosis

    b. Squaring of the vertebrae

    c. Osteophytes bridging the vertebrae

E. Pathology

  1. Laboratory findings

    a. HLA-B27 in 90% of patients

    b. Elevated ESR and CRP level

  2. Inflammation of ligamentous attachment sites

    a. Erosions, subchondral inflammation

    b. Ossification of joints such as the sacroiliac joint

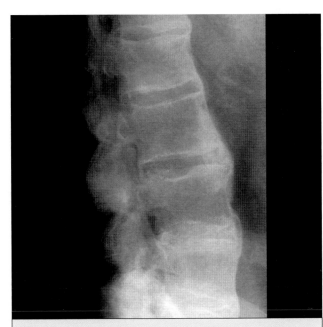

Figure 5 Lateral radiograph of the spine in a patient with ankylosing spondylitis. Note the anterior osteophytes bridging all the lumbar vertebrae.

3. Arthritis—pannus formation with lymphoid infiltration

F. Treatment: anti-TNF therapy

1. Infliximab (chimeric monoclonal antibody to TNF-α)

2. Etanercept (soluble p75 TNF receptor immunoglobulin G fusion protein)

VIII. Reactive Arthritis

A. Overview—Reactive arthritis (formerly called Reiter syndrome) occurs after an infection at another site in the body.

B. Genetics/etiology—Affected individuals are genetically predisposed (high incidence of HLA-B27).

C. Clinical presentation

1. An infection occurs 1 to 8 weeks before the onset of the arthritis.

2. Common extraskeletal involvement

a. Urethritis, prostatitis

b. Uveitis

c. Mucocutaneous involvement

3. Systemic symptoms are usually present: fatigue, malaise, fever, weight loss.

4. Arthritis is asymmetric.

5. Common sites include the knee, ankle, subtalar

joint, and metatarsophalangeal and interphalangeal joints.

6. Tendinitis/fasciitis common

a. Achilles tendon insertion

b. Plantar fascia

D. Radiographic appearance

1. Juxta-articular erosions

2. Joint destruction

E. Pathology

1. Synovial inflammation

2. Enthesitis

F. Treatment

1. Indomethacin

2. Recurrent joint symptoms and tendinitis are common.

IX. Systemic Lupus Erythematosus

A. Definition—Autoimmune disorder in which autoimmune complexes damage joints, skin, kidneys, lungs, heart, blood vessels, and nervous system.

B. Genetics/etiology

1. Multiple genes

2. HLA class II, HLA class III, HLA-DR, HLA-DQ

C. Clinical presentation

1. Multiple joint involvement

2. Osteonecrosis of the hips is common, especially in patients taking glucocorticoids.

D. Radiographic appearance

1. Unusual to have erosions or joint destruction

2. Osteonecrosis may be seen as a result of corticosteroid treatment.

E. Pathology—Anti-nuclear antibodies are present in 95% of patients.

F. Treatment

1. Analgesics

2. Antimalarials

X. Gout

A. Definition and demographics

1. Gout is a metabolic disorder caused by uric acid crystals in the synovium.

2. Affects older men and postmenopausal women

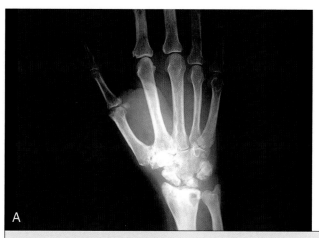
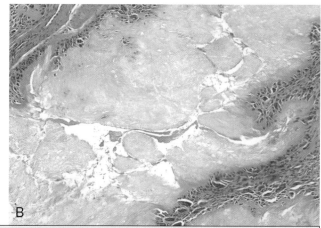

Figure 6 Gout. **A**, AP radiograph of the hand in a patient with gout showing a lucent lesion in the distal radius and erosive changes in the carpal bones. **B**, Hematoxylin and eosin stain of a patient with gout. Note the tophaceous areas are amorphous and white and are bordered by inflammatory cells.

B. Clinical presentation

   1. Severe pain in a single joint is common; joint is intensely painful, swollen, and erythematous.

   2. Often polyarticular in men with hypertension and alcohol abuse

C. Radiographic appearance (**Figure 6**, *A*)

   1. Periarticular erosions

   2. Peripheral margin of the erosion often has a thin overlying rim of bone (cliff sign).

D. Pathology

   1. Joint aspiration is the only definitive diagnostic procedure.

   2. Needle- and rod-shaped crystals with negative birefringence

   3. Joint white blood cell count usually <50,000 to 60,000/µL

   4. Serum uric acid often elevated (but not always)

   5. Hematoxylin and eosin staining shows amorphous material and inflammatory cells (**Figure 6**, *B*).

E. Treatment/outcome

   1. Nonsteroidal anti-inflammatory drugs

   2. Colchicine

   3. Hypouricemic therapy: allopurinol, probenecid

XI. Osteoporosis

A. Definition and demographics

   1. Characteristics

      a. Low bone mass

      b. Microarchitectural deterioration

      c. Fractures

   2. Peak bone mass is attained between 2 and 30 years of age, and failure to attain adequate bone mass at this time is one of the main determinants in the development of osteoporosis.

   3. World Health Organization definition

      a. Normal: within 1 SD of peak bone mass (T-score = 0 to –1.0)

      b. Low bone mass (osteopenia): 1.0 to 2.5 SDs below peak bone mass (T-score = –1.0 to –2.5)

      c. Osteoporosis: >2.5 SDs below peak bone mass (T-score = < –2.5)

B. Genetics/etiology

   1. Causes are multifactorial.

   2. Genetic predisposition is important.

   3. Genes that have been associated with the development of osteoporosis

      a. *COL1A1* (collagen 1α1): main bone collagen

      b. Vitamin D receptor

      c. LRP5: (low-density lipoprotein receptor-related protein)

C. Clinical presentation

   1. Patient usually presents with a fracture following minor trauma.

   2. Found on routine screening (bone mineral density)

   3. Most important risk factors

      a. Increasing age (geriatric patient)

      b. Female sex

c. Early menopause

d. Fair-skinned

e. Maternal/paternal history of hip fracture

f. Low body weight

g. Cigarette smoking

h. Glucocorticoid use

i. Excessive alcohol use

j. Low protein intake

k. Anticonvulsant or antidepressant use

D. Radiographic appearance

1. Osteopenia

2. Thinning of the cortices

3. Loss of trabecular bone

E. Pathology

1. Loss of trabecular bone

2. Loss of continuity of the trabecular bone

F. Treatment

1. Adequate calcium and vitamin D intake

2. Antiresorptive therapy for patients with osteoporosis

3. Parathyroid hormone therapy for patients with osteoporosis resistant to bisphosphonates

Top Testing Facts

1. Osteopetrosis is a rare disorder characterized by a failure of osteoclastic resorption with resultant dense bone with no medullary cavity (prone to fracture).

2. Oncologic osteomalacia is a paraneoplastic syndrome characterized by renal phosphate wasting and can be caused by a variety of bone and soft-tissue tumors (osteoblastoma, nonossifying fibroma, and phosphaturic mesenchymal tumor).

3. Hypercalcemia may occur as a complication of breast cancer, multiple myeloma, and lymphoma.

4. Paget disease is a remodeling disease characterized by disordered bone formation; it is treated with bisphosphonates.

5. Rheumatoid arthritis is a systemic inflammatory disorder characterized by morning stiffness and joint pain; 90% of patients are positive for rheumatoid factor.

6. Ankylosing spondylitis is an inflammatory disorder of the spine and sacroiliac joints characterized by HLA-B27 positivity; it is treated with anti-TNF therapy.

7. Gout is a metabolic disorder caused by uric acid crystals in the synovium resulting in periarticular erosions.

8. Osteoporosis is characterized by low bone mass (>2.5 SDs below the mean) and an increased risk of fracture.

Bibliography

Fauci AS, Langford CA (eds): *Harrison's Rheumatology.* New York, NY, McGraw-Hill, 2006, pp 69-104, 139-156, 259-268.

Favus MJ (ed): *Primer on the Metabolic Bone Diseases and Disorders of Mineral Metabolism*, ed 6. Washington, DC, American Society for Bone and Mineral Research, 2006.

McAlister WH, Herman TE: Osteochondrodysplasias, dysostoses, chromosomal aberrations, mucopolysaccharidoses, and mucolipodoses, in Resnik D, Kransdorf, M (eds): *Diagnosis of Bone and Joint Disorders*, ed 3. Philadelphia, PA, WB Saunders, 1995, pp 4200-4204.

Miclau T, Bozic KJ, Tay B, et al: Bone injury, regeneration, and repair, in *Orthopaedic Basic Science: Foundations of Clinical Practice*, ed 3. Rosemont, IL, American Academy of Orthopaedic Surgeons, 2007, pp 331-333.

Siris ES, Roodman GD: *Paget's Disease of Bone*, ed 6. Washington, DC, American Society for Bone and Mineral Research, 2006, pp 320-329.

4: Orthopaedic Oncology and Systemic Disease

Section 5

Sports Medicine

Section Editor

Kurt P. Spindler, MD

Chapter 45

Overuse Injuries

Christopher Kaeding, MD   Annunziato Amendola, MD

I. Stress Fractures

A. Epidemiology

1. Stress fractures are not uncommon in highly committed athletes.

2. Stress fractures have a predilection for certain bony locations; the vast majority are in the lower extremity, with the tibia and metatarsals being the most common.

3. Stress fractures do occur in the upper extremity; these tend to heal well with relative or absolute rest.

4. Stress fractures fortunately occur in <1% of the general athletic population, but running track athletes can have an incidence of 10% to 20%. The rate of recurrence may be approximately 10% for all athletes, but as high as 50% in runners.

B. Pathophysiology

1. The concept of a stress fracture was first described by Breithaupt in the 1850s, who called it a "march fracture" because it was observed in the metatarsals of marching soldiers.

2. Stress fractures can be considered a fatigue failure of bone; they result from the accumulation of microdamage that occurs with repetitive loading of bone.

3. Fatigue failure starts in an area of stress concentration and is termed "crack initiation."

4. If this initial microscopic crack is not repaired and repeated loading of the bone continues, the crack extends; this is referred to as "crack propagation."

5. Ultimately, if enough microdamage accumulates, the bone will fail macroscopically.

6. In vivo, bone responds to crack initiation and propagation with a reparative biologic response; this response appears to be dependent on age, nutritional status, hormonal status, and possibly genetic predisposition.

7. A dynamic balance exists between accumulation of microdamage and host repair processes.

a. When microdamage accumulates in excess of the reparative response, the result is a stress fracture.

b. Any factor that disrupts this dynamic balance can increase the risk of stress fracture.

c. Theoretically, any factor that increases stress on a bone will cause an increase in microdamage accumulation with each loading episode.

d. Likewise, any factor that impairs the reparative biologic response, such as poor vascularity or an altered hormonal milieu, may also increase the risk of developing a stress fracture.

C. Evaluation

1. Stress fractures typically present with an insidious onset of pain, but they may present with acute onset of pain.

2. A history of either a prolonged level of high activity or a recent rapid increase in activity level is usually present.

3. Without a history of significant repetitive loading episodes, an insufficiency fracture or pathologic fracture must be considered.

4. Physical examination may reveal pain to direct palpation or mechanical loading of the affected site.

5. Radiographs, bone scan, CT, and MRI are the imaging techniques of choice to evaluate stress fractures. Each has advantages.

a. Radiographs are frequently unremarkable or have very subtle findings; this is especially true early in the course of the fracture.

b. Bone scans are very sensitive in identifying the presence and location of stress fractures, but they do not reveal macroscopic fracture lines in the bone.

c. MRI can identify the bony edema associated with early stress fracture as well as reveal the presence of a fracture line. MRI has the additional advantage of showing the surrounding soft tissues.

d. Delineation of the location and extent of a fracture line is best achieved with CT.

5: Sports Medicine

Table 1

Locations of High-Risk Stress Fractures

Femoral neck—superolateral

Femoral neck—inferomedial*

Patella

Anterior tibial diaphysis

Medial malleolus

Talus

Tarsal navicular

Fifth metatarsal

Sesamoids

*Less risk of fracture than superolateral location. (Reproduced with permission from Kaeding CC, Yu JR, Wright R, Amendola A, Spindler KP: Management and return to play of stress fractures. Clin J Sport Med 2005;15:442-447.)

Table 2

Classification of Stress Fractures

	High Risk	Low Risk
Biomechanical environment	Tension	Compression
Natural history	Poor	Good
Management	Aggressive Complete fracture: surgery Incomplete fracture: strict non–weight-bearing or surgery	Conservative Symptomatic: activity modification Asymptomatic: no treatment needed, observation

(Reproduced with permission from Kaeding CC, Yu JR, Wright R, Amendola A, Spindler KP: Management and return to play of stress fractures. Clin J Sport Med 2005;15:442-447.)

D. Classification

1. Stress fractures at certain locations have a poor natural history and are termed high-risk stress fractures (**Table 1**).

2. Delayed recognition or undertreatment of high-risk stress fractures tends to result in fracture progression, nonunion, the need for surgery, and refracture.

3. Other fractures have a more benign natural history and are referred to as "low-risk" stress fractures; these fractures tend to heal with activity modification.

4. Recognizing the class of stress fracture is important for optimizing treatment (**Table 2**).

   a. Delayed recognition or undertreatment of a high-risk stress fracture can result in a prolonged recovery, surgery, or season/career-ending sequelae.

   b. Overtreatment of a low-risk stress fracture can result in undue loss of playing time and deconditioning.

5. One MRI classification of stress fractures is correlated with time to return to play.

E. Treatment principles

1. Treatment must alter the biomechanical and biologic environment such that the reparative processes exceed the accumulation of microdamage at the fracture site.

2. An evaluation of the athlete's biologic bone-healing capacity should be performed. This includes review of the athlete's nutritional, hormonal, and medication status.

3. The "female athlete triad" (amenorrhea, disordered eating, and osteoporosis) must be considered in any female athlete with stress fractures; appropriate evaluation/treatment should be initiated.

4. The fracture site must also be protected from future strain episodes through relative rest, absolute rest, bracing, technique modification, or surgical fixation.

   a. Relative rest involves decreasing the frequency or magnitude of strain episodes at the stress fracture site by modifying the athlete's training volume (intensity, duration, and frequency), technique, and equipment; through the use of a brace or orthosis; or by cross-training.

   b. Absolute rest removes all strain episodes from the fracture site. This is often done by making the athlete non–weight-bearing.

5. An assessment of biomechanical risk factors such as malalignment should be performed as well.

6. The use of biophysical enhancement technologies such as pulsed ultrasound and electrical stimulation in stress fractures is still under investigation.

7. With these principles in mind, the management of stress fractures depends on classifying each fracture as either high or low risk. This is summarized in **Figure 1**.

   a. High-risk stress fractures are typically treated with absolute rest or surgery.

   b. Serious consideration of risk must be done prior to allowing patients with high-risk stress fracture to continue to play; however, patients with low-risk stress fractures may do so with activity modification.

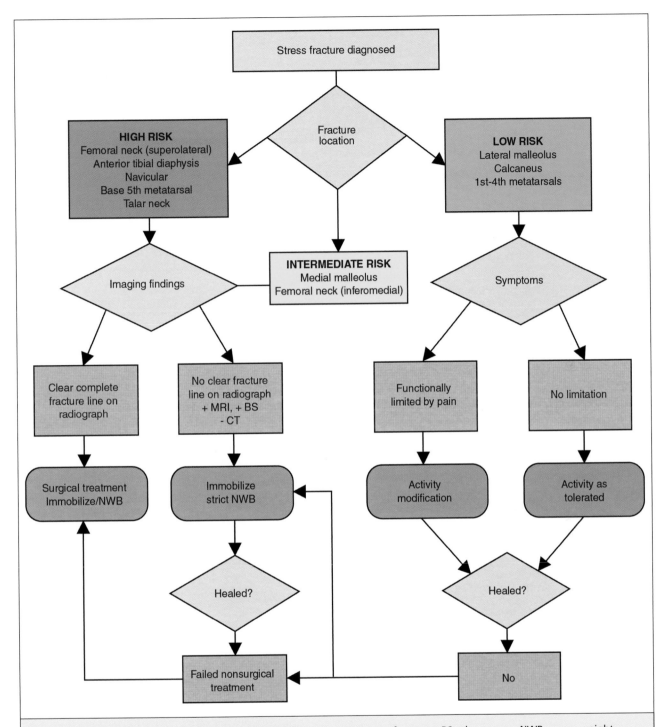

Figure 1 Treatment algorithm for management of lower extremity stress fractures. BS = bone scan, NWB = non–weight-bearing. *(Adapted with permission from Kaeding CC, Yu JR, Wright R, Amendola A, Spindler KP: Management and return to play of stress fractures.* Clin J Sport Med *2005;15:442-447.)*

II. Exercise-Induced Leg Pain and Compartment Syndrome

A. Epidemiology

1. It has been estimated that "shin splints" account for 10% to 15% of all running injuries.

2. Shin splints may account for up to 60% of leg-pain syndromes.

B. Etiology and differential are listed in **Table 3**.

C. Medial tibial stress syndrome

1. Definition—Tenderness over the posteromedial border of the tibia and dull aching to intense pain

Table 3

Etiology and Differential of Exercise-Induced Leg Pain and Compartment Syndrome

Tissue of Origin	Examples of Pathology
Bone	Tibial stress fracture, fibular stress fracture
Periosteum	Periostitis (medial tibial stress syndrome)
Muscle or fascia	Exertional compartment syndrome, fascial herniation
Tendon	Achilles, peroneal, or tibialis posterior tendinopathy
Nerve	Sural or superficial peroneal nerve entrapment
Blood vessel	Popliteal artery entrapment, intermittent claudication, or other insufficiency; venous insufficiency
Distant (referred)	Spinal radiculopathy

that is alleviated by rest, in the absence of any neurovascular abnormalities.

2. Imaging

   a. If the diagnosis is not clear, bone scan or possibly MRI should be diagnostic.

   b. Periostitis has a distinct scintigraphic/MRI appearance, with increased uptake along the posteromedial border of the tibia.

3. Treatment

   a. Nonsurgical

      i. Modification of activities

      ii. Modalities to decrease inflammation

         (a) Nonsteroidal anti-inflammatory medication

         (b) Local phonophoresis with corticosteroids

         (c) Ointments

         (d) Leg wraps

      iii. If pes planus needs correction, orthoses may help.

      iv. A dedicated program of strengthening of the invertors and evertors of the calf is very important in preventing recurrence; recurrence is common after patients resume heavy activity.

   b. Surgical

      i. The results of surgery are variable given the

absence of rigid diagnostic clinical criteria and variability in the surgery performed.

      ii. If nonsurgical treatment fails and the patient remains symptomatic, a fasciotomy of the deep posterior compartment with release of the painful portion of periosteum is recommended.

D. Exertional compartment syndrome

   1. Overview

      a. Anterior compartment involvement is more common and accounts for approximately 70% to 80% of cases.

      b. Posterior compartment involvement is less common and has been associated with less predictable surgical outcomes.

   2. Pathophysiology

      a. Experimental evidence has been unable to demonstrate a decrease in blood flow despite documented elevated compartment pressure and a consistent clinical presentation.

      b. MRI, MRI spectroscopy, and nuclear medicine blood flow studies all have been used with limited success.

      c. Muscle biopsies have provided conflicting results regarding the role of muscle ischemia in the generation of pain.

   3. Diagnosis—Although the diagnosis has long been considered to be one of exclusion, with a better understanding of the presentation the diagnosis is usually readily apparent.

      a. The patient characteristically has a normal physical examination, no pain at rest, and reproducible exercise-induced leg pain that is completely relieved by cessation of the offending activity.

      b. Investigation—Intracompartmental pressure measurements, rather than extensive imaging studies, are used to confirm the diagnosis.

      c. Measuring intracompartmental pressure

         i. Resting pressure, immediate postexercise pressure, and continuous pressure measurements for 30 minutes after exercise are most important for confirming the diagnosis.

         ii. A study is considered positive if the insertional pressure is ≥15 mm Hg, the immediate postexercise pressure is ≥30 mm Hg, or the pressure fails to return to normal or exceeds 15 mm Hg at 15 minutes postexercise.

   4. Treatment

      a. Nonsurgical

         i. Intracompartmental pressure normally rises

and falls with activity; therefore, nonsurgical modalities do not affect pressure.

  ii. Physical therapy, anti-inflammatory medications, and orthoses have generally been ineffective.

 b. Surgical—Indicated for patients who have appropriate clinical presentations with confirmatory pressure measurements and are unwilling to modify or give up their sport.

E. Fascial hernia

 1. Pathophysiology—A hernia can become symptomatic because of chronic exertional compartment syndrome, a compressive neuropathy, or ischemia of the herniated muscle tissue.

 2. Evaluation—A hernia at the exit of the superficial peroneal nerve or of one of its branches is common in "chronic compartment syndrome."

 3. Treatment

  a. Patients with asymptomatic hernias require no treatment.

  b. Symptomatic hernias should be managed initially with education, activity modification, and, possibly, use of support hose.

  c. Failure of these modalities may be an indication for decompressing the entire compartment with fasciotomy.

  d. Closure is contraindicated.

F. Peripheral neuropathy

 1. Pathophysiology

  a. The superficial peroneal nerve is a branch of the common peroneal nerve.

  b. The nerve is most commonly compressed as it exits the deep fascia to become subcutaneous, a point where localized tenderness may be encountered.

  c. In addition to muscle herniation, the nerve can also be compressed by the fascial edge or be subjected to repeated traction by recurrent inversion ankle sprains; 25% of patients note a history of trauma, particularly recurrent ankle sprains.

 2. Evaluation

  a. Patients may have activity-related pain and neurologic symptoms in the distal third of the leg or the dorsum of the foot and ankle.

  b. Weakness is not expected because the innervation of the peroneals is proximal to the site of compression.

 3. Treatment—If the neuropathy is caused by muscle herniation or compression on fascial edge, decompression can be performed.

III. Soft-Tissue Overuse

A. Pathophysiology

 1. Clinically, tendinosis is an overuse injury with recalcitrant symptoms of pain with activity.

 2. Histologically, tendinosis is a chronic intratendinous degenerative lesion of tendon.

 3. Puddu used the term *tendinosis* in 1976, noting it was troublesome in athletes.

 4. Tendinosis is not a failed healing response; there is no overt acute injury and no inflammatory phase as has been so well described in classic healing responses.

 5. Neovascularization has been described as a very early histologic finding in tendinosis.

 6. Tendon strain up to 6% is physiologic; strain in the 6% to 8% range can result in overuse injuries; and strain >8% can cause complete rupture of the tendon.

 7. In tendinosis, instead of the normal constructive adaptive response of repeated loading, the tendon no longer responds in a positive fashion, but starts to accumulate increasing amounts of poorly organized and dysfunctional matrix; it is this degenerative tissue that is the hallmark of tendinosis.

 8. Tendinosis occurs most commonly in the rotator cuff, patella tendon, Achilles tendon, posterior tibialis tendon, and common extensor origin at the elbow.

B. Classification—Blazina grading system of tendinitis:

 1. A grade I lesion on the Blazina scale is characterized by pain that occurs only after the activity.

 2. A grade II tendinitis lesion is characterized by pain that occurs during activity but does not affect performance.

 3. A grade III lesion is characterized by pain that occurs during the activity and affects performance, such that the athlete cannot train and perform at the desired level.

C. Treatment

 1. Nonsurgical

  a. Traditionally, initial treatment consists of rest and physical therapy. Many nonsurgical interventions have been advocated, including hyperbaric oxygen, nitric oxide, sclerotherapy, and extracorporeal shockwave, to name a few.

  b. Few controlled studies have been done.

  c. Eccentric exercises were shown in one controlled trial to be as effective as surgical débridement in treating patellar tendinopathy.

2. Surgical

    a. If nonsurgical measures fail in a grade 3 lesion and the tendinosis lesion is well established on MRI, surgery can be considered.

    b. Surgical intervention falls into two broad categories.

        i. The "excise and stimulate" group includes the open marginal or wide excision techniques.

        ii. The "stimulate a healing response" group includes using percutaneous needling, or open multiple longitudinal tenotomies.

    c. Both seek to induce a healing response in the tendinosis lesion by inflicting an acute traumatic event. This induced acute healing response will hopefully result in a repair of the degenerative lesion.

D. Results

1. Improvement in the patient's ability to perform activities of daily living is typical.

2. Unfortunately, relapse after the athlete returns to aggressive loading activity levels is not uncommon.

3. A randomized controlled trial found eccentric exercise as effective as surgery in treatment of patellar tendinopathy.

Top Testing Facts

1. The tibia and metatarsals are frequently affected with stress fractures.

2. Stress fractures result from "crack propagation" that exceeds the bone's reparative biologic response.

3. High-risk stress fractures usually involve the tension side of bone, have a poor natural history, and are aggressively managed, including with surgery.

4. Shin splints (medial tibial stress syndrome) are responsible for 10% to 15% of all running injuries.

5. The anterior compartment is most commonly involved in exertional compartment syndrome.

6. The diagnosis of exertional compartment syndrome can be made if the patient has both reproducible exercise-induced leg pain and an immediate postexercise intracompartmental pressure ≥30 mm Hg.

7. The treatment for athletes with exertional compartmental syndrome who are interested in returning to sport is surgical release of the involved compartment.

8. Tendinosis, a soft-tissue overuse injury, is considered a failed adaptive response.

9. The Blazina grading system uses a pain scale to stage tendinitis as well as functional limitation into three grades.

10. A randomized controlled trial found eccentric exercise as effective as surgery in treatment of patellar tendinopathy.

Bibliography

Bahr R, Fossen B, Loke S, Engebretsen L: Surgical treatment compared with eccentric training for patellar tendinopathy (jumper's knee): A randomized, controlled trial. *J Bone Joint Surg Am* 2006;88:1689-1698.

Boden BP, Osbahr DC: High-risk stress fractures: Evaluation and treatment. *J Am Acad Orthop Surg* 2000;8:344-353.

Boden BP, Osbahr DC, Jimenez C: Low-risk stress fractures. *Am J Sports Med* 2001;29:100-111.

Chambers HG: Medial tibial stress syndrome: Evaluation and management, in Drez D Jr, DeLee JC (eds): *Operative Techniques in Sport Medicine: Compartment Disorders: Classification, Pathophysiology, Diagnosis, and Treatment*. Philadelphia, PA, WB Saunders, 1995, pp 247-277.

Hamilton B, Purdam C: Patellar tendinosis as an adaptive process: A new hypothesis. *Br J Sports Med* 2004;38:758-761.

Khan KM, Fuller PJ, Brukner PD, et al: Outcome of conservative and surgical management of navicular stress fracture in athletes: Eighty-six cases proven with computerized tomography. *Am J Sports Med* 1992;20:657-666.

Pedowitz RA, Hargens AR, Mubarak SJ, et al: Modified criteria for the objective diagnosis of chronic compartment syndrome of the leg. *Am J Sports Med* 1990;18:35-40.

Rampersaud YR, Amendola A: The evaluation and treatment of exertional compartment syndrome, in Drez D Jr, DeLee JC (eds): *Operative Techniques in Sport Medicine: Compartment Disorders: Classification, Pathophysiology, Diagnosis, and Treatment*. Philadelphia, PA, WB Saunders, 1995, pp 267-273.

Wright RW, Fisher DA, Shively HA, et al: Refracture of proximal 5th metatarsal (Jones) fractures after intramedullary screw fixation in athletes. *Am J Sports Med* 2000;28:732-736.

Chapter 46

Neurologic Injuries Related to Sports Participation

John E. Kuhn, MD

I. Stingers/Burners

A. Overview/epidemiology

1. Stingers (also called burners) are transient unilateral upper extremity neurologic injuries seen in contact sports.

2. In the 1970s, 50% of football players had experienced at least one stinger during their careers; this number dropped to an incidence of 3.7% to 7.7% and prevalence of 15% to 18% by 1997, likely related to rule and equipment changes.

3. Having one stinger increases by threefold the risk of having another.

B. Pathoanatomy

1. The most common mechanism of injury is downward displacement of the shoulder and lateral flexion of the neck to the contralateral shoulder, producing brachial plexus traction.

2. Lateral head-turning toward the affected side may cause nerve root compression and may be a source of symptoms.

3. A direct blow to the supraclavicular fossa at the Erb point may cause injury as well and may be equipment related.

C. Evaluation

1. History

a. Patients experience a transient, unilateral tingling, burning, or numbing sensation in a circumferential, not dermatomal, distribution.

b. Ipsilateral sensory symptoms and motor weakness are typical findings in an acute stinger injury.

c. A C6 nerve root distribution is commonly involved, but the upper trunk of the brachial plexus and other cervical root involvement also has been described.

d. Symptoms typically resolve after 1 to 2 minutes.

e. Neck pain should not be a presenting symptom.

2. Physical examination

a. With chronic or repeated injury, atrophy may be noted.

b. The physical examination should assess the neck for stiffness, spasm, or pain.

c. A positive Spurling test and tenderness with percussion of the supraclavicular fossa may be present.

3. Differential diagnosis and natural history

a. Electromyographic (EMG) studies are indicated if symptoms do not resolve after 3 weeks. EMG will demonstrate abnormalities in the roots, cords, trunks, and peripheral nerves.

b. It is important to rule out other injury such as cervical fracture, dislocation, or spinal cord contusion.

c. Patients should be reexamined frequently.

d. Long-term muscle weakness with persistent paresthesias may result from severe or repeated stingers in 5% to 10% of patients.

e. Patients with cervical pain or findings should undergo a thorough workup of the neck.

D. Treatment

1. By definition, stingers are transient injuries and do not require formal treatment.

2. Systemic steroids have not been shown to be of benefit and may be harmful.

3. Return to play is allowed after rest and rehabilitation when the patient is symptom-free.

4. Players with residual muscle weakness, cervical abnormalities, restricted cervical motion, or abnormal EMG studies should be withheld from contact sports.

5. In football, equipment modifications to shoulder pads may reduce recurrence.

II. Long Thoracic Nerve Injury

A. Overview/epidemiology—Injury to the long thoracic nerve is uncommon but has been reported in nearly every sport.

B. Pathoanatomy

1. The long thoracic nerve arises from C5-C7, with a C8 contribution in 8% of individuals. It travels anterior to the scalenus posterior muscle and travels distally and laterally under the clavicle over the first or second rib. It runs along the mid-axillary line over a distance of 22 to 24 cm.

2. Repetitive stretch injury is the cause of most of these injuries, which are typically neurapraxic.

3. Positions with the head tilted or rotated away and the arm overhead put the nerve at risk.

4. A fascial band from the inferior brachial plexus to the proximal serratus anterior muscle may contribute to traction injury.

5. Direct trauma to the thorax also may injure the nerve.

6. Compression of the nerve can occur at many sites.

C. Evaluation

1. History

   a. Patients commonly report pain at the shoulder, neck, or scapula that is exacerbated by activity or tilting the neck.

   b. Weakness is noted when lifting away from the body or with overhead activity.

   c. Winging prominence may be noted when sitting against a chair back.

2. Physical examination

   a. Static and dynamic winging of the scapula is seen, with weakness when testing shoulder strength.

   b. The position of the resting scapula is superior and toward the midline as the trapezius dominates.

   c. Resisted forward elevation or having the patient perform a push-up will accentuate the winging.

3. Ancillary studies

   a. EMG and nerve conduction velocity (NCV) studies will confirm the diagnosis and delineate severity.

   b. These studies also are used to follow recovery.

D. Treatment

1. Most long thoracic nerve palsies recover spontaneously.

2. Physical therapy to strengthen compensatory muscles and braces that help to hold the scapula to the chest may provide some comfort.

3. Recovery typically occurs within 1 year but may take 2 years in some patients.

4. If symptoms warrant and there is no spontaneous recovery, muscle transfers are considered. (Sternal head of pectoralis major to inferior border of scapula is most popular.)

III. Suprascapular Nerve Injury

A. Overview/epidemiology

1. Suprascapular nerve injury is an uncommon cause of shoulder pain.

2. Infraspinatus impairment is found in 45% of volleyball players, and 1% to 2% of painful shoulder disorders are related to suprascapular nerve compression.

B. Pathoanatomy

1. The suprascapular artery lies above the transverse scapular ligament, and the suprascapular nerve lies below the transverse scapular ligament.

2. The suprascapular nerve is from the upper trunk of the brachial plexus, with C5 and C6 (and occasionally C4) roots.

3. It travels laterally across the posterior cervical triangle to reach the scapular notch close to the posterior border of the clavicle.

4. Entrapment occurs in three places:

   a. The suprascapular notch, by the transverse scapular ligament.

   b. The spinoglenoid notch, by the spinoglenoid ligament.

   c. The spinoglenoid notch, by a spinoglenoid notch ganglion cyst from the shoulder (usually associated with a small posterosuperior labral tear).

C. Evaluation

1. History—Patients present with a poorly localized dull ache over the lateral shoulder with weakness.

2. Physical examination may detect atrophy of the infraspinatus and sometimes supraspinatus, with weakness in external rotation.

3. MRI may demonstrate a ganglion cyst at the spinoglenoid notch or supraspinatus fossa. Pa-

tients with MRI scans that demonstrate a cyst in the spinoglenoid notch may have compression of the infraspinatus branch of the suprascapular nerve and may present with weakness in external rotation. The affected muscle is the infraspinatus.

4. An athlete who presents with shoulder pain, weakness in external rotation, and normal MRI scans may still have suprascapular nerve entrapment by the transverse scapular ligament or the spinoglenoid notch ligament.

5. EMG and NCV studies will isolate the lesion to the suprascapular notch (supraspinatus and infraspinatus) or spinoglenoid notch (supraspinatus is spared).

D. Treatment

1. Nonsurgical treatment can be used for athletes with a presumed microtraumatic source of injury.

2. Symptoms have been reported to resolve in 6 to 12 months after diagnosis.

3. Nonsurgical treatment usually includes rest and stretching of the posterior capsule of the shoulder.

4. Nonsurgical treatment is used for 4 to 6 weeks, followed by a repeat EMG study to assess recovery.

5. Surgery is indicated for masses compressing the nerve or for failure of nonsurgical treatment.

6. Surgery entails release of the transverse scapular ligament, release of the spinoglenoid ligament, or removal of the spinoglenoid notch ganglion cyst, either open or arthroscopically.

IV. Axillary Nerve Injury

A. Overview/epidemiology

1. Isolated injuries are uncommon and represent less than 1% of sports injuries; however, approximately 48% of patients with an anterior dislocation will have EMG changes in the axillary nerve. Older patients are at higher risk for neurologic injury with shoulder dislocation.

2. Quadrilateral space syndrome is very rare, affecting young, active adults between 20 and 40 years of age and commonly described in baseball players.

   a. The boundaries of the quadrilateral space are the long head of the triceps medially, the humeral shaft laterally, the teres minor muscle superiorly, and the teres major and latissimus dorsi inferiorly.

   b. The quadrilateral space contains the axillary nerve and the posterior circumflex humeral artery.

B. Pathoanatomy

1. The axillary nerve originates from C5 and C6 from the posterior cord of the brachial plexus. It travels below the coracoid process obliquely along the anterior surface of the subscapularis, then dives to the inferior border of the subscapularis. The nerve travels posteriorly adjacent to the inferomedial capsule, then through the quadrilateral space with the posterior circumflex humeral artery.

2. It innervates the teres minor and the deltoid from back to front.

3. The distance from the acromion to the nerve at the mid deltoid is 6 cm.

4. Injury can be from contusion, stretch (as in a dislocation), or entrapment in the quadrilateral space, or it may be iatrogenic (during a deltoid-splitting approach or vigorous retraction during surgery).

C. Evaluation

1. History and physical examination

   a. Patients may be asymptomatic or may describe easy fatigability and weakness.

   b. The physical examination will demonstrate deltoid atrophy. Weakness will also be noted, particularly in abduction, forward punching, and external rotation.

   c. Numbness in the sensory distribution of the axillary nerve, which is a spot on the lateral side of the arm over the deltoid, may be present.

2. Ancillary studies

   a. EMG and NCV studies will confirm diagnosis and assess severity. These studies also are used to follow recovery.

   b. Patients with quadrilateral space syndrome have more vague symptoms, and the physical examination may be nonspecific.

   c. In quadrilateral space syndrome, EMG is frequently not helpful; instead, an arteriogram with the arm in abduction and external rotation may show a lack of flow in the posterior circumflex humeral artery.

D. Treatment

1. Treatment of axillary nerve injury is typically nonsurgical.

2. As the nerve regenerates, the posterior deltoid and teres will recover before the anterior deltoid.

3. Surgery is indicated in symptomatic patients with no evidence of recovery after 3 to 6 months.

4. Surgery can include neurolysis, neurorrhaphy, nerve grafting, nerve transfer, and neurotization.

5: Sports Medicine

5. For patients with quadrilateral space syndrome, resection of fibrous bands around the nerve is usually curative if nonsurgical treatment has failed.

V. Lateral Femoral Cutaneous Nerve Injury

A. Overview/epidemiology

1. The lateral femoral cutaneous nerve originates from L2 and L3 in the lumbar plexus.

2. It lies on the surface of the iliopsoas and exits the pelvis under the inguinal ligament, passing just medial to the anterior superior iliac spine.

3. It supplies cutaneous innervation to the front of the thigh to the knee.

B. Pathoanatomy

1. Entrapment is known as meralgia paresthetica. The injury also is seen in patients with tight belts or trousers.

2. The lateral femoral cutaneous nerve can be injured during surgery, especially when harvesting bone graft or during anterior approaches to the hip.

C. Evaluation

1. Patients report pain or numbness in the anterolateral thigh.

2. In athletes, it is common that no identifiable cause is found.

3. A positive Tinel sign is frequently seen on examination.

4. Local nerve block with lidocaine can be diagnostic.

5. Plain radiographs or MRI can rule out other causes.

6. NCV studies demonstrate prolonged latency or decreased conduction velocity.

D. Treatment

1. Nonsurgical treatment includes heat, physical therapy, local steroid injections, and nonsteroidal anti-inflammatory drugs.

2. If symptoms remain and are disabling, surgical release of the fascial bands constricting parts of the inguinal ligament to decompress the nerve has been successful.

3. Transection of the nerve leaves hypoesthesia and possible painful neuromas.

Top Testing Facts

1. Ipsilateral sensory symptoms and motor weakness are typical findings in an acute stinger injury.

2. Injury to the long thoracic nerve results in a scapula that is positioned superior and toward the midline when at rest. Winging of the scapula will be noted with strength testing.

3. The suprascapular artery lies above the transverse scapular ligament, and the suprascapular nerve lies below the transverse scapular ligament.

4. An athlete who presents with shoulder pain, weakness in external rotation, and normal MRI scans may still have suprascapular nerve entrapment by the transverse scapular ligament or the spinoglenoid notch ligament.

5. Patients with MRI scans that demonstrate a cyst in the spinoglenoid notch may have compression of the infraspinatus branch of the suprascapular nerve and may present with weakness in external rotation. The affected muscle is the infraspinatus.

6. Subtle axillary nerve injury is common in anterior dislocations. Older patients are at higher risk for neurologic injury with shoulder dislocation. The axillary nerve often is injured.

7. The boundaries of the quadrilateral space are the long head of the triceps medially, the humeral shaft laterally, the teres minor muscle superiorly, and the teres major and latissimus dorsi inferiorly. The quadrilateral space contains the axillary nerve and the posterior circumflex humeral artery.

8. The axillary nerve is 6 cm from the lateral acromion at the mid deltoid region.

9. Recovery of the injured axillary nerve begins in the posterior deltoid, followed by the middle head. The anterior head of the deltoid is the last to recover.

10. The lateral femoral cutaneous nerve is a terminal branch of the second and third lumbar roots.

Bibliography

Bigliani LU, Dalsey RM, McCann PD, April EW: An anatomic study of the suprascapular nerve. *Arthroscopy* 1990;6: 301-305.

Castro FP: Stingers, cervical cord neuropraxia, and stenosis. *Clin Sports Med* 2003;22:483-492.

Kuhn JE, Plancher KD, Hawkins RJ: Scapular winging. *J Am Acad Orthop Surg* 1995;3:319-325.

McCrory P, Bell S: Nerve entrapment syndromes as a cause of pain in the hip, groin, and buttock. *Sports Med* 1999;27:261-274.

Moore TP, Fritts HM, Quick DC, Buss DD: Suprascapular nerve entrapment caused by supraglenoid cyst compression. *J Shoulder Elbow Surg* 1997;6:455-462.

Romeo AA, Rotenberg DD, Bach BR: Suprascapular neuropathy. *J Am Acad Orthop Surg* 1999;7:358-367.

Safran MR: Nerve injury about the shoulder in athletes: Part 1. Suprascapular nerve and axillary nerve. Am *J Sports Med* 2004;32:803-819.

Safran MR: Nerve injury about the shoulder in athletes: Part 2. Long thoracic nerve, spinal accessory nerve, burners/stingers, thoracic outlet syndrome. *Am J Sports Med* 2004; 32:1063-1076.

Steinmann SP, Moran EA: Axillary nerve injury: Diagnosis and treatment. *J Am Acad Orthop Surg* 2001;9:328-335.

Visser CP, Coene LN, Brand R, Tavy DL: The incidence of nerve injury in anterior dislocation for the shoulder and its influence on functional recovery. A prospective clincial and EMG study. *J Bone Joint Surg Br* 1999;81:679-685.

5: Sports Medicine

Chapter 47
Medical Aspects of Sports Participation

Robert Warne Fitch, MD   Mark E. Halstead, MD

I. Preparticipation Physical Examination

A. Objectives

1. The goal of the preparticipation physical examination (PPE) is to identify injuries or medical conditions that place the athlete at risk during participation in athletics.

2. Focus of the PPE

   a. To detect life-threatening conditions that may be exposed during activity

   b. To detect current injuries that may need treatment prior to seasonal play

   c. To provide a forum to discuss preventive care

   d. To meet legal and insurance requirements for the institution

B. History

1. Medical history alone may identify up to 75% of conditions that would prohibit sports participation in athletes.

2. For many lethal conditions, physical examination findings may be normal. Family history and specific focus on past symptoms may provide the only clues to an underlying disorder.

3. History should include past medical problems, including recent and chronic illness and injuries.

4. Medication and supplement use should be reviewed to determine appropriate management of illness as well as identify use of banned substances.

5. Cardiovascular history

   a. The cardiovascular history should include family history of sudden death, Marfan syndrome, long QT syndrome, hypertrophic cardiomyopathy (HCM), etc.

   b. Exertional symptoms of syncope, dizziness, chest pain, palpitations, or shortness of breath should raise concern.

6. Neurologic history

   a. The neurologic history should include previous head injuries, concussions, seizures, burners/stingers, and spinal trauma.

   b. Patients with these prior conditions may be at increased risk for additional injury.

7. Athletes with prior history of heat-related illness should be screened for risk factors and counseled on preventive measures.

8. Female athletes should be questioned on history of stress fractures, missed or abnormal menses, and disordered eating habits (female athlete triad).

C. Physical examination

1. The musculoskeletal examination should focus on areas of previous injury.

2. A focused cardiovascular examination is important.

   a. Blood pressures must be interpreted on the basis of patient's age, sex, and height.

   b. In general, pressures >140/90 should be further evaluated.

3. Symmetric pulses in all four extremities should be noted.

4. Auscultation of the heart should be performed with the patient standing, squatting, and supine. Murmurs that worsen with standing or the Valsalva maneuver, any diastolic murmur, and systolic murmurs greater than 3/6 in intensity should be evaluated further before clearance to play.

5. Routine screening with 12-lead electrocardiography and echocardiography is not recommended by the American Heart Association. However, these tests can be useful in assessing athletes thought to be at higher risk based on history or physical examination.

II. On-Field Management

A. Unconscious athlete

1. Immediate assessment should include evaluation of the patient's airway, breathing, and circulatory status (ABCs), with spinal immobilization.

2. A cervical spine injury should be assumed in any unconscious athlete.

3. If a player is found lying prone, he or she should be log-rolled into the supine position in a controlled effort directed by the person maintaining airway and cervical alignment.

4. Face masks should be removed to allow access to the airway; however, the helmet and shoulder pads should be left in place.

5. The helmet should be removed only if the head and cervical spine are not stabilized with the helmet in place, or if the airway cannot be maintained with the helmet in place. Shoulder pads should be removed with the helmet to prevent spinal malalignment.

6. The patient should be log-rolled or placed on a spine board using the five-man lift and secured in position with straps. The head and neck should be stabilized on either side with blocks or towels.

7. Standard ACLS (advanced cardiac life support) and ATLS (advanced trauma life support) protocols including rescue breathing, cardiopulmonary resuscitation (CPR), and use of the AED (automated external defibrillator) should be performed in the apneic and pulseless patient.

B. Neck injury

1. Spinal injuries should be assumed in the unconscious or altered level-of-consciousness athlete. Spinal injuries should be suspected in the athlete with neck pain, midline bony tenderness on palpation, neurologic signs or symptoms, or a severe distracting injury.

2. On-field assessment should include the ABCs with spinal stabilization until proven otherwise.

3. The posterior neck should be palpated for step-offs, deformities, and/or tenderness.

4. Transient quadriplegia is a neurapraxia of the cervical cord that can occur with axial loading of the neck in flexion or extension.

   a. Symptoms are bilateral upper and lower extremity pain, paresthesias, and weakness that by definition are transient and recover typically within minutes to several hours.

   b. Athletes with transient quadriplegia should have the spine stabilized until additional imag-

ing can be obtained to rule out fractures and spinal cord abnormalities.

5. Decisions regarding return to play after an episode remain controversial. The use of MRI or CT myelogram to rule out functional stenosis or loss of cerebrospinal fluid around the cord has been advocated.

C. Head injury

1. Approximately 300,000 sports-related brain injuries occur in the United States every year.

2. Traumatic head injury is the leading cause of death due to trauma in sports.

3. Severe head injuries in the unconscious or severely impaired athlete, including subdural hematomas (most common), epidural hematomas, subarachnoid hemorrhages, and intracerebral contusions, should be ruled out with a noncontrasted head CT.

4. A concussion is defined by the American Academy of Neurology as "a trauma induced alteration in mental status that may or may not be associated with a loss of consciousness."

5. Headache and dizziness are the most common symptoms in concussion; however, the clinical presentation can be extremely varied.

6. Loss of consciousness occurs in fewer than 10% of concussions.

7. On-field evaluation should include assessment of ABCs with spinal precautions, level of consciousness, symptoms, balance, memory (antegrade and retrograde), sensory and motor function, and thought process.

8. Athletes with severe, persistent, or worsening symptoms should be triaged to a medical center for further evaluation.

9. Concussion grading scales and other guidelines for return to play have been published but not validated. New guidelines suggesting a stepwise return to physical activity based on recurrence of symptoms have been suggested.

10. Experts agree that all symptomatic players should be withheld from activity and return-to-play decisions should be individually based.

11. Use of neuropsychological testing for evaluation of concussion and assistance with return-to-play decisions is promising and can be a helpful adjunct.

D. Orthopaedic emergencies

1. Orthopaedic injuries are the most common injuries encountered in athletes.

2. It is important to fully evaluate the athlete for potentially life-threatening injuries that may be rec-

ognized late due to focusing on obvious deformities to the extremities.

3. Fractures

a. No athlete should return to play if a fracture is suspected because a nondisplaced injury could potentially become displaced or open.

b. Fractures can be splinted in the position in which they are found, but if vascular compromise exists, reduction of dislocations and fractures should be performed on the field with gentle traction, and the extremity should be splinted in the position providing best vascular flow.

c. Open fractures should be suspected when a laceration is seen overlying the deformity.

d. Open fractures should be covered with moist, sterile dressings and splinted. These injuries require emergent care, including intravenous antibiotics and irrigation and débridement in the operating room.

4. Dislocations

a. Dislocations can be reduced by experienced personnel on the field; however, the athlete should always be referred for imaging to assess for fractures.

b. A thorough neurovascular examination is imperative prior to and after the reduction.

c. Knee dislocations in athletes are rare; however, they should be suspected in the injured knee with multidirectional instability.

d. Many will spontaneously reduce prior to evaluation, requiring a high index of suspicion.

e. Early on-field reduction with axial traction is imperative.

f. Rapid transport to a medical facility for orthopaedic and vascular consultation, including vascular studies, is mandatory.

E. Thorax injuries

1. Pneumothorax

a. May be spontaneous or traumatic. Spontaneous pneumothorax occurs more often in sports involving intrathoracic pressure changes (weight lifting and scuba diving).

b. Symptoms of pneumothorax include chest pain, shortness of breath, and diminished breath sounds on auscultation.

c. Field treatment includes transportation to the emergency room in a position of comfort with supplemental oxygen.

2. Tension pneumothorax

a. Can develop as progressive accumulation of air remains trapped within the pleural space

b. This can lead to increased intrathoracic pressure, resulting in decreased ability to ventilate, and can limit cardiac output.

c. Patients may present as hypotensive and hypoxic, with tracheal deviation and venous jugular distention.

d. Unrecognized tension pneumothorax can lead to cardiopulmonary arrest.

e. Immediate needle decompression should be performed using a 14-gauge angiocatheter placed anteriorly along the midclavicular line in the second intercostal space.

f. Patients require rapid transport to a medical facility for definitive thoracostomy tube placement.

3. Cardiac contusion

a. Can result after blunt anterior chest trauma

b. The right ventricle is most often affected because of its anterior position.

c. Patients present with persistent chest pain and tachycardia.

d. Suspected patients should be referred for electrocardiogram (ECG) and telemetry monitoring, as arrhythmias are common.

F. Abdominal injuries

1. Abdominal and pelvic injuries

a. Typically result from blunt trauma, most commonly affecting the liver and spleen

b. These patients may have abdominal pain and potentially referred pain to the shoulder (Kehr sign).

2. Injuries to the kidney

a. May occur with flank or posterior trauma

b. Hematuria may or may not be present, but its absence does not exclude injury.

c. Abdominal pain may not be present because the kidneys are located in the retroperitoneum.

d. A high index of suspicion based on mechanism may be required for the diagnosis.

3. Bowel and pancreatic injuries

a. Can occur with blunt trauma compressing the organs against the vertebral column

b. Presentation may be delayed and often missed initially on CT scan.

c. Laboratory tests and/or serial abdominal examinations may be necessary for diagnosis.

5: Sports Medicine

4. On-field examinaion

   a. A single on-field examination is inadequate to exclude injury.

   b. Athletes with a concerning mechanism, persistent or worsening pain, rebound tenderness, or abnormal vital signs should be sent for CT scan and/or continued observation.

III. Medical Conditions in Sports

A. Sudden death

   1. Hypertrophic cardiomyopathy

      a. HCM is the most common cause of cardiac sudden death in athletes.

      b. It is characterized by nondilated left ventricular hypertrophy, causing obstruction of the left ventricular outflow tract.

      c. Often asymptomatic, it should be considered in athletes with dyspnea on exertion, chest pain, a family history of sudden cardiac death, or with a systolic murmur that becomes louder upon standing.

      d. Death from HCM is believed to be due to fatal arrhythmias.

      e. Diagnosis can be made with echocardiography.

      f. Current recommendations are that athletes with HCM should be excluded from most competitive sports, with few exceptions.

   2. Coronary artery abnormality (CAA)

      a. The second most common cause of sudden cardiac death is CAA.

      b. The most frequent CAA is an anomalous origin of the left main coronary artery; this origin allows for the artery to be compressed under increased cardiac pressure, which restricts circulation to that artery and causes subsequent ischemia to the heart.

      c. Occasionally the athlete may experience chest pain, palpitations, or syncope that is related to exercise, but most often CAAs are asymptomatic with a normal physical examination.

      d. Diagnosis is by coronary angiography or MR angiography.

   3. Long QT syndrome

      a. Long QT syndrome is a congenital or acquired repolarization abnormality that can lead to sudden cardiac death via the development of ventricular tachycardia and torsades de pointes (a cardiac arrhythmia).

      b. Athletes may be asymptomatic but may have syncope or near-syncope with exercise.

      c. If exercise symptoms exist or there is a family history of sudden cardiac death, one should consider an ECG to evaluate for long QT syndrome.

      d. Diagnosis is based on the correct QT interval, but there is still controversy as to the interval duration that is considered worrisome.

      e. Sports participation is determined by phenotype, genotype, and the presence of a pacemaker.

   4. Commotio cordis

      a. Commotio cordis is caused by a blow to the anterior wall of the chest, near the heart, with objects such as a hockey puck, baseball, or a karate kick, which can lead to fatal ventricular fibrillation.

      b. Most episodes occur in children and adolescents.

      c. Survival rates are often low unless prompt CPR and, more important, early defibrillation, can be initiated.

      d. Attempts to prevent commotio cordis with chest protectors have not yielded a decline in commotio cordis; however, softer "safety" baseballs may potentially lower the risk.

B. Top five dermatologic conditions

   1. Tinea infections

      a. Tinea infections are superficial fungal infections caused by dermatophytes.

      b. Location on the body determines the naming of the lesion, such as tinea capitis (head), corporis (body), cruris (groin), and pedis (foot).

      c. Direct close contact with dermatophytes, coupled with breaks in the skin, can lead to infection.

      d. Diagnosis can be confirmed by scraping the scaly edge of lesions and using microscopic examination with potassium hydroxide preparation, looking for characteristic hyphae.

      e. Tinea corporis is also referred to as ringworm.

      f. Tinea cruris, pedis, and corporis are often treated with topical antifungals, with systemic antifungals reserved for more severe cases, while tinea capitis is treated with systemic antifungals.

      g. Tinea corporis is common in wrestlers and must be screened for prior to competition.

      h. Treatment is generally needed for 48 hours prior to return to competition.

2. Methicillin-resistant *Staphylococcus aureus* (MRSA)

   a. Community-acquired MRSA is an emerging problem in sports.

   b. MRSA often produces painful boils, pimples, or "spider-bite" type lesions.

   c. Initial treatment can be with topical mupirocin for small lesions.

   d. Larger lesions often require incision and drainage, with trimethoprim/sulfa as the usual first-line oral antibiotic agent.

   e. More severe infections may require hospitalization, surgical débridement, and intravenous antibiotics.

   f. Prevention can be accomplished by avoiding sharing of personal items (razors, towels, and soaps), good hygiene, and protecting compromised skin.

3. Herpes gladiatorum

   a. Herpes gladiatorum is caused by herpes-simplex type 1 virus and is transmitted by direct skin-to-skin contact.

   b. Infection occurs in 2.6% to 7.6% of wrestlers and affects primarily the head, neck, and shoulders.

   c. Treatment is with oral acyclovir or valacyclovir.

   d. Lesions close to the eye can progress to the more serious herpetic conjunctivitis.

   e. Return to play is often allowed once lesions have scabbed and crusted over.

4. Acne mechanica/folliculitis

   a. Acne mechanica is a type of acne seen in athletes that is caused by friction, heat, pressure, and occlusion of the skin.

   b. It is frequently seen in sports requiring protective pads (eg, shoulder pads), including lacrosse, hockey, and football.

   c. Lesions appear as red papules in area of occlusion.

   d. Treatment is often more difficult than for traditional acne.

   e. Washing immediately after exercise can be beneficial, as well as wearing moisture-wicking clothing.

   f. Pharmacologic treatment can be with keratinolytics such as tretinoin, but most cases will resolve once the season is over.

5. Subungual hemorrhage

   a. Subungual hemorrhages are common in sports. They result from acute trauma, such as having a toe stepped on, or from repetitive trauma, such as a toe being forced continually into the toe box of a shoe.

   b. Acutely these hemorrhages can be quite painful. Treatment can consist of evacuating the hematoma by creating a hole in the nail with an electrocautery device or a heated, sterile 18-gauge needle.

   c. Chronic hemorrhages can lead to nail dystrophy.

C. Exercise-induced bronchospasm

   1. Definition—Exercise-induced bronchospasm (EIB) occurs during or after exercise and is characterized by coughing, shortness of breath, wheezing, and chest tightness.

   2. Factors/conditions contributing to EIB

      a. Exercise in cold weather

      b. Exercise during viral respiratory illnesses

      c. Polluted air environment (including in indoor skating rinks from ice-resurfacing machines, or heavily chlorinated pools)

      d. Exercise during allergy seasons

      e. Intense exercise

   3. Diagnosis

      a. Diagnosis often can be suspected from the patient's history and physical examination.

      b. Office spirometry can be helpful in diagnosing underlying asthma, especially with an FEV_1 (forced expiratory volume) of <90%.

      c. Exercise challenge testing while observing the patient's symptoms and the patient's response to exercising in his or her own sport can be helpful.

      d. The International Olympic Committee recommends the eucapnic voluntary hyperventilation test, which is both sensitive and specific for EIB.

      e. Testing with a mannitol inhalation challenge is a newer and potentially more sensitive method than the traditional methacholine inhalation challenge used for asthma diagnosis.

   4. Treatment

      a. Avoidance of environmental and exercise triggers can be effective but often impractical.

      b. Adequate warm-up can help reduce symptoms.

      c. Pharmacologic treatment often begins with beta-2 receptor agonists, such as inhaled albuterol, prior to exercise.

5: Sports Medicine

d. Oral leukotriene modifiers are also effective in controlling symptoms of EIB.

e. For persistent symptoms, the addition of inhaled corticosteroids can be beneficial.

D. Heat illness

1. Heat cramps

a. Heat cramps are characterized by painful muscle cramping, most commonly seen in the calves, thighs, shoulders, and abdomen.

b. Cramps may occur as a result of a mild dilutional hyponatremia from excessive water intake or significant salt loss through sweating.

c. Treatment is through rest, cooling, intravenous fluids, or oral rehydration, and replacing salt losses.

d. Prevention can be through use of electrolyte sport drinks and potentially through adding some salt consumption during exercise.

2. Heat exhaustion

a. Heat exhaustion is the most common form of heat illness.

b. Findings can include significant fatigue, profuse sweating, core temperatures <40.5° C, headache, nausea, vomiting, heat cramps, hypotension, tachycardia, and syncope.

c. Treatment is by removal from the heat, oral or intravenous rehydration, and rapid cooling.

3. Heat stroke

a. Heat stroke is the most severe of the heat illnesses.

b. Findings in heat stroke are lack of sweating, core temperatures >40.5° C, and mental status changes.

c. Heat stroke is a medical emergency, and rapid whole-body cooling is a necessity.

d. The most rapid cooling can be achieved by whole-body immersion in an ice bath.

e. Basic life support and ACLS protocols must be followed.

f. Failure to recognize and treat heat stroke can lead to end-organ failure and death.

4. Heat syncope

a. Heat syncope can occur with a rapid rise from a prolonged seated or lying position in the heat, resulting in orthostatic syncope from inadequate cardiac output and hypotension.

b. Treatment of heat syncope is accomplished by laying the athlete supine with legs elevated and replacement of any fluid deficits from dehydration.

E. Cold exposure

1. Hypothermia

a. Hypothermia is defined as core body temperature <35° C (95° F), with milder being >32° C and moderate to severe <32° C.

b. Athletes with prolonged exposure to the cold, such as cross-country skiers, are more likely to be affected.

c. Mild hypothermia treatment is through removal from the cold exposure into a warmer environment, removal of wet clothing and replacing with dry clothes, drinking hot liquids, use of warmed blankets, and use of rewarming devices.

d. Moderate to severe hypothermia should be cared for in a controlled medical environment because organ dysfunction and electrolyte imbalances can lead to more serious issues if rewarming is undertaken improperly.

2. Frostbite

a. Frostbite is a localized freezing of tissues and can occur in any exposed body part, most commonly the extremities.

b. Superficial frostbite is a milder form of the condition and is characterized by a burning sensation in the affected area that can progress to numbness. Treatment can be initiated as soon as possible by thawing.

c. Deep frostbite is a more significant problem that is quite painful initially and then also goes numb. Thawing and treatment of deeper affected areas should be done in a hospital or emergency room setting.

3. Prevention of cold illness—Preventing cold exposure-related problems can be achieved by increasing the body's heat production (through eating and increasing muscle activity), proper use of clothing through layering and using wind barriers, and considering avoiding outdoor activities in extreme cold conditions.

IV. Ergogenic Aids

A. Legal

1. Creatine

a. Creatine is one of the most popular nutritional supplements derived from the amino acids glycine, arginine, and methionine.

b. Most creatine is stored in muscle and in its phosphorylated form contributes to the resynthesis of adenosine triphosphate.

c. Several studies have been conducted for anaerobic activities and have produced conflicting results on the beneficial effects of creatine on sports performance.

d. No study has shown an improvement in on-the-field performance.

e. Short-term side effects reported include cramping, dehydration, and possible renal effects.

f. Long-term effects of creatine are unknown.

2. Caffeine

a. Consumed daily by athletes and nonathletes alike throughout the world, caffeine can be used to enhance athletic performance.

b. Doses as low as 2 to 3 mg/kg have been documented to improve performance.

c. Caffeine is banned by the International Olympic Committee, but doses of up to 9 mg/kg are necessary to achieve the maximum allowable doses.

d. Caffeine is thought to improve performance by reducing fatigue and increasing alertness.

e. Athletes must exercise caution in using caffeine because daily dietary intake plus the lack of regulation of supplements can potentially lead to an unexpected positive test.

3. Amino acids

B. Illegal

1. Anabolic steroids

a. Anabolic steroids are believed to be widely abused in athletes of all ages, with use reported in up to 10% of adolescent athletes.

b. Steroids are synthetically derived to have similar effects to natural testosterone and can be given orally or through an injection.

c. Side effects include development of atherosclerotic disease, decreased high-density lipoprotein cholesterol, aggression and mood disturbances, testicular atrophy, masculinization in females, gynecomastia in males, acne, and an increased risk for hepatitis and human immunodeficiency virus infections in those sharing needles to inject steroids.

d. Most side effects are believed to be reversible with cessation of use but may require a prolonged period to return to normal.

e. Anabolic steroids are banned by college, Olympic, and most professional teams.

f. Most of these same organizations test for anabolic steroids, looking for a testosterone to epitestosterone ratio greater than 6:1.

2. Erythropoietin

a. Erythropoietin (EPO) acts to stimulate hemoglobin production, which in turn increases the body's oxygen-carrying capacity.

b. This ability has made EPO widely desirable among elite endurance athletes such as cyclists and cross-country skiers.

c. Several studies have documented increases in hematocrit and VO_{2max} in time to exhaustion.

d. Side effects of EPO use include increasing blood viscosity, which can lead to stroke, thromboembolic events, and myocardial infarctions.

e. EPO is currently illegal in all sports.

f. Testing does exist, but the substance can still be difficult to detect.

3. Human growth hormone

a. Human growth hormone (HGH) is a peptide secreted by the anterior pituitary and acts to stimulate the release of insulinlike growth factors.

b. Studies on athletes are essentially nonexistent.

c. Those studies that have been conducted are in patients with endocrine dysfunction and demonstrate increases in muscle size but not in strength.

d. Resistance to continued use is also thought to occur.

e. Side effects include water retention, development of myopathic muscles, carpal tunnel syndrome, and insulin resistance.

f. There are currently no available accurate tests for HGH.

Bibliography

Amaral JF: Thoracoabdominal injuries in the athlete. *Clin Sports Med* 1997;16:739-753.

Cordoro KM, Ganz JE: Training room management of medical conditions: Sports dermatology. *Clin Sports Med* 2005;24: 565-598.

Lugo-Amador NM, Rothenhaus T, Moyer P: Heat-related illness. *Emerg Med Clin North Am* 2004;22:315-327.

Marx RG, Delany JS: Sideline orthopedic emergencies in the young athlete. *Pediatr Ann* 2002;31:60-70.

5: Sports Medicine

McAlindon RJ: On field evaluation and management of head and neck injured athletes. *Clin Sports Med* 2002;21:1-14.

McCrory P, Johnston K, Meeuwisse W, et al: Summary and agreement statement of the 2nd international conference on concussion in sport, Prague 2004. *Br J Sports Med* 2005;39: 196-204.

Parsons JP, Mastronarde JG: Exercise-induced bronchoconstriction in athletes. *Chest* 2005;128:3966-3974.

Paterick TE, Paterick TJ, Fletcher GF, Maron BJ: Medical and legal issues in the cardiovascular evaluation of competitive athletes. *JAMA* 2005;294:3011-3018.

Tokish JM, Kocher MS, Hawkins RJ: Ergogenic aids: A review of basic science, performance, side effects and status in sports. *Am J Sports Med* 2004;32:1543-1553.

Wingfield K, Matheson GO, Meeuwisse WH: Preparticipation evaluation: An evidence-based review. *Clin J Sport Med* 2004;14:109-122.

Top Testing Facts

1. The preparticipation physical examination (PPE) may be normal in athletes with an underlying condition that places them at risk during athletics. A detailed family history and past history of exertional symptoms may provide the only clues to a potentially lethal disorder.

2. Cardiac murmurs that worsen with standing or the Valsalva maneuver, any diastolic murmur, and systolic murmurs greater than 3/6 in intensity should be evaluated further before clearance to play.

3. A cervical spine injury should be assumed in any unconscious athlete.

4. Face masks should be removed to allow access to the airway in an unstable patient; however, the helmet and shoulder pads should be left in place during transport.

5. Experts agree that all symptomatic players with a concussion should be withheld from activity and return-to-play decisions should be individually based.

6. Knee dislocations in athletes are rare; however, they should be suspected in the injured knee with multidirectional instability. A vascular study should be performed if this injury is suspected.

7. A single abdominal examination is inadequate to exclude injury. Athletes with a concerning mechanism, persistent or worsening pain, rebound tenderness, or abnormal vital signs should be sent for CT scan and/or continued observation.

8. Hypertrophic cardiomyopathy is the most common cause of sudden cardiac death in athletes.

9. Heat stroke is a medical emergency and treatment must be initiated promptly.

10. Exercise-induced bronchospasm is frequently managed by limited environmental aggravators and use of beta-2 agonists, such as albuterol, prior to exercise.

Chapter 48

Sports Rehabilitation

Timothy E. Hewett, PhD   Bruce D. Beynnon, PhD   Jon Divine, MD   Glenn N. Williams, PhD, PT, ATC

I. Definitions

A. Muscle exercise types

1. Isoinertial exercises

   a. Isoinertial exercises, often incorrectly referred to as isotonic exercises, involve applying a muscle contraction throughout a range of motion against a constant resistance or weight.

   b. These exercises are beneficial in that they strengthen both the primary and synergistic muscles, as well as provide stress to the ligaments and tendons throughout varying ranges of motion.

2. Isotonic exercises

   a. Isotonic exercises involve applying a muscle contraction throughout a range of motion against a constant muscle force.

   b. These types of muscle contractions are rarely used and may involve the use of free weights, such as dumbbells or weight devices.

3. Isometric exercises

   a. Isometric exercise can be defined as a process by which a muscle is contracted without appreciable joint motion.

   b. These exercises are used often as the first form of strengthening after injury or with individuals who are immobilized.

   c. These exercises can help improve static strengthening and minimize the extent of muscular atrophy.

4. Isokinetic exercises

   a. Isokinetic exercise refers to a type of strengthening protocol in which the speed of a muscle contraction is fixed but the resistance varies depending on the force exerted throughout a range of motion.

   b. Maximum muscle loading is postulated to occur throughout the entire range of motion.

   c. These exercises are performed using machines that automatically adjust the resistance throughout the range of motion, including active dynamometers.

   d. Isokinetic testing is used frequently to assess the progress of rehabilitation as well as to objectively determine whether full muscle strength has been regained following an injury.

B. Muscle contraction types

1. Concentric muscle contractions are contractions in which the individual muscle fibers shorten during force production and the origin and insertion of a particular muscle group move closer to one another.

2. Eccentric muscle contractions are contractions in which the individual muscle fibers lengthen during force production and the origin and insertion of a particular muscle group move apart from one another.

C. Training types

1. Sport-specific

   a. Sport-specific exercise is characterized by or related to a specific sport.

   b. An example of sport-specific training exercise for hockey is rollerblading, or in-line skating.

2. Periodization

   a. Periodization is a planned workout scheme in which the volume and/or the intensity of training is varied over a set period of time.

   b. Periodization of training can generally be divided into phases throughout the year, such as conditioning, precompetition, competition, and rest.

3. Plyometrics

   a. Plyometrics is a form of resistance training that involves the eccentric loading of a muscle followed by immediate concentric unloading of a muscle to create a fast, forceful movement.

   b. Plyometrics trains the muscles, connective tissue, and nervous system to effectively carry out the stretch-shortening cycle.

   c. This training modality emphasizes spending as little time as possible in contact with the ground and may include exercises such as bounding and hopping drills, jumping over hurdles, and depth jumps.

D. Joint motion

1. Active range of motion

a. Active range of motion is the process by which the individual moves a joint or muscle group without help from another person or machine.

b. Active range of motion allows for assessment of a patient's willingness to perform the movement, muscle strength, and joint range.

2. Passive range of motion is the process by which another person or machine moves a joint or muscle group of an individual.

E. Types of stretching

1. Active stretching

a. Active stretching is also referred to as static-active stretching.

b. An active stretch is one in which a position is held with no assistance other than using the strength of the agonist muscles.

c. The tension of the agonists in an active stretch helps to relax the muscles being stretched (the antagonists) and is referred to as reciprocal inhibition.

d. Many of the movements (or stretches) found in various forms of yoga are active stretches.

e. Active stretches are usually difficult to hold and maintain for more than 10 seconds and rarely are held longer than 15 seconds.

2. Passive stretching

a. Passive stretching is a stretching technique in which the muscle being stretched is relaxed without any movement to increase the range of motion; instead, an outside agent creates an external force, either manually or mechanically.

b. This position is then held with some other part of the body, with the assistance of a partner or some other apparatus.

c. A seated hurdler's stretch for the hamstrings is an example of a passive stretch.

3. Proprioceptive neuromuscular facilitation (PNF)

a. PNF is any type of stretching technique combining passive stretching and isometric stretching.

b. The technique involves a three-step process in which a muscle group is passively stretched, then isometrically contracted against resistance while in the stretched position, and then is passively stretched again by postisometric relax-

ation through the resulting increased range of motion.

c. PNF stretching usually employs the use of a partner to provide resistance against the isometric contraction and then later to passively take the joint through its increased range of motion.

F. Open versus closed chain exercises

1. Open chain exercises are movements, usually with some type of resistance, in which the hand or foot is not in direct contact with a solid object, such as the floor or a wall.

2. In open chain exercises, the foot, or end of the kinetic chain, is moved freely.

3. Closed chain exercises are exercises in which the end of the kinetic chain or foot is fixed to the ground or a wall or is otherwise weight bearing and not able to move freely.

4. In practical terms, open chain exercises involving the knee, such as leg extensions, are postulated to create greater shear force across the knee and its ligaments, especially the anterior cruciate ligament (ACL); closed chain exercises, such as leg presses or squats, are postulated to result in greater compression force at the knee and ACL, which is hypothesized to lead to decreased strain on the ACL during the postsurgical rehabilitation process.

G. Modalities

1. Ultrasound

a. Ultrasound is used to apply thermal (deep heat) energy from 2 to 5+ cm below the skin surface, or nonthermal deep massage by using acoustic energy (0.8 to 3.0 MHz) transfer using a round-headed wand or probe that is put in direct contact with the patient's skin.

b. Sound waves are absorbed by various tissues, causing the production of heat.

c. The greatest rise in temperature occurs in tissues with high protein content, such as muscle, tendon, and nerve.

d. Relatively little increase in adipose tissue temperature occurs with ultrasound treatment.

e. Most ultrasound treatments are from 3 to 5 min in duration.

f. Contraindications for ultrasound use include bleeding disorders, cancer, or a cardiac pacemaker.

g. Ultrasound should not be used for most acute injuries with edematous or necrotic tissue.

2. Pulsed ultrasound

a. Pulsed ultrasound is used when localized deep-tissue massage is desired to reduce edema in an acute injury situation.

   b. Pulsed ultrasound does not result in increased deep localized heating.

3. Phonophoresis—a noninvasive method of delivering medications to tissues below the skin using ultrasound

4. Neuromuscular electrical stimulation (NMES)

   a. NMES is a therapeutic modality technique using a wide variety of electrical stimulators, including burst-modulated alternating current ("Russian stimulator"), twin-spiked monophasic pulsed current, and biphasic pulsed current stimulators.

   b. NMES has been used for muscle strengthening, maintenance of muscle mass and strength during prolonged periods of immobilization, selective muscle retraining, and control of edema.

   c. NMES may be beneficial early in the rehabilitation phase when swelling is persistent and reflexively inhibiting muscle activation.

   d. Contraindications to the use of NMES include use in patients with a demand-type pacemaker, or use over the carotid sinus, across the heart, or over the abdomen of a pregnant woman.

5. Transcutaneous electrical nerve stimulation (TENS) is another form of electrical stimulation that has been used to control a wide variety of both acute and chronic pain symptoms.

6. High-voltage stimulation (HVS)

   a. HVS is the delivery of a monophasic pulse of short duration across the skin and into acutely injured, swollen tissue.

   b. HVS works by acting on negatively charged plasma proteins, which leak into the interstitial space and result in edema.

   c. In the setting of an acute injury with edema, a negative electrode is placed over the edematous site and a positive electrode at a distant site.

   d. A monophasic, high-voltage stimulus is applied, creating an electrical potential that disperses the negatively charged proteins away from the edematous site, resulting in reduced swelling.

   e. Injuries commonly treated with HVS are acute ankle and knee sprains as well as postoperative joint effusions.

   f. HVS is often applied concurrently with the more common methods of acute swelling reduction—ice, elevation, and compression.

   g. Contraindications to the use of HVS are similar to electrical stimulation.

7. Ice, or cryotherapy

   a. Cryotherapy is the modality used to cool tissue.

   b. Cryotherapy techniques are done at temperatures ranging from 0°C to 25°C.

   c. Depending on the application method and duration, cryotherapy results in decreased local metabolism, vasoconstriction, reduced swelling/edema, decreased hemorrhage, reduced muscle efficiency, and pain relief secondary to impaired neuromuscular transmission.

8. Heat

   a. Heat is any superficial modality that provides pain relief by using external warming methods, ranging from 37°C to 43°C.

   b. Traditionally categorized by method of primary heat transfer

     i. Conduction (hot packs, paraffin baths)

     ii. Convection (hydrotherapy, moist air)

     iii. Conversion (sunlight, heat lamp)

   c. Indications for the application of heat may include painful muscle spasms, abdominal muscle cramping, menstrual cramps, and superficial thrombophlebitis.

9. Iontophoresis

   a. Iontophoresis involves the delivery of a charged medication through the skin and into underlying tissue via direct current electrical stimulation; this results in a transdermal form of medicine delivery.

   b. The charged molecules are placed under an electrode of the same polarity and repelled into the area to be treated.

   c. Many ionic drugs are available, including dexamethasone, lidocaine, and acetate.

   d. Dexamethasone is the medication most commonly used for treating locally inflamed tissues due to tendinitis, bursitis, or arthritis.

   e. Currently, iontophoresis is used in the medical management of inflamed superficial tissues such as lateral epicondylitis, shoulder tendinitis, patella tendinitis, etc.

II. Rehabilitation Phases of Common Sports Injuries

A. Rehabilitation of the anterior cruciate ligament

  1. Initial phase after ACL tear or ACL reconstruction

   a. Early rehabilitation after ACL injury and reconstruction is similar in that the goal is to minimize pain and inflammation while obtaining good quadriceps muscle activation and full extension range of motion.

b. Ice and compression are used to treat pain and inflammation with either a commercially available joint cooling system or crushed ice with a compressive wrap.

c. Elevation is also important in minimizing swelling because placing the limb in a dependent position leads to pooling of edema in the distal leg.

d. Patients should use an assistive device during ambulation until good quadriceps function and a minimally antalgic gait are achieved.

2. Quadriceps function

a. Acquiring good control of the quadriceps as soon as possible is critical.

b. Beginning the day of injury or surgery, the patient should contract the quadriceps muscles as tightly as possible while the knee is in full extension with a small bolster under the Achilles tendon.

c. Straight-leg raises should begin only after the patient can perform a strong quadriceps contraction in which the heel lifts symmetrically with the opposite side, because straight-leg raises can be performed with relatively poor quadriceps function using the hip flexors.

d. Some patients have severe quadriceps inhibition. In this situation, high-intensity electrical stimulation or assisted eccentric lowering exercises may be helpful in improving activation.

3. Range of motion

a. Efforts should be directed toward obtaining extension range of motion equal to the opposite side as quickly as possible.

b. Although having a strong quadriceps muscle and early ambulation in full weight bearing are the most effective methods of obtaining full extension, patients sometimes still struggle with gaining full extension.

c. In these circumstances, low-load, long-duration stretching is helpful in inducing tissue creep and gaining motion.

d. This exercise should not be painful because this will induce counterproductive muscle guarding.

e. In extremely challenging cases, an extension promotion brace or drop-out casting is helpful.

4. Tailoring rehabilitation

a. Rehabilitation programs should be tailored to

the individual, although general principles apply to all patients.

b. Aquatic therapy may be helpful.

c. Strength and control of the entire lower extremity and core are important.

d. Because ACL injury and reconstruction have a particularly severe impact on the quadriceps muscles, this muscle group needs to be treated especially aggressively.

e. The optimal approach includes the combined use of open and closed kinetic chain exercises.

f. Closed kinetic chain exercises should be the primary method of strength training.

g. Rehabilitation exercises need to be performed with an appropriate volume, intensity, and frequency to provide the stimulus for strength improvement.

h. Neuromuscular training using cushions, disks, balance boards, perturbation training, and/or commercially available devices is used to progressively improve dynamic joint stability.

i. Cardiovascular training is advised to promote general health and deliver optimal blood supply to healing tissues.

5. Return to play

a. The decision on when it is "safe" to resume running is case dependent.

b. Running is generally safe 8 to 12 weeks after injury/surgery as long as it is in a straight line and progresses gradually.

c. Agility exercises and multidirectional training generally begin about 12 weeks after injury/surgery.

d. Continued aggressive strengthening is important because most patients still have quadriceps atrophy and strength deficits at the time they are released to sports participation.

e. The return-to-sports decision should be based on a confluence of signs, including patient-based outcomes measures, examination, and indicators of neuromuscular status such as functional tests and strength tests.

f. Thresholds for strength and hop tests should be reasonable (80% to 85% of the opposite side) and considered in light of the big picture of a patient's status because the validity of such tests as predictors of short-term function is questionable.

B. Ankle ligament injury rehabilitation

1. Lateral ligaments

a. Ankle ligament trauma, the most common

sports injury, can involve sprains of the lateral, medial, and/or syndesmosis ligaments.

b. One of the most well-established treatment modalities for acute injury of the ankle ligaments is RICE (rest, ice-cooling, compression, and elevation).

c. Cooling decreases tissue temperature, which in turn reduces blood flow and metabolism.

d. Cooling also appears effective in reducing swelling and limiting pain up to 1 week after the index injury.

e. For minor (grade I) and moderate (grade II) tears of the lateral ankle ligament complex, early mobilization of the injured ankle is recommended, with protection provided by the combination of a brace and an elastic wrap; this approach provides protection from reinjury and compression and has been shown to produce excellent short- and intermediate-term outcomes in >95% of patients.

f. For severe (grade III) sprains of the lateral ligaments, functional treatment produces similar excellent short- and intermediate-term outcomes.

g. A subgroup of severe sprains does not respond well to functional treatment; patients with these injuries may become candidates for surgical repair if recurrent giving-way episodes of the ankle are experienced.

h. After swelling is controlled, weight-bearing status is restored, and ankle range of motion is reestablished, a rehabilitation program that includes sensory-motor, strength training, and sport-specific exercises is recommended.

   i. For minor, moderate, and severe ankle ligament sprains, a 10-week sensory-motor training program that includes balance exercises should be completed.

   ii. During the sensory-motor training program, muscle strengthening and sports specific exercises should be implemented and progressed.

i. Loss of strength and its subsequent recovery takes time and is dependent on the severity of the index injury.

j. Return to play is usually indicated when full ankle range of motion is restored, full muscle strength is regained, sensory-motor control of the ankle is reestablished, and the joint is pain-free during activity with no swelling as a result of activity.

2. Syndesmosis injuries

   a. It has been estimated that up to 20% of pa-tients presenting with the more severe lateral ankle ligament sprains have an associated injury to the distal tibiofibular articulation, or syndesmosis (ie, the anterior inferior tibiofibular, interosseous tibiofibular, and/or posterior inferior tibiofibular ligaments).

   b. These injuries can range from minor tears of the syndesmosis (which are considered stable) to significant injuries that involve disruption of the syndesmosis combined with fracture of the fibula (which are unstable).

   c. It is important to educate the patient with regard to the longer time interval required for rehabilitation and recovery of injury to the syndesmosis ligament complex in comparison with isolated injury to the lateral ankle ligaments.

   d. Treatment of injuries to the syndesmosis without a fracture of the fibula requires particular attention to maintaining anatomic reduction of the ankle mortise and syndesmosis.

   e. If the syndesmotic injury is considered stable, the treatment should include the use of RICE combined with a posterior splint with the ankle in a neutral position and non–weight bearing for at least 4 days.

   f. This is followed by partial weight bearing with crutches and the use of a walking boot or ankle stirrup brace and then progression to full weight bearing as tolerated.

   g. After obtaining control of swelling, restoration of weight-bearing status, and reestablishing ankle range of motion, the same sensory-motor, progressive strength training, and sport-specific exercise program described for the treatment of lateral ankle ligament sprains is recommended.

   h. Treatment of syndesmotic tears within 12 weeks of injury that are considered to be unstable may require reduction of the syndesmosis with screw fixation.

   i. Rehabilitation of these severe injuries includes protection for 12 weeks followed by the program described for stable syndesmotic injuries.

   j. Treatment of chronic (>12 weeks after the index injury) syndesmotic injuries may require reconstruction of the syndesmosis.

C. Shoulder instability rehabilitation

1. Rehabilitation of the patient with shoulder instability is highly dependent on the type of instability (traumatic versus atraumatic or acquired), the direction of instability (anterior, posterior, or multidirectional), the treatment approach (nonsurgical versus surgical), and, in surgical patients, the procedure used (open versus arthroscopic techniques).

2. The goal early after a traumatic instability event or shoulder surgery is to minimize pain and inflammation.

3. Crushed ice or a commercially available joint-cooling system is the primary method of treating pain and inflammation.

4. Minimization of the effects of immobilization is a priority.

   a. This is accomplished by performing gentle passive range of motion in the "safe" range of motion.

   b. Range of motion should increase progressively within the "safe" limits for the specific procedure.

5. Surgeons should clearly determine whether there are any unusual risk factors and what the "safe" limits are for each patient throughout the rehabilitation process.

6. Rehabilitation programs should be tailored so that they are specific to an individual's unique circumstances.

7. Submaximal isometric exercises are performed within the "safe" range of motion early in the rehabilitation process to minimize muscle atrophy.

8. Electrical stimulation and/or biofeedback training is often used as adjunct atrophy-prevention methods.

9. When it is "safe," range of motion is progressed using wand exercises, joint mobilization, and low-load, long-duration stretching that promotes gentle creep of the tissues.

10. Developing a stable platform for shoulder movement through scapular stabilization exercise is a prerequisite to aggressive rotator cuff strengthening.

11. Most shoulder strength programs begin with resistance training using exercise bands, cords, and free weights.

12. As strength and control develop, patients are progressed to various resistance-training devices and plyometrics.

13. Neuromuscular control is facilitated by performing reactive training and various exercises that perturb shoulder stability.

14. Care should be taken to promote appropriate responses to perturbations rather than rigid cocontraction because this strategy of joint stabilization is inconsistent with agile movement and skilled performance.

15. The final stages of rehabilitation should involve sport-specific training and the development of skill in sport-specific tasks.

16. Interval training programs, video analysis, and the input of coaches are helpful in obtaining high success rates when treating overhead athletes.

17. Although adjunct measures of patient status such as strength testing can be helpful, return to sports participation is dependent on the ability to perform sport-specific tasks in a pain-free manner and patient-based outcomes.

III. Prevention of Common Sports Injuries

A. ACL tear

1. Female athletes have a rate of ACL injury that is two to eight times that of male athletes.

2. Unfortunately, surgical intervention does not change the odds of developing knee osteoarthritis after injury.

3. Researchers have developed ways for clinicians to identify athletes at risk for ACL injury and have begun to use training programs designed for ACL injury prevention.

4. Efforts to prevent ACL injury in female athletes should focus on the factors that make females more susceptible to injury and develop interventions to aid in the prevention of these injuries.

5. A meta-analysis by Hewett and associates attempted to quantitatively combine the results of six independent studies drawn from a systematic review of the published literature regarding ACL injury interventions in female athletes.

   a. All three studies that incorporated high-intensity plyometrics reduced ACL risk, but the studies that did not incorporate high-intensity plyometrics did not reduce ACL injury risk.

   b. Conclusions from this meta-analysis include that neuromuscular training may assist in the reduction of ACL injuries in females athletes under the following conditions.

      i. Plyometrics and technique training are incorporated into a comprehensive training protocol.

      ii. Balance and strengthening exercise may be used as adjuncts but may not be effective if used alone.

      iii. The training sessions are performed more than once per week.

      iv. The training program lasts a minimum of 6 weeks.

B. Ankle ligament sprains

1. The fundamental premise of prevention of ankle ligament injuries is that they occur not randomly but in patterns that reflect the process of the underlying causes.

   a. Consequently, it is important to understand the risk factors for these common injuries.

   b. Not only does this facilitate the development of prevention programs, but it also allows the identification of those at increased risk of injury so an intervention can be targeted at them.

2. One of the most significant risk factors for a lateral ankle ligament sprain is a previous ankle injury.

3. In addition, reduced dorsiflexion, poor proprioception, increased postural sway, and strength imbalances of the muscles that span the ankle have been associated with increased risk of sustaining an inversion ankle ligament injury.

4. Recognizing that one of the most important risk factors for an ankle ligament injury is a prior ankle ligament tear, adequate rehabilitation following an ankle injury before returning to sports participation is an important consideration.

   a. This includes the concept of progressive strength training of the muscles that span the ankle complex and sensory-motor training of the lower extremity.

   b. Sensory-motor training programs that include a minimum of 10 minutes of balance training 5 days a week for at least 10 weeks, with activities such as single-leg stance on an unstable balance pad or balance board training, can have a dramatic effect on improving sensory motor control.

5. The risk of sustaining an ankle ligament injury (or reinjury) can be minimized with the use of taping or bracing.

   a. There is evidence that taping is of value in preventing ankle injuries, but a taped ankle loses as much as 40% of the ankle range of restrictiveness following 10 minutes of exercise.

   b. Because of the problems associated with taping, the use of ankle bracing has increased in recent times.

Top Testing Facts

1. Bench press with the use of free weights is an isoinertial exercise.

2. Isotonic exercises apply a muscle contraction throughout a range of motion against a constant muscle force.

3. Isometric exercises involve muscle contraction without appreciable joint motion.

4. Isokinetic exercises occur when the speed of a muscle contraction is fixed but the resistance varies depending on the force exerted through the range of motion.

5. Plyometric exercises such as bounding and hopping are effective in ACL injury prevention programs.

6. Initial treatment of ankle sprain should be RICE.

7. PNF involves a three-step stretching technique combining passive stretching and isometric stretching.

8. Female athletes have a risk of ACL tears that is two to eight times that of their male counterparts.

9. Closed chain exercises are exercises in which the foot is fixed to the ground or a wall.

10. Periodization is a planned workout in which the volume and/or intensity of training is varied over time.

11. Shoulder rehabilitation for instability is highly dependent on the type and direction of instability and any surgical intervention.

Bibliography

Beynnon BD, Renstrom PA, Haugh L, Uh BS, Barker H: A prospective, randomized clinical investigation of the treatment of first time ankle sprains. *Am J Sports Med* 2006;34: 1401-1412.

Beynnon BD, Vacek PM, Murphy D, Alosa D, Paller D: First-time inversion ankle ligament trauma: The effects of sex, level of competition, and sport on the incidence of injury. *Am J Sports Med* 2005;33:1485-1491.

Escamilla RF, Fleisig GS, Zheng N, Barrentine SW, Wilk KE, Andrews JR: Biomechanics of the knee during closed kinetic chain and open kinetic chain exercises. *Med Sci Sports Exerc* 1998;30:556-569.

Hayes K, Callanan M, Walton J, Paxinos A, Murrell GA: Shoulder instability: Management and rehabilitation. *J Orthop Sports Phys Ther* 2002;32:497-509.

5: Sports Medicine

Hewett TE, Ford KR, Myer GD: Anterior cruciate ligament injuries in female athletes: Part 2. A meta-analysis of neuromuscular interventions aimed at injury prevention. *Am J Sports Med* 2006;34:490-498.

Hewett TE, Myer GD, Ford KR: Decrease in neuromuscular control about the knee with maturation in female athletes. *J Bone Joint Surg Am* 2004;86:1601-1608.

Nyland J, Nolan MF: Therapeutic modality: Rehabilitation of the injured athlete. *Clin Sports Med* 2004;23:299-313.

Prentice WE: *Therapeutic Modalities for Sports Medicine and Athletic Training*, ed 5. Boston, MA, McGraw-Hill, 2002.

Verhagen E, van der Beek A, Twisk J, Bouter L, Bahr R, van Mechelen W: The effect of a proprioceptive balance board training program for the prevention of ankle sprains: A prospective controlled trial. *Am J Sports Med* 2004;32:1385-1393.

Wright RW, Preston E, Fleming BC, et al: ACL reconstruction rehabilitation: A systematic review (Part I). *J Knee Surg* 2008;21(3):217-224.

Wright RW, Preston E, Fleming BC, et al: ACL reconstruction rehabilitation: A systematic review (Part II). *J Knee Surg* 2008;21(3):225-234.

5: Sports Medicine

Section 6

Trauma

Section Editor

Kenneth J. Koval, MD

Chapter 49

Gunshot Wounds and Open Fractures

Kenneth J. Koval, MD

I. Gunshot Wounds

A. Epidemiology

1. One third to one half of US households contain firearms.

2. Two thirds of weapons are loaded and stored within reach of children.

3. Firearm-related deaths totaled 30,136 in 2003 and 69,825 in 2005.

B. Ballistics

1. Low-velocity firearms are defined as <2,000 ft/sec and include all handguns.

2. High-velocity firearms are defined as >2,000 ft/sec and include all military rifles and most hunting rifles.

3. Shotguns can inflict either high- or low-energy injuries. Their wounding potential depends on three factors.

   a. Chote (shot pattern)

   b. Load (size of the individual pellet)

   c. Distance from target

C. Energy

1. The kinetic energy (KE) of a moving object is proportional to its mass (m) and the square of its velocity (v^2) and is defined by the equation: $KE = 1/2 \ (mv^2)$.

2. The energy delivered by a missile to a target is dependent on three factors.

   a. The energy of the missile on impact (striking energy)

   b. The energy of the missile on exiting the tissue (exit energy)

   c. The behavior of the missile while traversing the target (eg, tumbling, deformation, fragmentation)

D. Tissue parameters

1. The wounding potential of a bullet depends on its caliber, mass, velocity, range, composition, and design, as well as characteristics of the target tissue.

2. The degree of injury created by the missile depends on the specific gravity of the traversed tissue. The higher the specific gravity of the tissue, the greater the tissue damage.

3. A missile projectile achieves a high kinetic energy due to its high velocity.

   a. The impact area is relatively small, resulting in a small area of entry.

   b. A momentary vacuum is created by its resultant soft-tissue shock wave, which can draw adjacent material, such as clothing and skin, into the wound.

4. The direct passage of the missile through the target tissue defines the permanent cavity. The permanent cavity is small, and the surrounding tissues are subjected to crush.

5. A temporary cavity (cone of cavitation) is created by a stretch-type injury from the dissipation of imparted kinetic energy (ie, shock wave). It is larger than the permanent cavity; its size distinguishes high-energy from low-energy wounds.

6. Gases are compressible, whereas liquids are not.

   a. Penetrating missile injuries to the chest may produce destructive patterns only along the direct path of missile.

   b. Similar injuries to fluid-filled structures (eg, liver, muscle) produce considerable displacement of the incompressible liquid with shock-wave dissipation, resulting in much larger momentary cavities. This may lead to regions of destruction apparently distant to the immediate path of the missile with resultant soft-tissue compromise.

E. Clinical evaluation

1. Specific evaluation of the gunshot injury is based on the location of injury and patient presentation. A thorough physical examination must be performed to rule out the possibility of neurovascular damage.

2. Radiographic evaluation is necessary to assess for retained missile fragments, amount of fracture comminution, and the presence of other foreign bodies (eg, gravel).

3. Missile fragments often can be found distant to the site of missile entry or exit.

F. Treatment

1. Low-velocity wounds are treated based on fracture type

   a. Outpatient nonsurgical treatment

      i. Antibiotics (first-generation cephalosporin), tetanus toxoid, antitoxin

      ii. Irrigation and débridement of the entrance and exit skin edges

   b. Indications for surgical débridement

      i. Retention of bullet fragments in the subarachnoid or joint space

      ii. Vascular disruption

      iii. Gross contamination

      iv. A missile that is palpable on the palm or sole

      v. Massive hematoma, severe tissue damage, compartment syndrome, or gastrointestinal contamination

   c. Fractures generally are treated similar to a closed fracture.

2. High-velocity and shotgun wounds should be treated like high-energy injuries with significant soft-tissue damage

   a. Administration of antibiotics (first-generation cephalosporin), tetanus toxoid, antitoxin

   b. Extensive and often multiple surgical débridements

   c. Fracture stabilization

   d. Delayed wound closure with possible skin grafts or flaps for extensive soft-tissue loss

3. Gunshot wounds that pass through the abdomen and exit through the soft tissues with bowel contamination deserve special attention. These require débridement of the intra-abdominal and extra-abdominal missile paths, along with administration of broad-spectrum antibiotics covering gram-negative and anaerobic pathogens.

G. Complications

1. Retained missile fragments

   a. These generally are well tolerated and do not warrant a specific indication for surgery.

   b. Surgical exploration is necessary if symptoms develop (ie, pain, loss of function), the wound is in a superficial location (especially on the palms or soles) or in an intra-articular or subarachnoid location.

2. Foreign bodies in the wound

   a. Gunshot injuries are not necessarily "sterile injuries," with contamination secondary to skin flora, clothing, and other foreign bodies that may be drawn into the wound at the time of injury.

   b. Meticulous débridement and copious irrigation minimize the possibility of wound infection, abscess formation, and osteomyelitis.

3. Neurovascular damage

   a. The incidence of neurovascular damage is much higher in high-velocity injuries, secondary to shockwave energy dissipation.

   b. Temporary cavitation may result in traction or avulsion injuries to neurovascular structures remote from the immediate path of the missile.

4. Contamination with lead breakdown products

   a. Synovial or cerebrospinal fluid is caustic to lead components of bullet-missiles, resulting in lead break-down products that may produce severe synovitis and low-grade lead poisoning.

   b. Intra-articular or subarachnoid retention of missiles or missile fragments are indications for exploration and missile removal.

II. Open Fractures

A. Definition—An open fracture is a fracture that communicates with an overlying break in the skin.

B. Clinical evaluation

1. Initial assessment focuses on Airway, Breathing, Circulation, Disability, and Exposure (ABCDE).

   a. Because one third of patients with open fractures have multiple injuries, evaluation for life-threatening injuries must be addressed first, followed by injuries to the head, chest, abdomen, pelvis, and spine.

   b. Injuries to all four extremities must next be assessed, including a complete soft-tissue and neurovascular examination.

2. Surgical exploration of the open wound in the emergency setting is not indicated if surgical intervention is planned. Exploration risks further contamination with limited capacity to provide useful information and may precipitate further hemorrhage. However, if a surgical delay is expected, open wounds can be irrigated in the emergency department with sterile normal saline solution.

3. Compartment syndrome must be considered a possibility with all extremity fractures.

   a. Pain out of proportion to the injury, pain to passive stretch of fingers or toes, a tense extremity, and decreased sensation are all clues to the diagnosis.

   b. In the appropriate clinical setting, a strong suspicion based on clinical findings or if the patient is unconscious warrants monitoring of compartment pressures.

   c. Compartment pressures within 30 mm Hg of the diastolic blood pressure indicate compartment syndrome and the need for emergent fasciotomy.

C. Radiographic evaluation

1. A radiographic trauma survey includes a lateral cervical spine and AP views of the chest, abdomen, and pelvis.

2. Extremity radiographs should be ordered as indicated by clinical examination.

3. Additional studies such as CT (with and without contrast), cystography, urethrography, intravenous pyelogram, and angiography are ordered as clinically indicated.

4. Angiography should be obtained based on clinical suspicion of vascular injury and the following indications.

   a. Knee dislocations with an ankle-brachial index (ABI) <0.9

   b. A cool, pale foot with poor distal capillary refill

   c. High-energy injury in an area of compromise (eg, trifurcation of the popliteal artery)

   d. Documented ABI <0.9 associated with a lower extremity injury

D. Classification of open fractures

1. Gustilo and Anderson—Based on the size of the open wound, amount of muscle contusion and soft-tissue crush, fracture pattern, amount of periosteal stripping, and vascular status of the limb. This classification has been shown to have poor interobserver reproducibility.

   a. Grade I: Clean skin opening of <1 cm, usually from inside to outside with minimal muscle

contusion. The fracture pattern usually is simple transverse or short oblique.

   b. Grade II: A laceration >1 cm long, with extensive soft-tissue damage and minimal to moderate crushing component. The fracture pattern usually is simple transverse or short oblique with minimal comminution.

   c. Grade III: Extensive soft-tissue damage, including the muscles, skin, and neurovascular structures. These are high-energy injuries with a severe crushing component.

      i. IIIA: Extensive soft-tissue damage but adequate osseous coverage; there is no need for rotational or free flap coverage. The fracture pattern can be comminuted and segmental.

      ii. IIIB: Extensive soft-tissue injury with periosteal stripping and bone exposure requiring soft-tissue flap closure. These injuries usually are associated with massive contamination.

      iii. IIIC: Indicates a vascular injury requiring repair.

2. Tscherne—Takes into account wound size, level of contamination, and fracture mechanism.

   a. Grade I: Associated with a small puncture wound without associated muscle contusion and negligible bacterial contamination. These injuries result from a low-energy mechanism of injury.

   b. Grade II: Associated with a small skin laceration, minimal soft-tissue contusion, and moderate bacterial contamination. These injuries can result from a variety of mechanisms of injury.

   c. Grade III: Has a large laceration with heavy bacterial contamination and extensive soft-tissue damage. These injuries are frequently associated with arterial or neural injury.

   d. Grade IV: Incomplete or complete amputation with variable prognosis based on location of and nature of injury.

E. Nonsurgical treatment

1. Emergency department—occurs after the initial trauma survey and resuscitation for life-threatening injuries

   a. Control bleeding by direct pressure rather than limb tourniquets or blind clamping.

   b. Perform a careful clinical and radiographic examination.

   c. Initiate parenteral antibiotics and tetanus prophylaxis.

   d. Assess skin and soft-tissue damage and place a saline-soaked sterile dressing on the wound.

Table 1

Requirements for Tetanus Prophylaxis

Immunization History	dT	TIG	dT	TIG
Incomplete (<3 doses) or not known	+	-	+	+
Complete but >10 years since last dose	+	-	+	-
Complete and <10 years since last dose	-	-	-*	-

dT = diphtheria and tetanus toxoids; TIG = tetanus immune globulin; + = prophylaxis required; – = prophylaxis not required
* = required if >5 years since last dose

e. Reduce and splint all fractures.

f. Prepare the patient for emergent surgical débridement and osseous stabilization. Intervention within 8 hours after injury has been reported to result in a lower incidence of wound infection and osteomyelitis. However, there has been a move to delay operating on lower energy open fractures in the middle of the night and to treat the injury first thing in the morning.

2. Antibiotic coverage

a. Gustilo grades I and II open fractures usually are treated with a first-generation cephalosporin for 72 hours after each débridement.

b. Gustilo grade III open fractures are treated with a first-generation cephalosporin and an aminoglycoside.

c. Farm injuries are treated similar to grade III injuries with the addition of penicillin.

3. Tetanus prophylaxis

a. Should be initiated in the emergency room.

b. The current dose of toxoid is 0.5 mL, regardless of patient age.

c. For immune globulin, the dose is 75 U for patients younger than 5 years, 125 U for patients between 5 and 10 years, and 250 U for patients older than 10 years.

d. Both shots are administered intramuscularly, each from a different syringe and into a different site.

e. Requirements for tetanus prophylaxis are shown in **Table 1**.

F. Surgical treatment

1. Adequate irrigation and débridement is the most important step in open fracture management.

a. The wound should be extended proximally and distally to expose and explore the zone of injury.

b. Meticulous débridement should begin with the skin and subcutaneous fat and extended down to bone.

2. The fracture surfaces should be exposed, with re-creation of the injury mechanism.

a. Tendons, unless severely damaged or contaminated, should be preserved.

b. Bone fragments should be discarded only if they are devoid of soft-tissue attachments.

c. Extension into adjacent joints mandates exploration, irrigation, and débridement.

3. Pulsatile lavage irrigation, with or without antibiotic solution, should be performed.

4. Intraoperative cultures are considered not necessary.

5. Fasciotomy should be considered, especially in the forearm or leg.

6. Wound closure

a. Historically, traumatic wounds should not be closed. More recently, however, some trauma centers have been closing the open wound after débridement with close observation for signs or symptoms of sepsis.

b. If the wound is left open, it should be dressed with a saline-soaked gauze, synthetic dressing, a vacuum-assisted closure (VAC) sponge, or an antibiotic bead pouch.

7. Serial débridement(s) may be performed every 24 to 48 hours as necessary until there is no evidence of necrotic tissue.

G. Fracture stabilization

1. Provides protection from additional soft-tissue injury, maximum access for wound management, and maximum limb and patient mobilization.

2. The type of fracture stabilization (internal or external fixation) depends on the fracture location and degree of soft-tissue injury.

H. Soft-tissue coverage and bone grafting

1. Wound coverage is indicated once there is no further evidence of tissue necrosis.

a. Types include primary closure, split-thickness skin graft, and rotational or free muscle flap.

b. The type of soft-tissue coverage depends on the severity and location of the soft-tissue injury.

2. Bone grafting can be performed when the wound is clean, closed, and dry.

a. The timing of bone grafting after free flap coverage is controversial.

b. Some advocate bone grafting at the time of coverage; others wait until the flap has healed (normally 6 weeks).

I. Limb salvage versus amputation

1. In Gustilo grade III injuries, the choice between limb salvage and amputation is controversial.

2. Indications for immediate or early amputation

a. Nonviable limb, irreparable vascular injury, warm ischemia time of more than 8 hours, or a severe crush injury with minimal remaining viable tissue

b. Attempts at limb salvage leave the limb so severely damaged that function will be less satisfactory than that afforded by a prosthetic replacement.

c. The severely damaged limb constitutes a threat to the patient's life, especially in patients with severe, debilitating, or chronic disease.

d. The severity of the injury would demand multiple surgical procedures and prolonged reconstruction time that is incompatible with the personal, sociologic, and economic consequences the patient is willing to withstand.

e. The patient presents with severe multiple trauma in which the salvage of a marginal extremity may result in a high metabolic cost or large necrotic/inflammatory load that could precipitate pulmonary or multiple organ failure.

J. Complications

1. Infection

a. Open fractures may result in cellulitis or osteomyelitis despite aggressive serial débridements, copious lavage, appropriate antibiosis, and meticulous wound care.

b. Higher grade open fractures are at increased risk for infection.

c. Gross contamination at the time of injury is causative, although retained foreign bodies, soft-tissue compromise, and multiple-system injury also are risk factors.

2. Compartment syndrome

a. Devastating complication that can result in severe loss of function.

b. A high index of suspicion is required, with serial neurovascular examinations accompanied by compartment pressure monitoring, as needed.

c. Prompt identification of impending compartment syndrome and fascial release are essential to minimize the risk of long-term disability.

Top Testing Facts

1. The distinction between low- and high-velocity gunshot wounds is the speed of the projectile: low-velocity is <2,000 ft/sec; high-velocity is >2,000 ft/sec.

2. Shotgun blasts can inflict either high- or low-energy injuries, depending on chote (shot pattern), load (pellet size), and distance from the target.

3. Low-velocity gunshot wounds can be treated similar to a closed fracture, with antibiotics and débridement of the entrance and exit skin edges.

4. Indications for surgical débridement of low-velocity gunshot wounds include bullet fragments in the subarachnoid or joint space, vascular disruption, gross contamination, a palpable bullet fragment on the palm or sole, massive hematoma, severe tissue damage, compartment syndrome, or gastrointestinal contamination.

5. High-velocity gunshot wounds should be treated like high-energy injuries.

6. Open fractures should be treated with emergent surgical débridement and fracture stabilization.

7. Gustilo grades I and II open fractures can be treated with a first-generation cephalosporin, grade III with cephalosporin and an aminoglycoside, and farm injuries similar to grade III with the addition of penicillin.

8. Intraoperative cultures are not considered necessary for open fractures.

9. For open fractures, fracture stabilization provides protection from further soft-tissue injury.

10. For Gustilo grade III fractures, the indications for limb salvage versus amputation are controversial.

Bibliography

Bosse MJ, McCarthy ML, Jones AL, et al: The Lower Extremity Assessment Project (LEAP) Study Group: The insensate foot following severe lower extremity trauma. An indication for amputation? *J Bone Joint Surg Am* 2005;87:2601-2608.

Brumback RJ, Jones AL: Intraobserver agreement in the classification of open fractures of the tibia: The results of a survey of 245 orthopaedic surgeons. *J Bone Joint Surg Am* 1994; 76:1162-1166.

6: Trauma

Cole JD, Ansel LJ, Schwartzberg R: A sequential protocol for management of severe open tibial fractures. *Clin Orthop Relat Res* 1995;315:84-103.

Gustilo RB, Anderson J: Prevention of infection in the treatment of one thousand and twenty-five open fractures of long bones: Retrospective and prospective analyses. *J Bone Joint Surg Am* 1976;58:453-458.

Herscovici D Jr, Sanders RW, Scaduto JM, Infante A, DiPasquale T: Vacuum-assisted wound closure (VAC therapy) for the management of patients with high-energy soft tissue injuries. *J Orthop Trauma* 2003;17:683-688.

Keating JF, Blachut PA, O'Brien PJ, Meek RN, Broekhuyse H: Reamed nailing of open tibial fractures: Does the antibiotic bead pouch reduce the deep infection rate? *J Orthop Trauma* 1996;10:298-303.

MacKenzie EJ, Bosse MJ, Kellam JF, et al: LEAP Study Group: Factors influencing the decision to amputate or reconstruct after high-energy lower extremity trauma. *J Trauma* 2002;52:641-649.

McQueen MM, Gaston P, Court-Brown CM: Acute compartment syndrome: Who is at risk? *J Bone Joint Surg Br* 2000; 82:200-203.

Swan KG, Swan RC. *Gunshot Wounds: Pathophysiology and Management, ed 2.* Chicago, Year Book Medical Publishers, 1989.

Volgas DA, Stannard JP, Alonso JE: Ballistics: A primer for the surgeon. *Injury* 2005;36:373-379.

Chapter 50

Evaluation of the Trauma Patient
Philip Wolinsky, MD

I. Definition and Epidemiology

A. Definition—A major trauma victim is an individual who has potentially life- and/or limb-threatening injuries and requires hospitalization.

B. Epidemiology

1. Trauma is the fourth leading cause of death in the United States overall, but it is the leading cause of death in adults younger than 44 years. In 1999, 54 deaths per 100,000 people occurred as result of an injury; 8 of every 10 deaths in adults between the ages of 15 and 24 years result from injuries.

2. Worldwide, injuries cause 1 in 10 deaths.

3. Each year, 1.5 million individuals are admitted to hospitals and survive to discharge after an injury, representing 8% of all hospital discharges. Of emergency department visits, 38% occur for injury treatment.

4. The total lifetime costs for traumatic injuries that occur in 1 year have been estimated to be $260 billion; 41% of this cost is due to lost productivity of the injured individuals (1995 dollars).

5. The elderly (age ≥65 years) are at the highest risk for fatal or nonfatal injures requiring hospitalization. The incidence of injuries that result in death is 113 in 100,000 for patients age 65 years and older, and 169 in 100,000 for patients age 75 years and older.

6. Fatal injuries

   a. Major mechanisms of injury for traumatic injury and deaths in 1999 are listed in Table 1.

   b. Leading causes of traumatic death

      i. Central nervous system injuries: 40% to 50%

      ii. Hemorrhage: 30% to 35%

   c. Nonaccidental deaths represent 31% of traumatic deaths: of these, 63% are suicides, and 37% are homicides.

7. Nonfatal injuries

   a. The leading cause of nonfatal injuries is falls (representing 39% of hospitalizations).

Table 1	
Mechanisms of Injury in Accidental Deaths*	
Mechanism of Injury	**% of deaths**
Motor vehicle accidents	31
Gunshot wounds	19
Poisonings	13
Falls	9

*Data are from 1999.

   b. Injuries to the extremities are the leading reason for hospitalization (47%) and emergency department visits after nonfatal trauma. About 33% of extremity injuries that require hospitalization have an Abbreviated Injury Scale (AIS) score of 3 or above. These are moderately severe to severe injuries that may have a long recovery period and can result in permanent impairment.

II. Mortality and the Golden Hour

A. Three peak times of death after trauma

1. About 50% occur within minutes, from either a neurologic injury or massive hemorrhage.

2. Another 30% occur within the first few days after injury, most commonly from a neurologic injury.

3. The final 20% die days to weeks after injury as a result of infection and/or multiple organ failure.

B. The Golden Hour

1. Defined as the period of time during which life- and/or limb-threatening injuries should be treated so that the treatment results in a satisfactory outcome.

2. The Golden Hour can range from minutes for a compromised airway to hours for an open fracture.

3. Approximately 60% of preventable in-hospital deaths occur during the Golden Hour.

6: Trauma

III. Prehospital Care and Field Triage

A. General principles

1. Rapid assessment to identify life-threatening injuries

2. Proper field triage is critical to avoid wasting resources; only 7% to 15% of trauma patients require the resources of a level I or II trauma center.

3. Appropriate intervention to address life-threatening conditions (airway, breathing, circulation, external hemorrhage control)

4. Rapid transport

B. Goals of field triage

1. To match a patient's needs with the resources of a particular hospital

2. To transport all seriously injured patients to an appropriate hospital

3. To determine what resources will be needed at the time of arrival of the patient

4. To identify whether the patient is a major trauma victim

5. To monitor the rates of overtriage and undertriage

C. Components of field triage

1. Rapid decision making based on physiologic, anatomic, mechanism of injury (to assess the amount of energy absorbed at the time of injury), and comorbidity factors

   a. Physiologic criteria include assessment of vital signs such as blood pressure, heart rate, respiration rate and effort, level of consciousness, and temperature. These changes or trends may take time to see, particularly in younger patients.

   b. Anatomic criteria include observations based on physical examination, such as penetrating injuries to the head, neck, or torso; obvious fractures; burns; and amputations. These assessments, however, can be difficult in the field, particularly in a patient with an altered level of consciousness.

   c. Mechanisms of injury that may result in major injuries include falls of more than 15 feet; motor vehicle accidents in which a fatality has occurred, a passenger has been ejected, extrication has taken longer than 20 minutes, or a pedestrian was struck; motorcycle accidents in which the vehicle was traveling faster than 20 mph; or an obvious penetrating injury. Use of the mechanism of injury alone to assess injury severity may result in a high overtriage rate, but combining it with physiologic or anatomic data improves triage.

   d. Comorbidity factors include increased patient age, presence of chronic disease, and acute issues such as drug and alcohol intoxication.

2. Numerous scoring systems have been developed for field triage that use all or parts of these data.

D. Components of field assessment

1. Goals

   a. Should be quick and systematic

   b. Patients with potentially life-threatening injures must be quickly transported to the closest appropriate hospital; definitive care for internal hemorrhage cannot be provided at the scene.

2. Primary survey (ABCDE—*A*irway, *B*reathing, *C*irculation, *D*isability, *E*xposure)

   a. Performed just as in Advanced Trauma Life Support (ATLS) to establish priorities for management

   b. Treatment is initiated as problems are identified (same as ATLS).

3. Indications for field intubation

   a. Glasgow Coma Scale total score <8 (inability to maintain an airway)

   b. Need for ventilation

   c. Potentially threatened airway (inhalation injuries, expanding neck hematoma, etc.)

   d. Ventilation required if respiration rate is less than 10 breaths per minute.

4. External bleeding is controlled with direct pressure.

5. Initiation of intravenous fluids in the field remains controversial. In general, transport should not be delayed just to start fluids.

6. Secondary survey

   a. Performed after any acute issues have been addressed, perhaps during transport.

   b. AMPLE history (*A*llergies to medications, *M*edications the patient is taking, *P*ertinent medical history, *L*ast time eaten, *E*vents leading to the injury)

   c. Head-to-toe examination

7. Extremity trauma

   a. Bleeding associated with fractures can be life-threatening.

   b. External hemorrhage is controlled with direct pressure.

   c. Immobilization of the extremity helps control internal bleeding.

d. For critical injuries, immobilization with a backboard is sufficient; if not, individual fractures should be splinted.

e. A traction splint should be used for suspected femur fractures because it stabilizes the fracture and controls pain.

8. Amputations

a. Clean the amputated parts by rinsing them with lactated Ringer solution.

b. Cover with sterile gauze moistened with Ringer solution and place in a plastic bag.

c. Label the bag and place it in another container filled with ice.

d. Do not allow the part to freeze.

e. Transport the part with the patient.

IV. Trauma Scoring Systems

A. Components of present scoring systems include physiologic data, anatomic data, a combination of the two, and specialized data.

B. Although no single scoring system has been universally adapted, each has advantages and disadvantages.

C. Types of physiologic scores

1. Acute Physiology and Chronic Health Evaluation (APACHE)

a. Combines preexisting systemic diseases with current physiologic issues

b. Frequently used for the evaluation of medical and surgical patients in intensive care units, but not good for patients with acute trauma

c. One drawback for trauma care is that it requires data obtained after 24 hours of hospitalization.

2. Systemic Inflammatory Response Syndrome Score (SIRS)

a. Scores heart and respiratory rates, temperature, and white blood cell count

b. Predicts mortality and length of hospital stay for trauma patients

D. Types of anatomic scores

1. Glasgow Coma Scale

a. An attempt to score the function (level of consciousness) of the central nervous system

b. Components (**Table 2**)

2. Abbreviated Injury Scale (AIS)

a. Developed to accurately rate and compare injuries sustained in motor vehicle accidents.

b. Injuries scored from 1 (minor injuries) to 6 (fatal within 24 hours).

c. A total of 73 different injuries can be scored, but there is no mechanism to combine the individual injury scores into one score.

3. Injury Severity Score (ISS)

a. The sum of the squares of the three highest AIS scores of six regions provides an overall severity score (includes head and neck, face, thorax, abdomen, pelvis, extremities).

b. Each region is scored on a scale from 1 (minor injury) to 6 (almost always fatal).

c. An AIS score of 6 is automatically assigned an ISS value of 75, which represents a nonsurvivable injury.

d. A score of 15 or higher is frequently used as the definition of major trauma and correlates well with mortality.

e. Because ISS scores only one injury per body region, it does not reflect patient morbidity associated with multiple lower extremity fractures.

Table 2

Glasgow Coma Scale

Parameter	Score					
	6	5	4	3	2	1
Eye opening			Spontaneous	To voice	To pain	None
Verbal response		Oriented	Confused	Inappropriate	Incomprehensible	None
Motor response	Obeys command	Localized pain	Withdraws from pain	Flexion to pain	Extension to pain	None

6: Trauma

4. New Injury Severity Score (NISS)

   a. This modification of the ISS sums the squares of the AIS scores of the three most significant injuries, even if they occur in the same anatomic area.

   b. Better predictor of survival than the ISS

   c. One study looking at orthopaedic blunt trauma patients found the NISS to be superior to the ISS.

D. Combined systems

   1. Trauma and Injury Severity Score (TRISS)

      a. Tries to predict mortality based on postinjury anatomic and physiologic abnormalities

      b. Uses age, the Revised Trauma Score (RTS) calculated in the emergency department, the ISS (calculated using discharge diagnosis), and whether the injury mechanism was blunt or penetrating.

      c. The data from any institution can then be compared to the mortality data from the Major Trauma Outcomes Study conducted by the American College of Surgeons in 1990.

   2. Harborview Assessment for Risk of Mortality (HARM)—Consists of 80 variables, including ICD-9 codes, comorbidities, mechanism of injury, self-inflicted versus accidental injury, combined injuries, and age.

V. Initial Hospital Workup and Resuscitation

A. Goals

   1. Diagnosis and treatment of life-threatening injures takes priority over a sequential, detailed, definitive workup.

   2. ATLS, which provides a systematic method to evaluate trauma patients, was developed to teach this concept and ultimately improve patient survival.

B. Components of ATLS

   1. Primary survey

      a. A systematic effort to quickly identify immediately life-threatening injuries

      b. Treatment and resuscitation are performed simultaneously as problems are identified.

      c. Consists of evaluation of ABCDEs, which may need to be repeated because patient reevaluation is constantly occurring during this step.

   2. Secondary survey

      a. Performed later as part of a head-to-toe physical examination and detailed medical history

      b. Intended to diagnose and treat injuries that are not an immediate threat to life when the patient's vital signs are normalizing

      c. Additional radiographs, CT, and laboratory tests are performed during this phase.

C. Shock

   1. Hypovolemic shock is the most common type in trauma patients.

   2. Signs and symptoms

      a. Decreased peripheral or central pulses; peripheral vasoconstriction is an early compensatory mechanism for shock.

      b. Pale and/or cool, clammy extremities; a tachycardic patient who has cool, clammy skin is in hypovolemic shock until proven otherwise.

      c. Heart rate >120 to 130 beats/min in adult trauma patients should be assumed to be caused by shock.

      d. Altered level of consciousness may indicate a brain injury, hypovolemic shock, or both; the key to preventing secondary brain injury is to prevent (or treat, if present) hypoxia and hypotension.

      e. Relying on systolic blood pressure measurements alone can be misleading; because of compensatory mechanisms, up to 30% of blood volume can be lost before a patient becomes hypotensive (**Table 3**).

      f. Pulse pressures may decrease with loss of as little as 15% of blood volume.

      g. Urine output, although useful to judge resuscitation, is not used during the primary survey.

D. Shock resuscitation

   1. Initial bolus of 2 L of crystalloid that can be repeated once if vital signs are not restored to normal

   2. Patients who respond well to fluid resuscitation likely had a 10% to 20% blood volume deficit; patients who do not respond have a higher volume deficit.

   3. As the second bolus is being given, blood should be obtained.

E. Initial radiographic evaluation

   1. Views include a chest radiograph, lateral view of the cervical spine, and AP view of the pelvis.

   2. The AP pelvis and chest radiographs can identify potential bleeding sources.

   3. Focused Assessment for the Sonographic Evaluation of the Trauma Patient (FAST) may be needed for patients with persistent hypotension; like a ra-

Table 3

Symptoms of Hypovolemic Shock by Hemorrhage Class

Hemorrhage Class	Blood Volume Loss (%)	Blood Loss	Symptoms
I	15	750 cc	Minimal
II	15-30	750-1,500 cc	Tachycardia, tachypnea, mild mental status changes, decreased pulse pressure
III	30-40	1,500-2,000 cc	Decreased systolic BP
IV	> 40	>2 L	

diographic evaluation, FAST is quickly obtained and can be performed in the trauma bay.

4. FAST is accurate for detecting free intraperitoneal fluid and looking for blood in the pericardial sac and dependent regions of the abdomen, including the right and left upper quadrants and pelvis, but it cannot detect isolated bowel injuries and does not reliably detect retroperitoneal injuries.

F. Patient may require diagnostic peritoneal lavage.

VI. Associated Injuries

A. Neck injuries

1. Any patient with an injury above the clavicle who is unconscious or has a neurologic deficit is assumed to have a cervical spine injury.

2. Immobilize the neck until it has been proven that no injury exists.

B. Pelvic (retroperitoneal) versus intra-abdominal bleeding

1. These two injuries may coexist.

2. If diagnostic peritoneal lavage is performed in the presence of a pelvis fracture, it should be supraumbilical and performed early, before the pelvic hematoma can track anteriorly.

3. Diagnostic peritoneal lavage has a 15% false-positive rate in this setting; false-negatives are rare.

4. Unstable pelvis fractures should be stabilized early. Pelvic binders or bed sheets are a simple, quick, and effective means to accomplish this.

C. Head injuries

1. Autoregulation of cerebral blood flow is altered after a head injury, and blood flow may become dependent on the mean arterial blood pressure.

2. Secondary brain injury may develop if hypoperfusion or hypoxia occurs after the initial insult.

3. Whether early definitive fracture surgery has an adverse effect on neurologic outcome remains subject to debate. At least one study that used neuropsychologic testing showed that this is not the case.

4. Early surgery leads to more blood and fluid requirements and may require invasive monitoring to ensure that adequate cerebral blood flow is maintained during surgery.

VII. Decision to Operate: Surgical Timing

A. Early considerations

1. Before the 1970s, definitive fracture surgery was performed on a delayed basis.

2. The philosophy of early total care became accepted as it became clear that early stabilization of long bone fractures in patients with multiple trauma (ISS ≥ 18) decreased pulmonary complications and perhaps mortality in the most severely injured patients.

B. Current considerations

1. At present it is unclear which subgroups of patients might be at risk from early surgery, particularly those with femoral shaft fractures stabilized with reamed intramedullary nails.

2. The initial focus was on patients with thoracic injuries, but the current consensus is that the extent of the pulmonary injury is related to the severity of the initial injury to the thorax.

3. Although still controversial, there is evidence that patients with "occult hypotension" have higher complication rates with early definitive surgery, as do those who are clearly underresuscitated.

6: Trauma

C. Damage control orthopaedics

1. Long bones are temporarily stabilized with external fixation and converted to definitive fixation after the patient has been resuscitated.

2. Complication rates with this approach are lower compared with early definitive fixation.

D. Hypothermia

1. Must be detected and corrected before definitive fracture fixation

2. Leads to increased mortality in trauma patients

3. Hypothermic: <35°C

4. International normalized ratio (INR) > 1.5

5. "Severe" head injury

VIII. Determination of Extent of Resuscitation

A. Determining which patients are in compensated shock and which patients have been fully resuscitated often is difficult.

B. The distinction, however, is critical because inadequate resuscitation may allow local inflammation to progress to systemic inflammation, which can cause distant organ dysfunction, including adult respiratory distress syndrome (ARDS) and/or multiple organ failure.

C. Patients with abnormal perfusion also may be at risk for the "second hit" phenomenon, in which a primed immune system has a supranormal response to a second insult, which may include surgical blood loss.

D. Vital signs including blood pressure, heart rate, and urine output are abnormal in patients with uncompensated shock but can normalize with compensated shock.

E. There is level 1 evidence that the base deficit or lactate level on admission is predictive of complication rates and mortality, but standard hemodynamic parameters are not.

F. There is level 2 evidence that following the base deficit and/or lactate (time to normalization) is predictive of survival and can be used to guide resuscitation.

G. Patients at risk for complications after early definitive treatment

1. Obvious shock: systolic blood pressure of <90 mm Hg

2. Abnormal base deficit or lactate level

a. Depends not only on the absolute value but also the trend

b. Normalizing is a good sign, whereas getting worse or failing to improve may indicate ongoing bleeding.

Top Testing Facts

1. A major trauma victim is an individual who has potentially life- and/or limb-threatening injuries and requires hospitalization.

2. The goal of prehospital care is to minimize preventable deaths.

3. Field triage requires rapid decisions based on physiologic, anatomic, mechanism of injury, and comorbidity factors.

4. During the initial treatment of a trauma patient, the diagnosis and treatment of critical injuries takes priority over a sequential, detailed, definitive workup.

5. The primary survey is a systematic effort to quickly identify life-threatening injuries.

6. The most common source of shock in a trauma patient is hypovolemic shock.

7. Resuscitation begins with a bolus of 2 L of crystalloid that can be repeated once if the vital signs are not restored to normal.

8. It is difficult to determine which patients are in compensated shock and which patients have been fully resuscitated.

9. Initial radiographic evaluation includes chest radiograph, lateral C-spine, and AP pelvis.

10. The base deficit or lactate level on admission is predictive of complication rates and mortality.

Bibliography

Balogh ZJ, Varga E, Tomka J, et al: The new injury severity score is a better predictor of extended hospitalization and intensive care admission than the injury severity score in patients with multiple orthopedic injuries. *J Orthop Trauma* 2003;17:508-512.

Crowl AC, Young JS, Kahler DM, et al: Occult hypoperfusion is associated with increased morbidity in patients undergoing early fracture fixation. *J Trauma* 2000;48:260-267.

Englehart MS, Schreiber MA: Measurement of acid-base resuscitation endpoints: Lactate, base deficit, bicarbonate, or what? *Curr Opin Crit Care* 2006;12:569-574.

Harwood PJ, Giannoudis PV, Probst C, et al: The risk of local infective complications after damage control procedures for femoral shaft fracture. *J Orthop Trauma* 2006;20:181-188.

Harwood PJ, Giannoudis PV, van Griensven M, et al: Alterations in the systemic inflammatory response after early total care and damage control procedures for femoral shaft fracture in severely injured patients. *J Trauma* 2005;58:446-454.

McKee MD, Schemitsch EH, Vincent LO, et al: The effect of a femoral fracture on concomitant closed head injury in patients with multiple fractures. *J Trauma* 1997;42:1041-1045.

Moore E, Feliciano DV, Mattox KL (eds): *Trauma*, ed 5. New York, NY, McGraw-Hill, 2004.

Moore FA, McKinley BA, Moore EE, et al: Guidelines for shock resuscitation. *J Trauma* 2006;61:82-89.

Nowotarski PJ, Turen CH, Brumback RJ, Scarboro JM: Conversion of external fixation to intramedullary nailing for fractures of the shaft of the femur in multiply injured patients. *J Bone Joint Surg Am* 2000;82:781-788.

Osler T, Baker SP, Long W: A modification of the injury severity score that both improves accuracy and simplifies scoring. *J Trauma* 1997;43:922-926.

Pape HC, Hildebrand F, Pertschy S, et al: Changes in the management of femoral shaft fractures in polytrauma patients: From early total care to damage control orthopedic surgery. *J Trauma* 2002;53:452-462.

Poole GV, Tinsley M, Tsao AK, et al: AIS scale does not reflect the added morbidity of multiple lower extremity fractures. *J Trauma* 1996;40:951-955.

Schulman AM, Claridge JA, Carr G, et al: Predictors of patients who will develop occult hypoperfusion following blunt trauma. *J Trauma* 2004;57:795-800.

Shafi S, Elliot AC, Gentilello L: Is hypothermia simply a marker of shock and injury severity or an independent risk factor for mortality in trauma patients? *J Trauma* 2005;59:1081-1085.

Tisherman SA, Baie P, Bokhari F, et al: Clinical practice guideline: Endpoints of resuscitation. *J Trauma* 2004;57:898-912.

6: Trauma

Chapter 51

Hand and Wrist Fractures and Dislocations, Including Carpal Instability

Steven L. Moran, MD   Marco Rizzo, MD   Alexander Y. Shin, MD

I. Fractures of the Hand

A. General principles of fixation

1. Compression screws are stronger than Kirschner-wires (K-wires), which provide no compression.

2. Plates are stronger than screws alone. Screws have resistance to bending only in the plane of the screw and little resistance to rotational or shear stress.

   a. Compression plates resist bending and rotational forces better than neutralization or buttress plates.

   b. Dorsal plates are best at resisting dorsally applied bending forces.

   c. Plate bending strength is directly proportional to the thickness cubed and inversely proportional to the length cubed.

3. Lag screws

   a. Lag screws are indicated when fracture length is at least twice the bone diameter.

   b. Screws provide maximal compression when placed perpendicular to the fracture.

   c. Screws should be placed two screw head diameters apart.

B. Determinants of fracture stability (all fractures)

1. Fracture pattern (transverse-stable, oblique, and spiral-unstable)

2. Integrity of periosteal envelope

3. Muscle forces

4. External forces

C. Treatment goals (all fractures)

1. Stabilizing the fracture

2. Repairing injured soft tissue

3. Mobilizing adjacent joints and soft tissues, particularly tendons

4. Restoring articular congruity

D. Incidence of hand fractures by location

1. Distal phalanx: 45% to 50%

2. Metacarpal: 30% to 35%

3. Proximal phalanx: 15% to 20%

4. Middle phalanx: 8%

E. Predictors of poorer outcome following fracture fixation

1. Open fractures

2. Intra-articular fractures

3. Associated nerve injury

4. Associated tendon injury

5. Crush injury

II. Fractures of the Metacarpals

A. Anatomy and biomechanics

1. Most metacarpal diaphyseal fractures are apex dorsal as a result of the pull of the interossei, which results in flexion of the distal fragment.

2. The hand can adjust dorsal angulation by compensating with metacarpophalangeal (MCP) hyperextension and carpometacarpal (CMC) motion. CMC motion is greatest at the little finger (30°), followed by the ring finger (20°). The long and index fingers have minimal CMC motion and thus can tolerate less angular deformity.

3. Rotational deformity is poorly tolerated; >5° can lead to finger scissoring.

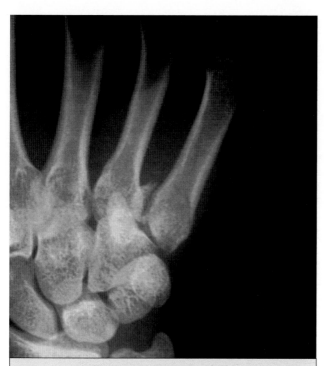

Figure 1 PA view of the hand demonstrates a base of the fifth metacarpal fracture, or "reverse Bennett" fracture. Note the subluxation of the base of the little finger metacarpal on the ulnar aspect of the hamate.

4. Normal physiologic rotation during digital flexion is 10° to 15° of pronation in the index and long fingers and 10° to 15° of supination in the ring and little fingers.

5. Shortening of 3 to 4 mm is tolerated. There is 7° of extensor lag per 2 mm of metacarpal shortening. MCP hyperextension usually can compensate for up to 4 mm of shortening.

6. Metacarpal shortening or angulation >30° can result in shortening of the intrinsics, which can lead to decrease in extensor excursion.

B. Fractures of the metacarpal diaphysis

1. Radiographic evaluation

   a. PA and lateral views are indicated.

   b. Acceptable angulation in metacarpal diaphyseal fractures:

      i. 20° at the index and long fingers

      ii. 40° at the ring and little fingers

      iii. More displacement is tolerable at the ring and little fingers because of the motion of the CMC joints at these fingers. The second and third CMC joints are relatively fixed.

2. Treatment

   a. Most metacarpal diaphyseal fractures can be treated nonsurgically.

b. Surgical treatment of these fractures is variable and may include percutaneous K-wire(s) placed longitudinally or transversely into the adjacent metacarpal, plate fixation, or intramedullary rods.

   i. K-wire fixation minimizes soft-tissue injury.

   ii. Plate fixation is usually performed dorsally.

   iii. Early mobilization is required to reduce the incidence of tendon adhesions.

c. Treatment of metacarpal diaphysis bone loss

   i. Distraction-fixation is used to restore length and alignment.

   ii. Soft-tissue coverage is crucial.

   iii. Secondary iliac crest bone graft can be used in fractures that are significantly contaminated.

   iv. An intramedullary wire or polymethylmethacrylate spacer can be used with secondary bone graft.

d. Malunion may be treated with opening or closing wedge osteotomies or derotational osteotomies in conjunction with internal fixation.

C. Fractures of the metacarpal base

1. Mechanism of injury/pathoanatomy

   a. Fractures of the metacarpal base can represent CMC fracture-dislocations.

   b. Fracture-dislocations are often associated with high-energy trauma, which may produce axial carpal injuries.

   c. Fracture-dislocations of the CMC joint of the little finger are sometimes called a "Tenneb" (*Bennett* spelled backward), "reverse Bennett," or "baby Bennett" fracture. The metacarpal diaphysis is displaced proximally and ulnarly as a result of the pull of the extensor carpi ulnaris (ECU) tendon (**Figure 1**).

2. Evaluation

   a. Oblique radiographs must be obtained to assess displacement.

   b. Sagittal CT also is helpful.

3. Treatment

   a. Congruent joint reduction is important to maintain mobility of the fourth and fifth CMC joints.

   b. Treatment of these fractures may be accomplished through closed reduction by longitudinal traction and K-wire fixation.

   c. More comminuted fractures may require external fixation.

d. In patients with posttraumatic arthritis, arthrodesis or hemi-arthroplasty can be considered.

D. Fractures of the metacarpal neck (boxer's fracture)

1. Acceptable angulation is similar to metacarpal diaphyseal fractures.

2. Excessive palmar displacement of the metacarpal head can lead to claw deformity, palmar mass, and extensor tendon lag.

E. Fractures of the metacarpal head

1. Evaluation—A Brewerton view (20° of MCP flexion) is needed for adequate visualization.

2. Surgical treatment—A dorsal approach is preferred.

III. Metacarpophalangeal Dislocations

A. Dorsal MCP dislocations

1. The most frequently involved digit is the index finger.

2. The thumb is also commonly involved.

B. Simple dislocation (subluxation)

1. Simple dislocations can be inadvertently converted to complete dislocation if improperly reduced.

2. Simple traction and hyperextension should not be used to reduce these dislocations. Instead, the finger should be flexed to take tension off the flexor tendons, and the base of the proximal phalanx should be pushed volarly and distally to slide the displaced volar plate over the metacarpal head.

C. Complex dislocation (complete dislocation)

1. Evaluation—The patient presents with the digit held in slight extension and a prominence in the palm.

2. Pathoanatomy—The metacarpal head is caught between the volar plate, flexor tendon, lumbrical, and A1 pulley.

3. Treatment

a. These dislocations are irreducible by closed means.

b. A volar approach puts digital nerves at risk of injury.

c. Dorsal approach—A longitudinal incision is made to split the volar plate. A freer elevator is used to push the volar plate in the palmar direction.

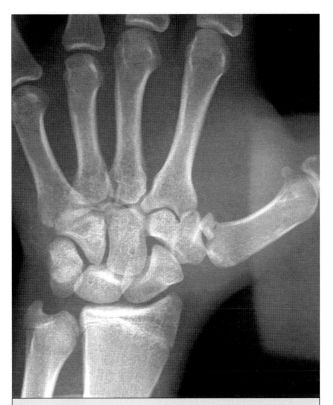

Figure 2   PA view of the hand demonstrates a Bennett fracture.

D. Fractures of the thumb metacarpal

1. Epidemiology and mechanism of injury

a. >80% of these fractures involve the base of the metacarpal.

b. These fractures are caused by an axially directed force through a partially flexed metacarpal.

2. Extra-articular fractures

a. Up to 30° of angulation is acceptable because of the mobility of the saddle joint.

b. Treatment is with a thumb spica cast and percutaneous K-wires as needed.

3. Bennett fracture—Base of the first metacarpal fracture (**Figure 2**)

a. Epidemiology—The Bennett fracture is the most common thumb fracture.

b. Mechanism of injury—The volar oblique ligament is attached to the volar ulnar fragment of the base; the abductor pollicis longus displaces the distal metacarpal proximally, and the adductor pollicis displaces the metacarpal into adduction. The metacarpal base is displaced dorsally and into supination.

c. Evaluation—The fracture is best visualized on the true lateral and hyperpronated AP (Robert) views.

d. Treatment

i. Closed reduction can be obtained with longitudinal traction with extension/abduction/pronation of the metacarpal as well as ulnarly based pressure over the base of the metacarpal. Percutaneous K-wire fixation may be used from the thumb metacarpal into the trapezium or into the index metacarpal.

ii. Open reduction is indicated if there is more than 2 to 3 mm of joint surface displacement or central impaction and a large fragment are present.

4. Rolando fracture

a. Rolando fractures are three-part Y or T intra-articular fractures.

b. Treatment

i. Open reduction and internal fixation (ORIF) (eg, interfragmentary screw, L- or T-plate)

ii. Alternative treatment includes external fixator and external traction device.

IV. Fractures of the Proximal and Middle Phalanx

A. Fractures of the proximal phalanx

1. Anatomy and biomechanics

a. Most transverse proximal phalanx fractures are apex palmar.

b. The central extensor tendon pulls the distal fragment dorsal, and the interossei insertion flexes the proximal fragment.

c. The proximal phalanx dorsal cortex is denser than the palmar cortex.

d. Proximal phalangeal fractures have less stability than metacarpal fractures because of multiple tendon forces acting on fragments.

e. Shortening of the proximal phalanx produces an extensor lag at the proximal interphalangeal (PIP) joint, with each millimeter of bone loss equaling 12° of extensor lag.

B. Fractures of the middle phalanx

1. Anatomy and biomechanics

a. Angulation depends on fracture position.

b. Proximal middle phalanx fractures are apex dorsal because of the pull of the central slip.

c. Distal middle phalanx fractures displace palmarly as a result of the pull of the superficialis insertion.

Table 1

Treatment for Fractures of the Proximal and Middle Phalanges

Type of Fracture	Treatment
Closed, displaced, stable	Consider buddy taping
Closed, displaced, unstable after reduction	Percutaneous K-wire Longitudinal K-wire for transverse/short oblique fractures Transverse K-wires for spiral/long oblique fractures Cast 3 to 4 weeks Begin motion in buddy tape in 24 to 48 hours
Closed, displaced, comminuted, unstable	Consider external fixator
Closed, displaced, unable to reduce	ORIF Transverse, short oblique fractures: tension band Long oblique, spiral fractures: lag screw Comminuted fractures: plate

d. Middle phalanx fractures may take longer to heal than fractures of the proximal phalanx and metacarpal because there is proportionately less cancellous bone in the diaphysis of the middle phalanx.

2. Complications—Shortening of the middle phalanx following fracture may result in distal interphalangeal joint extension lag.

C. Fractures of the proximal phalanx base—Extra-articular base fracture

1. Closed reduction and cast immobilization can be attempted with stable fractures, and the MCP joint should be flexed >60°.

2. Multiple tendon forces act on these fractures, so percutaneous K-wire fixation may provide more reliable fixation.

3. With complex trauma, including flexor tendon laceration, internal fixation with a minicondylar plate can allow early mobilization.

D. Fractures of the diaphysis of the proximal and middle phalanges

1. Angulation is usually volar apex as a result of the pull of the central slip and lateral bands.

2. Treatment—The type of fracture determines treatment (**Table 1**).

E. Fractures of the neck of the proximal and middle phalanges

1. Epidemiology and pathoanatomy

a. These fractures are uncommon in adults.

b. In children, phalangeal neck fractures may displace and rotate 90° (apex dorsally).

c. With complete displacement, the volar plate may become entrapped in the fracture.

2. Treatment

a. Treat with closed reduction and percutaneous K-wire.

b. Obtain lateral radiograph to verify reduction.

F. Condylar fractures of the proximal and middle phalanx

1. Evaluation—Evaluate angulation and malrotation with flexion fluoroscopy.

2. Treatment

a. Displaced condylar fractures require surgical reduction.

b. Internal fixation requires two screws, two wires, or a combination of both.

c. The PIP joint can be exposed by incising between the lateral band and the central tendon.

V. PIP Joint Dislocations and Fracture-Dislocations

A. Epidemiology

1. Dorsal—These PIP joint dislocations are common. They are often associated with volar plate avulsion or fracture of the volar base of the middle phalanx.

2. Lateral—These dislocations are uncommon.

3. Volar—These are rare.

B. Dorsal PIP joint dislocations and fracture-dislocations

1. Mechanism of injury: hyperextension and axial compression

2. Anatomy

a. The accessory collateral ligaments insert onto the volar plate.

b. The proper collateral ligaments insert onto the condyles.

c. Fracture-dislocations involving >40% of the volar base of the joint surface often disrupt both accessory and proper collateral ligaments, leading to an unstable fracture-dislocation.

3. Treatment of dorsal fracture-dislocations

a. Stable—Dorsal extension block splint with

joint in 60° to 70° of flexion, decreasing flexion 15° to 20° weekly.

b. Unstable—The usual options are:

i. ORIF

ii. Agee force couple or other dynamic skeletal traction

iii. Closed reduction and percutaneous K-wire fixation of the PIP joint in the reduced position

iv. Volar plate arthroplasty

4. Complications—Dorsal PIP joint dislocations may lead to pseudoboutonnière deformity.

C. Volar PIP joint fracture-dislocations

1. These injuries often involve a rotatory mechanism that disrupts the extensor mechanism and one central slip. The condyle can be trapped by the lateral band, preventing reduction.

2. If the central slip is disrupted, treatment must include initial immobilization of the finger in extension (in contradistinction to dorsal dislocations).

3. Volar PIP joint dislocations can lead to boutonnière deformity.

VI. Thumb MCP dislocations

A. Ulnar collateral ligament disruption (gamekeeper thumb)

1. Mechanism of injury and pathoanatomy

a. This injury results from a hyperabduction injury at the thumb MCP joint.

b. The adductor aponeurosis lies directly above the ulnar collateral ligament insertion on the ulnar aspect of the thumb. In many patients the avulsed ligament, with or without a bony fragment, may become displaced above the adductor aponeurosis, preventing reduction (Stener lesion).

2. Treatment

a. Partial tears without instability may be treated with immobilization for 4 to 6 weeks.

b. Complete tears and injuries associated with significant instability should be treated with surgical repair.

c. Chronic injuries may be treated with ligament reconstruction using tendon graft, MCP fusion, or adductor advancement.

VII. Fractures of the Distal Phalanx

A. Types of fractures

1. Tuft

2. Diaphyseal

3. Volar (mallet profundus tendon avulsion)

4. Dorsal (finger)

5. Epiphyseal injury (Seymour fracture)

B. Tuft fractures

1. Closed tuft fractures may be treated with a protective splint.

2. Open tuft fractures may require débridement and soft-tissue repair.

3. Widely displaced fractures require open reduction and possible internal fixation with K-wires.

4. Hypersensitivity may be present because of crushing of digital nerve terminal branches.

5. Fibrous unions of comminuted distal tuft fractures are often asymptomatic.

6. Subungual hematomas are commonly associated with tuft fractures.

   a. The hematoma should be decompressed for pain relief.

   b. Open repair of the nail plate will result in fewer nail deformities.

   c. Consider prophylactic antibiotics, as subungual hematomas can represent "open" fractures.

C. Fractures of the diaphysis of the distal phalanx

1. These fractures are usually stable and can be treated with a splint.

2. Longitudinal K-wires are used as needed.

D. Fractures of the base of the distal phalanx

1. These fractures are unstable as a result of the pull of the extensor and flexor tendons.

2. Dorsal apex angulation is typical.

3. The fracture fragment is avulsed from the extensor tendon insertion.

4. Mild deformity is well tolerated.

5. Treatment for most patients is splinting for 6 to 8 weeks.

E. Epiphyseal fractures (Seymour fracture)

1. Open epiphyseal fractures occur in children (typical mechanism: finger caught in car door).

2. The fracture results in nail matrix disruption. The plate may be avulsed lying dorsal to the proximal nail fold. The nail bed also may become interposed in fracture, resulting in nonunion or osteomyelitis.

F. Traumatic mallet finger

1. Indications for ORIF of traumatic mallet fingers

   a. Subluxation of the distal phalanx (volar subluxation seen with dorsal articular fracture fragment)

   b. Incongruity of the articular surface

2. Relative indications

   a. Articular fragment >40%

   b. Gap in articular surface >2 mm

VIII. Carpal Fractures

A. Scaphoid fractures

1. Epidemiology—The scaphoid is the most frequently fractured carpal bone.

2. Anatomy

   a. Half of the bone is covered by articular cartilage.

   b. Blood supply is through the palmar and dorsal vessels. The dorsal vessels supply the proximal pole and are at risk of injury with proximal pole fractures.

3. Mechanism of injury: Axial load across a hyperextended wrist

4. Evaluation

   a. Physical examination—The following findings are suggestive of a scaphoid fracture:

   i. Pain over the anatomic snuffbox

   ii. Pain with axial compression of first metacarpal

   iii. Tenderness at the scaphoid tuberosity

   b. Imaging

   i. Radiographs may initially appear normal.

   ii. When initial radiographs are normal, the patient can be casted and undergo one of the following: MRI within 24 hours (MRI allows for immediate identification of fractures and ligamentous injuries in addition to assessment of vascular status of the bone); bone scanning in 72 hours (bone scans obtained at 72 hours have an 85% to 93% positive predictive value); or repeat plain radiographs in 14 to 21 days.

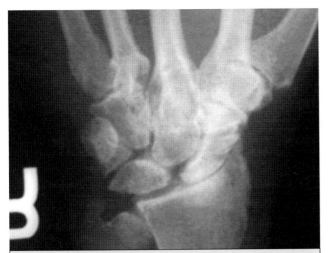

Figure 3 Radiograph of a patient with scapholunate advanced collapse (SLAC).

Table 2

Stages of Kienböck Disease

Stage	Characteristics
1	Changes evident only on bone scan
2	Increased sclerosis on plain radiographs
3a	Lunate collapse and/or fragmentation in the absence of increased radioscaphoid angle
3b	Lunate collapse and fragmentation with carpal instability as evidenced by radioscaphoid angle >60°
4	Pancarpal arthritis

5. Treatment

  a. Nonsurgical

    i. Nondisplaced scaphoid waist fractures, as verified by CT, can be treated with cast immobilization. A long arm-thumb spica cast has been shown to produce the smallest amount of internal scaphoid motion.

    ii. Distal pole scaphoid fractures, which occur commonly in children, almost always heal with nonsurgical treatment.

  b. Surgical

    i. Indications for surgery include displacement, evidence of a dorsal intercalated segment instability (DISI) deformity (radiolunate angle >15°), associated perilunate ligamentous injuries, and proximal pole fractures.

    ii. Procedures—Internal fixation with a compression screw has been found to produce results superior to K-wires alone. Proximal pole fractures can be treated successfully with immediate internal fixation. Avascularity and displacement result in the highest risk factor for nonunion. Treatment of nonunions has been reported with the use of vascularized bone grafts (1,2 intercompartmental recurrent branch of the radial artery) and internal fixation of the scaphoid. Vascularized pedicle grafts may be taken from either the dorsal or volar portion of the distal radius.

6. Complications

  a. Delay in acute fracture treatment beyond 28 days significantly increases risk of nonunion.

  b. Untreated scaphoid nonunions have the propensity to degenerate into a collapse or humpback deformity. Over time, this results in an increase in the radiolunate angle with degenerative changes occurring first at the radial styloid, radioscaphoid fossa, and eventually within the midcarpal joint. This degenerative pattern has been referred to as SNAC (scaphoid nonunion advanced collapse) (**Figure 3**) and is treated in a manner similar to scapholunate advanced collapse (SLAC).

B. Lunate injuries and Kienböck disease

  1. Injuries

    a. Traumatic dislocation of the lunate is more common than fracture.

    b. Large fracture fragments may be successfully treated with screw fixation (surgical approach is either volar through the carpal tunnel or dorsal).

    c. Volar avulsion fractures should raise suspicion of volar ligament disruption.

  2. Kienböck disease

    a. Definition—Kienböck disease is idiopathic osteonecrosis of the lunate.

    b. Etiology

      i. The etiology is unclear, but the shape of the lunate as well as the ulnar variance have been implicated. Positive ulnar variance has been linked to ulnar impaction, whereas ulnar negative variance has been linked to the development of Kienböck disease.

      ii. In cadaveric studies, 20% of lunates have been found to have a single artery supplying most of the bone. In patients with comparable anatomy, trauma may predispose them to progressive avascularity and collapse.

    c. Course of the disease—Kienböck disease follows a predictable course of lunate collapse with progressive arthritis (**Table 2**).

    d. Treatment—Treatment depends on the stage of the disease and the surgeon's preference.

6: Trauma

i. Stage 2 or 3a—Historically, for ulnar negative variance and stage 2 or 3a disease, a radial shortening osteotomy has provided good pain relief. Other options include capitate shortening and open and closing wedge osteotomies of the radius. Scaphotrapezial-trapezoid or scaphocapitate fusion may also be used for stage 3a disease. More recent options have included vascularized bone grafting from the dorsal distal radius, which has also shown good success with the possibility of revascularizing the lunate.

ii. Stage 3b disease is treated with proximal row carpectomy, wrist fusion, or total wrist arthroplasty.

iii. Stage 4 disease is treated with wrist fusion or total wrist arthroplasty.

C. Triquetrum fractures

1. Dorsal ridge fractures

a. Dorsal ridge fractures are not uncommon and can be associated with avulsions of the dorsal intercarpal ligaments, which insert on the triquetral ridge.

b. These fractures may often be treated with casting or splinting.

2. Volar fractures

a. Volar fractures of the triquetrum are more concerning.

b. These fractures can lead to lunotriquetral (LT) instability.

3. Body fractures

a. Fractures of the body of the triquetrum often can be treated with cast immobilization.

b. Volar body fractures may be associated with perilunate injuries.

D. Capitate fractures

1. Like the scaphoid, the capitate is covered mainly by cartilage, and the blood supply to the proximal pole can be compromised during transverse fractures. In such cases the proximal pole may develop osteonecrosis, requiring salvage with grafting or resection.

2. Scaphocapitate syndrome refers to a greater arc injury pattern where force passes from the scaphoid to the capitate neck, resulting in both scaphoid and capitate fractures. In this syndrome, the capitate head may be displaced 180°, requiring ORIF through a dorsal approach.

E. Hamate fractures

1. The most common presentation is a fracture of the hook of the hamate, which usually results

from a golf club, baseball bat, or racket sport injury.

2. Fractures may be treated with screw reduction or excision of the fragment, which avoids the possible complication of nonunion with reduction and closed casting.

IX. Wrist Instability and Dislocations

A. Anatomy and biomechanics

1. Radial wrist and scaphoid stabilizers

a. The scapholunate interosseous ligament (SLIL) is perceived as the primary stabilizer of the scapholunate joint. It is composed of three distinct portions:

i. The proximal or membranous portion, which has no significant strength

ii. The dorsal portion, which is the strongest portion and prevents translation

iii. The palmar portion, which acts as a rotational constraint

b. Distal scaphoid stabilizers include the scaphotrapezial interosseous ligaments (STIL).

c. The radioscapholunate ligament (ligament of Testut) is a volar intra-articular neurovascular structure and provides little mechanical stability.

d. The palmar stabilizers include the radioscaphocapitate ligament, long radiolunate ligament, and short radiolunate ligament. These ligaments are all thought to be secondary stabilizers of the scaphoid.

e. The dorsal stabilizers are the dorsal radiotriquetral ligament and the dorsal intercarpal ligament.

B. Pathomechanics

1. Mayfield described the four classic stages of progressive perilunate instability of the wrist (**Table 3**).

2. Reverse perilunate injury/dislocation also has been described and suggested by several authors as a mechanism of isolated LT ligament injury (**Table 3**).

C. Evaluation

1. Imaging

a. Radiographs

i. Carpal instability can be described by abnormalities seen on radiographs.

ii. Standard views: PA, lateral, ulnar deviation PA, and supinated clenched-fist

Table 3

Stages of Progressive Perilunar Instability and Reverse Perilunar Instability

Mayfield's Stages of Progressive Perilunar Instability

Stage	Characteristics
I	Scapholunate dissociation or scaphoid fracture
II	Capitolunate dislocation
III	Lunotriquetral dissociation or triquetral fracture
IV	Lunate dislocation

Stages of Reverse Perilunar Instability

Stage	Characteristics
I	Lunotriquetral dissociation
II	Capitolunate dislocation
III	Scapholunate dissociation

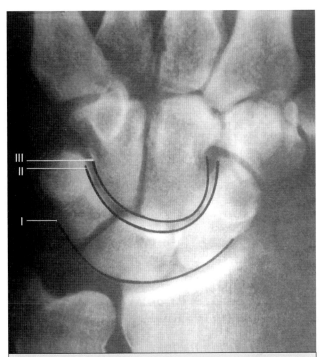

Figure 4   Carpal arcs of Gilula. I = smooth arc outlining the proximal surfaces of the scaphoid, lunate, and triquetrum; II = smooth arc outlining the distal surfaces of the scaphoid, lunate, and triquetrum; III = arc outlining the proximal surfaces of the capitate and hamate. *(Reproduced from Blazar PE, Lawton JN: Diagnosis of acute carpal ligament injuries, in Trumble TE [ed]:* Carpal Fracture-Dislocations. *Rosemont, IL, American Academy of Orthopaedic Surgeons, 2001, p 24.)*

b. Arthrography

  i. Historically, arthrography was the gold standard for the diagnosis of ligamentous injuries, but for the most part it has been replaced by diagnostic arthroscopy.

  ii. With arthrography, contrast medium is injected into the midcarpal, radiocarpal, and radioulnar joints. If dye flows between any of the compartments, an intercarpal ligament tear is indicated. Attritional changes seen with advancing age may lead to spurious findings.

2. Direction—Description of the abnormal stance of the carpus regardless of etiology.

  a. DISI: lunate extension

  b. (VISI) (volar intercalated segmental instability): lunate flexion

  c. Ulnar translocation means the carpus is displaced ulnarward (>50% of lunate lies ulnar to lunate fossa).

  d. Dorsal translocation refers to the carpus that unnaturally displaced dorsally (ie, malunited and dorsally angulated distal radius fracture).

3. History—Determining the time from injury helps determine treatment options.

  a. Acute: within 1 week of injury

  b. Subacute: 1 to 6 weeks after injury

  c. Chronic: more than 6 weeks after injury

4. Constancy

  a. Predynamic instability—No malalignment, only sporadic symptomatic dysfunction, normal radiographs.

  b. Dynamic instability—Malalignment demonstrated on stress radiographs.

  c. Static instability—Permanent alteration in carpal alignment, abnormal plain radiographs.

5. Radiographic parameters—The following measurements can be used to assess ligamentous stability using plain radiographs and fluoroscopy.

  a. Carpal arcs of Gilula—Gilula described three parallel arcs observed on PA radiographs: the first arc corresponds to the proximal articular surface of the proximal row, the second corresponds to the distal articular surface of the proximal row, and the final arc represents the proximal articular surface of the distal carpal row. Disruption of one of these arcs suggests a carpal fracture or ligamentous injury (**Figure 4**).

6: Trauma

Table 4

Intercarpal Angles and Distances

Parameter	Mean Value	Abnormal Value/Significance
Scapholunate angle	46°	<30° or >60°
Radiolunate angle	0°	>15° dorsal suggests DISI deformity. >15° palmar suggests VISI deformity.
Capitolunate angle	0° (range, 30° dorsal to 30° palmar)	>30° in either volar or dorsal direction
Intercarpal distance		>2 mm between the scaphoid and lunate Increased distance, or diastasis, between the scaphoid and lunate or lunate and triquetrum may indicate an SLIL or LTIL injury.

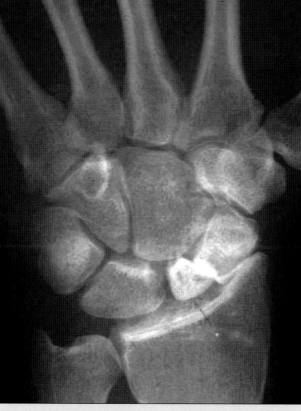

Figure 5   Radiograph of a patient with scaphoid nonunion advanced collapse (SNAC).

b. Carpal height ratio—This ratio is calculated by dividing the carpal height by the length of the third metacarpal. The normal ratio is 0.54 ± 0.03. In disease processes such as scapholunate dissociation, SLAC wrist, and Kienböck disease, collapse of the midcarpal joint produces a decrease in this ratio.

c. Intercarpal angles and distances—Significant deviation from normal values can indicate a disruption of the SLIL or LT interosseous ligament (**Table 4**).

d. Early ligamentous injuries may produce no abnormalities on plain radiographs. If the mechanism and physical exam suggest ligamentous injury, further studies are indicated.

D. Scapholunate ligament injuries

1. Epidemiology—Scapholunate ligament injuries are the most common form of traumatic carpal instability.

2. Pathomechanics—Disruption in the scapholunate relationship can lead to the following:

a. Unopposed extension forces on the lunate imparted by the triquetrum, leading to DISI deformity.

b. Abnormal scaphoid motion and dorsal subluxation of the scaphoid from the radial fossa during wrist flexion, leading to eventual wrist arthritis.

c. Migration of the capitate proximally between the scaphoid and capitate, leading to stage III SLAC arthritis (**Figure 5**).

3. Evaluation

a. Physical examination

i. Positive scaphoid shift test or Watson maneuver—The wrist is moved from ulnar to radial deviation with the examiner's thumb pressing against the scaphoid tubercle. Patients with partial tears will have increase in pain dorsally over scapholunate articulation. With complete tears, an audible clunk may be heard as the scaphoid is actively subluxated with dorsal pressure and spontaneously reduces into the radial fossa when the thumb is removed.

ii. The scaphoid shift test may be falsely positive in up to one third of individuals because of ligamentous laxity without injury, so both sides should always be checked.

Table 5

Geissler Classification of Carpal Instability

Grade	Characteristics
I	Attenuation or hemorrhage of the interosseous ligament as seen from the radiocarpal space No incongruency of carpal alignment in the midcarpal space
II	Attenuation or hemorrhage of interosseous ligament as seen from the radiocarpal space Incongruency or step-off of carpal space May be slight gap (less than width of probe) between carpal bones
III	Incongruency or step-off of carpal alignment as seen from both radiocarpal and midcarpal space Probe may be passed through gap between carpal bones
IV	Incongruency or step-off of carpal alignment as seen from both radiocarpal and midcarpal space Gross instability with manipulation A 2.7-mm arthroscope may be passed through gap between carpal bones

b. Radiographs—PA and lateral views should be obtained.

   i. Scapholunate angle: 46° is normal; >60° is considered abnormally elevated

   ii. Diastasis between the scaphoid and lunate: >2 mm is abnormal.

   iii. "Signet ring" sign: As the scaphoid flexes, the distal pole will appear as a ring on PA radiographs.

   iv. Radiolunate angle: >15° dorsal indicates a DISI deformity.

   v. Disruption of Gilula lines—With advanced carpal instability, the capitate migrates into the proximal carpal row, causing a disruption of the Gilula lines and a change in the carpal height ratio with the wrist held in neutral flexion/extension and neutral deviation.

   vi. The clenched-fist view may show early SLIL changes (dynamic instability) with widening of the scapholunate interval or increase in the scapholunate angle as the capitate is driven down into the scapholunate interspace.

   vii. Even complete division of the SLIL will not always produce an abnormality on plain radiographs because of the substantial number of secondary stabilizers of the scaphoid in addition to the SLIL.

c. Arthrography—May show communication between the midcarpal and radiocarpal joint with a dye leak seen at the SLIL indicating a tear.

d. Arthroscopy

   i. Arthroscopy is now the gold standard for diagnosis of instability patterns. It allows for direct inspection of SLIL ligament in addition to evaluation of supporting extrinsic ligaments.

   ii. Arthroscopic instability is graded by the Geissler classification (**Table 5**).

   iii. Midcarpal arthroscopy is the key to assessing the stability of the scapholunate joint. From the midcarpal perspective, the normal scapholunate joint is smooth, without a step-off or diastasis.

e. Stages of scapholunate instability (**Table 6**)

4. Treatment—Treatment of scapholunate injuries depends on whether the injury is acute, chronic, or chronic with arthritis (SLAC).

a. Acute injuries—Treatment includes open repair and cast immobilization.

b. Chronic injuries (dynamic or static)

   i. Indications for open repair—Satisfactory ligament remains for repair; the scaphoid and lunate remain easily reducible; no degenerative changes within the carpus.

   ii. Soft-tissue procedures

     (a) Dorsal capsulodesis or tenodesis prevents dynamic or static scaphoid flexion.

     (b) The Brunelli procedure uses a strip of the flexor carpi radialis brought palmarly through a bone tunnel in the distal scaphoid. The tendon is then brought dorsally and proximally and attached to the distal radius in an attempt to limit scaphoid flexion and stabilize the SLIL and STIL ligaments. A modification of the Brunelli procedure involves attaching the flexor carpi radialis to the lunate.

     (c) Ligament reconstruction—Attempts have been made to reconstruct the SLIL with bone-ligament-bone constructs from the carpus, foot, and extensor retinaculum.

     (d) Arthrodesis—Scaphotrapezial or scaphocapitate arthrodesis can be used to stabilize the scaphoid.

c. Chronic injuries with arthritis (SLAC changes)—See **Table 7**.

6: Trauma

Table 6

Stages of Scapholunate Instability

Stage	Pathoanatomy	Findings
Predynamic instability	Partial tear or attenuation of SLIL	Radiographs normal
Dynamic instability	Partial or complete tear of SLIL	Stress radiographs abnormal Arthroscopy abnormal (Geissler type II or III)
Static instability	Early: Complete SLIL tear with attenuation or attrition of supporting wrist ligaments Late: Lunate extends as a result of its sagittal plane shape and the unopposed extension force of the intact LT interosseous ligament and becomes fixed in dorsiflexion.	Early: Radiographs positive for scaphoid changes; scapholunate gap >3 mm, scapholunate angle >60 Arthroscopy abnormal (Geissler type IV) Late: Lateral radiograph shows DISI deformity (radiolunate angle >15°)
SLAC wrist	With long-standing abnormal positioning of the carpal bones, arthritic changes occur. Arthritic changes are first seen at the styloscaphoid and radioscaphoid joints and move to the midcarpal joint in a standard progression.	1. Stage 1: arthritis noted at radial styloid 2. Stage 2: arthritis noted at radiocarpal joint 3. Stage 3: arthritis noted at capitolunate interface

SLAC = scapholunate advanced collapse; SLIL = scapholunate interosseous ligament; LT = lunotriquetral; DISI = dorsal intercalated segment instability.

Table 7

Treatment of SLAC Changes

Stage	Characteristics	Treatment
I	Early arthritic changes, present only at radial styloid	STT fusion combined with radial styloidectomy for pain relief Scaphocapitate fusion with radial styloidectomy
II	Arthritis present at radioscaphoid joint	Four-corner fusion or proximal row carpectomy*
III	Arthritis present at the capitolunate joint	If the capitate is too arthritic to allow a proximal row carpectomy, options may be limited to: Four-corner fusion Total wrist fusion Total wrist arthroplasty

STT = scaphotrapezial-trapezoid
* There is ongoing debate as to the benefits of four-corner fusion over proximal row carpectomy and vice versa; however, no studies to date clearly show superiority of one procedure over another.

E. Lunotriquetral ligament injuries

1. Fixed carpal collapse (VISI) seen on radiographs represents static instability and is classified as LT ligament dissociation.

2. Anatomy of the LT ligament

    a. Like the scapholunate ligament, the LT interosseous ligaments are C-shaped ligaments, spanning the dorsal, proximal, and palmar edges of the joint surfaces.

    b. The palmar region of the LT is the thickest and strongest region.

    c. The dorsal LT ligament region is most important in rotational constraint.

3. Pathomechanics

    a. With loss of the integrity of the lunotriquetral ligament, the triquetrum tends to extend and the scaphoid and lunate attempt to flex.

    b. A complete LT ligament dissociation is not sufficient to cause a static carpal collapse into a VISI stance.

4. Physical examination

    a. Ulnar deviation with pronation and axial compression will elicit dynamic instability with a painful snap if a nondissociative midcarpal joint or LT ligament injury is present.

    b. Useful tests include the LT ballottement, shear, and compression tests.

5. Radiographic evaluation

    a. With LT ligament tears, radiographs are often normal.

b. LT dissociation

   i. LT dissociation results in a disruption of the smooth arcs formed by the proximal and distal joint surfaces of the proximal carpal row (carpal arcs of Gilula I and II) and the proximal joint surfaces of the distal carpal row (carpal arc of Gilula III).

   ii. LT dissociation also results in proximal translation of the triquetrum and/or LT overlap. Unlike scapholunate injuries, no LT gap occurs. The longitudinal axis of the triquetrum, defined as a line passing through the distal triquetral angle and bisecting the proximal articular surface, forms a 14° angle (range, +31° to −3°) with the lunate longitudinal axis, defined as a line passing perpendicularly to a line drawn from the distal dorsal and volar edges of the lunate. LT dissociation results in a negative angle (mean value, −16°).

   iii. If a VISI deformity is present with LT dissociation, the scapholunate and capitolunate angles will be altered. The scapholunate angle may be diminished from its normal 47° to 40° or less but is often normal. The lunate and capitate, which are normally co-linear, will collapse in a zigzag fashion, resulting in an angle greater than 10°.

6. Arthroscopy

   a. Arthroscopy is performed through the ulnocarpal and midcarpal portals.

   b. Arthroscopy is diagnostic for LT injuries.

7. Treatment

   a. Surgical treatment for LT injuries—Treatment options include LT ligament repair, LT ligament reconstruction, and LT arthrodesis. A comparison of results and outcomes following arthrodesis, ligament repair, and reconstruction has demonstrated superior results with LT ligament repair or reconstruction.

   b. Treatment for attritional LT instability secondary to ulnar positive variance

      i. Attritional LT instability secondary to ulnar positive variance refers to LT instability secondary to a long ulna that chronically impacts the triquetrum, resulting in a LT tear with instability. This is often associated with a degenerative (nonrepairable) tear of the triangular fibrocartilage complex.

      ii. Ulnar shortening is an attractive alternative in these cases.

F. Perilunate dislocations

   1. Epidemiology and mechanism of injury

      a. Perilunate dislocations are rare injury patterns.

      b. They are usually associated with significant trauma (eg, a fall from a height).

   2. Pathoanatomy

      a. The lunate often remains bound to the carpus by stout radiolunate ligaments, but the carpus dislocates around it. The capitate may move dorsally to cause dorsal perilunate dislocation (common) or palmarly to cause palmar perilunate dislocation (rare).

      b. Lunate dislocation occurs when the lunate dislocates from radial fossa palmarly (palmar lunate dislocation, common) or dorsally (dorsal lunate dislocation, rare).

      c. Fractures may pass through any bone found within the "greater arc" of the wrist and include the distal radius, scaphoid, trapezium, capitate, hamate, and triquetrum.

      d. "Lesser arc" injuries pass only through ligamentous structures, with no corresponding fractures.

   3. Evaluation

      a. Diagnosis can be delayed because some radiographic findings may be subtle; 25% of these injuries are missed during initial presentation.

      b. The physical examination may reveal significant swelling, ecchymosis, and decreased range of motion.

      c. The chance of acute carpal tunnel syndrome can be as high as 25%.

      d. Radiographs

         i. PA views will show disruption of the carpal arcs of Gilula and overlapping of carpal bones (**Figure 6, A**).

         ii. Lateral views will show dislocation of the capitate or lunate (**Figure 6, B**).

      e. Scintigraphy, CT, and MRI are usually not required to make the diagnosis.

   4. Treatment

      a. Acute presentation

         i. Closed reduction may be preformed initially for pain relief, but surgery is the definitive treatment.

         ii. Lunate dislocations usually require an extended carpal tunnel approach initially for lunate reduction if the lunate cannot be reduced by closed means.

      b. Delayed presentation

         i. Outcomes are worse than for injuries repaired acutely.

6: Trauma

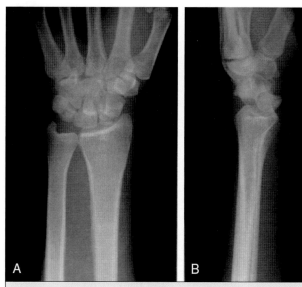

Figure 6 PA **(A)** and lateral **(B)** views of a transscaphoid perilunate dislocation. Note the disruption of the carpal arcs of Gilula on the PA view.

ii. Treatment options include ORIF, proximal row carpectomy, and total wrist fusion.

iii. Studies have shown that in patients treated 6 weeks or longer after injury, ORIF provided the most reliable improvement in function and pain.

X. Fractures of the Distal Radius

A. Overview

1. Fractures of the distal radius are among the most common fractures seen in the emergency department.

2. Patients of advanced age who have osteoporosis have an increased fracture risk with low-energy falls.

3. Fracture patterns vary depending on the mechanism of injury.

4. Principles of treatment—The goal of surgery is to restore the anatomy of the radius and its relationship with the carpus and the distal ulna.

B. Management of distal radius fractures

1. Options include closed reduction and cast immobilization, closed reduction and percutaneous pinning with or without external fixation, and ORIF.

2. Surgical treatment indications

a. Loss of reduction following attempt at closed treatment and/or excessive shortening ≥5 mm; dorsal articular tilt ≥15° (ie, apex volar angulation); loss of radial inclination >10°

b. 2 mm or more of articular displacement

c. Volar oblique fracture (Smith fracture)

d. Intra-articular volar shear fracture (Barton fracture)

e. Die-punch fracture

f. Significant dorsal comminution involving more than one third of the anteroposterior dimension of the radius

g. Open fractures

h. Multiple trauma (relative indication)

3. Closed treatment

a. Long-arm sugar-tong splint or cast in the initial period (up to 2 weeks) with the wrist in neutral position to avoid median nerve compression

b. Graduation to short arm cast after swelling diminishes

c. Total length of immobilization: approximately 6 weeks

4. Surgical treatment procedures

a. Closed reduction and percutaneous pinning with or without external fixation

i. A combination of 0.62- and 0.45-in K-wires is used to maintain reduction.

ii. The wires are inserted from the radial styloid to the intact radial metaphysis or diaphysis, with care taken to avoid injury to the superficial branch of the radial nerve. Limited incisions and protective devices minimize risk.

iii. Subchondral pins help to maintain the articular surface reduction.

iv. Kapandji pins (through the dorsal aspect of the fracture and directed proximally and volarly) are used to buttress and maintain the reduction (volar tilt).

b. External fixator

i. External fixation provides ligamentotaxis.

ii. Beware of overdistraction, which can lead to complex regional pain syndrome, stiffness, or limited finger ROM. Full passive finger ROM following fixator placement suggests that the amount of distraction is appropriate.

iii. Full incisions over the radius and index metacarpal at the time of fixator pin placement minimize the risk of iatrogenic nerve injury.

iv. Adjustable fixators allow for modifications of the wrist position after securing the device.

v. The fixator and pins typically remain in place no longer than 4 to 6 weeks.

vi. Bone graft can be used to structurally support bone defects.

c. Open reduction and internal fixation

i. ORIF allows for earlier rehabilitation and recovery.

ii. Locking plates provide a stronger construct than nonlocked plates or external fixation and are able to maintain the tendency of the fracture to fall dorsally.

iii. Approach is through a volar incision between the flexor carpi radialis and radial artery.

iv. Potential pitfalls include intra-articular distal screw/peg placement; injury to the radial artery, median nerve, or lateral antebrachial cutaneous nerve; and carpal tunnel syndrome.

v. Dorsal plating has both advantages and disadvantages. Advantages include the fact that the plate is on the biomechanically favorable side of the fracture and fewer neurovascular structures are at risk. Disadvantages include the possibility of tendon adhesions and rupture, which have been reported with previous plate designs, and the potential need to remove the plate following fracture healing.

C. Smith fracture—This volarly displaced fracture of the distal radius ("reverse Colles") is an inherently unstable fracture pattern.

1. Classification

a. Type 1: Extra-articular

b. Type II: Intra-articular (similar to volar Barton fracture pattern)

c. Type III: Juxtaphyseal fracture pattern

2. Surgical treatment—ORIF with a volar buttress plate.

D. Fractures of the radial styloid ("chauffeur" fractures)

1. These fractures may be associated with scapholunate ligament injuries because the intra-articular fracture line extends into the joint at that level. Therefore, in the setting of isolated radial styloid fractures, intercarpal ligament injuries must be suspected.

2. Treatment

a. Nonsurgical—If the fracture is completely nondisplaced, it may be treated nonsurgically

b. Surgical—Intra-articular displacement (or diastasis) greater than 1 to 2 mm is an indication for surgery. Compression screw fixation with partially threaded 3.5 or 4.0 cancellous screws can effectively compress the fragments and maintain the reduction. Alternative fixation options include K-wires and plate and screw fixation.

E. Distal radioulnar joint

1. The distal radioulnar joint must be assessed following stabilization of the radius.

2. Preoperative comparison with the unaffected side is helpful.

F. Malunions

1. Malunions following distal radius fracture are associated with pain and disability.

2. Indications for surgery

a. Loss of radial height ≥5 mm

b. Loss of >10° of radial inclination

c. Dorsal tilt ≥15°

3. Surgical procedures

a. Surgery must correct all three parameters: radial height, radial inclination, and volar tilt.

b. The osteotomy should be made in the sagittal plane, parallel to the joint surface.

c. Autogenous (iliac crest) bone graft is preferred.

d. Fixation options include dorsal plating and locked volar plating.

Top Testing Facts

1. In index and long finger MCP fractures, 15° to 20° of angulation is acceptable; in fractures of the ring and little fingers, 30° to 40° of angulation is acceptable.

2. The main deforming force in a Bennett fracture is provided by the abductor pollicis longus. In a "baby Bennett" fracture, it is the extensor carpi ulnaris.

3. In complex MCP dislocations, the metacarpal head is caught between the volar plate, flexor tendon, lumbrical, and A1 pulley.

4. Bennett fractures are best viewed on the Robert (hyperpronated) view.

5. Dorsal PIP joint dislocations may lead to pseudoboutonnière deformity. Volar PIP joint dislocations may lead to boutonnière deformity.

6. Nondisplaced scaphoid waist fractures, as verified by CT, can be treated with cast immobilization in a long arm-thumb spica cast, which has been shown to produce the smallest amount of internal scaphoid motion. Indications for surgery include any displacement, a radiolunate angle >15°, associated perilunate ligamentous injuries, and proximal pole fractures.

7. The SLAC pattern of arthritis progresses from the radioscaphoid joint to the scaphocapitate joint to the capitolunate joint.

8. Surgical indications for distal radius fractures include loss of reduction following attempt at closed treatment and/or excessive shortening (≥5 mm), dorsal angulation ≥15°, loss of radial inclination >10°, or ≥2 mm articular displacement.

9. In the setting of isolated radial styloid fractures, intercarpal ligament injuries must be suspected.

Bibliography

Cooney WP III, Linscheid RL, Dobyns JH: Carpal instability: Treatment of ligament injuries of the wrist. *Instr Course Lect* 1992;41:33-44.

Mack GR, Bosse MJ, Gelberman RH, Yu E: The natural history of scaphoid non-union. *J Bone Joint Surg Am* 1984;66:504-509.

Mayfield JK, Johnson RP, Kilcoyne RK: Carpal dislocations: Pathomechanics and progressive perilunar instability. *J Hand Surg [Am]* 1980;5:226-241.

Sheetz KK, Bishop AT, Berger RA: The arterial blood supply of the distal radius and ulna and its potential use in vascularized pedicled bone grafts. *J Hand Surg [Am]* 1995;20:902-914.

Chapter 52

Fractures of the Humeral Shaft and Distal Humerus

Frank A. Liporace, MD

I. Fractures of the Humeral Shaft

A. Epidemiology

1. Humerus fractures account for 3% of all fractures and most commonly occur in the middle third of the bone.

2. They exhibit a bimodal age distribution with peak incidence in the third decade of life for males and the seventh decade for females.

3. In the younger age group, high-energy trauma is more frequently the cause. Lower energy mechanisms are more common in the elderly.

B. Anatomy

1. The anatomy of the humerus varies throughout its length (**Figure 1**).

   a. The shaft is generally cylindrical and provides origin and insertion points for the pectoralis, deltoid, biceps, coracobrachialis, brachialis, and triceps.

   b. These origins and insertions determine the displacement of the major fracture fragments.

   c. Distally, the humerus becomes triangular, and its intramedullary canal terminates approximately 2 to 3 cm proximal to the olecranon fossa.

   d. Medial and lateral septae delineate the posterior and anterior compartments of the arm.

2. The main neurovascular structures of the arm and forearm traverse the soft tissues overlying the humerus. Posteriorly, the spiral groove houses the radial nerve. Its location is approximately 14 cm proximal to the lateral-distal articular surface and 20 cm proximal to the medial-distal articular surface.

C. Surgical approaches

1. Anterolateral approach—May be considered for proximal third to middle third shaft fractures.

   a. The radial nerve can be identified between the brachialis and brachioradialis and traced proximally.

   b. Alternatively, for more proximal fractures, the brachialis (innervated by the radial and musculocutaneous nerves) can be split to spare its innervation and protect the radial nerve during retraction.

2. Posterior approach—Effective for most of the humerus, from the deltoid insertion and distally. The deltoid prevents extension of this approach proximally to the shoulder.

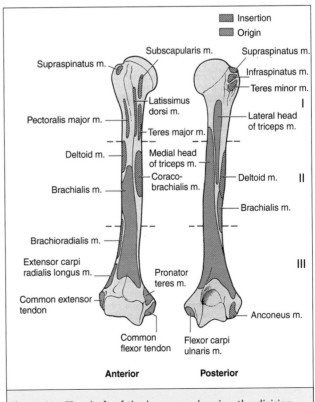

Figure 1 The shaft of the humerus, showing the division into three surfaces. (*Adapted with permission from Browner BD, Jupiter JB, Levine AM, Trafton PG (eds):* Skeletal Trauma, *ed 2. Philadelphia, PA, WB Saunders Company, 2002, p 1524*).

a. The radial and ulnar nerves can be identified through this approach. The interval between the lateral and long heads of the triceps is used, with elevation of the medial (deep) head off the posterior aspect of the shaft.

b. The ulnar nerve emerges medially from deep to the medial head of the triceps. It courses distally through the cubital tunnel. It can be palpated along the medial aspect of the triceps along the distal third of the humerus.

3. Anterior, anteromedial, and direct lateral approaches—These have been described and may be used based on wound considerations, other injuries (ie, need for associated vascular repair), or the need for other approaches based on concomitant injuries.

D. Mechanism of injury and associated injuries

1. Distal humerus fractures may be due to high- or low-energy trauma. In patients with osteoporosis or osteopenia, the bone mineral density is decreased, so less force is required for injury (eg, a fall from a standing position).

2. Torsional, bending, axial, or a combination of these forces can be responsible for humerus fractures. Direct impact or blast injury (eg, gunshot wounds) can cause these fractures as well.

3. With any long-bone injury, associated proximal or distal articular fractures or dislocations may be present, necessitating a complete radiographic examination of the bone, including the joints above and joint below.

4. With high-energy situations, forearm and wrist radiographs are warranted to rule out a "floating elbow" (humeral fracture with associated both-bone forearm fracture).

5. Many neurovascular structures course the upper arm, so associated neurovascular injury may occur.

E. Clinical evaluation

1. Patients typically present with pain, swelling, and deformity (most frequently shortening and varus).

2. Fracture pattern is related to mechanism of injury and bone quality. Therefore, a careful history is imperative to match these factors in cases in which pathologic processes are suspected and would require further workup.

3. Careful neurovascular examination is important because radial nerve injury is a common associated finding.

F. Radiographic studies

1. Standard radiographic series of AP and lateral radiographs should be acquired.

2. When obtaining the transthoracic lateral view, rotating the patient will prevent rotation of the dis-

tal fragment and avoid risk of further soft-tissue or nerve injury.

3. Radiographic series should include the shoulder and elbow ("joint above and joint below") to rule out further associated injuries.

4. Traction views may aid in preoperative planning for severely comminuted fractures that meet surgical indications.

5. Advanced imaging studies need be considered only when concomitant intra-articular injury is present or a pathologic process is suspected based on history and initial radiographic evaluation.

G. Classification—Several different systems have been used to classify humeral shaft fractures.

1. OTA classification system—Uses a combination of numbers and letters to describe the fracture: bone number (humerus = 1); location (diaphysis = 2); fracture pattern (simple = A, wedge = B, complex = C); and severity (1 through 3) (**Figure 2**).

2. Descriptive classification system—Based on relative location to the pectoralis and deltoid. This provides information as to the relative direction and displacement of the main fracture fragments.

3. Classification system based on the fracture characteristics (transverse, oblique, spiral, segmental, comminuted)—can aid in determining treatment.

H. Nonsurgical treatment

1. This is the treatment of choice for most humeral shaft fractures. A recent review of 922 patients showed that closed treatment with a functional brace resulted in a fracture union rate >98% in closed fractures and >94% in open fractures; 98% exhibited <25° of angulation and had <25° of restricted shoulder motion at the time of brace removal.

2. Closed treatment may involve initial coaptation splinting followed by a functional brace or a hanging arm cast.

a. The coaptation splint is used for 7 to 10 days, followed by application of a fracture brace in the office.

b. Weekly radiographs are obtained for 3 weeks to ensure appropriate maintenance of reduction; thereafter, they are obtained at 3- to 4-week intervals.

c. Immediately upon fracture brace application, the patient is encouraged to do pendulum exercises for shoulder mobility. Elbow, wrist, and hand exercises also are encouraged.

d. The patient is instructed to adjust the tension of the fracture brace twice per week and to sleep in a semi-erect position until 4 to 6 weeks postinjury.

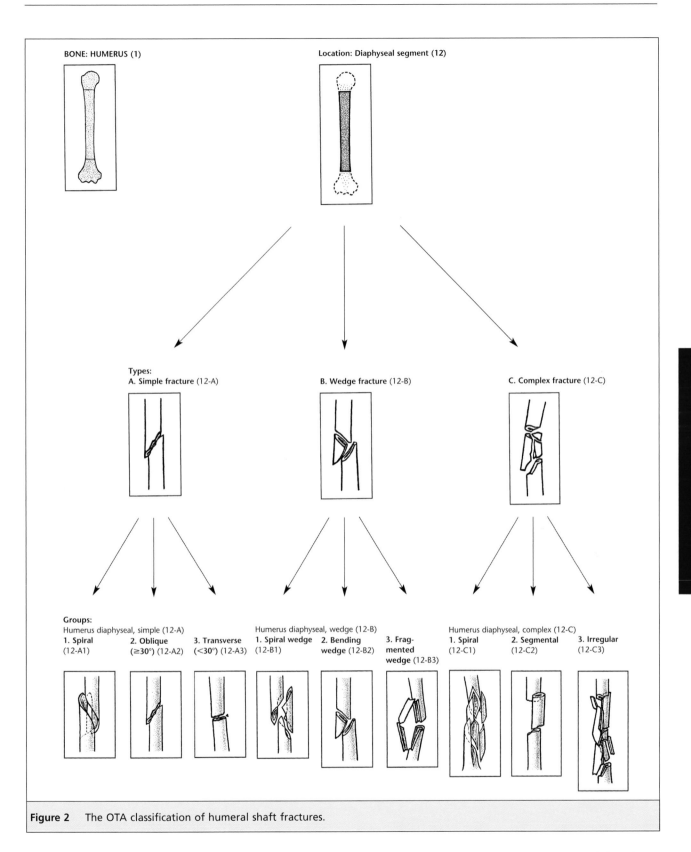

Figure 2 The OTA classification of humeral shaft fractures.

e. The fracture brace is worn for 10 to 12 weeks, until there is no pain with palpation at the fracture site, >90° of painless shoulder and elbow motion, and bridging callus is seen radiographically on 3 of 4 cortices.

3. Hanging arm casts may be considered for shortened oblique, spiral, and transverse fractures. The cast should extend from 2 cm proximal to the fracture, across the 90° flexed elbow, and to the wrist; the forearm should be in neutral rotation.

6: Trauma

Table 1

Indications for Surgical Treatment of Humeral Shaft Fractures

Absolute Indications	Relative Indications
Concomitant vascular injury	Multiply injured patient
Severe soft-tissue injury	Concomitant head injury
Open fractures	Inability to maintain an
Floating elbow	acceptable reduction
Concomitant displaced	closed
humeral articular injuries	Segmental fractures
Pathologic fractures	Transverse or short oblique
	fractures in a young
	athlete

Suspension straps are attached to loops on the forearm aspect of the cast to aid in alignment.

4. No consensus exists on acceptable alignment, but it has been proposed that 20° apex anterior or posterior angulation and 30° varus/valgus, 15° malrotation, and 3 cm shortening are acceptable.

I. Surgical treatment

1. Absolute and relative indications for surgical treatment are listed in **Table 1**.

2. Outcomes—Open fractures have been shown to have a 12% infection rate without fixation and a 10.8% infection rate with fixation.

3. Surgical procedures

   a. Open reduction and plate fixation

      i. This is the most common surgical treatment of humeral shaft fractures.

      ii. Plate and screw constructs offer union rates ≥94%, with low infection rates (0% to 6%), low incidence of iatrogenic nerve injury (0% to 5%), and the ability for the multiply injured patient to weight bear through the injured extremity.

      iii. Conventional plating is traditionally done with a broad 4.5-mm plate with three or four screws per side for axial and torsional stability.

      iv. For bending stability when using a long plate, screw placement should include "near-near" and "far-far" relative to the limits of the fracture.

      v. In osteoporotic bone, locked plating has been shown to improve stability and resistance to torsional stresses.

   b. Intramedullary nailing

      i. Advocated by some as an alternative to plate fixation

      ii. Originally, nonlocking flexible nails were used and inserted in either an antegrade or retrograde fashion, but the newer interlocking nails have become more common and allow for better rotational control.

      iii. Intramedullary nails can be useful in the medically unstable patient to avoid a large exposure, with segmental fractures, with the multiply injured patient to limit positioning changes, and with pathologic fractures.

      iv. Intramedullary nails have been shown to withstand higher axial and bending loads than plates, although plated humerus fractures have been shown to clinically allow for full weight bearing and have not shown a higher incidence of malunion or nonunion.

      v. Intramedullary nailing of humerus fractures has been shown to result in a higher incidence of shoulder pain.

      vi. A recent meta-analysis comparing plating and nailing of humeral shaft fractures has shown that plating results in less need for revision, a lower nonunion rate, and fewer shoulder problems.

   c. External fixation

      i. Indications—Staged external fixation is indicated with severe soft-tissue injury, bone defects, vascular injury with acute repair, the medically unstable patient, and infected nonunions.

      ii. When applying external fixation, care must be taken with respect to neurovascular structures in the arm.

      iii. Typically, the elbow joint is spanned with two lateral pins placed proximal to the fracture in the humeral diaphysis and two pins in the ulna or radius, depending on whether a forearm injury is present.

      iv. The ulna is the preferred location for pin placement when possible because of its subcutaneous location, limited risk to neurovascular structures, and ability to maintain pronation-supination during the period of external fixation.

      v. An open approach is recommended for the humeral pins because of the variability of nerve course in the region. An open approach also should be used if the distal pins are applied to the radius.

4. Surgical pearls

   a. To decrease shoulder pain, an anterior starting point for antegrade intramedullary nailing has been suggested.

i. The interval between the anterior and middle third of the deltoid is split and an inline-splitting incision of the rotator cuff is made. This allows a direct path to the intramedullary canal and an easier side-to-side tendon closure.

ii. The surgeon must be aware that the humeral canal ends 2 to 3 cm proximal to the olecranon fossa and it narrows distally, which can result in a risk for fracture distraction when impacting the nail.

b. When plating from a posterior approach, the radial nerve must be identified.

i. The radial nerve can be located by bluntly dissecting deep to bone at a point approximately 2 cm superior to the proximal aspect of the triceps fascia.

ii. The ulnar nerve can be located if necessary by finding the intermuscular septum that separates the posterior and anterior compartments approximately 2 to 3 cm proximal to the flare of the medial epicondyle.

J. Rehabilitation

1. Humeral shaft fractures treated nonsurgically should undergo rehabilitation as described previously in the nonsurgical treatment section (section I.H).

2. Surgically treated fractures can be splinted for 3 to 7 days to rest the soft tissues. Subsequently, active and passive range of motion (ROM) of the shoulder, elbow, wrist, and hand can progress.

3. Resistive strengthening exercises may begin at 6 weeks postoperatively or if nonsurgical treatment is done, when callus with no motion or pain at the fracture sight is evident.

K. Complications

1. Radial nerve palsy

a. Humeral fractures are often associated with radial nerve palsies, whether from the time of injury, attempted closed reduction, or during surgical intervention.

b. A recent meta-analysis of 4,517 fractures found an overall 11.8% incidence of concomitant radial nerve palsies in transverse and spiral fractures, with the middle and mid-distal third most frequently involved.

i. Overall, the recovery rate was 88.1%, whether the palsy was primary or secondary to iatrogenic intervention.

ii. Statistically different rates of recovery were reported for complete (77.6%) versus incomplete (98.2%) and closed (97.1%) versus open (85.7%) injuries.

iii. The onset of spontaneous recovery was evident at an average of 7.3 weeks, with full recovery at an average of 6.1 months.

iv. When nerve exploration was required, it was conducted at an average of 4.3 months.

v. Barring open injury, vascular injury, segmental fracture, or floating elbow, no difference in recovery between early and late exploration could be deduced.

c. With a concomitant nerve injury, in patients who do not require surgical treatment of the fracture, electromyography/nerve conduction velocity studies should be acquired 6 weeks postinjury. In patients who require surgical treatment, exploration is done at the time of surgery.

d. With secondary palsies that occur during fracture reduction, it has not been clearly established that surgery will improve the ultimate recovery rate when compared with results of nonsurgical management. Delayed surgical exploration should be done after 3 to 4 months if no evidence of recovery is apparent using electromyography or nerve conduction velocity studies.

2. Vascular injury is rare with humeral shaft fractures and may be the result of a penetrating injury (eg, industrial accident, gunshot wound). Revascularization should be attempted within 6 hours.

3. Interlocking with humeral nails can place the axillary nerve at risk proximally and the lateral antebrachial cutaneous nerve, median nerve, or brachial artery at risk distally. This risk can be minimized by using a limited open approach with careful blunt dissection to bone when applying interlocking screws for intramedullary humeral nails.

4. With intramedullary nailing, when passing the reamer through an area of comminution, consider turning off the reamer and pushing it through this area manually to avoid damage to the radial nerve.

5. When radial nerve dysfunction is present preoperatively and intramedullary nailing is chosen, consideration should be given to a limited open approach to ensure that the fracture is clear of neurovascular structures.

6. Nonunions—Although union rates are relatively high with humeral shaft fractures, nonunions do occur.

a. Motion, avascularity, gap, and infection are all potential causes of nonunion.

b. With osteopenia and osteoporosis, stability can be difficult to achieve with standard compression plating.

7. Infected nonunions

a. Eradication of the infection is important to help achieve union.

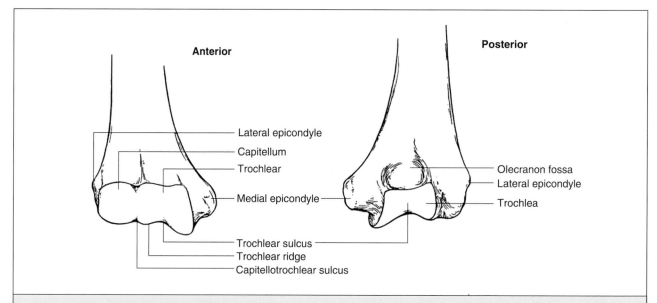

Figure 3   Anterior and posterior views of the anatomy of the distal articular surface of the humerus. The capitellotrochlear sulcus divides the capitellar and trochlear articular surfaces. The lateral trochlear ridge is the key to analyzing humeral condyle fractures. In type I fractures, the lateral trochlear ridge remains with the intact condyle, providing medial-to-lateral elbow stability. In type II fractures, the lateral trochlear ridge is a part of the fractured condyle, which may allow the radius and ulna to translocate in a medial-to-lateral direction with respect to the long axis of the humerus. *(Reproduced with permission from Koval KJ, Zuckerman JD (eds):* Handbook of Fractures, ed 2. *Philadelphia, PA, Lippincott Williams & Wilkins, 2002, p 98.)*

b. In select cases of severe infection, temporary or definitive external fixation along with resection of affected tissue and antibiotic treatment may be required.

c. Whether required by atrophic nonunion or infection, resection and shortening of up to 4 cm can be tolerated.

8. Nerve conduction velocity studies can be considered after 6 weeks to help determine a baseline for prognosis and severity of nerve injury.

9. Ultrasound has also been suggested as a modality for nerve evaluation but is very dependent on the quality of the technician, radiologist, and ultrasound machine.

II. Distal Humerus Fractures

A. Epidemiology

1. Intercondylar fractures are the most common distal humerus fracture pattern.

2. Extension supracondylar fractures account for >80% of all supracondylar fractures.

3. Fractures of the capitellum constitute approximately 1% of all elbow injuries.

4. Fractures of a single condyle (lateral more common than medial) account for 5% of all distal humerus fractures.

B. Anatomy (**Figure 3**)

1. The elbow is a constrained, hinged joint. The ulna rotates around the axis of the trochlea, which is positioned in relative valgus and external rotation.

2. The capitellum articulates with the proximal radius and is involved with forearm rotation, not elbow flexion/extension. Posteriorly, the capitellum is nonarticular and allows for distal posterolateral hardware placement.

3. Medially, the medial collateral ligament originates on the distal surface of the medial epicondyle. The ulnar nerve resides in the cubital tunnel in a subcutaneous location.

4. Laterally, the lateral collateral ligament originates on the lateral epicondyle, deep to the common extensor tendon.

C. Classification

1. Classifications of fractures of the distal humerus were traditionally descriptive and based on the number of columns involved and the location of the fracture (ie, supracondylar, transcondylar, condylar, and bicondylar)(**Table 2**).

2. The OTA classification system divides these fractures into type A (extra-articular), type B (partial articular), and type C (complete articular).

a. Each category is subclassified based on the degree and location of fracture comminution.

Table 2

Descriptive and Anatomic Classifications of Distal Humerus Fractures

I. Intra-articular Fractures	II. Extra-articular/Intracapsular Fractures	III. Extracapsular Fractures
Single-column fractures Medial (high/low) Lateral (high/low) Divergent	High transcolumnar fractures Extension Flexion Abduction Adduction	Medial epicondyle
Two-column fractures T pattern (high/low) Y pattern H pattern λ pattern (medial/lateral)	Low transcolumnar fractures Extension Flexion	Lateral epicondyle
Capitellar fractures		
Trochlear fractures		

b. It has been shown that the OTA classification has substantial agreement with regard to fracture type (A, B, and C) but is less reliable with regard to subtype.

D. Surgical approaches

1. Extra-articular and partial articular fractures are typically approached through a posterior triceps-splitting or triceps-sparing approach.

   a. With a triceps-splitting approach, a posterior incision is made and carried deep to the triceps, which is subsequently split between the long and lateral heads and distally at its ulnar insertion.

   b. The triceps-sparing approach involves mobilization of the ulnar nerve and subsequent elevation of the entire extensor mechanism in continuity, progressing from medial to lateral. Upon completion of the procedure, reattachment of the extensor mechanism through drill holes in the ulna and to the flexor carpi ulnaris fascia is required.

   c. An alternative approach is the posterior triceps-preserving approach. It involves mobilization of the triceps off the posterior humerus from the medial and lateral aspects of the intermuscular septum. The ulnar nerve (medially) and the radial nerve (laterally and proximally) need to be identified and preserved.

2. Simple fractures often can be stabilized through one of these approaches with either lag screws alone or screws and an antiglide plate.

3. With an isolated lateral column or capitellar fracture, a Kocher approach may be considered.

   a. Either a posterior skin incision or an incision going from the lateral epicondyle to a point

6 cm distal to the olecranon tip can be used. The incision can be extended proximally as needed.

   b. For capitellar exposure, the interval of the anconeus and extensor carpi ulnaris can be opened.

4. Complete articular fractures can be repaired using one of the above approaches if adequate articular reduction and fixation can be achieved. With increasing complexity of the articular injury, they may require direct visualization through a trans-olecranon osteotomy.

   a. It is necessary to find and free the ulnar nerve before performing an olecranon osteotomy. A chevron-style osteotomy pointing distally is made at the level of the nidus of the olecranon.

   b. Some believe in drilling and tapping the proximal ulna for larger screw insertion before osteotomizing the olecranon to facilitate later fixation.

   c. Once the osteotomy is complete, the entire extensor mechanism can be reflected proximally to allow visualization of the entire distal humerus.

   d. Fixation of the osteotomy can be performed using Kirschner wires and a tension band, long large-fragment intramedullary screw fixation with a tension band, a plate, or two small-fragment lag screws that penetrate the anterior ulnar cortex distal to the site of the osteotomy.

   e. An olecranon osteotomy is a potential site for nonunion, hardware discomfort, and need for future procedures.

5. Patients with open distal humerus injuries have been shown to have worse functional and ROM scores.

6: Trauma

6. Regardless of the approach used for fixation, the goals of fixation are anatomic articular reduction, stable internal fixation, and early range of elbow motion.

   a. In patients with irreconstructible or missing segments of the articular surface, care must be taken to avoid decreasing the dimensions of the trochlea and limiting the ability for flexion and extension.

   b. Once articular reduction is accomplished, stable fixation of the distal end to the metadiaphyseal component with restoration of the mechanical axis is performed.

E. Mechanism of injury

   1. Distal humerus fractures can result from low-energy falls (common in the elderly) or high-energy trauma with extensive comminution and intra-articular involvement (eg, gunshot wounds, motor vehicle accidents, falls from a height).

   2. The amount of elbow flexion at the time of impact can affect fracture pattern.

   3. A transcolumnar fracture results from an axial load directed through the forearm with the elbow flexed 90°.

   4. With the elbow in a similar position but with direct impact on the olecranon, an olecranon fracture with or without distal humerus fracture may result.

   5. With the elbow in >90° of flexion, an intercondylar fracture may result.

   6. Potential associated injuries include elbow dislocation, floating elbow (humerus and forearm fracture), and concomitant "terrible triad" injuries (olecranon, coronoid, radial head/neck fractures).

F. Clinical evaluation

   1. Patients typically present with elbow pain and swelling. Crepitus and/or gross instability with attempted range of elbow motion is often observed.

   2. Excessive motion testing should not be done because of the risk of further neurovascular injury.

   3. A careful neurovascular examination should be performed because all neurovascular structures to the forearm and hand cross the area of injury and sharp bone fragments can cause damage, especially to the radial nerve, ulnar nerve, and brachial artery.

   4. Serial compartment examinations may be required because of extreme cubital fossa swelling or in the obtunded patient to avoid missing a volar forearm compartment syndrome with resultant Volkmann contracture.

G. Radiographic evaluation

   1. AP and lateral radiographs of the humerus and elbow are required.

   2. When concomitant elbow injuries are present, forearm and wrist radiographs may be needed.

   3. To aid in preoperative planning, traction radiographs, oblique radiographs, and CT scans may be of value.

   4. Recently, a blinded study comparing evaluation of distal humerus fractures based on two-dimensional CT scans and plain radiographs versus three-dimensional CT scans showed that three-dimensional CT scans improved the intraobserver and interobserver reliability of two commonly used classification systems.

H. Supracondylar fractures—These are OTA type A fractures that are distal metaphyseal and extra-articular.

   1. Nonsurgical treatment is reserved for nondisplaced or minimally displaced fractures or for comminuted fractures in elderly low-demand patients.

      a. A splint is applied for 1 to 2 weeks before initiation of ROM exercises.

      b. At 6 weeks, with progressive evidence of healing, immobilization may be discontinued completely.

      c. Up to 20° loss of condylar-shaft angle may be acceptable.

   2. Surgical treatment is indicated for most displaced fractures as well as those associated with an open injury or vascular injury.

      a. Open reduction and internal fixation (ORIF) is typically done, with plates placed on the medial and lateral columns.

      b. Biomechanically, 90-90 plating (medial and posterolateral), bicolumnar plating (medial and lateral), and locked plating constructs have been shown to be effective in supplying adequate stability.

   3. ROM exercises may be initiated once the soft tissues allow.

I. Transcondylar fractures

   1. Epidemiology—Transcondylar fractures traverse both columns, reside within the joint capsule, and are typically seen in elderly patients.

   2. Mechanism of injury—These fractures occur with a flexed elbow or a fall on an outstretched hand with the arm in abduction or adduction.

   3. Clinical evaluation—The examiner must be wary of a Posadas fracture, which is a transcondylar

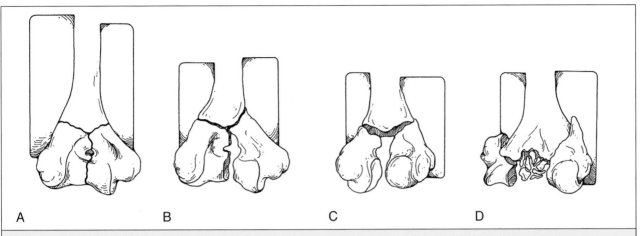

Figure 4   Intercondylar fractures. **A,** Type I undisplaced condylar fracture of the elbow. **B,** Type II displaced but not rotated T-condylar fracture. **C,** Type III displaced and rotated T-condylar fracture. **D,** Type IV displaced, rotated, and comminuted condylar fracture. *(Reproduced with permission from the Mayo Foundation.)*

Table 3

Two-column Intercondylar Distal Humerus Fractures

Type	Description
High T fracture	A transverse fracture line divides both columns at or proximal to the olecranon fossa.
Low T fracture	Similar to the high T fracture except the transverse component is through the olecranon fossa, making treatment and fixation more difficult.
Y fracture	Oblique fracture lines cross each column and join in the olecranon fossa, extending vertically to the joint surface.
H fracture	The trochlea is a free fragment and at risk for osteonecrosis. The medial column is fractured above and below the medial epicondyle, whereas the lateral column is fractured in a T or Y configuration.
Medial λ fracture	The most proximal fracture line exits medially. Laterally, the fracture line is distal to the lateral epicondyle, rendering a very small fragment left for fixation on the lateral side.
Lateral λ fracture	The most proximal fracture line exits laterally. Medially, the fracture line is distal to the medial epicondyle, rendering a very small fragment left for fixation on the medial side.
Multiplane fracture	This represents a T fracture with concomitant coronal fracture lines.

fracture with anterior displacement of the distal fragment with concomitant dislocation of the radial head and proximal ulna from the fragment.

4. Treatment

   a. Nonsurgical and surgical management follow recommendations and principles similar to those for supracondylar fractures.

   b. Total elbow arthroplasty may be considered in the elderly with very distal fractures and poor bone quality.

J. Intercondylar fractures (**Figure 4**)

   1. Epidemiology—Intercondylar fractures are the most common distal humerus fracture; frequently they are comminuted.

2. Classification

   a. According to the OTA classification, these are type C fractures.

   b. **Table 3** lists the descriptive types.

3. Pathoanatomy—The medial flexor mass and lateral extensor mass are responsible for rotation and proximal migration of the articular surface.

4. Treatment

   a. Treatment is primarily surgical, using medial and lateral plate fixation according to the principles and fixation types described previously.

   b. In some bicondylar fractures with simple fracture lines and adequate bone quality, lag screw or columnar screw fixation may be used alone

6: Trauma

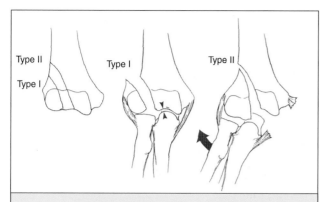

Figure 5 Milch lateral column fractures. Type I fractures: the lateral trochlear ridge remains attached, preventing dislocation of the radius and ulna; Type II fractures: the lateral trochlear ridge is a part of the fractured lateral condyle, resulting in dislocation of the radius and ulna. *(Reproduced with permission from Koval KJ, Zuckerman JD (eds): Handbook of Fractures, ed 2. Philadelphia, PA, Lippincott Williams & Wilkins, 2002, p 98.)*

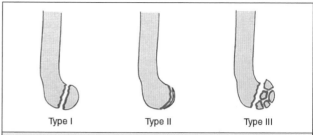

Figure 6 Fractures of the capitellum. Type I: Hahn-Steinhal fragment; type II: Kocher-Lorenz fragment; type III: comminuted and multifragmented. *(Reproduced with permission from Browner BD, Jupiter JB, Levine AM, Trafton PG (eds): Skeletal Trauma, ed 2. Philadelphia, PA, WB Saunders, 2002, p 1511.)*

or in concert with plate constructs if fracture morphology or osteopenia dictates.

c. The goal is stable fixation to allow early range of elbow motion.

d. In younger patients with extremely comminuted, distal, intra-articular fractures, minifragment fixation can help stabilize smaller fragments.

e. With older, medically unfit, or demented patients, "bag of bones" nonsurgical treatment has been described. This involves approximately 2 weeks of immobilization in 90° of elbow flexion followed by gentle ROM to ultimately achieve a minimally painful, functional pseudarthrosis.

f. Total elbow arthroplasty may be used in elderly patients. In a recent review of 49 elderly patients with distal humerus fractures treated with total elbow arthroplasty, the average flexion arc was 24° to 131° and the Mayo elbow performance score averaged 93 out of a possible 100.

K. Condylar fractures

1. Classification

a. These represent OTA type B (partial articular) fractures of the distal humerus.

b. They can be divided into low or high medial/lateral column fractures.

i. The following characteristics make a condylar fracture "high": the involved column includes most of the trochlea; the forearm follows the displacement of the fractured column.

ii. Because of the larger size of "high" column fractures, internal fixation is more straightforward and can frequently be achieved using lag screws with or without unilateral plating.

iii. Lateral column fractures are more common.

iv. Milch tried to determine fracture stability based on pattern (**Figure 5**). It was suggested that type I fractures (lateral wall of trochlea attached to main mass of humerus) were "stable" relative to type II fractures (lateral wall of trochlea attached to displaced fracture fragment).

2. Treatment

a. Surgical treatment is recommended for all but nondisplaced fractures.

b. Nonsurgical—The elbow is positioned in 90° of flexion with the forearm in supination or pronation for lateral or medial column fractures, respectively.

L. Capitellum fractures

1. Classification—Capitellum fractures can be classified into three types (**Figure 6**).

a. Type I (Hahn-Steinhal fragment): These involve a large osseous component of the capitellum that can include some involvement of the trochlea.

b. Type II (Kocher-Lorenz fragment): These are separations of articular cartilage with minimal attached subchondral bone.

c. Type III: These are severely comminuted multifragmentary fractures.

2. Treatment

a. Type I fractures usually require ORIF. Minifragment screw fixation from posterior to anterior or countersunk minifragment screws from anterior to posterior can be used. Alternatively, headless screws may be used.

b. Typically, type II fractures and irreconstructible parts of type III fractures are excised.

3. Complications—If instability is present or creeping substitution of devascularized fragments is unsuccessful, arthritis, osteonecrosis, decreased motion, cubital valgus, and tardy ulnar nerve palsy can result.

M. Trochlear fractures

1. Epidemiology—These fractures in isolation are extremely rare. When they occur, a high index of suspicion for an associated elbow dislocation that caused a shearing of the articular surface is warranted.

2. Treatment

a. Nondisplaced fractures may be treated with 3 weeks of immobilization followed by ROM exercises.

b. Displaced fractures require ORIF or excision if not reconstructible.

N. Epicondylar fractures

1. Epicondylar fractures may occur on the medial or lateral aspect of the elbow.

2. Treatment

a. Epicondylar fractures that are nondisplaced and have a stable elbow joint to ROM may be treated nonsurgically.

b. In children, medial epicondyle fractures with up to 5 mm of displacement may be treated nonsurgically if no concomitant instability or nerve deficits exist.

c. If significantly displaced or with concomitant elbow instability or ulnar nerve symptoms, ORIF with screws or Kirschner wires is recommended.

d. Consider excision in patients who present late with a painful nonunion or fragment that cannot be reconstructed.

O. Fracture of the supracondylar process

1. Anatomy

a. The supracondylar process is a bony protrusion on the anteromedial surface of the distal humerus and represents a congenital variant.

b. The ligament of Struthers courses a path from the supracondylar process to the medial epicondyle.

c. Fibers of the pronator teres or the corachobrachialis may arise from this ligament.

2. Treatment

a. Fracture of the supracondylar process is most frequently treated nonsurgically.

b. Excision is required only if there is an associated brachial artery injury or median nerve compression.

P. Surgical pearls

1. When approaching the distal humerus from a posterior location, the ulnar nerve should be identified. Approximately 2 cm proximal to the superior aspect of the medial epicondyle, the nerve can be palpated as it emerges in the area of the intermuscular septum. Subsequently, it can be dissected to the first motor branch to the flexor carpi ulnaris.

2. If surgical dissection must be carried proximally or laterally, the radial nerve can be found in one of two ways.

a. Blunt deep dissection approximately 2 cm proximal to the fascia of the confluence of the triceps mechanism will allow the radial nerve to be palpated in the spiral groove.

b. Posterolaterally, the radial nerve can be found by retracting the triceps medially to expose the lateral brachial cutaneous nerve that branches off the radial nerve on the posterior aspect of the lateral intermuscular septum. This can be traced proximally to identify the radial nerve proper.

3. When performing an olecranon osteotomy, one should make sure that the apex of the chevron points distally to ensure a larger proximal fragment. This minimizes the risk of its fracture with later osteotomy repair.

4. The olecranon osteotomy can be initiated with an oscillating saw but should be completed with an osteotome to avoid taking a curf that would result in decreasing the olecranon arc upon repair of the osteotomy.

5. Transient sensory ulnar nerve symptoms may occur. Patients should be warned of this preoperatively.

6. Although the ulnar nerve may be transposed, some return it to its native location providing there is no tethering or abrasive hardware in its path.

7. When operating on a severely comminuted distal humerus fracture in an elderly individual, with the possibility of poor bone quality or a very distal fracture, one should be prepared to perform a total elbow arthroplasty. If attempting internal fixation, choose a surgical exposure that will not negatively affect arthroplasty placement if the fracture cannot be reconstructed.

Q. Rehabilitation

1. Postoperatively, the elbow should be immobilized at 90° of flexion, with a wound check at 2 to 3 days.

6: Trauma

2. Active and passive ROM of the shoulder, elbow, wrist, and hand is usually initiated within a few days of surgery. If the soft tissue is tenuous, the elbow motion is deferred until 7 to 10 days postoperatively, but the other therapy is initiated.

3. Typically, with a posterior approach, resistive exercises, especially extension, are delayed for 6 weeks.

R. Outcomes—Closed injuries treated with ORIF can ultimately expect approximately 105° arc of motion and the return of approximately 75% of flexion and extension strength. Loss of elbow extension is typically greater than loss of flexion.

S. Complications

1. Fixation failure and malunion are more common with inadequate fixation.

2. Nonunion can occur at either the distal humerus fracture or the olecranon osteotomy. When appropriate principles are followed, the incidence is relatively low. With higher energy trauma and greater soft-tissue injury, the risk is higher.

3. Infection is a relatively uncommon complication (0% to 6%) and has been described most commonly with grade 3 open fractures.

4. Ulnar nerve palsy can be very debilitating. Iatrogenic injury, inadequate release, impingement due to bony causes or hardware, and postoperative fibrosis may all be causes.

5. Posttraumatic arthritis can result from inappropriate articular reduction or a devastating initial injury. Revision surgery, allograft, or total elbow arthroplasty may all be considered in such instances.

Top Testing Facts

1. Most humeral shaft fractures can be treated nonsurgically.

2. Indications for surgical management of humeral shaft fractures include vascular injury, severe soft-tissue injury, open fracture, floating elbow, concomitant intra-articular elbow injury, and pathologic fractures.

3. Extension-type supracondylar fractures account for most supracondylar fractures

4. Intramedullary nailing of humeral shaft fractures is associated with a higher rate of shoulder pain.

5. The "terrible triad" of elbow injuries involves fractures of the olecranon, coronoid, and radial head/neck.

6. For patients with a concomitant radial nerve injury who do not require surgical treatment, electromyography/nerve conduction velocity studies should be performed 6 weeks postinjury. For those who require surgical treatment, exploration is done at the time of surgery.

7. Total elbow arthroplasty should be considered in low-demand elderly individuals who sustain a complex distal humerus fracture.

8. The ligament of Struthers extends from the supracondylar process to the medial epicondyle.

9. In general, intercondylar fractures are managed surgically with medial and lateral plate fixation.

10. The chevron-type olecranon osteotomy should be pointed distal to minimize fracturing of the olecranon fragment.

Bibliography

Ali A, Douglas H, Stanley D: Revision surgery for nonunion after early failure of fixation of fractures of the distal humerus. *J Bone Joint Surg Br* 2005;87:1107-1110.

Anglen J: Distal humerus fractures. *J Am Acad Orthop Surg* 2005;13:291-297.

Bhandari M, Devereaux PJ, McKee MD, et al: Compression plating versus intramedullary nailing of humeral shaft fractures—A meta-analysis. *Acta Orthop* 2006;77:279-284.

Doornberg J, Lindenhovius A, Kloen P, et al: Two and three-dimensional computed tomography for the classification and management of distal humeral fractures: Evaluation of reliability and diagnostic accuracy. *J Bone Joint Surg Am* 2006;88:1795-1801.

Frankle MA, Herscovici D Jr, DiPasquale TG, et al: A comparison of open reduction and internal fixation and primary total elbow arthroplasty in the treatment of intraarticular distal humerus fractures in women older than age 65. *J Orthop Trauma* 2003;17:473-480.

Gardner MJ, Griffith MH, Demetrakopoulos D, et al: Hybrid locked plating of osteoporotic fractures of the humerus. *J Bone Joint Surg Am* 2006;88:1962-1967.

Hierholzer C, Sama D, Toro JB, et al: Plate fixation of un-united humeral shaft fractures: Effect of type of bone graft on healing. *J Bone Joint Surg Am* 2006;88:1442-1447.

McKee MD, Jupiter JB, Bosse G, et al: Outcome of ulnar neurolysis during post-traumatic reconstruction of the elbow. *J Bone Joint Surg Br* 1998;80:100-105.

Sarmiento A, Zagorski JB, Zych GA, et al: Functional bracing for the treatment of fractures of the humeral diaphysis. *J Bone Joint Surg Am* 2000;82:478-486.

Shao YC, Harwood P, Grotz MR, et al: Radial nerve palsy associated with fractures of the shaft of the humerus: A systematic review. *J Bone Joint Surg Br* 2005;87:1647-1652.

Tingstad EM, Wolinsky PR, Shyr Y, et al: Effect of immediate weightbearing on plated fractures of the humeral shaft. *J Trauma* 2000;49:278-280.

6: Trauma

Chapter 53

Pelvic, Acetabular, and Sacral Fractures
Robert V. Cantu, MD

I. Pelvic Fractures

A. Epidemiology

1. Most fractures occur in young adults involved in high-energy accidents such as motor vehicle accidents or falls from a height.

2. Pelvic fractures are often associated with other life-threatening injuries.

3. A smaller percentage of fractures occur in older patients with osteoporosis who sustain lower energy injuries, most commonly from a fall from a standing height. Patients with osteoporosis are also prone to insufficiency fractures of the pelvis.

B. Anatomy

1. The pelvis is formed by two innominate bones and the sacrum. Each innominate bone is formed from three ossification centers that fuse to become the ilium, ischium, and pubis (**Figure 1**).

2. The anterior portion of the pelvic ring is joined by the ligaments of the symphysis pubis.

3. The posterior pelvic ligaments join the sacrum to the innominate bones and include the sacrospinous, sacrotuberous, anterior and posterior sacroiliac ligaments. These are some of the strongest ligaments in the body and take considerable force to disrupt. The iliolumbar ligaments connect the ilium to the L5 transverse process.

4. The sciatic nerve is formed from the lumbosacral plexus and includes the roots of L4, L5, S1, S2, and S3.

   a. The L5 nerve root runs over the sacral ala approximately 2 cm medial to the sacroiliac joint.

   b. The sciatic nerve exits the pelvis through the greater sciatic notch and typically runs deep to the piriformis muscle and then superficial to the remaining external rotators.

5. The common iliac artery divides into the external and internal iliac arteries.

   a. The external iliac artery exits the pelvis under the inguinal ligament, becoming the femoral artery, and the internal iliac artery divides into an anterior and posterior artery.

   b. The anterior division gives off several branches: the inferior gluteal artery exits the pelvis through the greater sciatic notch and supplies the gluteus maximus muscle, the internal pudendal artery exits the pelvis through the sciatic notch, the obturator artery runs anteriorly exiting the pelvis through the obturator foramen.

   c. The posterior division of the internal iliac artery gives off three main branches: the superior gluteal artery runs across the SI joint and exits the pelvis through the greater sciatic notch, supplying the gluteus medius/minimus and tensor fascia lata muscles. The other two branches include the iliolumbar and lateral sacral arteries.

6. Other important vascular structures in the pelvis include the posterior venous plexus and the corona mortis.

   a. The posterior venous plexus is a large collection of veins that join to drain into the internal iliac veins. Injury to the plexus accounts for most of the bleeding in many pelvic fractures.

   b. The corona mortis is an anastomotic connection between the obturator and the external iliac systems. It can be either venous or arterial. The anastomosis runs across the superior pubic ramus, on average approximately 6 cm lateral to the pubic symphysis.

C. Surgical approaches

1. When performing an anterior approach to the sacroiliac (SI) joint, it is important to carefully dissect over the joint to avoid injury to the L5 root.

2. When performing a posterior Kocher-Langenbeck approach, the sciatic nerve should be identified and carefully retracted. The external rotators, with the exception of the piriformis, can be placed between the retractors and the nerve to provide some protection.

6: Trauma

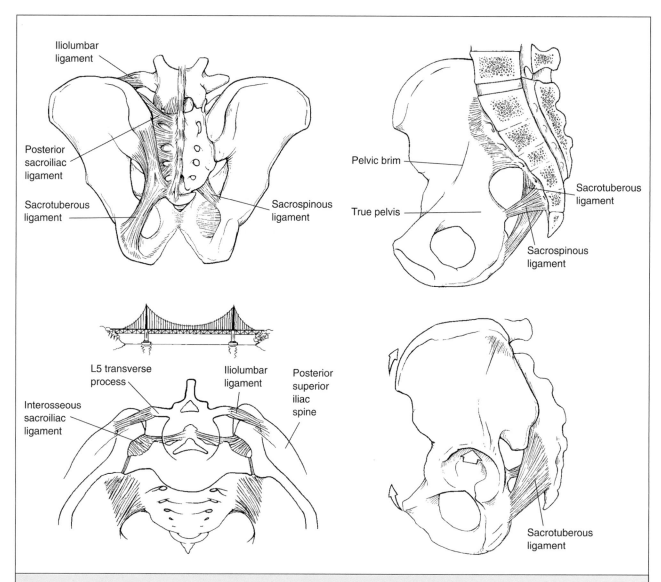

Figure 1   Anatomy of the pelvis, showing bony structure and ligamentous connections. *(Reproduced from Tile M: Acute pelvic fractures: I. Causation and classification. J Am Acad Orthop Surg 1996;4:143-151.)*

3. The obturator artery is at risk with the ilio-inguinal approach to the acetabulum.

4. The superior gluteal artery is at risk with the posterior approach to the acetabulum or pelvis. If the artery is injured as it exits the notch, it can retract and angiography may be necessary to control bleeding.

5. It is important to look for and if necessary ligate the corona mortis during the ilioinguinal or modified Stoppa approach to the acetabulum.

D. Pelvic stability

1. Pelvic stability is determined primarily by the degree of injury to the posterior pelvis.

2. Stability has been described in both rotational and vertical planes.

a. An injury that disrupts only the symphysis pubis but not the posterior ligaments or sacrum should be stable to both rotation and vertical force.

b. An injury that disrupts the symphysis pubis and some of the posterior ligaments (sacrospinous, sacrotuberous, anterior sacroiliac) but not the posterior sacrospinous ligaments will be unstable to rotational force, but stable to vertical force.

c. An injury that also disrupts the anterior and posterior sacroiliac ligaments or results in a distracted fracture through the sacrum will be unstable in both planes.

E. Mechanism of injury

1. High-energy injuries can result in unstable fracture patterns.

2. Fractures resulting from a fall from a height are usually stable and often involve a minimally displaced superior and inferior ramus fracture in the front of the pelvis and an impacted sacral fracture in the back.

F. Clinical evaluation

1. Hemodynamic status

    a. Hemorrhage is a leading cause of death in patients with pelvic fractures.

    b. Patients with a pelvic fracture who present with hypotension have a marked increase in mortality compared with those who are hemodynamically stable.

    c. There are three main sources for hemorrhage resulting from pelvic fractures: vascular, osseous, and visceral. Hemorrhage most often results from venous and osseous bleeding. Venous bleeding can lead to the formation of a large retroperitoneal hematoma. This bleeding may not be readily apparent on physical examination, but will be seen on CT scan of the pelvis.

    d. Patients who present with tachycardia or hypotension should receive 2 L of crystalloid, according to ATLS guidelines. If hemodynamic stability is not restored, blood transfusion with type O-negative blood should be initiated immediately. Consideration should be given to angiography to evaluate possible arterial sources of bleeding.

    e. Diagnostic peritoneal lavage performed in a patient with a pelvic fracture should be done supraumbilically because infraumbilical lavage can give a false-positive result because of tracking hematoma.

2. Neurologic injury

    a. A detailed neurologic examination is required for all patients with a pelvic fracture.

    b. The lumbosacral trunk and sciatic nerve are at risk with fractures and dislocations of the sacrum and sacroiliac joint. Careful assessment of the L5 nerve root (motor = extensor hallucis longus function, sensory = first web space on the dorsum of the foot) and the S1 nerve root (motor = gastrocnemius function, sensory = dorsum of foot minus first web space) should be performed. Motor strength should be graded from 0 to 5, as partial nerve palsy is common.

    c. Although less commonly injured, the femoral nerve (L2, L3, L4; motor = quadriceps) and the obturator nerve (motor = hip adductors) function should be examined.

    d. Pelvic fractures can also injure the pudendal nerve (S2, S3, S4), resulting in decreased perineal sensation and sexual dysfunction.

3. Gastrointestinal injury

    a. Abdominal examination is performed to assess for tenderness or swelling.

    b. All patients with a pelvic fracture also require a rectal examination. If a rectal injury is suspected, especially in patients with open pelvic fractures, rigid sigmoidoscopy is also required.

4. Genitourinary injury

    a. Evaluation begins with inspection on physical examination. If blood is present at the urethral meatus, a retrograde urethrogram should be performed before attempting insertion of an indwelling urinary catheter.

    b. The male urethra is less mobile and more prone to injury than the female urethra. The bulbous urethra is the part most commonly injured.

    c. Other potential signs of urethral injury include a high-riding prostate on physical examination in males, and an elevated bladder on intravenous pyelogram.

    d. Bladder injuries are common with pelvic fractures and should be looked for on CT scan or cystogram.

G. Radiographic evaluation

1. Radiographic evaluation begins with the AP view of the pelvis. Inlet and outlet views can be obtained to assess for AP and vertical displacement, respectively (**Figure 2**).

2. CT is helpful to further define the fracture, especially in the sacrum and posterior pelvis, which may be obscured by bowel gas on plain radiographs (**Figure 3**).

H. Fracture classification

1. The Tile classification scheme consists of three types based on the fracture stability (**Table 1**).

    a. Type A fractures are stable in both rotation and vertical directions.

    b. Type B fractures are unstable to rotation but remain stable vertically.

    c. Type C fractures are unstable in both rotation and vertical directions.

2. The Young-Burgess classification is based on the mechanism of injury and also consists of three main types (**Figure 4**).

    a. Anteroposterior compression (APC) fractures result from a force in the front or back of the pelvis. APC fractures are subdivided into three types and are sometimes referred to as the "open book" type injury.

    b. Lateral compression (LC) fractures result from

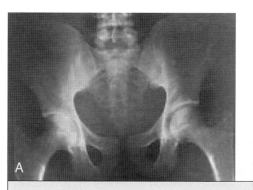
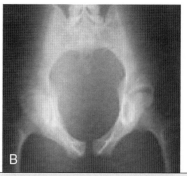
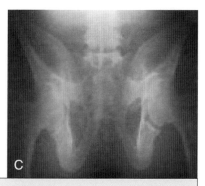

Figure 2 AP **(A)**, inlet **(B)**, and outlet **(C)** views of the pelvis. *(Reproduced with permission from Tile M (ed): Fractures of the Pelvis and Acetabulum, ed 2. Baltimore, MD, Williams & Wilkins, 1995.)*

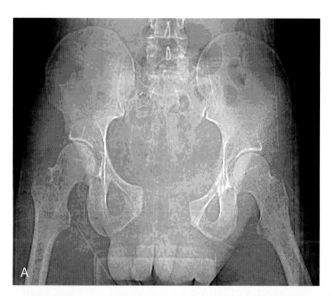

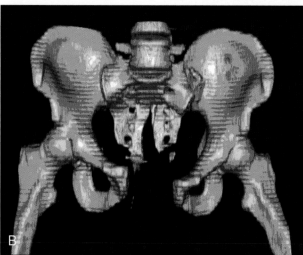

Figure 3 Comparison of plain radiograph **(A)** with CT scan **(B)**. The CT scan more clearly defines the posterior (sacral) fracture.

Table 1

Tile Classification of Pelvic Ring Lesions

Type A: Stable (posterior arch intact)

A1: Avulsion injury
A2: Iliac-wing or anterior-arch fracture due to a direct blow
A3: Transverse sacrococcygeal fracture

Type B: Partially stable (incomplete disruption of posterior arch)

B1: Open-book injury (external rotation)
B2: Lateral-compression injury (internal rotation)
B2-1: Ipsilateral anterior and posterior injuries
B2-2: Contralateral (bucket-handle) injuries
B3: Bilateral

Type C: Unstable (complete disruption of posterior arch)

C1: Unilateral
C1-1: Iliac fracture
C1-2: Sacroiliac fracture-dislocation
C1-3: Sacral fracture
C2: Bilateral, with one side type B, one side type C
C3: Bilateral

a laterally directed force to the pelvis and also have three subtypes.

c. Vertical shear (VS) fractures result from a vertically directed force through the pelvis such as in a fall from a height and are unstable injuries.

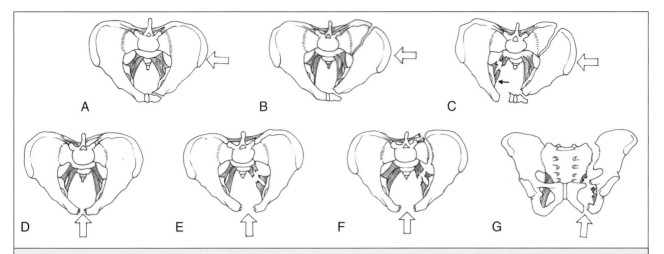

Figure 4 Young-Burgess classification of pelvic fractures. The arrows indicate the direction of the force causing the injury. **A** through **C** represent lateral compression injuries; **D** through **F** depict the increasing injury to the ligaments of the pelvis with anteroposterior compression injuries; and **G** shows a vertical shear injury, which ruptures the pelvis anteriorly and posteriorly. *(Reproduced from Beaty JH (ed):* Orthopaedic Knowledge Update 6. *Rosemont, IL, American Academy of Orthopaedic Surgeons, 1998, p 236.)*

d. A fourth type of fracture in the Young-Burgess classification involves a combination of any two patterns.

I. Treatment

1. Initial management

   a. Initial treatment depends on fracture stability and the hemodynamic status of the patient. ATLS protocols should be followed for all patients with traumatic pelvic injuries.

   b. Unstable fracture patterns in hypotensive patients require emergent stabilization in an effort to control ongoing hemorrhage.

   c. Multiple devices have been used to stabilize pelvic fractures: bedsheets, pneumatic anti-shock garments (PASGs), pelvic binders, C-clamps, and external fixators. Bedsheets are readily available but require care to ensure that they are wrapped and held tightly around the pelvis. Towel clips are recommended to hold the sheet tightly rather than tying a knot. PASGs are effective in stabilizing fractures but are used less frequently because of potential complications such as compartment syndrome and respiratory compromise. The advent of pelvic binders has made quick and effective provisional stabilization of pelvic fractures relatively easy.

      i. Rapid provisional fixation of unstable pelvic fractures can be performed in the trauma bay with application of the pelvic binder.

      ii. Pelvic binders can remain in place during further diagnostic test such as angiography; if necessary, a portion of the binder can be cut to allow for vascular access.

   d. Fluid resuscitation of hypotensive patients begins with placement of two large-bore IVs (16 gauge or higher) and infusion of 2 L of crystalloid. If the patient remains hypotensive or only transiently responds to fluids, then blood transfusion is indicated. Any coagulopathy should be corrected with appropriate transfusion of fresh frozen plasma and platelets.

   e. If a patient remains hemodynamically unstable after fluid resuscitation and pelvic stabilization, emergent angiography should be considered. Although arterial bleeding is found in only 10% to 15% of patients, when it occurs emergent embolization can be lifesaving.

2. Definitive management—nonsurgical

   a. Stable pelvic fractures (Tile type A or Young-Burgess APC1 or LC1) are treated nonsurgically.

   b. Ambulation using crutches or a walker is allowed when other injuries allow.

   c. Repeat radiographs should be obtained once the patient has been out of bed to verify that there have been no changes in pelvic alignment.

3. Definitive management—surgical

   a. External fixation

      i. Anterior pelvic external fixation can be used as definitive treatment of injuries that primarily involve the anterior pelvis but not for unstable posterior injuries. An example is the APC II injury, where external fixation can close down the anterior diastasis. Since the posterior SI ligaments are intact, they provide support to the posterior pelvis, similar to the binding on a book.

    ii. The pins for the external fixator can be placed in the iliac wing, or alternatively, a single pin can be placed on each side in the supra-acetabular region (Hannover frame). With either construct, the bars connecting the pins should leave room for abdominal expansion. The Hannover construct requires use of a C-arm to ensure that the pins are above the acetabulum.

    iii. An external fixator is more commonly used for temporary fixation. An anterior external fixator can provide stability to the front of the pelvis but cannot reduce the posterior pelvis when the SI joint is dislocated or there is a diastased fracture through the sacrum.

    iv. The stabilization afforded by the external fixator can help limit hemorrhage in a hemodynamically unstable patient but requires conversion to definitive internal fixation when the patient's condition is more stable.

  b. Open reduction and internal fixation

    i. Anterior symphyseal injury can be treated with symphyseal plating. A Pfannenstiel incision is used, and reduction clamps are applied to the symphysis. A 3.5-mm reconstruction plate can be contoured to fit along the superior aspect of the symphysis.

    ii. Multiple approaches can be used for open reduction and internal fixation of posterior pelvic injuries. Displaced SI joint injuries can be approached anteriorly, using a retroperitoneal approach. Following reduction of the SI joint, two short 3.5- or 4.5-mm plates can be used for fixation. The L5 nerve root runs approximately 2 cm medial to the SI joint and should be carefully retracted during fixation.

    iii. Percutaneous iliosacral screws can be placed for SI joint dislocations or sacral fractures, provided closed reduction of any displacement other than pure diastasis can be achieved. Partially threaded screws can be used to close down diastasis of the SI joint, but care is required to avoid overcompressing sacral fractures that extend into the sacral foramen. SI screws can be placed with the patient either prone or supine. A radiolucent operating table and excellent fluoroscopic visualization are mandatory.

    iv. Posterior plating of the pelvis requires the patient to be in the prone position. With transiliac posterior plating, vertical incisions are made over each SI joint. The SI joints are exposed and reduced with clamps. A reconstruction plate is contoured and placed subcutaneously and secured with screws into each iliac wing. Transiliac bars can be used in a similar fashion but tend to be more prominent and result in a higher risk of soft-tissue irritation and breakdown.

    v. A more recent construct for posterior pelvic fixation is the triangular synthesis. This involves placing a pedicle screw at the L5 level and screws in the ilium and sacrum connected by bars. Biomechanical studies have shown this to be the most stable construct for posterior fixation.

J. Miscellaneous pelvic fractures and other conditions

  1. Open pelvic fractures

    a. Open pelvic fractures result from high-energy mechanisms and consequently have an increased risk for associated injuries and mortality.

    b. Initial treatment follows ATLS guidelines, focusing on resuscitation and control of hemorrhage.

    c. Rectal and pelvic examinations, including a speculum examination in women, should be performed to rule out hidden lacerations.

    d. Tetanus booster and broad-spectrum antibiotics should be given.

    e. A diverting colostomy is performed for open wounds in close proximity to the rectum to prevent contamination.

  2. Fractures with neurologic injury

    a. Neurologic injury occurs in approximately 10% to 15% of patients with pelvic fracture. The extent and permanence of neurologic injury is the most important predictor of long-term outcomes for these patients.

    b. If a patient has a neurologic deficit and a CT scan shows entrapment of the nerve root(s) in the sacral foramen, posterior decompression should be considered.

    c. Electromyography can be obtained at 6 weeks after the injury as a baseline from which to measure recovery.

    d. Final outcome of a neurologic injury can take 18 months or longer.

  3. Fractures with genitourinary injury

    a. Treatment of an extraperitoneal bladder injury is broad-spectrum antibiotic treatment and urinary catheter drainage for 10 to 14 days. A cystogram is performed before catheter removal to ensure that the rupture has healed.

b. Peritoneal bladder ruptures require surgical repair. Any bony spicules penetrating the bladder should be removed.

4. Hypovolemic shock

a. Treatment begins with placement of two large-bore IVs and infusion of 2 L of crystalloid (normal saline solution). If the patient remains hypotensive or shows only a transient response to the fluids, transfusion should be started with type O-negative blood.

b. While fluid resuscitation is underway, any unstable pelvic fracture should be stabilized. Options include a sheet, a C-clamp, a PASG, an external fixator, or a pelvic binder.

c. Angiography should be considered as arterial pelvic bleeding can lead to rapid exsanguination.

K. Rehabilitation

1. Assuming stable fixation, patients are mobilized with touchdown weight bearing on the affected side. Range-of-motion exercises are begun as soon as symptoms allow.

2. After 4 to 6 weeks, weight bearing is advanced and strengthening exercises are started. Outpatient physical therapy may continue for an additional 6 weeks to 3 months to restore strength, balance, and proper gait pattern.

3. Final functional outcome can take 6 months to a year, sometimes longer if a neurologic injury is present.

L. Complications

1. Thromboembolic disease is a major concern for patients with pelvic fractures because of a high incidence of deep venous thrombosis (DVT) (35% to 50%) and pulmonary embolism (up to 10%). Fatal pulmonary embolism can occur in up to 2% of patients. Patients should be treated with chemical prophylaxis for DVT until ambulatory status is restored.

2. If other injuries preclude chemical prophylaxis, consideration should be given to placement of an IVC filter.

3. Iatrogenic nerve injury is a risk, especially with posterior fixation of pelvic fractures. If percutaneous iliosacral screws are used, a preoperative CT should be obtained to ensure a "safe zone" for screw placement.

4. With open treatment, self-retaining retractors should be used with caution because both neurologic and vascular injury have been reported.

5. Fracture nonunion in these patients is rare; malunion is more common, especially with vertically displaced fractures. Treatment of either is

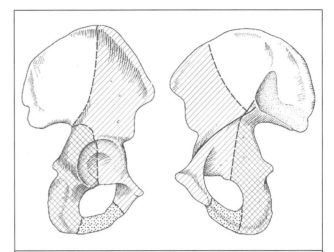

Figure 5   Anatomy of the acetabulum, showing the location of the anterior column (area with lines), posterior column (cross-hatched area), and ischiopubic rami (speckled area). *(Reproduced with permission from Letournel E, Judet R (eds): Fractures of the Acetabulum, ed 2. Berlin, Germany, Springer-Verlag, 1993.)*

challenging, with long surgical times and large volume of blood loss common.

6. Superficial wound infections often can be treated with appropriate antibiotics. Deep infection requires surgical irrigation and débridement.

II. Acetabular Fractures

A. Epidemiology

1. Acetabular fractures most often occur in young adults involved in high-energy motor vehicle collisions or falls from a height.

2. As with pelvic fractures, acetabular fractures also can occur in older patients with osteoporotic bone, usually from a low-energy fall.

B. Anatomy

1. The acetabulum or hip socket is part of the innominate bone and is formed from the ilium, ischium, and pubis.

2. The bony anatomy was described by Letournel as an inverted Y.

a. The anterior column begins superiorly with the anterior portion of the iliac wing and includes the anterior wall, the pelvic brim, and the superior pubic ramus.

b. The posterior column begins superiorly with the superior and inferior sciatic notch and includes the posterior wall, the ischial tuberosity, and most of the quadrilateral plate (**Figure 5**).

6: Trauma

C. Surgical approaches—Type depends on location of the fracture.

1. The ilioinguinal approach is used to access the anterior wall and anterior column and the quadrilateral plate.

   a. The incision begins approximately 2 cm above the symphysis pubis and extends laterally to the ASIS and continues along the iliac crest.

   b. Three "windows" have been described with the ilioinguinal approach.

      i. The first or medial window lies medial to the external iliac artery and vein.

      ii. The second or middle window lies between the external iliac vessels and the iliopsoas muscle.

      iii. The third or top window lies lateral to the iliopsoas.

   c. Anatomic structures at risk include the femoral nerve, artery, and vein, which can be injured either during the approach or by retractors placed in the middle window.

   d. In men, the spermatic cord is at risk in the first window. The bladder also lies deep in the medial window and should be carefully retracted.

   e. The lateral femoral cutaneous nerve runs near the ASIS, and some authors recommend sacrificing the nerve because prolonged retraction can lead to a painful stretch injury.

   f. The iliopectineal fascia runs between the femoral nerve and the external iliac artery. The fascia is incised during the approach.

   g. The obturator artery and nerve lie deep in the medial window. The corona mortis is an anastomotic connection between the external iliac and obturator artery or vein. If encountered, the corona mortis should be ligated.

2. The Kocher-Langenbeck approach is used to access the posterior column or posterior wall of the acetabulum.

   a. The incision begins approximately 5 cm anterior to the posterior superior iliac spine and carried distally in a curved fashion to the greater trochanter and then another 5 to 10 cm in line with the femoral shaft.

   b. The fascia lata is incised, and the gluteus maximus muscle fibers are bluntly divided up to the level of the inferior gluteal nerve. The sciatic nerve lies posterior to the external rotators of the hip and should be identified.

   c. The piriformis, superior and inferior gemellus, obturator externus, and obturator internus are incised approximately 1 cm from their inser-

tion on the greater trochanter to preserve the ascending branch of the medial femoral circumflex artery, which runs deep to these tendons before joining the femoral arterial ring at the base of the femoral neck. The quadratus femoris muscle is left intact also to protect the medial femoral circumflex artery.

   d. Minimal dissection of the joint capsule, which is often torn, is performed to preserve the remaining blood supply to the posterior wall fragments.

3. Other approaches include the extended iliofemoral, the triradiate, the Watson-Jones, the modified Stoppa, and the Hardinge.

C. Mechanism of injury

1. Like pelvic fractures, most acetabular fractures result from high-energy mechanisms, most commonly motor vehicle accidents or falls from a height.

2. Fracture pattern depends on the position of the femoral head in the acetabulum at the time of impact and the direction of the force applied.

D. Clinical evaluation

1. Patients with acetabular fractures often have multiple injuries and the initial approach to evaluation should follow ATLS guidelines.

2. Careful assessment of the ipsilateral lower extremity to rule out fracture or ligamentous injury of the knee should be performed.

3. The soft tissues overlying the greater trochanter should be carefully inspected for signs of a Morel-Lavallee lesion, a closed degloving injury resulting in a hematoma and liquefied fat forming between the subcutaneous tissues and the fascial layer.

4. Sciatic nerve function should be carefully assessed in the ipsilateral extremity, especially with fractures involving the posterior wall.

E. Radiographic evaluation

1. AP views of the pelvis, including Judet views (45° internal and external views) should be obtained.

2. Six radiographic lines should be assessed for any loss of continuity: the iliopectineal line (anterior column), the ilioischial line (posterior column), the anterior rim of the acetabulum (anterior wall), the posterior rim of the acetabulum (posterior wall), the dome (roof) of the acetabulum, and the teardrop (radiographic U) (**Figure 6**).

   a. The iliac oblique view better demonstrates the ilioischial line (posterior column) and the anterior rim (anterior wall).

   b. The obturator oblique view better demonstrates the iliopectineal line (anterior column) and the posterior rim (posterior wall).

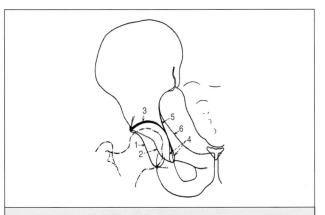

Figure 6 Radiographic evaluation of the acetabulum showing the location of the six radiographic lines: (1) posterior wall, (2) anterior wall, (3) roof, (4) radiographic U, (5) ilioischial line, (6) iliopectineal line. (*Adapted with permission from Letournel E, Judet R (eds): Fractures of the Acetabulum, ed 2. Berlin, Germany, Springer-Verlag, 1993, p 259.*)

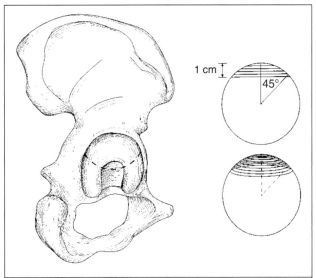

Figure 7 Roof arc measurement corresponding to the superior 1 cm on CT scan. (*Adapted with permission from Olson SA, Matta JM: The computerized tomography subchondral arc: A new method of assessing acetabular articular continuity after fracture (a preliminary report).* J Orthop Trauma 1993;7:402-413.)

3. CT scan better defines acetabular fractures, particularly in identifying the location and displacement of fractures and loose fragments in the hip joint. CT also helps with preoperative planning.

4. Involvement of the acetabular dome can be assessed by using roof arc measurements.

   a. On the AP pelvis and Judet views, roof arc is measured by the angle formed by a straight line drawn though the center of the acetabulum and a line to the highest point of the fracture in the acetabulum. A roof arc angle less than 45° corresponds with a fracture in the weight-bearing dome of the acetabulum.

5. On a CT scan, the area within the 45° roof arc also corresponds with the superior 10 mm of the acetabulum (**Figure 7**).

F. Fracture classification

   1. The Letournel-Judet classification includes five simple and five complex or associated fracture patterns.

      a. The simple patterns include posterior wall, posterior column, anterior wall, anterior column, and transverse.

      b. The associated patterns include posterior column and posterior wall, transverse with posterior wall, T type, anterior column and posterior hemitransverse, and both column (**Figure 8**).

   2. Transverse, transverse with posterior wall, T type, anterior column and posterior hemitransverse, and both-column fractures involve both columns of the acetabulum. Both-column fractures differ from other types in that the articular surface is separated from the ilium. With the other four fracture types, a portion of the articular surface remains in continuity with the ilium.

3. For both-column fractures, the "spur" sign above the acetabulum on an obturator oblique radiograph is diagnostic.

G. Treatment

   1. Nonsurgical

      a. Nondisplaced fractures or displaced fractures that do not involve the dome of the acetabulum are treated nonsurgically. The dome of the acetabulum has been defined as the area within the 45° roof arc or the superior 10 mm on a CT scan.

      b. An exception to this rule is posterior wall fractures, which may not involve the dome but nevertheless can result in hip instability if a large fragment is involved.

      c. Some both-column fractures have extensive comminution, but the fragments remain minimally displaced around the femoral head. This so-called secondary congruence also allows for nonsurgical management.

      d. Other contraindications to open reduction and internal fixation include the following: associated medical conditions that prevent surgery; advanced osteoporosis or degenerative joint disease, making hip arthroplasty the better option; and local or systemic sepsis (**Table 2**).

      e. Mobilization out of bed with toe touch weight bearing for 10 to 12 weeks.

6: Trauma

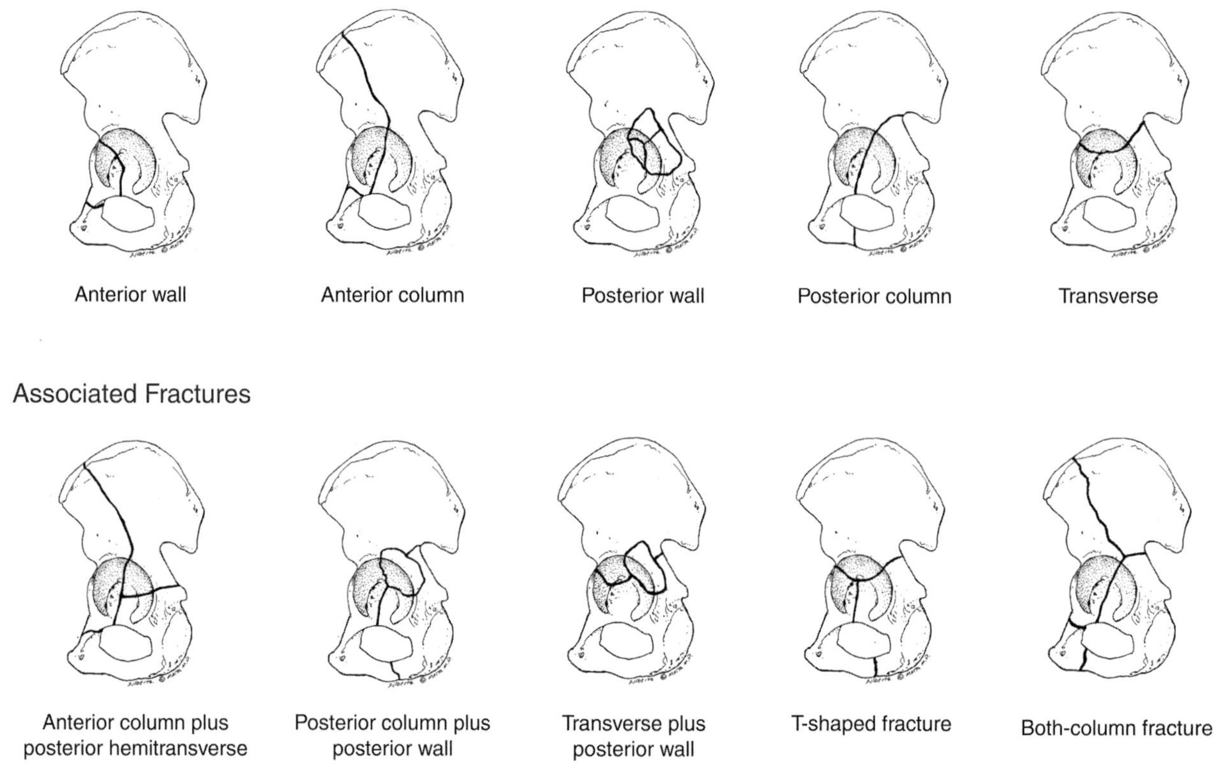

Elementary Fractures

Anterior wall   Anterior column   Posterior wall   Posterior column   Transverse

Associated Fractures

Anterior column plus   Posterior column plus   Transverse plus   T-shaped fracture   Both-column fracture
posterior hemitransverse   posterior wall   posterior wall

Figure 8 Letournel-Judet classification of acetabular fractures showing the five simple and five complex fracture patterns. *(Courtesy of Joel M. Matta, MD.)*

Table 2

Indications for Nonsurgical Management of Acetabular Fractures

Nondisplaced fractures or fractures with less than 2 mm of displacement

Displaced fractures below the level of the weight-bearing dome of the acetabulum but with a stable femoroacetabular relationship (congruency)

Both-column fractures having secondary congruence

Posterior wall fractures, the size and position of which do not affect hip joint stability

Advanced medical problems that make the risk of surgery outweigh its benefits of osteopenia or fracture fragmentation that make adequate reduction or stable fixation unlikely

---

2. Surgical

   a. Indications include fractures involving the dome of the acetabulum with at least 2 mm of displacement, fractures that result in instability of the hip joint, and fractures with trapped intra-articular fragments.

   b. The approach selected depends on pattern and location of the fracture. Fractures involving a single column or wall can be approached through a single approach (ilioinguinal or modified Stoppa for anterior fractures and Kocher-Langenbeck for posterior fractures).

   c. Both-column fractures may require both an anterior and a posterior approach or an extensile approach such as the extended iliofemoral (Table 3).

   d. Intraoperative traction of acetabular fractures can greatly assist fracture reduction.

   e. Marginal impaction is often seen with posterior wall fractures and should be elevated and bone grafted.

H. Rehabilitation

   1. Following stable fixation, patients should be mobilized as soon as possible. Weight bearing on the injured side is limited to touch down for 10 to 12 weeks.

Table 3		
Surgical Approaches Based on Acetabular Fracture Type		
Fracture Type	**Recommended Approach**	**Indicator(s)**
Transverse	Kocher-Langenbeck	Major displacement at posterior column
	Ilioinguinal	Major displacement at anterior column
		Fracture angle from high anterior to low posterior
	Extended approach	Major displacement transtectal
		Fracture healing evident (> 15 days old)
Transverse and posterior wall	Kocher-Langenbeck	Use in most patients
	Extended approach	Major displacement transtectal
		Fracture healing evident (> 15 days old)
		Extended posterior wall component
		Associated pubic symphysis disruption
	Simultaneous front and back	Alternative to extended approaches
		Inability to fully visualize a transtectal fracture line is an important limitation
T-shaped	Kocher-Langenbeck	Use in most patients
	Ilioinguinal	Minimal posterior displacement
	Extended approach	Major displacement transtectal
		Wide separation of columns
		Associated pubic symphysis disruption
		Fracture healing evident (> 15 days old)
	Simultaneous front and back	Alternative to extended approaches (as above)
	Sequential front and back	When selected approach fails to reduce the opposite column
Anterior column/wall and posterior hemitransverse	Ilioinguinal	Use in most patients
	Extended approach	Fracture healing evident (> 15 days old) and
		Wide displacement of posterior column
	Front and back choices	Alternatives to extended approaches
Both columns	Ilioinguinal	Use in most patients
	Extended approach	Posterior column is comminuted
		Fracture healing evident (> 15 days old)
		A displaced fracture line crosses the sacroiliac joint

2. With stable fractures or solid fixation, active and active-assist range of motion of the affected extremity is begun as soon as symptoms allow. Isometric quadriceps exercises and straight leg raises are begun early to minimize thigh atrophy.

3. Full weight bearing is delayed for 10 to 12 weeks, at which point progressive strengthening exercises are added. Aquatherapy can be helpful in transitioning to a fully ambulatory status.

I. Complications

1. As with pelvic fractures, DVT is a major concern for patients with acetabular fractures.

   a. Prevention includes use of pneumatic compression boots and chemical prophylaxis.

   b. Patients who cannot receive chemical prophylaxis should be considered for IVC filter placement.

6: Trauma

2. Iatrogenic nerve or vessel injury can result from surgical treatment.

   a. Maintaining the knee in flexion and the hip in extension during the Kocher-Langenbeck approach helps to decrease the tension on the sciatic nerve.

   b. Self-retaining retractors should be used with caution.

3. Heterotopic ossification is most common with the extended iliofemoral and Kocher-Langenbeck approaches and least common with the ilioinguinal approach.

   a. Patients at significant risk should be treated with either indomethacin (25 mg three times daily for 4 to 6 weeks) or radiation therapy (700 cGy) in a single dose. Radiation should be avoided in children or women of childbearing age.

   b. For maximum effectiveness, prophylaxis should be given preoperatively or within 48 hours after surgery.

4. The risk of osteonecrosis is highest when hip dislocation occurs concurrently with acetabular fracture.

   a. Dislocations should be reduced as soon as possible to limit thrombosis of stretched vessels supplying the femoral head.

   b. With surgical treatment, the ascending branch of the medial femoral circumflex artery should be preserved.

5. Untreated Morel-Lavallee lesions have a high rate of infection.

III. Sacral Fractures

A. Epidemiology

1. Sacral fractures are considered a fracture of the pelvic ring. They occur principally in young adults as a result of a high-energy accident.

2. Older patients also can sustain these fractures, most often the result of a low-energy fall. Insufficiency fractures of the sacrum also can develop in patients with osteoporosis.

B. Anatomy

1. The sacrum is the terminal extension of the spine. The sacrum forms an articulation on either side with the ilium known as the SI joint. The joint is held together tightly by the anterior and posterior SI ligaments.

2. The sacral nerve roots (S1-S4) exit the sacrum anteriorly through the sacral foramen. The L5 nerve root runs on top of the sacral ala, approximately 2 cm medial to the SI joint.

3. Sacral root injury is most common with zone 3 injuries.

C. Surgical approaches

1. Sacral fractures and SI joint-dislocations can be exposed from either an anterior or a posterior approach. Alternatively, fractures that can be closed reduced may be amenable to percutaneous fixation. Percutaneous treatment is reserved for fractures in which any vertical or AP displacement can be reduced in a closed manner.

2. The anterior approach uses the top window of the ilioinguinal incision. The iliac muscle is elevated off of the ilium, and the SI joint is exposed. Medial dissection is limited by the L5 nerve root.

3. Posterior approaches use vertical incisions over the SI joint or a single midline incision. The gluteus maximus muscle is elevated to expose the SI joint and the posterior sacrum.

D. Mechanism of injury

1. Most sacral fractures result from motor vehicle accidents or falls from a height.

2. Repetitive stress in older patients can lead to insufficiency fractures.

E. Clinical evaluation is the same as for pelvic ring injuries, except that additional emphasis on the neurologic examination is necessary because sacral fractures often are associated with sacral root injury.

F. Radiographic evaluation

1. Plain radiographs include AP pelvis and inlet/outlet views.

2. Because sacral fractures are often difficult to fully visualize on plain radiographs, CT is often helpful to better define the fracture and the degree of displacement.

G. Fracture classification

1. The Denis classification divides the sacrum into three zones (**Figure 9**).

   a. Zone 1 includes the alar region lateral to the foramen.

   b. Zone 2 includes the foraminal region.

   c. Zone 3 is the central portion located between the foramen.

2. Fractures are defined based on which zone they involve.

H. Treatment

1. Nonsurgical—fractures that have minimal displacement or are impacted are typically stable and can be treated nonsurgically.

2. Surgical

    a. Significantly displaced fractures benefit from surgical treatment. When reducing fractures, especially those involving zone 2, care should be taken to avoid overcompressing the fracture and the neural foramen because of the possibility of causing iatrogenic nerve dysfunction.

    b. Loose bone fragments in the neural foramen may require removal to decompress the sacral nerve root(s).

    c. Percutaneous fixation is unreliable in patients with osteoporotic bone.

I. Rehabilitation—essentially the same as described for pelvic fractures following a stable sacral fracture or one in which solid fixation is achieved.

J. Complications

    1. Iatrogenic sacral nerve root injury can result from improper hardware placement with either open or percutaneous techniques.

    2. Malreduction is a significant risk with vertically displaced fractures.

    3. As with any pelvic fracture, DVT is a risk and requires prophylaxis.

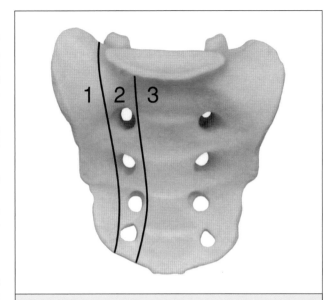

Figure 9 Denis classification of sacral fractures. *(Reproduced from Vaccaro AR, Kim DH, Brodke DS, et al: Diagnosis and management of sacral spine fractures.* Instr Course Lect *2004;53:375-385.)*

Top Testing Facts

Pelvic Fractures

1. Pelvic fractures in young adults result from high-energy injuries and are often associated with other life-threatening injuries.

2. Rapid, provisional fixation of unstable pelvic fractures can be performed in the trauma bay with application of the pelvic binder.

3. Pelvic binders can remain in place during further diagnostic tests such as angiography; if necessary, a portion of the binder can be cut to allow for vascular access.

4. Open pelvic fractures may require a diverting colostomy.

5. External fixators can be used for definitive treatment of anterior pelvic injuries but not unstable posterior injuries.

6. Diagnostic peritoneal lavage performed in a patient with a pelvic fracture should be done supraumbilical, as an infraumbilical lavage can give a false-positive result due to tracking hematoma.

7. Patients with pelvic fractures have a high incidence of DVT (35% to 50%) and pulmonary embolism (up to 10%).

Acetabular Fractures

1. The area within the 45° roof arc angle corresponds with the superior 10 mm of the acetabulum on CT scan.

2. Secondary congruence of both-column fractures may allow successful nonsurgical management.

3. Intraoperative traction of acetabular fractures can greatly assist fracture reduction.

4. Marginal impaction is often seen with posterior wall fractures and should be elevated and bone grafted.

5. Untreated Morel-Lavallee lesions have a high rate of infection.

6. Heterotopic ossification is common, especially with the extended iliofemoral and Kocher-Langenbeck approaches.

Sacral Fractures

1. Sacral fractures are often difficult to fully visualize on plain radiographs; thus, CT is helpful in defining the fracture.

2. Percutaneous treatment is reserved for fractures in which any vertical or AP displacement can be reduced in a closed manner.

3. Sacral root injury is most common with zone 3 injuries.

4. Overcompression of fractures involving zone 2 should be avoided.

5. Percutaneous fixation is unreliable in patients with osteoporotic bone.

6: Trauma

Bibliography

Barei DP, Bellabarba C, Mills WJ, Routt ML Jr: Percutaneous management of unstable pelvic ring disruptions. *Injury* 2001; 32(suppl 1):SA33-SA44.

Baumgaertner MR: Fractures of the posterior wall of the acetabulum. *J Am Acad Orthop Surg* 1999;7:54-65.

Bellabarba C, Schildhauer T, Vaccaro A, Chapman J: Complications associated with surgical stabilization of high-grade sacral fracture dislocations with spino-pelvic instability. *Spine* 2006;31(11S):S80-S88.

Borrelli J Jr, Goldfarb C, Ricci W, Wagner JM, Engsberg JR: Functional outcome after isolated acetabular fractures. *J Orthop Trauma* 2002;16:73-81.

Chiu FY, Chen CM, Lo WH: Surgical treatment of displaced acetabular fractures: 72 cases followed for 10 (6-14) years. *Injury* 2000;31:181-185.

Cole JD, Bolhofner BR: Acetabular fracture fixation via a modified Stoppa limited intrapelvic approach: Description of operative technique and preliminary treatment results. *Clin Orthop Relat Res* 1994;305:112-123.

Copeland CE, Bosse MJ, McCarthy ML, et al: Effect of trauma and pelvic function on female genitourinary, sexual, and reproductive function. *J Orthop Trauma* 1997;11:73-81.

Dalal SA, Burgess AR, Siegel JH: Pelvic fracture in multiple trauma: Classification by mechanism is key to pattern of organ injury, resuscitative requirements, and outcome. *J Trauma* 1989;29:981-1002.

Gansslen A, Hufner T, Krettek C: Percutaneous iliosacral screw fixation of unstable pelvic injuries by conventional fluoroscopy. *Oper Orthop Traumatol* 2006;18:225-244.

Gruen GS, Leit ME, Gruen RJ, Garrison HG, Auble TE, Peitzman AB: Functional outcome of patients with unstable pelvic ring fractures stabilized with open reduction and internal fixation. *J Trauma* 1995;39:838-845.

Henry SM, Pollak AN, Jones AL, Boswell S, Scalea TM: Pelvic fracture in geriatric patients: A distinct clinical entity. *J Trauma* 2002;53:15-20.

Mehta S, Auerbach JD, Born CT, Chin KR: Sacral fractures. *J Am Acad Orthop Surg* 2006;14:656-665.

Miranda MA, Riemfer BL, Butterfield SL, Burke CJ III: Pelvic ring injuries: A long term functional outcome study. *Clin Orthop Relat Res* 1996;329:152-159.

O'Neill PA, Riina J, Sclafani S, Tornetta P III: Angiographic findings in pelvic fractures. *Clin Orthop Relat Res* 1996;329: 60-67.

Routt ML Jr, Nork SE, Mills WJ: High-energy pelvic ring disruptions. *Orthop Clin North Am* 2002;33:59-72.

Chapter 54

Hip Dislocations and Femoral Head Fractures

*Robert F. Ostrum, MD

I. Hip Dislocations

A. Epidemiology

1. 90% of dislocations of the hip are posterior, most often secondary to motor vehicle accidents (MVAs) and knee-to-dashboard trauma with a posterior directed force.

2. Right hip involved much more often than left in MVAs

B. Anatomy/surgical approaches

1. Anatomy

a. Strong capsular ligaments—The anterior iliofemoral and posterior ischiofemoral ligament run from the acetabulum to the femoral neck (**Figure 1**).

b. The ligamentum teres runs from the acetabulum (cotyloid fossa) to the femoral head (fovea centralis).

c. The main arterial blood supply is from the superior and posterior cervical arteries, which are primarily derived from the medial circumflex artery (posterior); the lesser blood supply (10% to 15%) is through the artery of the ligamentum teres (**Figure 2**).

2. Surgical approaches—For irreducible dislocations, "go where the money is."

a. Posterior approach (Kocher-Langenbeck)—Allows access to posterior dislocations.

b. Anterior approach (Smith-Petersen)—Allows access to anterior dislocations and also better visualization of the anterior joint.

c. Anterolateral approach (Watson-Jones)—Allows access to the posterior hip through the same incision.

Robert F. Ostrum, MD, is a consultant for or an employee of DePuy and Biomet.

C. Mechanism of injury

1. Anterior dislocations

a. Result from an abduction and external rotation force

b. A flexed hip leads to an inferior (obturator) dislocation; an extended hip results in a superior (pubic) dislocation.

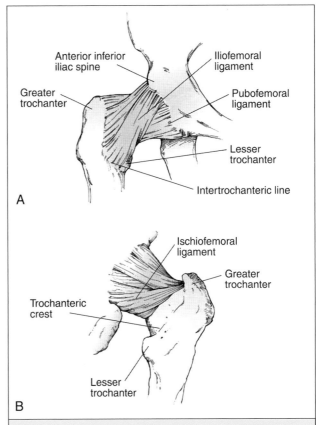

Figure 1   The hip capsule and its thickenings (ligaments) as visualized from anteriorly **(A)** and posteriorly **(B)**. *(Reproduced with permission from Bucholz RW, Heckman JD [eds]: Rockwood and Green's Fractures in Adults, ed. 5. Philadelphia, PA: Lippincott Williams and Wilkins, 2001, p 1557.)*

6: Trauma

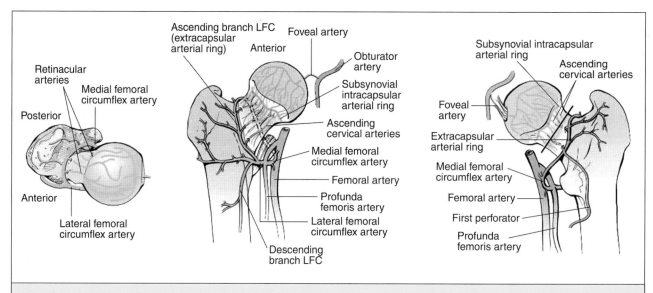

Figure 2   The vascular supply to the femoral head arises from the medial and lateral circumflex vessels, which create a ring giving rise to the cervical vessels. A minor contribution comes from the obturator artery via the ligamentum teres. *(Reproduced with permission from Bucholz RW, Heckman JD [eds]: Rockwood and Green's Fractures in Adults, ed. 5. Philadelphia, PA: Lippincott Williams and Wilkins, 2001, p 1558.)*

c. Femoral head impaction or osteochondral fractures are commonly seen.

2. Posterior dislocations

   a. Most commonly seen after dashboard injuries, where the knee hits the dashboard, resulting in a posteriorly directed force through the femur

   b. The presence of an associated fracture as well as the location and extent of the fracture are dictated by the flexion, abduction, and rotation of the hip joint at the time of the impact. Increased flexion and adduction favor a pure dislocation without fracture of the posterior wall.

D. Clinical evaluation

1. High incidence of associated injuries (up to 95%) in patients with a hip dislocation secondary to MVA

2. Anterior dislocations present with the leg in a flexed (inferior) or extended (superior), abducted, and externally rotated attitude.

3. Posterior hip dislocations present with the limb in an adducted and internally rotated position.

4. Common associated injuries include those around the ipsilateral knee secondary to direct trauma.

   a. Patella fractures

   b. Ligamentous tears and dislocations (posterior)

   c. Bone bruises

   d. Meniscal tears

5. Sciatic nerve injury may be seen in up to 8% to 20% of patients; a thorough neurologic examination should precede any attempts at reduction. Prereduction and postreduction neurologic examinations should be documented.

E. Imaging evaluation

1. Standard AP radiograph shows dislocation of the femoral head.

   a. The attitude of the limb and appearance of the femoral head can distinguish an anterior from a posterior dislocation.

   b. In posterior dislocations, the femoral head appears small and is located superiorly, whereas with anterior dislocations the femoral head appears larger and overlaps the medial acetabulum or the obturator foramen.

2. Judet views (iliac and obturator oblique)

   a. Can help with diagnosing the location of the dislocation but also assist in identifying associated transverse or posterior wall fractures

   b. The obturator oblique view gives the best picture of the posterior dislocation and the posterior wall.

3. CT scans are necessary following all reductions of hip dislocations.

   a. Important information gained from this study includes:

     i. Concentric reduction

     ii. Bony or cartilaginous fragments in the joint

     iii. Associated fractures

iv. Marginal impaction of the posterior wall

v. Avulsion fractures

vi. Femoral head or neck fractures

b. The percentage of posterior wall fracture can also be calculated. Assess need for internal fixation on postreduction CT scan. Identify size of posterior wall fragment and dome involvement. More than 25% involvement of the posterior wall is an indication for fixation.

4. Prereduction CT scans

a. Reserved for irreducible dislocations in an attempt to determine the block to reduction

b. Obtaining these CT scans before reduction in simple dislocations or fracture-dislocations provides little information and may lead to prolonged dislocation and concomitant osteonecrosis or sciatic nerve or cartilage injury.

F. Classification

1. Hip dislocations are classified as anterior or posterior.

2. Further clarification that also helps with prognosis is gained by using the Thompson-Epstein classification (**Table 1**).

G. Treatment

1. Preoperative—Abduction pillows are usually sufficient for postreduction stability while awaiting surgery. Skeletal traction is reserved for patients with instability or dome involvement.

2. Closed reduction

a. Prompt closed reduction as an emergent procedure should be the initial treatment.

b. Adequate pharmacologic muscle relaxation is necessary.

c. Reduction is performed by using traction in line with the thigh, with the extremity in an adducted attitude, and with countertraction exerted on the pelvis. Avoid forceful reduction, which can lead to femoral head or neck fractures.

d. Once reduction is successful, abduction with external rotation and extension should maintain reduction for posterior dislocations. For anterior dislocations, the limb is maintained in extension, abduction, and either neutral or internal rotation. Traction is indicated for unstable injuries or for those with dome involvement.

e. Irreducible dislocations are seen in 2% to 15% of patients with these injuries.

i. Irreducible anterior dislocations are due to buttonholing through the capsule or soft-tissue interposition.

Table 1

Thompson-Epstein Classification of Hip Dislocations

Type	Characteristics
I	Dislocation with or without minor fracture
II	Dislocation with single large fracture of the rim with or without a large major fragment
III	Dislocation with comminuted fracture of the rim with or without a large major fragment
IV	Dislocation with fracture of the acetabular floor
V	Dislocation with fracture of the femoral head

ii. In posterior dislocations, the piriformis, gluteus maximus, capsule, labrum, or a bony fragment can prevent reduction.

f. If one or two attempts at closed reduction with sedation are unsuccessful, then an emergent open reduction is necessary.

g. A CT scan should be done before open reduction to determine pathology.

h. Nonconcentric reductions can be missed even with careful scrutiny of postreduction radiographs of the hip. Postreduction CT is mandatory to assess the hip joint following reduction.

3. Surgical treatment

a. Indications

i. Irreducible dislocations

ii. Nonconcentric reductions

iii. Unstable hip joints

iv. Associated femoral or acetabular fractures

b. Stability determination

i. Stress testing under anesthesia is controversial.

ii. Do not assess hip stability after reduction with range of motion. No real parameters have been established for stability, and further damage to cartilage or nerves may occur.

c. Open reduction or internal fixation should be performed through an approach from the direction of the dislocation.

i. Posterior dislocations: Kocher-Langenbeck approach is used.

ii. Anterior dislocations: An anterior (Smith-Petersen) or anterolateral (Watson-Jones) approach is used.

H. Rehabilitation

1. Early mobilization

2. Avoid hyperflexion with posterior dislocations for 4 to 6 weeks.

3. Immediate weight bearing for simple dislocations

4. Delayed weight bearing with large posterior wall or dome fracture fixation

I. Complications

1. Posttraumatic arthritis develops in 15% to 20% of patients due to cellular cartilage injury, nonconcentric reduction of hip, articular displacement, marginal impaction. Posttraumatic arthritis can develop years after the initial injury.

2. Osteonecrosis develops in approximately 2% to 10% of patients reduced within 6 hours.

   a. The rate of osteonecrosis increases with a delay in reduction.

   b. Osteonecrosis usually appears within 2 years after the injury but is evident at 1 year in most patients.

3. Sciatic nerve injury affects the peroneal division.

   a. Seen in 8% to 19% of posterior dislocations

   b. More common with fracture-dislocations than simple dislocations

4. Redislocation reported in 1% of dislocations

5. Myositis around the hip is uncommon after posterior dislocation.

II. Femoral Head Fractures

A. Epidemiology

1. Femoral head fractures occur in 6% to 16% of patients with posterior hip dislocations.

2. May be the result of impaction, avulsions, or shear fractures

3. Anterior dislocations are more commonly associated with impaction of the femoral head.

4. Produced by contact of the femoral head on the posterior rim of the acetabulum at the time of dislocation

5. The location and size of the fracture and degree of comminution are a result of the position of the hip at the time of dislocation impact.

B. Anatomy/surgical approaches—Same as for hip dislocations, described in section I. B.

C. Mechanism of injury/clinical evaluation—Same as for hip dislocations, described in section I. C.

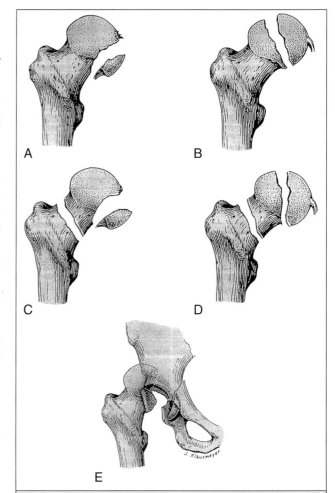

Figure 3 Pipkin classification of femoral head fractures. **A,** Infrafoveal fracture, Pipkin type 1. **B,** Suprafoveal fracture, Pipkin type II. **C** and **D,** Intrafoveal fracture or suprafoveal fracture associated with femoral neck fracture, Pipkin type III. **E,** Any femoral head fracture configuration associated with an acetabular fracture, Pipkin type IV. *(Reproduced with permission from Swionkowski MF: Intrascapular hip fractures, in Browner BD, Jupiter JB, Levine AM, Trafton PG [eds]: Skeletal Trauma: Basic Science, Management, and Reconstruction, ed 2. Philadelphia, PA, WB Saunders, p 1756.)*

D. Imaging evaluation

1. Radiographs—AP and Judet views of the acetabulum, both prereduction and postreduction.

2. CT scan—2-mm sections through the acetabulum. CT scans should be obtained postreduction only because delay in reduction caused by waiting for a CT scan can lead to further damage to the femoral head blood supply or possible sciatic nerve injury.

E. Classification—The Pipkin classification system is used for femoral head fractures (**Figure 3**)

F. Treatment—Based on fragment location, size, displacement, and hip stability (**Table 2**)

Table 2		

Treatment of Femoral Head Fractures Based on the Pipkin Classification

Type	Characteristics	Treatment
1	Infrafoveal, disruption of the ligamentum teres from the head fragment	Nonsurgical treatment is most common because this is not a weight-bearing fragment Non–weight-bearing, hip precautions, progressive weight bearing May need excision of small fragments, fixation of large fragments because they can heal as a malunion and limit hip motion
2	Suprafoveal, ligamentum teres attached to head fragment	Countersunk screws for open reduction and internal fixation Usually Smith-Petersen approach—Optimizes fracture visualization and fixation, minimizes complication rate Periacetabular capsulotomy to preserve femoral head blood supply
3	Associated femoral neck fracture	Simultaneous open reduction and internal fixation of femoral head and neck through a Watson-Jones or Smith-Petersen approach Consideration should be given to prosthetic replacement, especially in patients who are elderly, osteoporotic, or with comminution.
4	Associated acetabulum fracture	Posterior Kocher-Langenbeck approach for acetabular fixation, excision of small infrafoveal fragments through this approach Small posterior wall fragments may be treated nonsurgically and suprafoveal fractures can then be treated through an anterior approach. Use of anterior and posterior approaches together is controversial.

G. Rehabilitation

1. Immediate early range of motion of the hip with weight bearing delayed for 6 to 8 weeks is recommended.

2. Stress strengthening of the abductors and quadriceps

3. Radiographs after 6 months to evaluate for osteonecrosis and arthritis

H. Complications

1. Anterior approach associated with decreased surgical time, better visualization, improved fracture reduction, and no osteonecrosis but an increase in heterotopic ossification compared with posterior approach. Heterotopic ossification is extra-articular and rarely clinically significant.

2. Osteonecrosis related to a delay in hip dislocation reduction

   a. Impact of anterior surgical incision on osteonecrosis is unknown.

   b. Occurs in 0% to 23% of patients

   c. Patients should be counseled about this complication preoperatively.

3. Fixation failure associated with osteonecrosis or nonunion

4. Posttraumatic arthritis seen as a result of joint incongruity or initial cartilage damage

5. Decreased internal rotation is commonly seen after these femoral head fractures, but it may not be a clinical problem or cause disability.

Bibliography

Bhandari M, Matta J, Ferguson T, Matthys G: Predictors of clinical and radiological outcome in patients with fractures of the acetabulum and concomitant posterior dislocation of the hip. *J Bone Joint Surg Br* 2006;88:1618-1624.

Brumback RJ, Holt ES, McBride MS, Poka A, Bathon GH, Burgess AR: Acetabular depression fracture accompanying posterior fracture dislocation of the hip. *J Orthop Trauma* 1990;4:42-48.

Hak DJ, Goulet JA: Severity of injuries associated with traumatic posterior hip dislocations. *J Trauma* 1999;47:60-63.

Hougaard K, Thomsen PB: Traumatic posterior dislocation of the hip: Prognostic factors influencing the incidence of avascular necrosis of the femoral head. *Arch Orthop Trauma Surg* 1986;106:32-35.

Keith JE Jr, Brashear HR Jr, Guilford WB: Stability of posterior fracture-dislocations of the hip: Quantitative assessment using computed tomography. *J Bone Joint Surg Am* 1988;70:711-714.

6: Trauma

Moed BR, WillsonCarr SE, Watson JT: Results of operative treatment of fractures of the posterior wall of the acetabulum. *J Bone Joint Surg Am* 2002;84:752-758.

Sahin V, Karakas ES, Aksu S, Atlihan D, Turk CY, Halici M: Traumatic dislocation and fracture-dislocation of the hip: A long-term follow-up study. *J Trauma* 2003;54:520-529.

Schmidt GL, Sciulli R, Altman GT: Knee injury in patients experiencing a high-energy traumatic ipsilateral hip dislocation. *J Bone Joint Surg Am* 2005;87:1200-1204.

Stannard JP, Harris HW, Volgas DA, Alonso JE: Functional outcome of patients with femoral head fractures associated with hip dislocations. *Clin Orthop Relat Res* 2000;377:44-56.

Swiontkowski MF, Thorpe M, Seiler JG, Hansen ST: Operative management of displaced femoral head fractures: Case-matched comparison of anterior versus posterior approaches for Pipkin I and Pipkin II fractures. *J Orthop Trauma* 1992;6:437-442.

Thompson VP, Epstein HC: Traumatic dislocations of the hip: A survey of two hundred and four cases covering a period of twenty-one years. *J Bone Joint Surg Am* 1951;33:746-778.

Tornetta P, Mostafavi H: Hip dislocations: Current treatment regimens. *J Am Acad Orthop Surg* 1997;5:27-36.

Top Testing Facts

Hip Dislocations

1. Assess hip stability, intra-articular fragments, and concentric reduction on postreduction CT scan of the hip.

2. Check postreduction CT scan for marginal impaction of the posterior wall.

3. Assess need for internal fixation on postreduction CT scan. Identify size of posterior wall fragment and dome involvement. Anything over 25% involvement of the posterior wall is an indication for fixation.

4. Good relaxation is required with attempted closed reduction of posterior hip dislocations. Avoid forceful reduction, which can lead to femoral head or neck fractures.

5. Document the neurologic examination before and after reduction.

6. In most patients, osteonecrosis is evidenced at 1 year following injury. Arthritis can develop later.

7. Check the ipsilateral knee in posterior dislocations to assess for ligamentous or other injury.

Femoral Head Fractures

1. Assess good quality radiographs with Judet views pre- and postreduction for femoral head fractures. Diagnosis can be made on postreduction CT scan.

2. There is no need for prereduction CT scan, and leaving the hip dislocated for a longer period can lead to further damage to the femoral head blood supply or possible sciatic nerve injury.

3. It is important to identify whether the femoral head fracture is suprafoveal (weight bearing) or intrafoveal.

4. Usually a Smith-Petersen approach to the hip is used for fixation, with a periacetabular capsulotomy to preserve blood supply.

5. Femoral head fracture is easier to see and fix through an anterior approach with countersunk or headless screws.

6. With a large posterior wall fracture (Pipkin type 4), a Kocher-Langenbeck approach can be used with subluxation or dislocation of the femoral head. This will allow access to the femoral head for fracture reduction and fixation.

7. Small fragments or foveal avulsion fractures can be excised through a posterior approach when associated with a posterior wall fracture.

8. Decreased internal rotation is commonly seen after femoral head fractures, but this may not be a clinical problem or cause disability.

Chapter 55

Fractures of the Hip

Steven J. Morgan, MD

I. General Considerations

A. Epidemiology

1. Hip fractures occur most commonly in patients 70 years of age or older.

2. The risk of hip fracture increases with decreasing bone mass.

3. Hip fractures are more common in women than in men.

4. Intertrochanteric femur fractures account for approximately 50% of all proximal femur fractures.

5. Femoral neck fractures are slightly less common and account for approximately 40% of proximal femur fractures.

B. Anatomy

1. Fractures of the proximal femur are distinguished by their anatomic location in relationship to the joint capsule.

   a. Femoral neck fractures are considered intracapsular fractures, which are at higher risk of nonunion because they can be enveloped by synovial fluid. Because of the absence of periosteal or extraosseous blood supply, no callus forms during healing. Rather, fracture healing occurs by intraosseous bone healing.

   b. Intertrochanteric fractures are considered extracapsular fractures. Callus formation is common in these fracture patterns, and nonunion is rare because of the absence of synovial fluid and the presence of an abundant blood supply.

2. Vascular anatomy (**Figure 1**)

   a. The medial femoral circumflex artery is the main blood supply to the femoral head. This artery terminates in the posterior aspect of the extracapsular arterial ring.

   b. The lateral femoral circumflex artery gives rise to the anterior aspect of the arterial ring.

   c. The superior and inferior gluteal arteries also contribute branches to the ring.

   d. The ascending cervical arteries originate from the extracapsular arterial ring and are divided into four distinct groups based on their anatomic relationship to the femoral neck: lateral, medial, posterior, and anterior. The lateral group of ascending branches is the main blood supply to the femoral head.

   e. The ascending branches give off multiple perforator vessels to the femoral neck and terminate in the subsynovial arterial ring located at the margin of the articular surface of the femoral head. The lateral epiphyseal artery then penetrates the femoral head and is believed to be the dominant blood supply to the femoral head from this system. Fractures that disrupt the ascending blood flow to the lateral epiphyseal vessel have increased risk of osteonecrosis.

   f. The artery of the ligamentum teres arises from either the obturator or medial femoral circumflex artery. It does not provide sufficient blood supply to maintain the viability of the femoral head.

C. Surgical approaches

1. The anterior lateral (Watson-Jones) approach is used for open reduction and internal fixation (ORIF) of femoral neck fractures or hemiarthroplasty.

   a. This approach is based on the interval between the gluteus medius and the tensor fascia lata. There is no internervous plane because both muscles are innervated by the superior gluteal nerve.

   b. The superior gluteal nerve can be damaged if the intermuscular plane is extended to the iliac crest.

2. The anterior (Smith-Peterson) approach can be used for ORIF of the femoral neck or hemiarthroplasty. If used for ORIF, a separate lateral approach to the proximal femur is required for fixation placement.

   a. The superficial dissection is between the tensor fascia lata (superior gluteal nerve) and the sartorious (femoral nerve).

6: Trauma

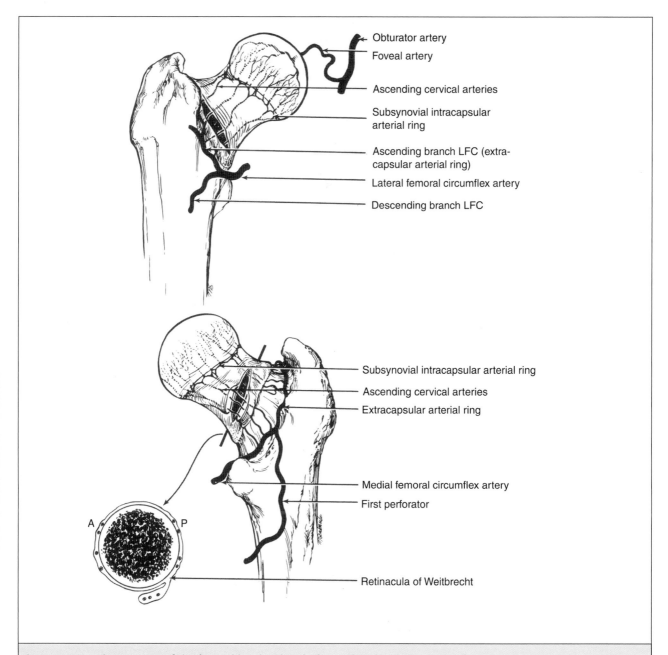

Figure 1 Vascular anatomy of the femoral head and neck. *(Reproduced with permission from DeLee JC: Fractures and dislocations of the hip, in Rockwood CA Jr, Green DP, Bucholz RW, Heckman JD [eds]: Rockwood and Green's Fractures in Adults, ed 4. Philadelphia, PA, Lippincott Williams & Wilkins, 2001, p 1662.)*

b. The deep dissection is between the gluteus medius (superior gluteal nerve) and the rectus femoris (femoral nerve).

c. The lateral femoral cutaneous nerve is at risk with this approach.

d. The ascending branch of the lateral femoral circumflex artery is encountered between the tensor and the sartorius and must be sacrificed.

3. The lateral (Hardinge) approach is used primarily for hemiarthroplasty. This approach splits both the gluteus medius and the vastus lateralis, reflecting the anterior third of these structures medially. The superior gluteal nerve and artery are at risk in this approach.

4. The posterior (Southern) approach is used primarily for partial or total hip arthroplasty (THA).

a. The approach splits the gluteus maximus muscle (inferior gluteal nerve) and the fascia lata.

b. The tendons of the piriformis, obturator internus, and the superior and inferior gemelli are transected at their point of insertion and retracted posteriorly.

c. The sciatic nerve is the main structure at risk with this exposure.

5. The lateral approach to the proximal femur is used for ORIF of intertrochanteric femur fractures.

  a. This is a direct lateral approach that splits the fascia lata and either elevates the vastus lateralis from posterior to anterior, or splits the muscle fibers.

  b. There is no internervous plane; the vastus lateralis is innervated by the femoral nerve.

D. Hip biomechanics

1. The average neck-shaft angle in the adult femur is 130° ± 7°. The average anteversion of the neck is 10° ± 7°.

2. Forces on the proximal aspect of the femur are complex. The osseous structure itself also is complex, consisting of both cortical and cancellous bone.

  a. The two prime trabecular groups of the proximal femur are the principal tensile group and the principal compressive group. There are also secondary compressive and tensile trabecular groups (**Figure 2**). These trabecular bone patterns are the result of bone response to stress, expressed as Wolff's law.

  b. The weakest area in the femoral neck is located in the Ward triangle.

  c. The calcar femorale is a medial area of dense trabecular bone that transfers stress from the femoral shaft to the inferior portion of the femoral neck.

  d. Fractures of the proximal femur follow the path of least resistance.

  e. The amount of energy absorbed by the bone determines the degree of comminution.

3. Standing position

  a. The center of gravity is located at the midpoint between the two hips.

  b. The weight of the body is supported equally by both hips.

  c. The force vector acting on the hip is vertical.

  d. The Y ligament of Bigelow resists hyperextension. Minimal muscle forces are required for balance in symmetric stance, and the joint reactive force or compressive force across the hip is approximately one half the body weight.

4. Single-leg stance

  a. The center of gravity moves away from the hip. To counter the eccentric lever arm created by the weight of the body, the hip abductors

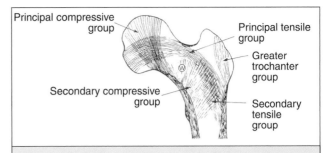

Figure 2   Trabecular groups of the proximal femur. W = the Ward triangle. *(Adapted with permission from Singh M, Nagrath AR, Maini PS: Changes in trabecular pattern of the upper end of the femur as an index of osteoporosis. J Bone Joint Surg Am 1970;52:457-467.)*

contract to maintain the pelvis in a level position. Because the lever arm created by the lateral offset of the greater trochanter is shorter than the lever arm created by the entire body opposite the hip, the magnitude of muscle contracture is greater than the weight of the body. This results in a compressive load across the hip of approximately 4 times the body weight.

  b. The resulting force vector in the standing phase is oriented parallel to the compressive trabeculae of the femoral neck.

  c. In repetitive load situations, the tensile forces can cause microfractures in the superior femoral neck.

    i. Failure of these microfractures to heal in conditions of repetitive loading results in stress fracture.

    ii. Frequency and degree of load influence the fatigue process.

5. Trendelenburg gait

  a. Trendelenburg gait is noted when the hip abductors are no longer sufficient to counter the forces in single-leg stance. Without compensation, the pelvis cannot be maintained in a level position. Weakness of the abductors can be caused by disuse, paralysis, or by a diminished lever arm as a result of decreased femoral offset.

  b. To compensate for the weakness of the abductors, the center of gravity can be shifted closer to the affected hip. This is done by shifting the upper body over the standing hip in single-leg stance, resulting in the classic waddling gait. Alternatively, a cane used in the opposite hand can diminish the load on the hip in single-leg stance by nearly 40%.

E. Mechanism of injury

1. Hip fractures in the elderly are generally the result of low-energy trauma. Frequently, the patient

6: Trauma

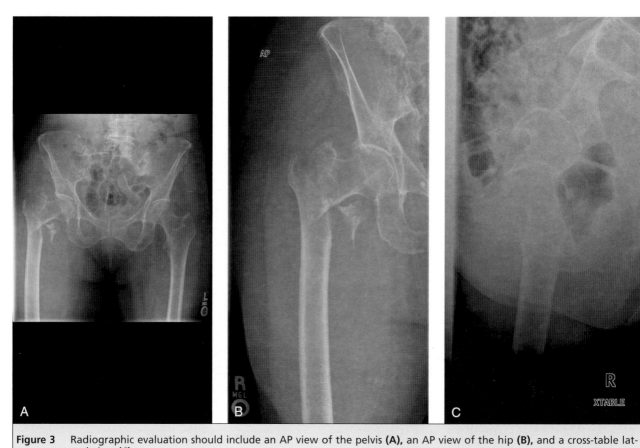

Figure 3 Radiographic evaluation should include an AP view of the pelvis **(A)**, an AP view of the hip **(B)**, and a cross-table lateral view **(C)**.

sustains the fracture as a result of a fall from a standing height.

   a. A fall to the side that impacts the greater trochanter is more likely to cause a fracture.

   b. External rotation of the distal extremity and the tethering of the anterior femoral capsule can result in posterior comminution of the femoral neck.

   c. One method of fracture prevention is training in fall prevention; protective padding has demonstrated efficacy but is often not practical.

2. Hip fractures in younger individuals are often the result of high-energy trauma that exerts an axial load on the femoral shaft either through the distal femur or through the foot with the hip and knee extended.

F. Clinical evaluation

1. The injured extremity is usually shortened and externally rotated. A careful examination of the extremity should be performed, with particular attention given to skin condition and neurologic status.

2. In the geriatric population, a careful evaluation for medical comorbidities should be undertaken.

The number of comorbidities is directly related to 1-year mortality figures: Patients with four or more comorbidities have been reported to have a higher 1-year mortality rate than patients with three or fewer.

3. In the high-energy trauma patient, a systematic search for other injuries should be undertaken as well as a careful secondary assessment of the injured extremity for associated fractures.

G. Radiographic evaluation

1. An AP radiograph of the pelvis, an AP of the hip, and a cross-table or frog lateral are required for diagnosis and preoperative planning (**Figure 3**).

2. Normal radiographs do not exclude a hip fracture; 8% of patients with hip pain have an occult fracture. MRI to evaluate for the presence of an occult fracture is recommended when it can be performed in the acute setting. Alternative imaging studies include CT and bone scan. The sensitivity of bone scan is increased by waiting 24 to 72 hours following injury.

H. Surgical indications

1. Most, if not all, fractures of the proximal femur should be stabilized surgically to prevent displacement and allow for early mobilization and weight

bearing. In the case of displaced fractures of the femoral neck in patients of advanced age or in patients with preexisting arthritis, arthroplasty should be considered.

2. In the young patient with high-energy trauma, every effort should be made to obtain and maintain an anatomic reduction of the proximal femur fracture with internal fixation.

3. Nonsurgical management should be considered only in nonambulatory patients and in patients who are deemed too medically ill for surgical intervention.

I. Timing of surgery

1. In the elderly patient with significant comorbidities, it is important to reverse easily correctible medical conditions before surgery, but surgery should be performed as soon as reasonably possible. Surgery should be performed when optimal medical support is available, preferably during normal surgical hours, because surgery performed in less optimal conditions is associated with increased risk of malreduction and other technical errors.

2. In the younger trauma population, femoral neck fractures should be addressed as soon as possible after other life-threatening injuries have been stabilized. Performing surgery without delay helps to preserve and maintain the blood flow to the femoral head, preventing or limiting the development of osteonecrosis.

J. Anesthesia considerations

1. The goal of the anesthetic technique selected is to eliminate pain, allow for appropriate intraoperative positioning, and achieve muscle relaxation to effect the reduction.

2. Spinal and general anesthetic techniques result in similar long-term outcomes, but spinal anesthesia may result in less postsurgical confusion, a reduced deep venous thrombosis (DVT) rate, and a diminished risk of early postsurgical death.

3. Spinal anesthetics are not successful in 20% of patients and must be converted to a general anesthetic.

K. Postoperative management

1. Postoperative management should focus on early mobilization of the patient and minimization of complications such as DVT, disorientation, bowel or bladder irregularities, and pressure sores.

2. Early hospital discharge with adequate outpatient medical and social assistance has been demonstrated to decrease overall cost and improve recovery. Inpatient rehabilitation stays have not been associated with improved functional outcomes for community ambulators.

3. Elderly patients should be allowed to weight bear as tolerated. This population autoregulates their weight bearing based on the stability of the fracture pattern and fixation.

4. In younger individuals who sustain a high-energy femoral neck fracture, early weight bearing should be avoided because of the associated soft-tissue injury and the possible risk of fixation failure.

5. Antibiotic prophylaxis should be given within 1 hour of surgery and continued no longer than 24 hours following surgery to prevent postoperative wound infection.

6. DVT is reported to occur in up to 80% of patients who sustain a proximal femur fracture. Mechanical devices and chemical prophylaxis should be used as prophylactic measures against DVT. The risk of DVT is substantially reduced with prophylaxis, although the exact type of prophylaxis and duration remain controversial.

II. Fractures of the Femoral Neck

A. Classification—Three main classification systems are used for fractures of the femoral neck.

1. Pauwels classification system

a. Not widely used, this system divides fractures into three groups based on the angle of the femoral neck fracture (**Figure 4**).

b. This system seems most applicable to high-energy femoral neck fractures.

c. Vertical fracture lines were believed to be at highest risk for nonunion and osteonecrosis; however, this system seems to have little predictive value.

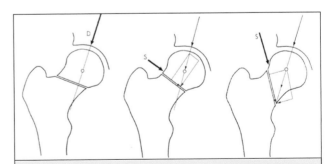

Figure 4　Pauwels classification of femoral neck fractures. **A,** in type I patterns, the fracture is relatively horizontal (<30°) and compressive forces caused by the hip joint reactive force predominate. **B,** In type II patterns, shear forces at the fracture are predicted. **C,** In type III patterns, when the fracture angle is 50° or higher, shear forces predominate. Arrows indicate joint reactive force. *(Adapted with permission from Bartonicek J: Pauwels' classification of femoral neck fractures. J Orthop Trauma 2001;15:359-360.)*

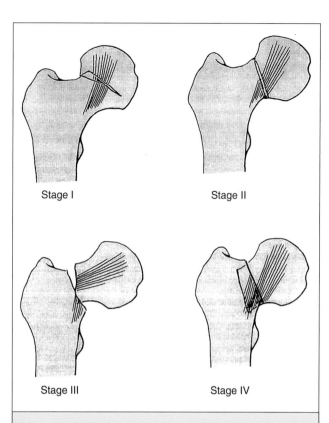

6: Trauma

Figure 5 Garden classification of femoral neck fractures. Stage I is an incomplete, impacted fracture in valgus malalignment (generally stable). Stage II is a nondisplaced fracture. Stage III is an imcompletely displaced fracture in varus malalignment. Stage IV is a completely displaced fracture with no engagement of the two fragments. The compression trabeculae in the femoral head line up with the trabeculae on the acetabular side. Displacement is generally more evident on the lateral view in stage IV. For prognostic purposes, these groupings can be lumped into nondisplaced/impacted (stages I and II) and displaced (stages III and IV), as the risks of nonunion and aseptic necrosis are similar within these grouped stages. *(Reproduced with permission from Swiontkowski MF: Intracapsular hip fractures, in Browner BD, Jupiter JB, Levine AM, Trafton PG [eds]:* Skeletal Trauma: Basic Science, Management, and Reconstruction, *ed 2. Philadelphia, PA, WB Saunders, 1998, p 1775.)*

2. Garden classification

   a. This system divides fractures into four types based on the degree of displacement (**Figure 5**).

   b. The interobserver agreement for this classification scheme as originally described is poor.

   c. Interobserver agreement increases significantly, however, when type I and type II fractures are combined and considered nondisplaced, and type III and type IV patterns are combined and considered displaced. The risk of nonunion and osteonecrosis is similar within the combined classification schemes.

3. AO/OTA classification

   a. This classification system subdivides fractures based on location in the femoral neck and degree of displacement.

   b. The femoral neck is divided into subcapital, transcervical, and basicervical regions.

   c. This system is used mostly for research purposes.

B. Nonsurgical treatment

1. Nonsurgical treatment is reserved for the nonambulatory patient or the patient in the terminal stages of life. In general, acute pain can be controlled with narcotic medication and will subside in the first few days to a week, allowing transfers in the nonambulatory patient that are tolerable for the staff and patient.

2. Nonsurgical treatment can be considered for a nondisplaced femoral neck fracture, but the reported incidence of late displacement is between 15% and 30%.

3. Compression-related stress fractures can also be considered for nonsurgical treatment, but close follow-up and restricted weight bearing are required.

C. Surgical treatment

1. Nondisplaced fractures

   a. The outcome is poor for displaced femoral neck fractures, so nondisplaced fractures should be stabilized to prevent late displacement. In surgically treated nondisplaced femoral neck fractures, the risk of late displacement is between 1% and 6%.

   b. Transcervical and subcapital fractures are best treated with percutaneous placement of three partially threaded compression screws. The screws should be started at or above the level of the lesser trochanter on the lateral cortex to minimize the risk of subsequent subtrochanteric fracture. Screws should be placed in the periphery of the femoral neck to gain the support of the residual cortical bone to resist shear forces and within 5 mm of the articular surface to gain purchase in the subchondral bone. Care should be taken not to penetrate the articular surface, and multiplanar fluoroscopy should be used to confirm that no intraarticular penetration has occurred.

   c. Basicervical fractures behave like intertrochanteric femur fractures and should be surgically stabilized with a sliding hip screw that allows controlled compression of the fracture. This fracture pattern has less inherent rotational stability than an intertrochanteric fracture, so an additional parallel screw should be placed to resist rotational forces.

2. Displaced fractures

   a. Open reduction and internal fixation

      i. In the young patient with high-energy trauma or in the active elderly patient without preexisting arthritis, reduction and fixation of the displaced femoral neck fracture with the previously described techniques should be attempted.

      ii. The key factor in preventing nonunion, loss of fixation, and osteonecrosis is the quality and maintenance of the reduction. Closed reduction can be attempted, but the reduction needs to be anatomic. If closed reduction is unsuccessful, open reduction with an anterolateral or anterior approach to the hip should be performed.

      iii. When closed reduction techniques are used in high-energy fractures, a capsular release may help to diminish the risk of osteonecrosis by relieving the capsular pressure on the ascending branches.

   b. Hemiarthroplasty

      i. Hemiarthroplasty should be considered in the low-demand individual of advanced physiologic age or chronologic age older than 80 years.

      ii. Short-term outcomes are similar for unipolar and bipolar prosthetic designs, but in patients followed for >7 years, those with a bipolar prosthesis appeared to have better function.

      iii. A cemented technique is preferable in most patients who are ambulatory. Uncemented technique is associated with greater postsurgical pain and higher revision rates. An uncemented prosthesis has usually been reserved for minimal ambulators.

   c. Total hip arthroplasty

      i. The primary indication for THA has been an arthritic, symptomatic hip joint.

      ii. Recent studies suggest that for displaced femoral neck fractures, functional outcomes are better with THA than with hemiarthroplasty. This topic remains controversial.

      iii. Pathologic fracture of the femoral neck is also an indication for THA.

D. Surgical pearls

   1. Pathologic fractures of the femoral neck should be treated with hemiarthroplasty or THA.

   2. Screw fixation below the level of the lesser trochanter increases the risk of subtrochanteric femur fracture.

3. In patients between the ages of 65 and 80, surgical decision making should be based on physiologic, not chronologic, patient age.

4. Reversible medical comorbidities in geriatric patients should be minimized promptly. Surgical delay beyond 72 hours has been reported to increase the risk of 1-year mortality.

E. Complications

   1. Osteonecrosis

      a. In nondisplaced fractures, the incidence of osteonecrosis can be as high as 15%. In displaced fractures fixed appropriately, the rate of osteonecrosis has been reported to range between 20% and 30%.

      b. Osteonecrosis alone is not necessarily of clinical significance unless late segmental collapse ensues. Segmental collapse can be seen as early as 6 to 9 months following injury, but it is most likely to be recognized in the second year following surgery. In most cases it can be excluded following the third year.

   2. Nonunion

      a. Nonunion rates are reported to be from 5% in the elderly to 30% in the young, high-energy trauma population.

      b. Nonunion is generally associated with more vertically oriented fracture patterns and loss of reduction with varus collapse.

      c. Nonunion repair is based on reorientation of the fracture line to a more horizontal position. A valgus osteotomy of the proximal femur is the treatment of choice in the physiologically young patient.

III. Intertrochanteric Fractures

A. Classification

   1. The Evans classification system divides intertrochanteric fractures into stable and unstable fracture patterns (**Figure 6**). The distinction between stable and unstable fractures is based on the integrity of the posterior medial cortex. The Evans classification also recognizes the reverse obliquity fracture pattern, which is prone to medial displacement of the distal fragment.

   2. All other intertrochanteric fracture classification schemes, including the AO/OTA classification, are variations on the Evans classification.

   3. No classification of intertrochanteric fractures has gained wide acceptance, and all demonstrate suboptimal observer agreement.

6: Trauma

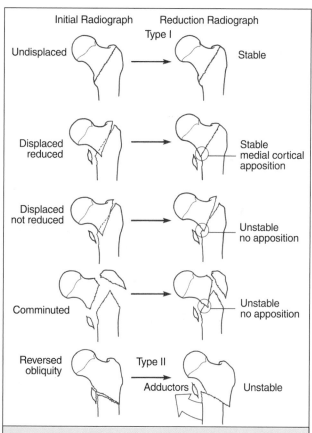

Figure 6   The Evans classification of intertrochanteric fracture. *(Adapted with permission from DeLee JC: Fractures and dislocations of the hip, in Rockwood CA Jr, Green DP, Bucholz RW, Heckman JD [eds]: Rockwood and Green's Fractures in Adults, ed 4. Philadelphia, PA, Lippincott Williams & Wilkins, 1996, p 1721.)*

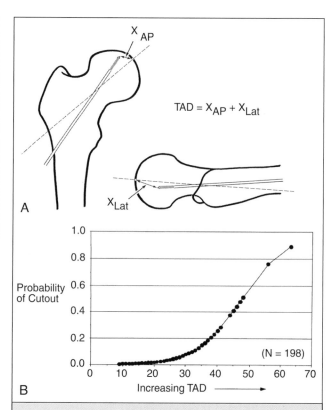

$$TAD = X_{AP} + X_{Lat}$$

Figure 7   The tip-apex distance (TAD) is estimated by combining the distance from the guide-pin tip to the apex of the femoral head on the AP and lateral fluoroscopic views **(A)**. The risk for cutout failure increases dramatically when the TAD exceeds 25 mm **(B)**. *(Reproduced from Baumgaertner MR, Brennan MJ: Intertrochanteric femur fractures, in Orthopaedic Knowledge Update: Trauma 2. Rosemont, IL, American Academy of Orthopaedic Surgeons, 2000, pp 125-131.)*

4. Intertrochanteric fractures may be best classified as either stable or unstable based on the ability to resist compressive loads.

5. In general, when the posterior medial cortex is comminuted, fractures are considered unstable secondary to the likelihood the fracture will collapse into varus and retroversion.

B. Nonsurgical treatment

1. Nonsurgical treatment should be reserved for the nonambulatory patient or the patient who is at significant risk for perioperative mortality related to anesthesia or surgery.

2. These patients should receive adequate analgesics and be mobilized to a chair.

3. Nonsurgical treatment is associated with an increased mortality rate and an increased risk for decubiti, urinary tract infection, contracture, pneumonia, and DVT.

C. Surgical treatment

1. General considerations

a. Surgical fixation of intertrochanteric fractures is based on reestablishing normal femoral neck-shaft alignment angle and allowing for controlled collapse of both stable and unstable fracture types.

b. Devices that allow controlled collapse have eliminated the need for restoring medial cortical contact either by direct reduction techniques or medial displacement osteotomies. Regardless of the device, the main technical factors that eliminate complications of treatment are accurate restoration of alignment and placement of the lag screw in the femoral head. The lag screw should be placed in the center aspect of the head and in the subchondral bone. Measurement of the tip-apex distance (TAD) is predictive of fixation failure (**Figure 7**). A TAD >25 mm has been associated with fixation failure.

2. Internal fixation techniques—The two main devices used for internal fixation are the sliding hip screw/side plate and the intramedullary hip screw.

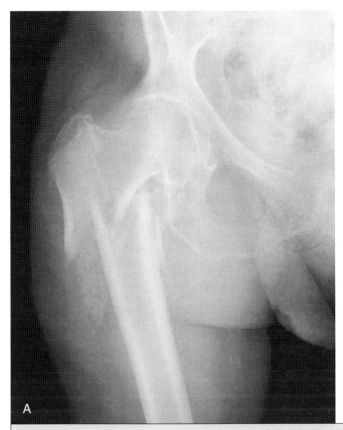 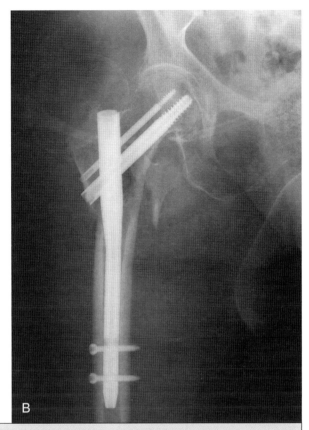

Figure 8   Reverse obliquity fracture. **A,** AP view showing a four-part comminuted intertrochanteric fracture with reverse obliquity. **B,** The same hip after treatment with an intramedullary hip screw. *(From Haidukewych GJ, Jacofsky DJ: Hip trauma, in Vaccaro AR [ed]: Orthopaedic Knowledge Update 8. Rosemont, IL, American Academy of Orthopaedic Surgeons, 2005, p 404.)*

Both devices have theoretical advantages, but no data indicate one device is superior to the other.

a. Sliding hip screw

  i. Advantages: ease of application, surgeon familiarity, availability, high success rate, minimal complications, cost

  ii. Disadvantages: open technique, increased blood loss, increased failure in reverse obliquity or subtrochanteric extension patterns, excessive collapse resulting in limb shortening and fracture deformity in unstable fracture patterns

b. Intramedullary hip screw

  i. Advantages: percutaneous application, limited blood loss, lateral buttress allowing limited collapse, increased resistance to varus forces

  ii. Disadvantages: periprosthetic fracture, increased incidence of screw cutout, cost

3. Arthroplasty

  a. Traditional arthroplasty is not effective for most intertrochanteric fractures secondary to the comminuted nature of the proximal femur.

  b. A calcar-replacing prosthesis or a proximal femoral component is frequently required for reconstruction.

  c. Secure fixation of the greater trochanter is problematic.

  d. Because of the extensive nature of proximal femoral replacement and the associated increased surgical stress, arthroplasty is not warranted in most fractures.

  e. Proximal femoral replacement should be reserved for salvage of failed ORIF or pathologic fractures.

D. Unusual fractures

  1. Reverse obliquity fracture

    a. The reverse obliquity fracture is an unstable fracture pattern that does not have an intact lateral cortex to support controlled compaction with a sliding hip screw (**Figure 8**).

    b. These fractures are best thought of as subtrochanteric femur fractures and therefore should be treated with either an intramedullary nail or a fixed-angle device such as a blade plate or dynamic condylar screw.

2. Fractures of the greater trochanter

   a. Fractures of the greater trochanter are usually the result of a direct blow.

   b. The primary deforming force is the external hip rotators, not the hip abductors.

   c. Most of these fractures can be treated nonsurgically, regardless of the degree of displacement, but in the younger, more active patient, repair should be considered for fracture displacement >1 cm.

3. Fractures of the lesser trochanter

   a. Isolated fractures of the lesser trochanter are rare; they are seen in adolescents and generally represent an avulsion of the trochanter by the iliopsoas.

   b. A more common etiology is a pathologic fracture as a result of tumor metastasis.

E. Complications

1. Loss of fixation

   a. Usually occurs during the first 3 months following fracture treatment and is the most common complication.

   b. Varus malalignment at the time of fracture fixation, advanced age, and osteopenia are all contributory factors to screw cutout of the femoral head.

   c. The most important predictor of cutout is the TAD. According to one study, a TAD <27 mm was not associated with screw cutout, but a TAD >45 mm was associated with a failure rate of 60%.

2. Nonunion

   a. Occurs in <2% of patients and is most commonly associated with unstable fracture patterns

   b. Nonunion can be associated with fixation failure and varus collapse.

   c. Failure of controlled impaction at the fracture site is also contributory.

   d. Revision internal fixation and valgus osteotomy versus proximal femoral replacement are the treatment options for this complication.

3. Malunion in the form of a varus deformity or a rotational deformity is common.

   a. Comminuted unstable fracture patterns are at greatest risk for an internal rotation deformity.

   b. Corrective osteotomy is the best salvage procedure for this condition.

IV. Subtrochanteric Femur Fractures

A. Classification

1. Seinsheimer

   a. The Seinsheimer classification system is a comprehensive scheme that subdivides the fracture patterns into eight groups (**Figure 9**).

   b. Interobserver agreement is relatively low, and the system is not widely used.

2. Russell-Taylor

   a. The Russell-Taylor classification system divides subtrochanteric fractures into four types, based on the involvement of the lesser trochanter and the piriformis fossa (**Figure 10**).

   b. This system provides guidance for treatment: whether to treat the fracture with a nail, the type of nail to use, and when nailing should be avoided.

   c. The Russell-Taylor classification has not been subjected to reliability tests.

B. Nonsurgical treatment—Nonsurgical treatment is appropriate only for the nonambulatory patient.

C. Surgical treatment

1. General considerations

   a. Evaluation of the anatomic location and orientation of the fracture pattern guides selection of the most appropriate device and its application for these fractures.

   b. The goals of internal fixation should be anatomic restoration of femoral alignment, maintenance of alignment, and minimization of the surgical insult.

2. Intramedullary nailing

   a. Intramedullary nailing can be used for all subtrochanteric femur fractures that do not extend to the piriformis fossa or greater trochanter.

   b. A standard nail with locking screws that do not enter the femoral head can be used in fractures that are below the level of the lesser trochanter as long as the device offers an oblique proximal locking option.

   c. For fractures that extend to or involve the lesser trochanter, a cephalomedullary nail is required for adequate fixation.

   d. Nailing can be performed in fractures that extend into the nail starting point, but it is not the preferred technique for most surgeons.

   e. The main pitfall of intramedullary nailing is varus deformity with the proximal fragment

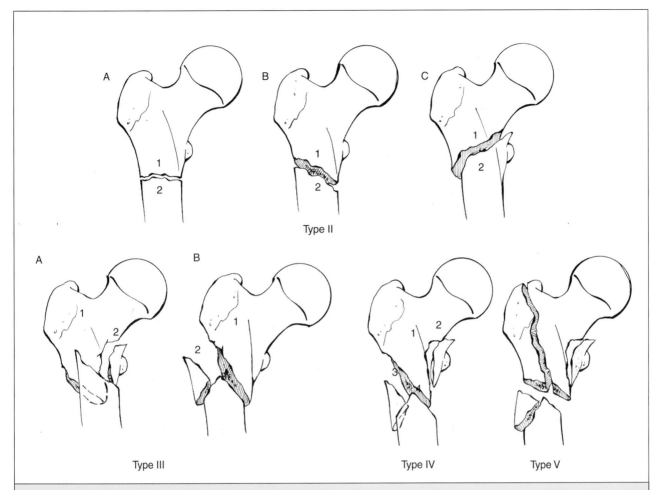

A   B   C

Type II

A   B   Type III   Type IV   Type V

Figure 9 Seinsheimer classification of subtrochanteric femur fractures. Type I fractures (not shown) are nondisplaced. (*Reproduced with permission from Leung K: Subtrochanteric fractures, in Bucholz RW, Heckman JD, Court-Brown C [eds]: Rockwood and Green's Fractures in Adults, ed 6. Philadelphia, PA, Lippincott Williams & Wilkins, 2006, p 1831.*)

also assuming a flexed position. Alignment must be restored before reaming and placement of the intramedullary nail.

f. Fracture reduction and intramedullary nailing can be facilitated by positioning the patient laterally on the fracture table. This allows the femur to be flexed in relation to the hip, matching the unopposed flexion of the proximal fragment.

g. Intramedullary nails are load-sharing devices, and early weight bearing can frequently be initiated.

3. Plate fixation

a. Plate fixation with a fixed-angle device such as a blade plate or a dynamic condylar screw can be used on all subtrochanteric femur fractures regardless of location, but the open nature of the technique and the associated blood loss make its practical use limited to the most proximal fractures.

b. The surgical approach is a direct lateral approach to the proximal femur.

c. Dissection of the medial fragments during fracture reduction should be avoided because of the relatively high rate of nonunion (30%) with excessive periosteal dissection.

d. Fixed-angle plates are load-bearing devices, and early weight bearing should be avoided.

D. Complications

1. The deforming forces involved in subtrochanteric fractures of the femur are significant; obtaining and maintaining an adequate reduction in subtrochanteric fractures while performing internal fixation can be difficult. Malunion in the form of varus and proximal fragment flexion is not uncommon.

2. Nonunion is associated with fracture comminution and excessive dissection in the area of the medial femur. Supplemental bone grafting is recommended when medial dissection is performed.

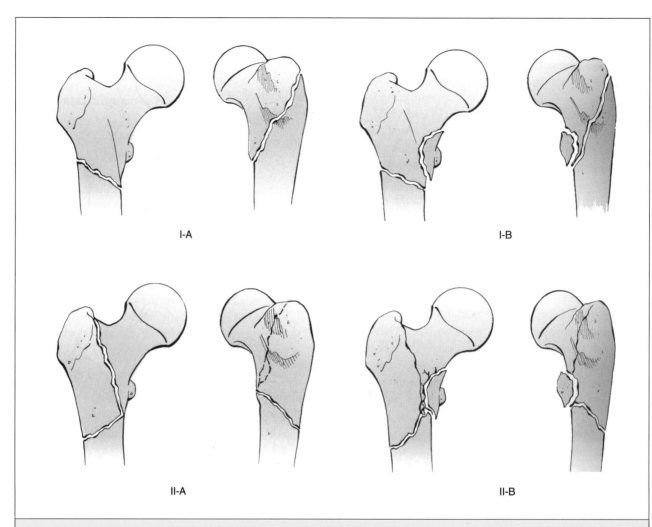

Figure 10   Russell-Taylor classification of subtrochanteric fractures. *(Reproduced with permission from Leung K: Subtrochanteric fractures, in Bucholz RW, Heckman JD, Court-Brown C [eds]: Rockwood and Green's Fractures in Adults, ed 6. Philadelphia, PA, Lippincott Williams & Wilkins, 2006, p 1832.)*

Top Testing Facts

Fractures of the Femoral Neck

1. Fractures of the femoral neck can result from direct or indirect force (fall onto the proximal thigh or a rotational force).

2. The main blood supply to the femoral head comes from the medial femoral circumflex artery.

3. The structure at risk during the anterior approach to the hip is the lateral femoral cutaneous nerve.

4. The Y ligament of Bigelow resists hip hyperextension.

5. Pathologic fractures of the femoral neck should be treated with hemiarthroplasty or THA.

6. Screw fixation below the level of the lesser trochanter increases the risk of subtrochanteric femur fracture.

Intertrochanteric Fractures

1. A TAD <25 mm should be maintained when placing the lag screw of a plate or nail device.

2. Lesser trochanteric fractures are often associated with tumor metastasis.

3. Reverse obliquity fractures should be treated with an intramedullary nail or a fixed-angle plate.

Subtrochanteric Fractures

1. When using an open technique, medial dissection should be avoided.

Bibliography

Adams CI, Robinson CM, Court-Brown CM, McQueen MM: Prospective randomized controlled trial of an intramedullary nail versus dynamic screw and plate for intertrochanteric fractures of the femur. *J Orthop Trauma* 2001;15:394-400.

Ahrengart L, Tornkvist H, Forander P, et al: A randomized study of the compression hip screw and Gamma nail in 426 fractures. *Clin Orthop Relat Res* 2002;401:209-222.

Baumgaertner MR, Curti SL, Linskog DM, Keggi JM: The value of the tip apex distance in predicting failure of fixation of peritrochanteric fractures of the hip. *J Bone Joint Surg Am* 1995;77:1058-1064.

Bhandari M, Devereux PJ, Swintowski MF, et al: Internal fixation compared with arthroplasty for displaced fractures of the femoral neck: A meta-analysis. *J Bone Joint Surg Am* 2003;85:1673-1681.

Haidukewych GJ, Berry DJ: Hip arthroplasty for salvage of intertrochanteric hip fractures. *J Bone Joint Surg Am* 2003; 85-A:899-904.

Haidukewych GJ, Israel TA, Berry DJ: Reverse obliquity of fractures of the intertrochanteric region of the femur. *J Bone Joint Surg Am* 2001;83:643-650.

Koval KJ, Sala DA, Kummer FJ, Zuckerman JD: Postoperative weight bearing after a fracture of the femoral neck or intertrochanteric fracture. *J Bone Joint Surg Am* 1998;80:352-356.

Marti RK, Schuller HM, Raaymakers EL: Intertrochanteric osteotomy for non-union of the femoral neck. *J Bone Joint Surg Br* 1989;71:782-787.

Oakes DA, Jackson KR, Davies MR, et al: The impact of the Garden classification on proposed operative treatment. *Clin Orthop Relat Res* 2003;409:232-240.

Ong BC, Maurer SG, Aharanoff GB, Zuckerman JD, Koval KJ: Uniopolar versus bipolar hemiarthroplasty: Functional outcome after femoral neck fracture at a minimum of 36 months of follow up. *J Orthop Trauma* 2002;16:317-322.

Rizzo PF, Gould ES, Leyden JP, Asnis SE: Diagnosis of occult fracture about the hip: Magnetic resonance imaging compared with bone scanning. *J Bone Joint Surg Am* 1993;75:395-401.

Szita J, Cserhati P, Bosch U, Manninger J, Bodzay T, Fekete K: Intracapsular femoral neck fractures: The importance of early reduction and stable osteosynthesis. *Injury* 2002;33:C41-C46.

Tanaka J, Seki N, Tokimura F, Hayashi Y: Conservative treatment of Garden stage I femoral neck fracture in elderly patients. *Arch Orthop Trauma Surg* 2002;122:24-28.

Trueta J, Harrison MHM: The normal vascular anatomy of the femoral head in adult man. *J Bone Joint Surg Br* 1953;35:442-461.

Vaidya SV, Dholakia DB, Chatterjee A: The use of a dynamic condylar screw and biologic reduction techniques for subtrochanteric femur fractures. *Injury* 2003;34:123-128.

Zuckerman JD, Skovorn ML, Koval KJ, Aharonoff G, Frankel VH: Postoperative complications and mortality associated with operative delay in older patients who have a fracture of the hip. *J Bone Joint Surg Am* 1995;77:1551-1556.

6: Trauma

Chapter 56

Fractures of the Femoral Shaft and Distal Femur

Lisa K. Cannada, MD

I. Fractures of the Femoral Shaft

A. Anatomy

1. The femur is the largest, strongest bone in the body and is enveloped by a thick mass of muscle (**Figure 1**).

2. The femoral shaft is defined as the diaphyseal portion of the bone, which extends from below the lesser trochanter to above the metaphyseal portion of the distal femur.

3. The bony anatomy of the femoral shaft includes an anterior bow.

4. Compartments of the thigh

   a. Anterior compartment with the quadriceps muscles

   b. Posterior compartment with the hamstrings

   c. Adductor compartment

5. Deforming forces after a fracture

   a. The abductors—gluteus medius and minimus—insert on the greater trochanter and abduct the proximal segment.

   b. The iliopsoas inserts on the lesser trochanter and flexes the proximal fragment.

   c. The adductor longus, adductor brevis, gracilis, and adductor magnus have a broad area of insertion on the distal femur and contribute to a varus force on the distal segment.

   d. The gastrocnemius originates on the distal femur and causes a flexion deformity with more distal femoral shaft fractures.

B. Surgical approaches

1. Antegrade insertion points include the piriformis fossa or greater trochanter.

   a. The incision is made approximately 6 cm proximal to the tip of the greater trochanter.

   b. The gluteus maximus fascia is incised, and the muscle is spread in line with the incision.

2. Retrograde insertion

   a. Midline incision with entry point in the center of the distal femoral condyle and approximately 10 mm anterior to the posterior cruciate ligament femoral insertion.

   b. On the lateral knee view, the starting point is at the anterior aspect of the Blumensaat line.

C. Mechanisms of injury

1. Femoral shaft fractures often are high-energy injuries, such as from a motor vehicle or motorcycle accident. The most common mechanism in motor vehicle accident is impact of the knee against the car's dashboard. Common associated injuries include pelvis/acetabulum fractures, hip fractures and/or dislocations, and fractures of the femoral head, distal femur, patella, and tibial plateau.

2. A small percentage occur as a result of repeated stress, such as that experienced by a young military recruit or runner following an increase in the intensity of physical training.

3. A fall from a standing height is a common mechanism in the elderly, underscoring the emphasis of osteoporotic fracture prevention.

4. Pathologic fractures may be the first presentation of metastatic cancer. Radiographs should be evaluated for possibility of bony lesions, especially when the injury is not consistent with the mechanism (eg, stepping off a curb).

5. Bilateral femur fractures have a mortality rate of up to 25%.

D. Clinical evaluation

1. Advanced Trauma Life Support (ATLS) principles should be initiated in these patients.

2. Physical examination

   a. Obvious thigh deformity with the limb shortened and swollen compared with the contralateral extremity.

6: Trauma

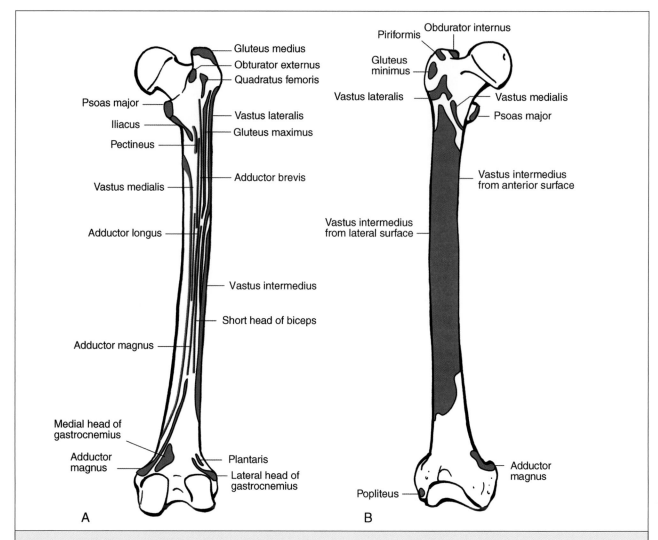

Figure 1 The primary muscular attachments on the anterior **(A)** and posterior **(B)** aspects of the femur. (*Reproduced with permission from Nork SE: Fractures of the shaft of the femur, in Bucholz RW, Heckman JD, Court-Brown C [eds]: Rockwood and Green's Fractures in Adults, ed 6. Philadelphia, PA, Lippincott Williams & Wilkins, 2001, p 1852.*)

b. The limb should be palpated for tenderness and deformity.

c. The distal extremity should be evaluated for pulses, sensation, and motor function.

d. The presence of ecchymosis, crepitus, and deformity indicates that the patient should be examined for additional injuries.

3. Additional injuries to the spine, pelvis, and ipsilateral lower extremity can occur, as can soft-tissue injuries, specifically ligamentous and/or meniscal injuries of the knee; therefore, patients with femur fractures should always be closely evaluated for associated injuries.

4. Ipsilateral femoral neck fracture also can occur but is still routinely missed (up to 50% of patients).

a. Initially these fractures are nondisplaced or minimally displaced in up to 60% of patients.

b. The femoral neck fracture often is oriented vertically.

E. Radiographic evaluation

1. An AP view of the pelvis and AP and lateral radiographs of the femur, including the knee joint, are indicated.

2. CT evaluation of the hip is recommended in trauma patients who have sustained a femoral shaft fracture to detect associated nondisplaced femoral neck fracture.

F. Fracture classification

1. The Winquist and Hansen classification is based on the amount of comminution and has implications regarding weight-bearing status and the use of interlocking screws (**Figure 2**).

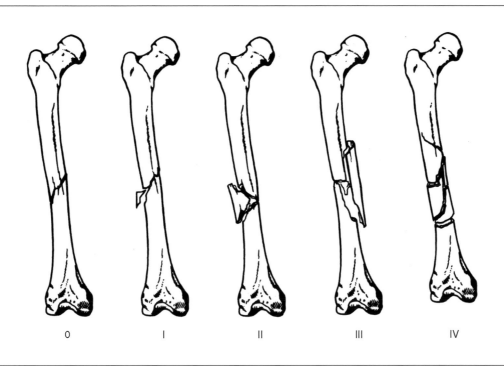

Figure 2   The Winquist and Hansen classification of femoral shaft fractures. Type 0—no comminution; type I—minimal or no comminution; type II—at least 50% of the cortices intact; type III—comminution of at least 50% to 100% of the circumference of the bone; Type IV—no cortical contact at the fracture site with circumferential comminution. (*Reproduced from Poss R [ed]:* Orthopaedic Knowledge Update 3. *Park Ridge, IL, American Academy of Orthopaedic Surgeons, 1990, pp 513-527*).

2. The AO/Orthopaedic Trauma Association (OTA) fracture classification/universal classification system is used more commonly for research purposes and is not very useful in guiding treatment (**Figure 3**).

G. Nonsurgical treatment

1. Early stabilization (within the first 24 hours) of femur fractures minimizes the complication rates and can decrease the length of stay.

2. Skeletal traction may be the definitive treatment in patients who are too sick for surgical treatment.

3. A long period of bed rest may be detrimental, however, and patients should be monitored closely.

   a. Patients should be closely evaluated for pin tract infection and decubiti secondary to prolonged immobilization.

   b. Serial radiographs should be obtained to monitor for distraction at the fracture site during treatment.

   c. Mechanical and chemical deep vein thrombosis (DVT) prophylaxis is important in these patients.

H. Surgical treatment

1. A statically locked, reamed intramedullary (IM) nail is the standard of care for femoral shaft fractures.

   a. An IM nail can be a load-sharing device, as opposed to a compression plate, which is a load-bearing device.

   b. Central placement of an IM nail within the femoral canal results in lower tensile and shear stresses on the implant.

   c. IM nailing has a number of benefits over plate and screws, including less extensive exposure and dissection, a lower infection rate, less quadriceps scarring, early functional use of the extremity, improved restoration of length and alignment with comminuted fractures, rapid fracture healing, and low refracture rate.

   d. The starting point should be based on surgeon preference.

   e. At least two interlocking screws, one proximal and one distal, should be used for all fractures.

2. Retrograde approach

   a. Indications for this approach include multiple-system trauma; trauma to the ipsilateral ex-

6: Trauma

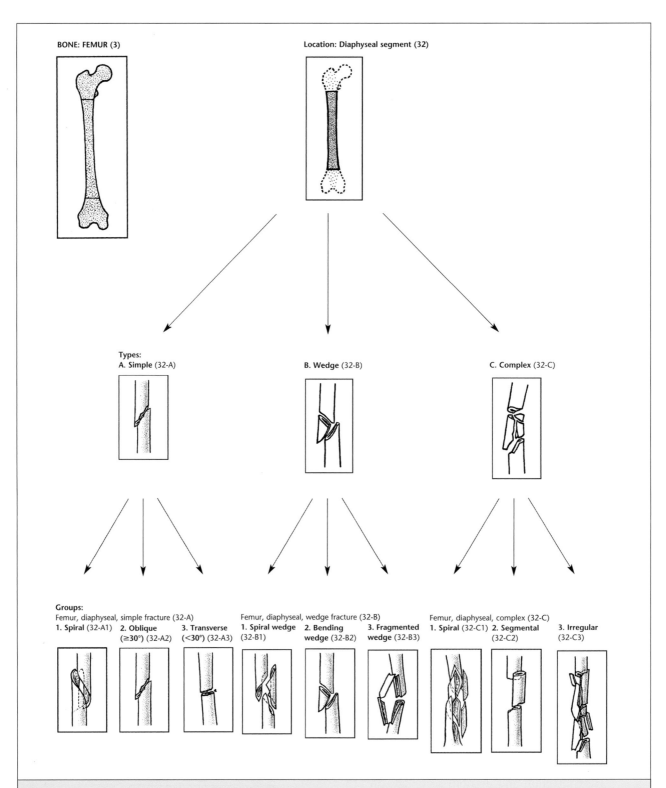

BONE: FEMUR (3)

Location: Diaphyseal segment (32)

Types:
A. Simple (32-A)

B. Wedge (32-B)

C. Complex (32-C)

Groups:
Femur, diaphyseal, simple fracture (32-A)
1. Spiral (32-A1)   2. Oblique (≥30°) (32-A2)   3. Transverse (<30°) (32-A3)

Femur, diaphyseal, wedge fracture (32-B)
1. Spiral wedge (32-B1)   2. Bending wedge (32-B2)   3. Fragmented wedge (32-B3)

Femur, diaphyseal, complex (32-C)
1. Spiral (32-C1)   2. Segmental (32-C2)   3. Irregular (32-C3)

Figure 3   The OTA classification of femoral shaft fractures. Type A fractures are simple fractures, type B are wedge fractures, and type C are complex fractures.

tremity, pelvis/acetabulum, and/or spine; bilateral femur fractures; and morbid obesity.

b. The overall union rate of retrograde nailing is comparable to that of antegrade nailing.

c. The approach has several advantages, including ease of entry point, the potential for quicker surgical times, and no need to set up the fracture table.

d. The recommended starting point for retrograde nailing is 10 mm anterior to the posterior cruciate ligament in the intercondylar notch and in line with the femoral canal.

e. The optimum starting point in the lateral plane is just anterior to the Blumensaat line.

f. A true lateral radiograph should be obtained preoperatively, with both femoral condyles overlapping and appearing as a single condyle. The radiograph should be reviewed preoperatively to assess for patella baja that may interfere with a percutaneous incision and require an arthrotomy (rare).

g. Surgical pearls

   i. Use a radiolucent triangle or bump strategically placed to assist with reduction.

   ii. Protect the prepatellar skin and patella during reaming by seating the reamer in bone before starting.

   iii. Before the patient wakes up, an AP pelvic radiograph should be obtained to rule out a femoral neck fracture; limb rotation and length should be evaluated and the knee should be checked for ligamentous injuries.

h. Complications include malalignment (proximal third fractures) and knee pain.

3. Piriformis entry point

   a. This entry point is in line with the mechanical axis of the femur.

   b. A too-anterior entry point increases the risk for femoral neck fracture secondary to hoop stresses.

   c. The piriformis entry point may result in more muscle and tendon damage and damage to the blood supply of the femoral head than the trochanteric entry point.

4. Trochanteric entry point

   a. This entry point has several advantages over a piriformis entry point, including that its more lateral location is easier to find, it may result in less abductor muscle damage, and fluoroscopic time and surgical time are shorter.

   b. Complications include iatrogenic fracture if a straight piriformis-type nail is used and iatrogenic comminution with malreduction.

I. Reamed versus nonreamed IM nailing

1. Reamed IM nailing is recommended over nonreamed nailing because it allows placement of a larger diameter nail with better cortical fit.

2. Previous concerns with reaming included increased incidence of adult respiratory distress syndrome (ARDS) and lung complications in patients who had associated pulmonary injury. However, a study comparing open reduction and internal fixation with reamed IM nailing in this patient population showed no increased incidence.

J. Flat table versus fracture table

1. Whether to use a fracture table or a fluoroscopic flat table is a decision to be made with all antegrade nailings. Studies support either choice.

2. Considerations include the fracture pattern, patient body habitus, the number of assistants available, associated injuries, and surgeon preference.

K. Plate and screws

1. Plate fixation of femur fractures is not commonly used and has few indications.

2. The best indication for compression plating is a fracture involving the distal metaphyseal-diaphyseal junction of the femur.

3. Complications of compression plating

   a. Failure of fixation

   b. Infection

   c. Nonunion

   d. Devitalization of fracture fragments with excessive periosteal stripping

   e. Stress shielding with possible refracture

L. External fixation

1. External fixation of femur fractures is often used as a form of damage control orthopaedics.

2. External fixation is useful for the unstable trauma patient and patients whose skin does not permit initial definitive fracture fixation.

3. Concerns regarding external fixation include

   a. Pin tract infection

   b. Timing of external fixation removal and conversion to IM nailing. The literature supports safe conversion to IM nailing within the first 2 weeks to minimize the risk for infection.

M. Ipsilateral femoral neck and shaft fractures

1. Radiographic evaluation

   a. Most femoral neck fractures that are associated with an ipsilateral shaft fracture are vertically oriented and nondisplaced or minimally displaced, making radiographic detection difficult.

   b. Fine-cut CT may help to detect femoral neck fractures before surgery.

2. Treatment

   a. The timing of discovery of the femoral neck fracture has implications for its treatment.

   b. No matter when the fracture is discovered, it is essential to obtain an anatomic reduction.

   c. Treatment options—One device or two devices may be used.

      i. With one device, either a cephalomedullary nail or a centromedullary nail with cannulated screws strategically placed using the "miss a nail" technique may be used.

      ii. With two devices, either a retrograde nail with cannulated screws or a retrograde nail with a sliding hip screw may be used. The optimal treatment option has yet to be decided.

N. Open femoral shaft fractures

   1. Open femoral shaft fractures should be treated with irrigation and débridement and primary intramedullary nailing.

   2. The infection rate of open fractures of the femur is significantly lower than that of open tibia fractures.

O. Rehabilitation

   1. With stable fracture fixation, early mobilization and weight bearing are permitted. Most patients are allowed to bear weight to varying degrees, with associated injuries, fracture pattern, implant selection, and surgeon preference dictating the exact postoperative therapy orders.

   2. Early active motion of the hip and knee joint is encouraged.

P. Complications

   1. Perioperative

     a. Fat embolism syndrome

      i. This usually occurs 24 to 72 hours after initial trauma in a small percentage of patients with long bone fractures.

      ii. It can be fatal in up to 15% of patients.

      iii. Classic symptoms include tachypnea, tachycardia, hypoxemia, mental status changes, and petechiae.

      iv. Treatment includes mechanical ventilation with high positive end-expiratory pressure levels.

      v. Prevention involves early (within 24 hours) stabilization of long bone fractures.

    b. Thromboembolism

      i. DVT is a concern in trauma patients, especially those with long bone trauma, pelvic and acetabular fractures, and spine trauma. It may lead to a fatal pulmonary embolism (PE).

      ii. A duplex ultrasound may be used to diagnose DVT.

      iii. In patients with suspected PE, a spiral CT scan, ventilation-perfusion scan, or pulmonary angiography (gold standard) may be used for diagnosis.

      iv. The symptoms of a PE include acute onset tachypnea, tachycardia, low-grade fevers, hypoxia, mental status changes, and chest pain.

      v. Preventive measures include chemical prophylaxis: warfarin, subcutaneous heparin, low-molecular weight heparin; sequential compression devices or foot pumps; and early surgical stabilization and subsequent mobilization, which are important, controllable measures.

    c. Adult respiratory distress syndrome

      i. ARDS is an acute respiratory failure with pulmonary edema.

      ii. It can result from multiple etiologies and is known to occur after trauma and shock.

      iii. The patient may be difficult to ventilate secondary to decreased lung compliance.

      iv. Other signs/symptoms include tachypnea, tachycardia, and hypoxemia.

      v. Treatment is with high positive end-expiratory pressure.

      vi. The mortality can be up to 50%.

      vii. From an orthopaedic surgeon's perspective, early stabilization of long bone fractures helps decrease the incidence of ARDS.

    d. Compartment syndrome

      i. Compartment syndrome after femur fractures is rare. It is important to consider the mechanism of injury; a crush injury or an injury with a prolonged extrication in which the dashboard console was crushing the leg compartments should be followed closely.

      ii. Compartment syndrome has been reported after IM nailing on the fracture table.

    e. Nerve palsy

      i. In femur fractures stabilized on the fracture table, pudendal nerve palsy may occur as a result of excessive traction and/or improper positioning with the perineal post.

ii. A peroneal nerve neurapraxia may also occur secondary to excessive traction.

f. Nonunion, delayed union, malunion

i. The rate of nonunion after treatment of femoral shaft fractures with a locked IM nail is low.

ii. Treatment is exchange nailing with a larger IM nail.

iii. With an infected nonunion (a rare complication), the use of chronic suppressive antibiotics until healing occurs is recommended, followed by implant removal.

iv. Delayed unions may occur because of technical concerns. Removal of the interlocking screw may allow compression across the fracture and allow union to occur.

v. Up to 20% of patients may have limb rotational deformities.

vi. Previously it was thought that internal rotation deformities were not well tolerated, but in most patients, rotational deformities of less than 20° are well tolerated.

g. Hardware failure and recurrent fracture

i. With reamed, statically locked IM nailing of femur fractures, the occurrence of hardware failure is low.

ii. The closer a fracture is to the interlocking screw placement, the higher the stresses on the hardware.

h. Heterotopic ossification

i. The insertion site for an antegrade nail involves soft-tissue disruption of the abductors. Thus, some patients may develop heterotopic ossification about the hip.

ii. Heterotopic ossification of minimal clinical significance has been reported to occur in up to 26% of patients with fractures stabilized using a piriformis starting point. The occurrence rate associated with a trochanteric starting point has not yet been reported.

II. Fractures of the Distal Femur

A. Epidemiology

1. Distal femur fractures are bimodally distributed.

2. There is a higher incidence in young, healthy males (often from high-energy trauma) and elderly, osteopenic females (from low-energy mechanisms).

B. Anatomy

1. The geometric cross-section of the femoral shaft transitions from cylindrical to trapezoidal, with the medial condyle extending further distally.

2. The distal femur is trapezoidal and is composed of cancellous bone.

3. The distal femur is in physiologic valgus.

4. It is important to keep in mind that the posterior half of both femoral condyles lies posterior to the femoral shaft.

5. Deforming forces after a fracture

a. The origin of the gastrocnemius characteristically pulls the distal fragment into flexion.

b. Closely evaluate preoperatively for a coronal plane Hoffa fracture.

C. Surgical approach

1. Depends on choice of reduction type (indirect or direct) and plate.

2. Minimally invasive surgical approaches include minimally invasive plate osteosynthesis (MIPO).

a. This approach is ideal for extra-articular fractures, which can be reduced indirectly.

b. A small lateral incision is made to facilitate plate placement, with stab incisions for screw placement.

3. Transarticular approach with retrograde plate fixation (TARPO) and lateral parapatellar arthrotomy

a. Can also be used with indirect reduction techniques

b. Can be useful for partial articular fractures

4. Lateral parapatellar approach

a. Affords excellent exposure of the femoral shaft and permits eversion of the patella.

b. One disadvantage is that a different incision is needed for future total knee arthroplasties (TKAs).

c. The advantage of the approach is that it affords good visualization of the joint surface.

d. The lateral parapatellar approach should be used for reduction of lateral Hoffa fragments.

D. Mechanism of injury

1. Fractures involving the supracondylar femur are often a result of the same high-energy mechanisms seen in fractures of the femoral shaft.

2. Low-energy mechanisms, such as minor falls, are common in the older population.

E. Clinical evaluation

1. Consider the mechanism of injury: with high-energy mechanisms, a full trauma evaluation should be completed.

2. The patient usually presents with pain, swelling, and deformity in the distal femur region.

3. Neurovascular structures lie close to these fractures, so neurovascular status should be assessed thoroughly.

4. The skin should be examined closely for open wounds.

5. In the elderly patient, preexisting medical conditions and degenerative knee joint disease should be considered.

F. Radiographic evaluation

1. AP and lateral radiographs of the distal femur are standard.

2. Radiographic evaluation of the ipsilateral lower extremity should be considered because of the risk of associated injuries.

3. Oblique views may be helpful to provide further details regarding the intercondylar anatomy; however, with use of CT scanning there is often no need for these additional radiographs.

4. Traction radiographs are helpful but may be too uncomfortable for the patient.

5. Contralateral views may be helpful in preoperative planning and templating.

6. CT provides details regarding intra-articular involvement and can identify coronal plane deformities with reconstruction views.

G. Classification—The OTA classification is the universally accepted system for characterizing injuries of the distal femur (**Figure 4**).

1. Type A fractures are extra-articular injuries.

2. Type B fractures are partially articular and involve a single condyle.

3. Type C fractures are intercondylar or bicondylar intra-articular injuries with varying degrees of comminution.

H. Nonsurgical treatment—Nonsurgical treatment is indicated only for nondisplaced distal femur fractures. Nonsurgical treatment of displaced supracondylar and intercondylar femur fractures is generally associated with poor results and should be reserved for patients who otherwise represent an unacceptable surgical risk.

I. Surgical treatment

1. The goal of surgical treatment should be stable fixation to permit early mobility.

2. The trend in recent years regarding periarticular fractures has changed from large, extensile approaches, subperiosteal dissection, circumferential clamps, absolute stability with compression by lag screws and use of short plates with multiple screws to the concept of biologic reduction techniques that emphasize limited lateral exposures and preservation of the soft-tissue attachments.

3. The locking plate has become quite popular. Multiple manufacturers offer locking plate systems.

a. The main advantages of the newer plating systems include the ability to place the implant percutaneously, less periosteal stripping, and application of a plate laterally without need for additional medial plate stabilization.

b. The locked nature of the screws in the femoral condyles allow for the placement of multiple "internal external fixators" that have been shown to be axially superior to earlier fixation techniques. The improved axial strength of the newer implants should not lead to a false sense of security, however.

c. Another advantage of the newer design plates is the submuscular advancement of the plate to the bone, which minimizes periosteal stripping and preserves the blood supply. The implants do not rely on direct contact of the plate to the bone for stability. The concept is called relative stability, and longer plates and fewer screws are used.

d. If using a long percutaneous plate, proximal visualization of the plate placement may be difficult. Consider making an incision to ensure proper placement proximally on the femur.

J. Surgical technique

1. The patient should be positioned supine on a radiolucent table.

2. Open fractures should be treated in accordance with open fracture treatment principles. Temporizing knee-spanning external fixators should be used until the soft tissue permits the placement of internal fixation.

3. Once the soft tissues have been stabilized, the surgical approach and tactic is dictated by the degree of articular comminution (**Table 1**).

a. Type A fractures

i. Plate fixation is a viable option and is associated with good results.

ii. Traditional plating options include dynamic condylar screw, a 95° blade plate, or a locking plate. Dynamic condylar screw or blade plating requires the use of a more invasive incision for direct reduction techniques.

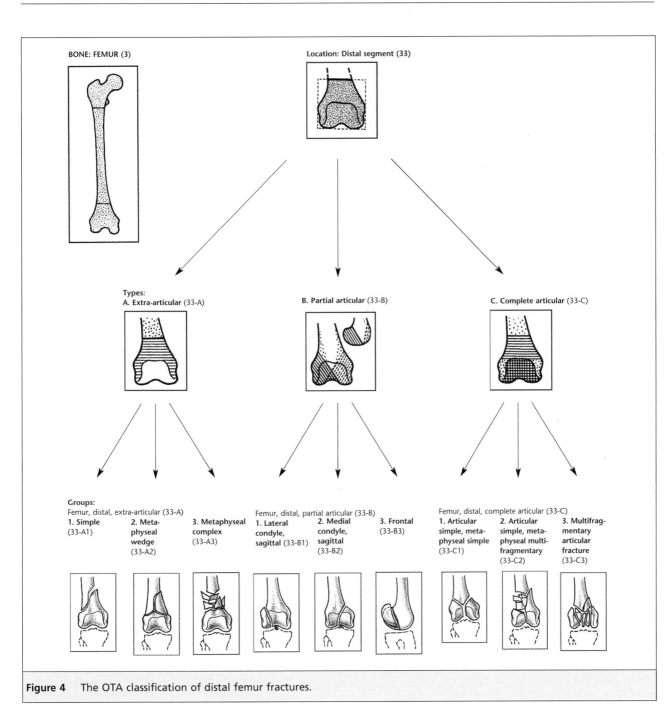

Figure 4   The OTA classification of distal femur fractures.

iii. Locked plating can be performed through a minimally invasive lateral approach to the distal femur, exposing only the portion of the distal lateral condyle necessary to facilitate placement of the implant.

b. Type B fractures

   i. Lag screw fixation

   ii. Plate fixation

c. Type C fractures

   i. Open reduction and internal fixation with plates

   ii. An anatomic articular reduction is critical for a good result.

K. IM nails

1. Retrograde IM nailing represents a good choice for distal femur fractures not involving the articular surface.

2. When attempting retrograde IM nailing of a distal femur fracture with extension into the articular surface, the articular surface should be stabilized with Kirschner wires and/or screws before nail placement.

Table 1

Possible Implants for Distal Femur Fractures as Determined by the AO/OTA Classification System.

Type A or C1/C2 Fractures

Dynamic condylar screw

95° blade plate

Antegrade femoral nail

Retrograde femoral nail

Locked internal fixator (lateral plate with locked distal screws)

Type B Fractures

Screw and/or plate fixation

Type C3 Fractures

Standard condylar buttress plate

Locked internal fixator (lateral plate with locked distal screws)

(Reproduced from Kregor PJ, Morgan SJ: Fractures of the distal femur, in Baumgaertner MR, Tornetta P III [eds]: Orthopaedic Knowledge Update: Trauma 3. Rosemont, IL, American Academy of Orthopaedic Surgeons, 2005, pp 397-408.)

3. There are few indications for a short retrograde nail.

L. External fixation—Bridging external fixation may be advantageous as a temporizing measure in open fractures or in fractures with significant comminution or soft-tissue compromise. When using a bridging external fixation, the external fixator pins should be placed away from the planned plate.

M. Associated vascular injury

1. Neurovascular status should be evaluated carefully because of the proximity of vascular structures to these fractures.

2. If the fracture is associated with a knee dislocation, angiography may be considered because the risk of vascular injury is significantly greater with associated dislocation.

N. Supracondylar fracture after TKA

1. Retrograde nail (if the implant permits)

2. Locking plate

   a. The locking plate is the fixation device of choice for very distal fractures in osteopenic bone.

b. The literature supports good results for locking plate fixation of periprosthetic fractures proximal to a TKA.

c. A locked plate should be considered for very distal periprosthetic supracondylar femur fractures.

O. Rehabilitation

1. Postoperative treatment should include the administration of intravenous antibiotics for 24 to 48 hours following closure of all wounds and the routine use of mechanical and chemical prophylaxis for DVT.

2. Patients are assisted out of bed on the first postoperative day and should be non–weight-bearing on the affected limb with the use of ambulatory assistive devices.

3. Active assisted range-of-motion exercises should be initiated in the early postoperative period. Early range-of-motion exercises are critical in that functionally poor results are most often attributed to knee stiffness, and little improvement is gained after 1 year.

P. Complications

1. The metaphyseal location and preponderance of cancellous bone in these fractures can lead to significant comminution, even with low-energy injury mechanisms. Therefore, meticulous attention to preoperative planning with full consideration of all patient factors (condition of the soft tissues, concomitant injuries, comorbidities, functional level before injury) is of paramount importance.

2. Even with locking plate fixation, failures have been reported. The need for bone grafting, therefore, should not be ignored in those fractures where it is warranted.

3. Nonunions

   a. The rate of nonunion has improved with the use of more biologically friendly techniques such as minimally invasive plate application.

   b. Nonunions should be treated with bone grafting and/or implant revision.

4. Infection

   a. Infection rates have improved with the use of soft-tissue friendly surgery.

   b. Infection should be managed with thorough débridement, cultures, and appropriate antibiotics, and consideration of removal of hardware if the fracture permits.

Top Testing Facts

Femoral Shaft Fractures

1. Always closely evaluate the patient with a femur fracture for associated injuries.

2. Early stabilization (within the first 24 hours) of femur fractures minimizes the complication rates and can decrease the length of stay.

3. Bilateral femur fractures have a mortality rate of up to 25%.

4. The infection rate for open femur fractures is significantly lower than that of open tibia fractures.

5. Rotation deformities may occur if the leg is not properly positioned on the fracture table.

6. A statically locked, reamed IM nail is the standard of care for femoral shaft fractures.

7. The starting point should be based on surgeon preference.

8. At least two interlocking screws, one proximal and one distal, should be used for all fractures.

9. Before the patient wakes up, AP pelvic radiographic imaging should be performed to rule out a femoral neck fracture; limb rotation and length should be evaluated and the knee should be checked for ligamentous injuries.

10. Conversion of an external fixator to an IM nail should occur within the first 2 weeks to minimize the risk of infection.

Distal Femur Fractures

1. The origin of the gastrocnemius characteristically pulls the distal fragment into flexion.

2. A bump or radiographic triangle strategically placed under the deformity may assist with reduction.

3. Closely evaluate preoperatively for a coronal plane Hoffa fracture.

4. If using a long percutaneous plate, proximal visualization of the plate placement on the femur may be difficult. Consider making an incision to ensure proper placement proximally on the femur.

5. When using a bridging external fixator, place the external fixator pins away from the planned plate location.

6. The goal of surgical treatment should be stable fixation to permit early mobility.

7. Even with locking plate fixation, failures have been reported. The need for bone grafting, therefore, should not be ignored in those fractures where it is warranted.

8. A locked plate should be considered for very distal periprosthetic supracondylar femur fractures.

Bibliography

Bolhofner BR, Carmen B, Clifford P: The results of open reduction and internal fixation of distal femur fractures using a biologic (indirect) reduction technique. *J Orthop Trauma* 1996;10:372-377.

Brumback RJ, Uwagie-Ero S, Lakatos RP, Poka A, Bathon GH, Burgess AR: Intramedullary nailing of femoral shaft fractures: Part II. Fracture-healing with static interlocking fixation. *J Bone Joint Surg Am* 1988;70:1453-1462.

Copeland CE, Mitchell KA, Brumback RJ, Gens DR, Burgess AR: Mortality in patients with bilateral femur fractures. *J Orthop Trauma* 1998;12:315-319.

Gliatis J, Megas P, Panagiotopoulos E, Lambiris E: Midterm results of treatment with retrograde nail for supracondylar periprostheic fractures of femur following total knee arthroplasty. *J Orthop Trauma* 2005;19:164-170.

Harwood PJ, Giannoudis PV, Griensven MV, Krettek C, Pape HC: Alterations in the systemic inflammatory response after early total care and damage control procedures for femoral shaft fracture in severely injured patients. *J Trauma* 2005;58:446-454.

Jaarsma RL, Pakvis DF, Verdonschot N, Biert J, van Kampen A: Rotational malalignment after intramedullary nailing of femoral fractures. *J Orthop Trauma* 2004;18:403-409.

Kregor PJ, Stannard JA, Zlowodzki M, Cole PA: Treatment of distal femur fractures using the less invasive stabilization system. *J Orthop Trauma* 2004;18:509-520.

Nork SE, Agel J, Russell GV, Mills WJ, Holt S, Routt ML Jr: Mortality after reamed intramedullary nailing of bilateral femur fractures. *Clin Orthop Relat Res* 2003;415:272-278.

Nowotarski PJ, Turen CH, Brumback RJ, Scarboro JM: Conversion of external fixation to intramedullary nailing for fractures of the shaft of the femur in multiply injured patients. *J Bone Joint Surg Am* 2000;82:781-788.

Ostrum RF, Agarwal A, Lakatos R, Poka A: Prospective comparison of retrograde and antegrade femoral intramedullary nailing. *J Orthop Trauma* 2000;14:496-501.

Ricci WM, Bellabarba C, Evanoff B, Herscovici D, Dipasquale T , Sanders R : Retrograde versus antegrade nailing of femoral shaft fractures. *J Orthop Trauma* 2001;15:161-169.

Stephen DJ, Kreder HJ, Schemitsch EH, Conlan LB, Wild L, Mckee MD: Femoral intramedullary nailing: A comparison of fracture table and manual traction: A prospective, randomized study. *J Bone Joint Surg Am* 2002;84:1514-1521.

Tornetta P, Creevy WR, Kain M: Avoiding missed femoral neck fractures: Improvement by using a standard protocol in cases of femoral shaft fractures. *J Bone Joint Surg Am* 2007; 89:39-43.

Vallier HA, Hennessey TA, Sontich JK, Patterson BM: Failure of LCP condylar plate fixation in the distal part of the femur: A report of six cases. *J Bone Joint Surg Am* 2006;88:846-853.

Watson JT, Moed BR: Ipsilateral femoral neck and shaft fractures: Complications and their treatment. *Clin Orthop Relat Res* 2002;399:78-86.

Chapter 57

Knee Dislocations and Patella Fractures

Robert V. Cantu, MD   Kenneth J. Koval, MD

I. Knee Dislocations

A. Epidemiology

1. Traumatic knee dislocations are rare, with an incidence of < 0.2% of orthopaedic injuries.

2. Actual incidence is likely higher due to underreporting because 20% to 50% of knee dislocations spontaneously reduce.

B. Anatomy

1. The knee is a hinge joint with three articulations: patellofemoral, tibiofemoral, and tibiofibular.

2. Normal range of motion of the knee ranges from up to 10° of extension to 140° of flexion with 8° to 12° of rotation through the flexion-extension arc.

3. Dynamic and static knee stability is conferred by the soft tissues (ligaments, muscles, tendons, and menisci) and the bony articulations.

4. The popliteal vascular bundle courses through a fibrous tunnel at the level of the adductor hiatus.

   a. Within the popliteal fossa, the popliteal artery gives off five branches: superior medial and lateral geniculate arteries, inferior medial and lateral geniculate arteries, and the middle geniculate artery.

   b. The popliteal artery runs deep to the soleus muscle through another fibrous tunnel. It is the tethering of the popliteal artery at the adductor hiatus and soleus that makes it prone to injury during dislocation (**Figure 1**).

5. The common peroneal nerve runs behind the fibular head and is also prone to injury (typically a stretch injury) with knee dislocation.

6. The posterolateral corner consists of the lateral collateral ligament (LCL), the popliteus tendon, the popliteofibular ligament, and the iliotibial band. It is often injured with knee dislocation and if not addressed can be a source of instability.

C. Mechanism of injury

1. High-energy mechanism typically is a motor vehicle accident in which the knee strikes the dashboard, causing an axial load to a flexed knee, or a fall from a height.

2. Lower energy mechanism typically is an athletic injury resulting in knee dislocation. A rotatory component to the dislocation is common. Morbid obesity (body mass index [BMI] >35) also is a risk factor for low-energy knee dislocations.

3. Hyperextension of the knee, with or without a varus or valgus stress, results in an anterior dislocation, whereas knee flexion with a posterior-directed force results in a posterior dislocation (dashboard injury).

4. Substantial soft-tissue injury is needed for knee dislocation. Typically at least three of the four ligaments are torn.

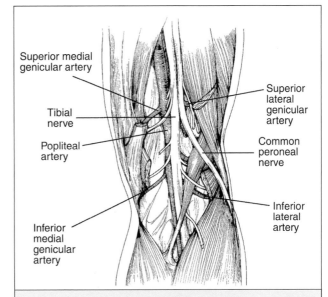

Figure 1   Posterior anatomy of the knee showing the relationship between the popliteal artery and the tibial and common peroneal nerves. (*Reproduced from Good L, Johnson RJ: The dislocated knee. J Am Acad Orthop Surg 1995;3:284-292.*)

6: Trauma

D. Clinical evaluation

1. Gross knee distortion is common on presentation unless the knee spontaneously reduces. Immediate reduction is indicated, without waiting for radiographs in the dislocated position.

2. Patients who sustain a knee dislocation that spontaneously reduces may have a relatively normal-appearing knee. Subtle signs of injury such as mild abrasions, a minimal effusion, or reports of knee pain may be the only abnormalities.

3. The extent of ligamentous injury is related to the degree of bony displacement. Ligamentous injury occurs with displacement of more than 10% to 25% of the resting length of the ligament. Certain tests can be used to assess ligamentous stability after joint reduction.

   a. Anterior cruciate ligament (ACL): Lachman test at 30° knee flexion

   b. Posterior cruciate ligament (PCL): Posterior drawer test at 90° knee flexion

   c. LCL/posterolateral corner (PLC): Varus stress at 30° and full extension, increased tibial external rotation at 30° flexion, increased posterior tibial translation at 30° flexion

   d. Medial collateral ligament (MCL): Valgus stress at 30° knee flexion

   e. LCL/PLC and cruciate (at least one cruciate ACL or PCL): Varus in full extension and at 30° flexion

   f. MCL and PCL: Increased valgus in full extension and at 30°

   g. PLC and PCL: Increased tibial external rotation at 30° and 90°, increased posterior tibial translation at 30° and 90°

E. Vascular injury

1. Careful neurovascular examination is critical, both before and after reduction, and serially thereafter because thrombosis due to an unsuspected intimal tear may cause delayed ischemia hours or even days after reduction.

   a. The popliteal artery is at risk during traumatic knee dislocations (in up to 60% of patients) because of the bowstring effect across the popliteal fossa, secondary to proximal and distal tethering.

   b. Although distal pulses and capillary refill may be detected as a result of collateral circulation, these are inadequate to maintain limb viability.

2. The mechanism of arterial injury varies with the type of dislocation.

   a. With anterior dislocations, the artery usually is injured as a result of traction, resulting in an intimal tear.

   b. With posterior dislocations, the artery frequently is completely torn.

3. Vascular examination includes evaluation of the dorsalis pedis and posterior tibial artery pulses.

   a. If the pulses are absent, immediate closed reduction should be considered. If still absent after reduction, emergent surgical exploration is indicated.

   b. If pulse returns after closed reduction, angiography should be considered versus observation. The maximum time for ischemia in the limb is 8 hours.

   c. If there are palpable pulses, the ankle brachial index (ABI) should be assessed. An ABI > 0.9 warrants observation, but if greater, angiography and/or surgical exploration is indicated (**Figure 2**).

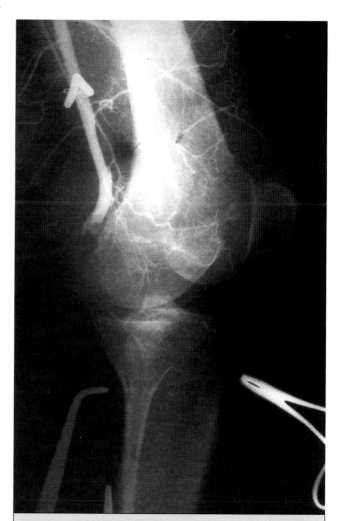

Figure 2 Intraoperative angiogram showing complete disruption of the popliteal artery following posterior knee dislocation. (*Reproduced from Good L, Johnson RJ: The dislocated knee.* J Am Acad Orthop Surg *1995;3:284-292.*)

F. Principles of treatment of vascular injuries

1. Vascular status (dorsalis pedis and posterior tibial artery pulses and capillary refill) must be evaluated and documented in any patient with a proven or suspected knee dislocation. The presence of arterial insufficiency or abnormality confirms a vascular injury.

2. Revascularization should be performed within 8 hours.

3. Spasm is an unacceptable explanation as a cause for decreased or absent pulses in an attempt to justify observation.

4. Consultation with a vascular surgeon is recommended to verify clinical findings and interpret studies.

G. Treatment of vascular injury

1. Following reduction, circulation should be reassessed, with immediate surgical exploration indicated if the limb is ischemic.

2. Urgent arteriography is indicated for patients with abnormal vascular status (diminished pulses, decreased capillary refill, ABI < 0.9) and a viable limb. Waiting for arteriography, however, should not delay surgical re-anastomosis.

3. Careful observation with serial examinations is indicated for patients with a normal vascular status (normal dorsalis pedis and posterior tibial artery pulses, normal capillary refill, ABI > 0.9).

4. MR arthrography/MRI is useful to evaluate non-occlusive (intimal) injury; however, their sensitivity and specificity are uncertain.

5. Arterial injury is treated with excision of the damaged segment and re-anastomosis with reverse saphenous vein graft.

H. Neurologic injury

1. Injury to the peroneal nerve is commonly associated with posterolateral dislocations, with injury varying from neurapraxia (usual) to complete transection (rare).

2. Primary exploration with grafting or repair is not effective; secondary exploration at 3 months also has been associated with poor results.

3. Bracing and/or tendon transfer may be necessary for treatment of muscular deficiencies.

I. Imaging

1. Radiographic evaluation

a. Because of the high incidence of neurovascular compromise associated with knee dislocation, immediate reduction is recommended before radiographic evaluation.

b. Following reduction, AP and lateral views of

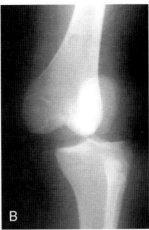
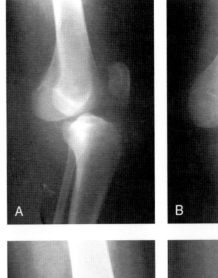
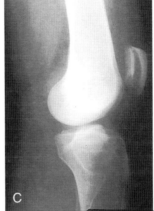
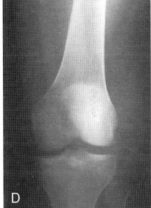

Figure 3 Pre- and post-reduction radiographs of an anterolateral knee dislocation. (*Reproduced from Rihn JA, Cha PS, Groff YJ, and Harner CD: The acutely dislocated knee: Evaluation and management. J Am Acad Orthop Surg 2004;12:334-346.*)

the knee should be obtained to assess the reduction and identify associated injuries. Dislocation is suggested by several findings (**Figure 3**).

i. Obvious dislocation

ii. Irregular or asymmetric joint space

iii. Lateral capsular (Segond) sign

iv. Ligamentous avulsions and osteochondral defects

2. Angiography

a. The use of angiography after knee dislocation is controversial.

b. Vascular compromise is an indication for emergent surgical intervention. Identifying intimal tears in a limb with an intact neurovascular status may be unnecessary because most do not result in thrombosis and vascular occlusion.

6: Trauma

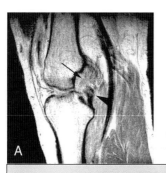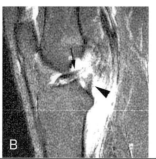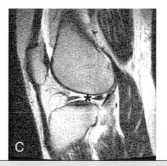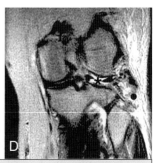

Figure 4   MRIs of the left knee of a patient who sustained a twisting injury from stepping in a hole during a softball game. T1-weighted **(A)** and T2-weighted **(B)** sagittal scans show disruption of the ACL (arrow) and PCL (arrowhead). **C,** T1-weighted sagittal image shows an injury to the lateral meniscus (asterisk), which appears to be elevated off the lateral tibial plateau. **D,** T2-weighted coronal image shows injuries to the lateral meniscus (asterisk) and PLC (black dot). (*Reproduced from Rihn JA, Cha PS, Groff YJ, Harner CD: The acutely dislocated knee: Evaluation and management.* J Am Acad Orthop Surg *2004;12:334-346.*)

c. Some authors advocate selective arteriography only if the ABI < 0.9. Regardless, the patient should be closely observed for evidence of vascular insufficiency.

3. Magnetic Resonance Imaging

   a. MRI is indicated for all knee dislocations and equivalents.

   b. MRI has value for preoperative planning, identifying avulsions and other ligamentous injuries, and identifying meniscal pathology and articular cartilage lesions (**Figure 4**).

J. Dislocation classification

1. Descriptive terms are based on displacement of the proximal tibia in relation to the distal femur.

   a. Anterior: Forceful hyperextension of the knee beyond −30°. This is the most common type of dislocation, affecting between 30% and 50% of patients. Associated injuries include PCL (and possibly ACL) tears, with high incidence of popliteal artery disruption with increasing degree of hyperextension.

   b. Posterior: Posteriorly directed force against proximal tibia of flexed knee (25%), also called a "dashboard" injury. Associated injuries include anterior and posterior ligament disruption and popliteal artery compromise with increasing proximal tibial displacement.

   c. Lateral: Valgus force (13%) that disrupts the medial supporting structures, often with associated tears of both cruciate ligaments.

   d. Medial: Varus force (3%) in which both lateral and posterolateral structures are disrupted.

   e. Rotational: Varus/valgus with rotatory component (4%) that usually results in buttonholing of the femoral condyle through the articular capsule.

2. Other descriptive terms include open versus closed, reducible versus irreducible, and "occult" fractures, which indicate a knee dislocation with spontaneous reduction.

K. Closed reduction

1. Immediate closed reduction is essential, even in the field and especially in the compromised limb. Direct pressure on the popliteal space should be avoided during or after reduction.

2. Reduction maneuvers for specific dislocations

   a. Anterior: Axial limb traction combined with lifting of the distal femur

   b. Posterior: Axial limb traction combined with extension and lifting of the proximal tibia

   c. Medial/lateral: Axial limb traction combined with lateral/medial translation of the tibia

   d. Rotatory: Axial limb traction combined with derotation of the tibia

3. Posterolateral dislocation is believed to be "irreducible" because of buttonholing of the medial femoral condyle through the medial capsule, resulting in a dimple sign over the medial aspect of the limb. This dislocation requires open reduction.

4. Arthroscopy can be used to assess residual laxity.

5. Following reduction, the knee is splinted at 20° to 30° of flexion. It is essential to maintain this reduction.

6. Initial stabilization can be done with either a knee immobilizer (in extension for 6 weeks) or external fixation.

   a. External fixation is better for grossly unstable knees that may subluxate in the brace.

   b. It also protects vascular repair and fasciotomy and allows skin care for open injuries.

c. External fixation is also indicated for obese or multiple trauma patients.

L. Surgical repair

1. Repair or reconstruction of the torn structures generally is recommended because nonsurgical treatment in active individuals often leads to poor results. Shorter periods of immobilization result in improved knee motion and residual laxity whereas longer periods may improve stability but limit motion. Recent clinical series have reported better results with surgical treatment. However, no prospective, controlled, randomized trials of comparable injuries have been performed.

2. Complete posterolateral corner disruption is best treated with early open repair. Reconstitution of the PLC is important; the PLC should always be repaired before the ACL.

3. Immediate surgical repair

   a. Unsuccessful closed reduction

   b. Residual soft-issue interposition

   c. Open injuries

   d. Vascular injuries

      i. These require external fixation and vascular repair typically with a reverse saphenous vein graft from the contralateral leg.

      ii. Amputation rates as high as 86% have been reported when there is a delay beyond 8 hours with documented vascular compromise to limb.

      iii. A fasciotomy should be performed at time of vascular repair for limb ischemia of longer than 6 hours.

4. Ligamentous repair is controversial: The current literature favors acute repair of lateral ligaments followed by early motion and functional bracing.

5. Timing of surgical repair depends on the condition of both the patient and the limb.

6. Meniscal injuries also should be addressed at the time of surgery.

M. Complications

1. Limited range of motion, most commonly related to scar formation and capsular tightness. This reflects the balance between sufficient immobilization to achieve stability versus mobilization to restore motion. If severely limiting, lysis of adhesions may be indicated to restore range of motion.

2. Ligamentous laxity and instability

3. Vascular compromise, which may result in atrophic skin changes, hyperalgesia, claudication, and muscle contracture

4. Nerve traction injury resulting in sensory and motor disturbances portends a poor prognosis, as surgical exploration in the acute (<24 hours), subacute (1 to 2 weeks), and long-term settings (3 months) has yielded poor results. Bracing or muscle tendon transfers may be necessary to improve function.

II. Patella Fractures

A. Epidemiology

1. Patella fractures represent 1% of all skeletal injuries.

2. The male to female ratio is 2:1.

3. The most common age group is 20 to 50 years old.

4. Bilateral injuries are uncommon.

B. Anatomy

1. The patella is the largest sesamoid bone in the body. The quadriceps tendon inserts on the superior pole, and the patellar ligament originates from the inferior pole of the patella.

2. There are seven articular facets. Of these, the lateral facet is the largest (50% of the articular surface). The articular cartilage may be up to 1 cm thick.

3. The medial and lateral extensor retinaculae are strong longitudinal expansions of the quadriceps and insert directly onto the tibia. If these remain intact in the presence of a patella fracture, then active extension will be preserved (**Figure 5**).

4. The function of the patella is to increase the mechanical advantage and leverage of the quadriceps tendon, help nourish the femoral articular surface, and protect the femoral condyles from direct trauma. The blood supply arises from the geniculate arteries, which form an anastomosis circumferentially around the patella.

C. Mechanism of injury

1. Direct: Trauma to the patella may produce incomplete, simple, stellate, or comminuted fracture patterns.

   a. Displacement may be minimal due to preservation of the medial and lateral retinacular expansions.

   b. Abrasions over the area or open injuries are common. Active knee extension may be preserved.

6: Trauma

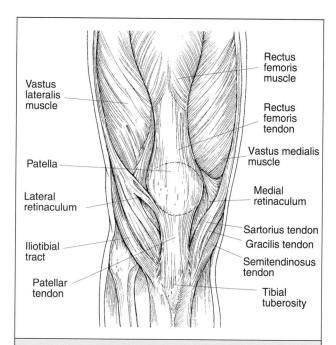

Figure 5 Anatomy of the extensor mechanism of the knee. *(Reproduced from Matava MJ: Patellar tendon ruptures. J Am Acad Orthop Surg 1996;4:287-296.)*

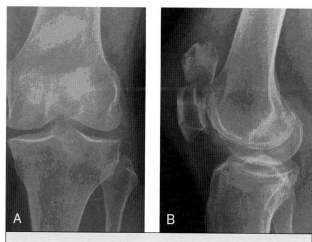

Figure 6 AP **(A)** and lateral **(B)** radiographs of a displaced patella fracture.

2. Indirect (most common): This is the most common mechanism, occurring secondary to forcible quadriceps contraction while the knee is in a semiflexed position (eg, in a stumble or fall).

   a. The intrinsic strength of the patella is exceeded by the pull of the musculotendinous and ligamentous structures.

   b. A transverse fracture pattern is most commonly seen with this mechanism, with variable inferior pole comminution.

c. The degree of fragment displacement suggests the degree of retinacular disruption. Active knee extension is usually lost.

3. Combined direct/indirect: The patient experiences direct and indirect trauma to the knee, such as in a fall from a height.

D. Clinical evaluation

1. Patients typically present with limited or no ambulatory capacity with pain, swelling, and tenderness of the involved knee. A defect at the patella may be palpable.

2. Open fracture must be ruled out because these constitute a surgical emergency; assessment may require instillation of 50 to 70 mL of saline solution into the knee to determine communication with overlying lacerations.

3. Active knee extension should be evaluated to assess injury to the retinacular expansions. This examination may be aided by decompression of hemarthrosis.

4. Associated lower extremity injuries may be present following high-energy trauma. The ipsilateral hip, femur, tibia, and ankle must be carefully examined, with appropriate radiographic evaluation, if indicated.

E. Radiographic evaluation—AP, lateral, and axial (sunrise) views of the knee should be obtained.

1. On the AP view, a bipartite patella (8% of population) may be mistaken for a fracture; these usually occur in the superolateral position and have smooth margins and are bilateral in 50% of individuals.

2. On the lateral view, displaced fractures usually are obvious (**Figure 6**).

3. The axial view (sunrise) may help identify osteochondral or vertical marginal fractures.

F. Fracture classification

1. Patella fractures are classified descriptively in one of the following ways: open or closed, nondisplaced or displaced.

2. They also are described based on the fracture pattern: transverse, vertical, marginal, comminuted, osteochondral, or sleeve (**Figure 7**).

G. Treatment

1. Nonsurgical treatment

   a. Indications include nondisplaced or minimally displaced (2 to 3 mm) fractures with minimal articular disruption (1 to 2 mm) and an intact extensor mechanism.

b. Treatment involves a cylinder cast or knee immobilizer for 4 to 6 weeks. Early weight bearing is encouraged, advancing to full weight bearing with crutches as tolerated. Early straight leg raises and isometric quadriceps strengthening exercises should be started within a few days.

c. After radiographic evidence of healing, progressive active flexion and extension strengthening exercises are begun with a hinged knee brace initially locked in extension for ambulation.

2. Surgical treatment

    a. Open reduction and internal fixation

        i. Indications for open reduction and internal fixation include >2 mm articular incongruity, >3 mm fragment displacement, or open fracture.

        ii. There are multiple methods of surgical fixation, including tension banding (using parallel longitudinal Kirschner wires or cannulated screws), circumferential cerclage wiring, and interfragmentary screw compression supplemented by cerclage wiring (**Figure 8**). Retinacular disruption should be repaired at the time of surgery.

        iii. Postoperatively, the patient should be placed in a splint for 3 to 6 days until skin healing, with early initiation of knee motion. Active-assist range-of-motion exercises should be started, progressing to partial and full weight bearing by 6 weeks. Severely comminuted or marginally repaired fractures, particularly in older patients, may necessitate immobilization for 3 to 6 weeks.

    b. Patellectomy

        i. Partial patellectomy—Indications include the presence of a large, salvageable fragment in the presence of smaller comminuted polar fragments in which restoring the articular surface or achieving stable fixation is considered impossible (**Figure 9**). The quadriceps or patellar tendons should be reattached without creating a patella baja or alta. Reattachment of the patellar tendon close to the articular surface will help to prevent patellar tilt.

        ii. Total patellectomy—Total patellectomy is reserved for patients with severe, extensive comminution and is rarely indicated. Peak torque of the quadriceps is reduced by 50%. Repair of medial and lateral retinacular injuries at the time of patellectomy is essential. Postoperatively, the knee should be immobilized in a long leg cast at 10° of flexion for 3 to 6 weeks.

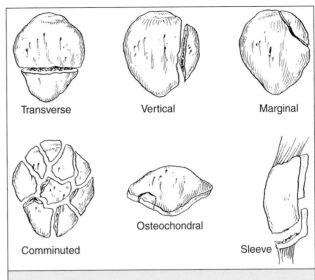

Figure 7   Classification of patella fractures on the basis of the configuration of fracture lines. *(Reproduced from Cramer KE, Moed BR: Patellar fractures: Contemporary approach to treatment. J Am Acad Orthop Surg 1997;5:323-331.)*

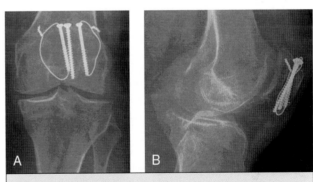

Figure 8   AP **(A)** and lateral **(B)** radiographs showing interfragmentary screw fixation and wiring of a patella fracture.

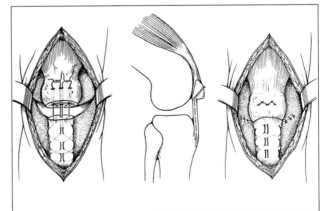

Figure 9   Technique of partial patellectomy. *(Reproduced from Cramer KE, Moed BR: Patellar fractures: Contemporary approach to treatment. J Am Acad Orthop Surg 1997;5:323-331.)*

6: Trauma

H. Complications

1. Postoperative infection related to open injuries may necessitate serial débridement. Relentless infection may require excision of nonviable fragments and repair of the extensor mechanism.

2. Fixation failure has an increased incidence in osteoporotic bone or failure to achieve compression at fracture site.

3. Refracture can occur in up to 5% of patients secondary to decreased inherent strength at the fracture site.

4. Nonunion occurs in up to 2% of patients. Most patients retain good function, although partial patellectomy can be considered for painful nonunion. Revision osteosynthesis should be considered in active, younger individuals.

5. Osteonecrosis (proximal fragment) can occur in association with greater degrees of initial fracture displacement. Treatment consists of observation only, with spontaneous revascularization occurring by 2 years.

6. Posttraumatic osteoarthritis develops in more than 50% of patients in long-term studies. Intractable patellofemoral pain may require Maquet tibial tubercle advancement.

7. Loss of knee motion secondary to prolonged immobilization or postoperative scarring can also occur.

8. Painful retained hardware may necessitate removal for adequate pain relief.

9. Loss of extensor strength and extensor lag is possible, and most patients will experience a loss of knee extension of approximately 5°, although this is rarely clinically significant.

Top Testing Facts

1. The actual incidence of knee dislocations is likely higher than reported because of spontaneous reduction.

2. Typically, at least three of the four main knee ligaments (ACL, PCL, LCL, MCL) are disrupted with knee dislocation.

3. Vascular injury is common with knee dislocation (reported range 20% to 60%).

4. Arteriography should be performed if the ABI is <0.9.

5. Timing and extent of ligament repair/reconstruction is controversial, but there is general agreement that repair of the lateral ligaments (including the PLC) should be performed in the acute period.

6. The patella is the largest sesamoid bone in the body.

7. The patella functions to increase the mechanical advantage of the quadriceps tendon.

8. Active knee extension should be assessed to determine the status of the retinacular extension around the patella.

9. Bipartite patella (present in 8% of the population; most often found in the superolateral region) may be mistaken for a fracture.

10. Nonsurgical treatment of patella fractures assumes an intact extensor mechanism.

Bibliography

Barnes CJ, Pietrobon R, Higgins L: Does the pulse examination in patients with traumatic knee dislocation predict a surgical arterial injury? A meta-analysis. *J Trauma* 2002;53:1109-1114.

Carpenter JE, Kasman R, Mathews LS: Fracture of the patella. *Instr Course Lect* 1994;43:97-108.

Chhabra A, Cha PS, Rihn JA, et al: Surgical management of knee dislocations. *J Bone Joint Surg Am* 2005;87:1-21.

Dedmond BT, Almedinders LC: Operative versus nonoperative treatment of knee dislocations: A meta-analysis. *Am J Knee Surg* 2001;14:33-38.

Harner CD, Waltrip RL, Bennett CH: Surgical management of knee dislocations. *J Bone Joint Surg Am* 2004;86:262-273.

Hegyes MS, Richardson MW, Miller MD: Knee dislocation-complications of nonoperative and operative management. *Clin Sports Med* 2000;19:519-543.

Mariani PP, Santoriello P, Iannone S, et al: Comparison of surgical treatment for knee dislocation. *Am J Knee Surg* 1999;12:214-221.

Niall DM, Nutton RW, Keating JF: Palsy of the common peroneal nerve after traumatic dislocation of the knee. *J Bone Joint Surg Br* 2005;87:664-667.

Owens BD, Neault M, Benson E, et al: Primary repair of knee dislocations: Results in 25 patients (28 knees) at a mean follow-up of four years. *J Orthop Trauma* 2007;21:92-96.

Pritchett JW: Nonoperative treatment of widely displaced patella fractures. *Am J Knee Surg* 1997;10:145-147.

Richter M, Bosch U, Wippermann B, et al: Comparison of surgical repair or reconstruction of the cruciate ligaments versus nonsurgical treatment in patients with traumatic knee dislocations. *Am J Sports Med* 2002;30:718-727.

Rihn JA, Groff YJ, Harner CD, et al: The acutely dislocated knee: Evaluation and management. *J Am Acad Orthop Surg* 2004;12:334-346.

Tzurbakis M, Diamantopoulos A, Xenakis T, et al: Surgical treatment of multiple knee ligament injuries in 44 patients: 2-8 years follow-up results. *Knee Surg Sports Traumatol Arthrosc* 2006;14:739-749.

6: Trauma

Chapter 58

Tibial Plateau and Tibia-Fibula Shaft Fractures

*Kenneth Egol, MD

I. Tibial Plateau Fractures

A. Epidemiology

1. As with most fracture patterns, the epidemiology of tibial plateau fractures is changing. In the past, tibial plateau fractures were more common in young patients following high-energy trauma, whereas now a larger percentage are a result of a low-energy fall in older patients with osteoporotic bone.

2. Tibial plateau fractures account for approximately 2% of all fractures, with bimodal incidence in both men and women and mean patient age of 48 years.

B. Anatomy (**Figure 1**)

1. Tibial plateau

   a. The medial tibial plateau, the larger of the two plateau bones, is concave and covered with hyaline cartilage.

   b. Both plateaus are covered by a fibrocartilaginous meniscus. The coronary ligaments attach the menisci to the plateaus, and the intermensical ligament connect the menisci anteriorly.

2. Tibial spines serve as attachment points for the anterior cruciate ligament (ACL), the posterior cruciate ligament (PCL), and the menisci.

3. Tibial shaft

   a. The tibial shaft is triangular in cross section.

   b. Proximally, the tibial tubercle is located anterolaterally about 3 cm and is the point of attachment for the patellar tendon.

   c. Laterally on the proximal tibia is the Gerdy tubercle, which is the point of insertion for the iliotibial band.

4. Soft-tissue structures

   a. The medial (tibial) collateral ligament inserts into the medial proximal tibia.

   b. The ACL and PCL provide anterior-posterior stability.

5. Neurovascular structures

   a. The common peroneal nerve courses around the neck of the fibula distal to the proximal tibia-fibula joint before it divides into its superficial and deep branches.

   b. The trifurcation of the popliteal artery into the anterior tibial, posterior tibial, and peroneal arteries occurs posteromedially in the proximal tibia.

   c. Vascular injuries to these structures are common following knee dislocation but also can occur in high-energy fractures of the proximal tibia.

6. Musculature

   a. The anterior compartment musculature attaches to the proximal lateral tibia.

   b. The proximal medial tibial surface is devoid of muscle coverage but serves as an attachment point for the pes tendons.

C. Mechanisms of injury

1. Tibial plateau fractures result from direct axial compression—usually with a valgus (more common) or varus (less common) moment—and indirect shear forces. Examples:

   a. High-speed motor vehicle accidents

   b. Falls from a height

   c. Collisions between the bumper of a car and a pedestrian (hence the term bumper injury)

2. The direction, magnitude, and location of the force, as well as the position of the knee at impact, determines the fracture pattern, location, and degree of displacement.

*Kenneth Egol, MD, or the department with which he is affiliated has received research or institutional support from Biomet, Smith & Nephew, Stryker, and Synthes and holds stock or stock options in Johnson & Johnson.

6: Trauma

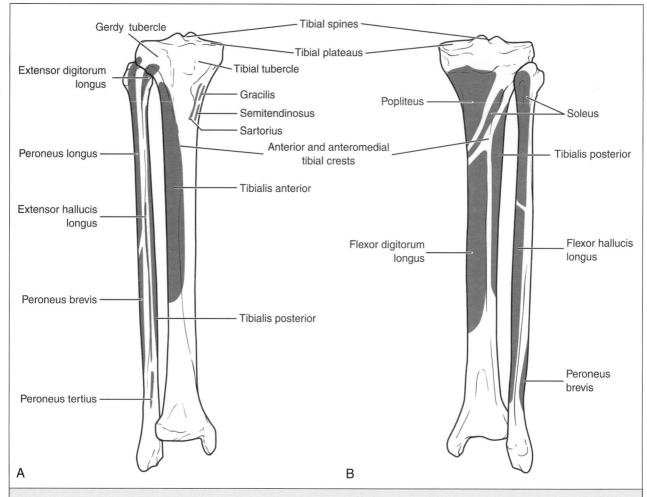

Figure 1 Anatomy of the tibia and fibula. Shaded areas indicate origins and insertions of the indicated muscles. **A,** Anterior view. **B,** Posterior view.

3. Associated injuries

   a. Meniscal tears are associated with up to 50% of tibial plateau fractures.

   b. Associated injury to the cruciate or collateral ligaments occurs in up to 30% of patients.

   c. Skin compromise may be present in high-energy fracture patterns.

D. Clinical evaluation

1. Physical examination

   a. One should palpate over the site of potential fracture or ligamentous disruption to elicit tenderness.

   b. Hemarthrosis typically is present; however, capsular disruption may lead to extravasation into the surrounding soft-tissue envelope.

   c. Any widening of the femoral-tibial articulation of more than 10° on stress examination compared with the other leg indicates instability.

2. Neurovascular examination

   a. If pulses are not palpable, Doppler studies should be performed.

   b. One should assess for signs and symptoms of an impending compartment syndrome (pain out of proportion to the injury, pallor, pulselessness, pain on passive stretch of the toes, or impaired neurologic status).

   c. Compartment pressures also should be measured if the patient is unconscious and has a tense, swollen leg.

   d. Ankle-brachial index (ABI) <0.9 requires consultation with a vascular surgeon.

3. Radiographic evaluation

   a. Plain radiographs—Should include a trauma series (AP, lateral, and oblique views) and a plateau view (10° caudal tilt).

   b. CT—Allows for improved assessment of fracture pattern, aids in surgical planning, and im-

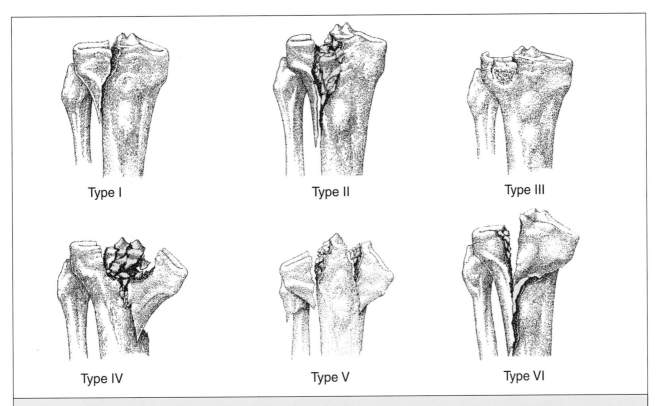

Figure 2   Schatzker classification of tibial plateau fractures. Type I: lateral plateau split; type II: lateral split-depression; type III: lateral depression; type IV: medial plateau fracture; type V: bicondylar injury; type VI: tibial plateau fracture with metaphyseal-diaphyseal dissociation. *(Reproduced from Watson JT, Knee and Leg: Bone Trauma, in Beaty JH [ed]: Orthopaedic Knowledge Update 6. Rosemont, IL, American Academy of Orthopaedic Surgeons, 1999, p 523.)*

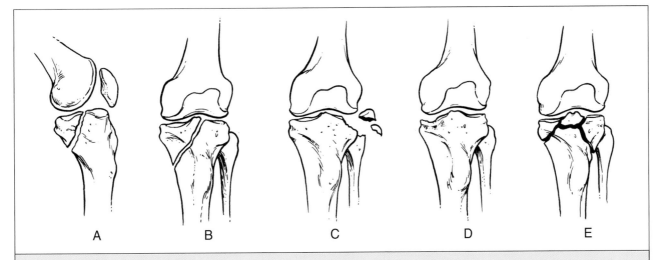

Figure 3   The Moore classification of tibial plateau fractures. **A,** Split fracture of the medial plateau in the coronal plane. **B,** An entire condyle fracture. **C,** Rim avulsion fracture. **D,** Pure compression fracture. **E,** Four-part fracture.

proves ability to classify fractures. CT should be ordered when better visualization of the bone fragments is required.

   c. MRI—Evaluates both bony and soft-tissue components of the injury in a noninvasive manner. Indications for ordering MRI for these injuries have not been well established.

E. Fracture classification

   1. The Schatzker classification is most commonly used (**Figure 2**).

   2. The Moore classification accounts for patterns not described in the Schatzker classification (**Figure 3**).

6: Trauma

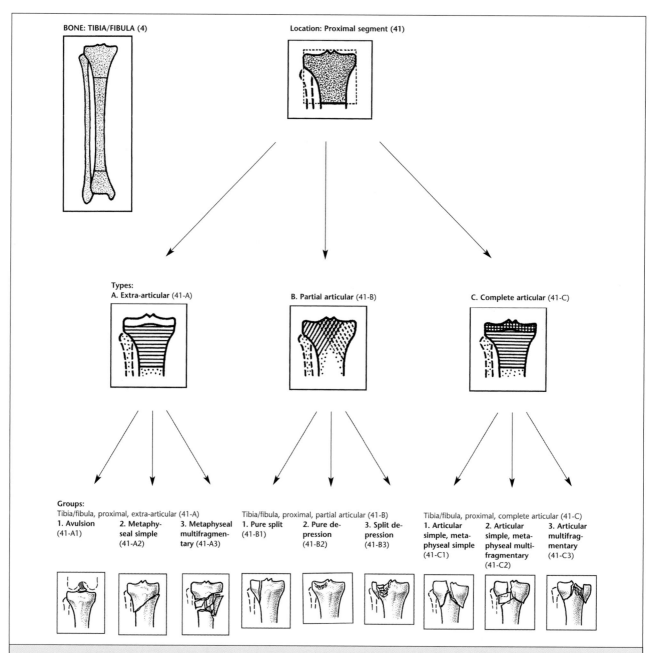

Figure 4 The OTA classification of proximal tibia/fibula fractures. Type A fractures are extra-articular, type B fractures are partial articular, and type C fractures are complete articular. A1: avulsion; A2: metaphyseal simple; A3: metaphyseal multifragmentary; B1: pure split; B2: pure depression; B3: split depression; C1: articular simple, metaphyseal simple; C2: articular simple, metaphyseal mulitfragmentary; and C3: articular multifragmentary.

3. The OTA classification is the internationally accepted classification system (**Figure 4**).

F. Nonsurgical treatment

1. Indicated for nondisplaced and stable fractures.

2. Patients are placed in a hinged fracture brace, and early range-of-motion exercises are initiated.

3. Partial weight bearing (30 to 50 lb) for 8 to 12 weeks is allowed, with progression to full weight bearing as tolerated thereafter.

4. If this approach fails to maintain the reduction, surgical treatment is indicated.

G. Surgical management

1. Indications

a. For closed fractures, the range of articular depression considered to be acceptable varies from ≤2 mm to 1 cm. Instability >10° of the nearly extended knee compared to the contralateral side is an accepted indication for surgical treatment of closed tibial plateau fractures.

b. For open fractures, irrigation and débridement are required, with either temporary fixation or immediate open reduction and internal fixation. Regardless of approach, the knee joint should not be left open.

c. If there will be a delay in surgical intervention, consider use of temporary spanning external fixation if the limb is shortened or subluxated.

2. Reduction techniques

a. Indirect techniques have the advantage of minimal soft-tissue stripping and fragment devitalization. Ligamentotaxis, however, will not work on fractures with centrally depressed articular fragments.

b. With direct techniques, depressed articular fragments may be elevated through a cortical window.

3. Fixation techniques

a. Arthroscopy can be used as a diagnostic tool to assess intra-articular structures in patients who sustain low-energy fractures; it also can be used as an adjunct to treatment in assessing the quality of fracture reduction.

b. Most fracture patterns are treated with a lateral approach and buttress plating.

c. A posteromedial approach is used to buttress posteromedial fragments.

d. Screws alone can be used for simple split fractures that are anatomically reduced, for depression fractures that are elevated percutaneously, and for fractures with fragments that are avulsed by soft-tissue attachments.

e. Plates may be placed percutaneously for fractures that extend to the metadiaphyseal region.

4. External fixation techniques

a. A hybrid technique can be used, consisting of placement of a pin or wire 10 to 14 mm below the articular surface to avoid penetration of the synovial recess posteriorly.

b. A circular frame is an alternative to a long percutaneous plate.

5. Identify and repair all meniscal damage intraoperatively.

6. Bicondylar tibial plateau fractures

a. Bicondylar fractures require dual plate fixation or unilateral fixation with a locking plate.

b. Anterior midline incision should be avoided for bicondylar fractures because of the high rate of wound slough.

H. Postoperative management

1. Continuous passive motion from 0° to 30° may be used. It is started a few days after surgery and

may be continued until the patient regains full range of knee motion.

2. Physical therapy should consist of active and active-assisted range-of-motion exercises, isometric quadriceps strengthening, and protected weight bearing.

3. Progressive weight bearing depends on the rate of fracture healing.

I. Complications

1. Early complications

a. Infection rates vary widely, from 1% to 38% of patients; superficial infections are more common (up to 38% of patients), whereas deep wound infections are less common (up to 9.5%). Pin tract infections are common when external fixation is used.

b. Thromboembolism is less common, with deep venous thrombosis developing in up to 10% of patients and pulmonary embolism in 1% to 2%.

2. Late complications

a. Painful hardware can occur.

b. Posttraumatic arthrosis may be related to chondral damage that occurs at the time of the injury.

c. Nonunion is rare.

d. Loss of reduction, collapse, and/or malunion can occur with failure to adequately buttress elevated fragments.

II. Tibia-Fibula Shaft Fractures

A. Epidemiology

1. Most tibial shaft fractures result from low-energy mechanisms of injury and account for 4% of fractures seen in the Medicare population. When these fractures occur in younger patients, a high-energy injury such as motor vehicle accident usually is the cause.

2. Isolated fibular shaft fractures are rare and usually the result of direct blow; they also can be associated with rotational ankle injuries (Maisonneuve fractures).

B. Anatomy

1. Bony structures

a. The anteromedial crest of the tibia is subcutaneous.

b. The proximal medullary canal is centered laterally.

c. The anterior tibial crest is made of dense cortical bone.

d. The fibular shaft is palpable proximal and distally. The fibula serves as the site of the muscular attachment for the peroneal musculature and the flexor hallucis longus, but it contributes little to load bearing (15%).

2. Musculature

a. The anterior compartment contains the tibialis anterior, extensor digitorum longus, extensor hallucis longus, the anterior tibial artery, and the deep peroneal nerve.

b. The lateral compartment contains the peroneus longus and brevis and the superficial peroneal nerve.

c. The superficial posterior compartment contains the gastrocnemius-soleus complex, the soleus, the popliteus, and the plantaris muscles, as well as the sural nerve and saphenous vein.

d. The deep posterior compartment contains the tibialis posterior, flexor digitorum longus, flexor hallucis longus, tibial nerve, peroneal nerve, and posterior tibial nerve.

3. Vascular structures

a. The nutrient artery supplies the inner two thirds of the cortex, and the periosteal vessels supply the outer third.

b. Popliteal artery branches located in the proximal tibia are the anterior and posterior tibial arteries and the peroneal artery.

C. Mechanism of injury

1. Tibia-fibula shaft fractures result from either torsional (indirect) or bending (direct) mechanisms.

2. Indirect mechanisms result in spiral fractures.

3. Direct mechanisms result in wedge or short oblique fractures (low energy) or increased comminution (higher energy).

4. Associated injuries include open wounds, compartment syndrome, ipsilateral skeletal injury (ie, extension to the plateau or plafond), and remote skeletal injury.

D. Clinical evaluation

1. Physical examination

a. One should inspect the limb for gross deformity, angulation, and malrotation.

b. Palpation for tenderness and swelling is important as well. The fact that the anterior tibial crest is subcutaneous makes identification of the fracture site easier.

2. Neurovascular examination

a. One should assess for signs and symptoms of impending compartment syndrome (tense compartment, pain out of proportion to the injury, pallor, paresthesia, pain on passive stretch, or pulselessness).

b. Intracompartmental monitoring is critical with a high index of suspicion for compartment syndrome.

c. Compartment syndrome release is indicated if the patient has one or more of the above signs and symptoms and an absolute pressure >40 mm Hg or <30 mm Hg difference between compartmental pressure and diastolic pressure.

d. Once the diagnosis is made, all four compartments must be released.

3. Radiographic evaluation

a. Plain radiographs should include a trauma series (AP, lateral, and oblique), with dedicated ankle or plateau views if the fracture extends to the surface of the joint. The entire tibia and fibula must be visualized, from knee to ankle.

b. With any fracture manipulation, postreduction views must also be obtained.

c. CT can be used to assess fracture healing or identify nonunion, but it plays no role in acute fracture management.

E. Fracture classification

1. Fractures are usually described based on the pattern, location, and amount of comminution.

2. The OTA classification includes types 42A (simple patterns—ie, spiral, transverse, oblique), 42B (wedge), and 42C (complex, comminuted) (**Figure 5**).

3. Soft tissue classification

a. Oestern and Tscherne for closed fractures (**Table 1**)

b. Gustilo for open fractures (**Table 2**)

F. Nonsurgical treatment

1. Indications

a. Low-energy stable tibia fractures (ie, axially stable fracture patterns)

b. Virtually all isolated fibular shaft fractures

2. Long leg casting is indicated, followed by functional bracing in a patellar tendon bearing brace or cast, with weight bearing as tolerated after 2 to 3 weeks. Cast wedging may be used, if needed.

3. At follow-up, shortening after closed treatment averages 4 mm, with nonunion in 1.1% of patients and <6° angulation.

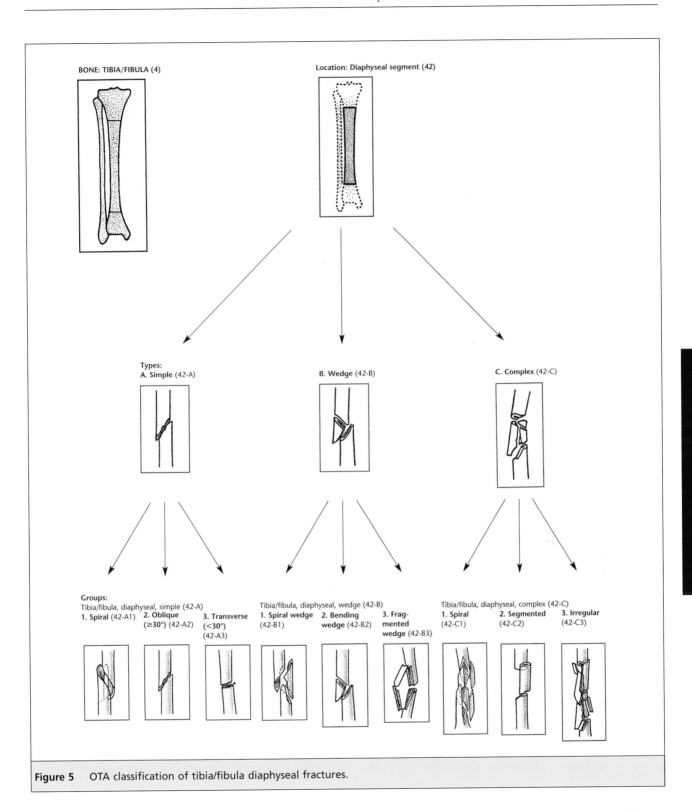

Figure 5 OTA classification of tibia/fibula diaphyseal fractures.

G. Surgical treatment

1. Indications

    a. Failure to maintain acceptable reduction parameters (<50% displacement, <10° angulation, <1 cm shortening, 10° rotational malalignment)

    b. Open fractures, fractures with associated compartment syndrome, inherently unstable patterns (segmental, comminuted, short), and patients with multiple injuries (eg, floating knee)

2. Intramedullary (IM) nailing

    a. Reamed IM nailing is the treatment of choice for unstable fracture patterns because it allows

Table 1

Oestern and Tscherne Classification of Closed-Fracture Soft-Tissue Injury

Grade	Description
0	Injuries from indirect forces with negligible soft-tissue damage
I	Superficial contusion/abrasion, simple fractures
II	Deep abrasions, muscle/skin contusion, direct trauma, impending compartment syndrome
III	Excessive skin contusion, crushed skin or destruction of muscle, subcutaneous degloving, acute compartment syndrome, and rupture of major blood vessel or nerve

(Reproduced with permission from Oestern HJ, Tscherne H: Pathophysiology and classification of soft tissue injuries associated with fractures, in Tscherne H, Gotzen L [eds]: Fractures With Soft Tissue Injuries. Berlin, Germany, Springer-Verlag, 1984, pp 1-9.)

Table 2

Gustilo Classification of Open Fractures

Type	Description
I	Clean wound less than 1 cm in length
II	Wound longer than 1 cm without extensive soft-tissue damage
III	Wound associated with extensive soft-tissue damage; usually longer than 5 cm Open segmental fracture Traumatic amputation Gunshot injuries Farmyard injuries Fractures associated with vascular repair Fractures more than 8 hours old
IIIA	Adequate periosteal cover
IIIB	Presence of significant periosteal stripping
IIIC	Vascular repair required to revascularize leg

(Adapted with permission from Bucholz RW, Heckman JD, Court-Brown C [eds]: Rockwood and Green's Fractures in Adults. Lippincott Williams & Wilkins, 2005, p 2084.)

for use of a larger diameter nail (with larger locking bolts) and results in increased periosteal perfusion. In addition, with a reamed IM nail, there is no significant concern for embolization of marrow contents.

b. A nonreamed IM nail is looser fitting and associated with less cortical necrosis. It is also associated with a higher rate of locking screw breakage than reamed IM nailing.

c. Use of blocking screws, a unicortical plate, a lateral starting point, and IM nailing in a semi-extended position may help prevent proximal fractures from extending into valgus.

d. Use of blocking screws and or fibular plating may help prevent distal fractures from going into valgus (if at the same level as a fibula fracture), or into varus (if the fibula is intact).

e. Open plating techniques typically have been associated with wound problems and nonunion.

f. Contraindications for IM nailing include a preexisting tibial shaft deformity that may preclude IM nail passage and a history of previous IM infection.

3. Plates and screws

a. Newer plate designs and minimally invasive techniques have allowed these implants to play a role in metadiaphyseal fractures or in tibial shaft fractures in which IM nailing is not possible (ie, following total knee arthroplasty, tibial plateau fixation).

b. Lateral placement may be preferred to anteromedial placement when there are soft-tissue concerns.

4. External fixation

a. This has gained popularity in open tibia fractures with soft-tissue compromise because of dissatisfaction of outcomes treated by traditional techniques.

b. Advantages are that it is low risk, provides access to wounds, provides a mechanically stable construct, and allows for radiographic evaluation.

c. Several types of frame constructs are available, including half-pin monolateral frames, which are considered safe and violate tissues on one side only; thin wire circular frames that allow for fixation in metaphyseal bone; and hybrid frames.

d. Construct stiffness is increased with increased pin diameter, number of pins on either side of the fracture, rods closer to the bone, and multiple plane construct.

5. Treatment of open fractures

a. Require emergent débridement and fracture stabilization.

b. Current evidence supports immediate closure of wounds, if possible.

c. Vacuum-assisted closure versus early flap (rotational versus free)

d. First-generation cephalosporin, with or without aminoglycoside, should be given in the emergency department.

e. Tetanus immunoglobin should be given if immune status is known and up to date; toxoid should be added if status is unknown or if patient has not had immunization for more than 10 years.

H. Rehabilitation

1. Following nonsurgical treatment of axially stable fractures, patients should be able to bear weight as tolerated after 1 to 2 weeks.

2. Following surgical treatment, weight-bearing status depends on the fracture pattern and implant type. With axially stable fracture patterns with bony contact, weight bearing as tolerated is allowed. With comminuted fractures, partial weight bearing is allowed until radiographic signs of healing.

3. Repeat radiographs should be obtained at 6 and 12 weeks.

4. External fixators should be dynamized before removal to ensure healing and prevent repeat fracture.

5. External bone stimulation has been shown to help in fracture healing.

I. Complications

1. Nonunion/delayed union

a. Nonunion—A fracture that has lost its capacity to unite.

b. Delayed union—A fracture that takes longer than expected to unite.

c. Treatment can consist of dynamization, exchange nailing, or bone graft.

2. Compartment syndrome—Failure to identify impending compartment syndrome is the most serious complication after tibia-fibula shaft fractures.

3. Knee pain occurs in up to 30% of patients following tibial nailing.

4. Infection—either superficial or deep. Deep infection usually is associated with open fractures (fracture hematoma communication) and may lead to osteomyelitis.

5. Painful hardware can occur because locking bolts and plates are usually placed on the subcutaneous border of the tibia.

6. Nerve injury, usually affecting the peroneal (most common) or the saphenous nerve, may occur. Peroneal nerve injury may occur secondary to pressure from the fracture table, whereas the saphenous nerve can be injured as a result of placement of the locking bolts.

7. Malalignment often is associated with late loss of reduction (ie, cast, external fixator) in proximal and distal metaphyseal fractures.

a. Immediate postoperative malalignment is preventable with careful surgical technique and awareness of this potential complication, particularly with nailing of proximal or distal tibia fractures.

b. Methods to prevent malalignment during tibial nailing include blocking screws, provisional plating, distractions, and fibular plating.

c. A more lateral proximal entry site should be considered to avoid valgus with a proximal one-third fracture.

Top Testing Facts

1. Skin compromise may be present in high-energy fracture patterns.

2. If there will be a delay in surgical intervention after tibial plateau fracture, consider use of temporary spanning external fixation if the limb is shortened or subluxated.

3. Identify and repair all meniscal damage intraoperatively.

4. Bicondylar tibial plateau fractures require dual plate fixation or unilateral fixation with a locking plate.

5. Anterior midline incision should be avoided for bicondylar tibial plateau fractures because of the high rate of wound slough.

6. Failure to identify impending compartment syndrome is the most serious complication after tibia-fibula shaft fractures.

7. Immediate postoperative malalignment is preventable with careful surgical technique and awareness of this potential complication, particularly with nailing of proximal or distal tibia fractures.

8. Methods to prevent malalignment during tibial nailing include blocking screws, provisional plating, distractors, and fibular plating.

9. A more lateral proximal entry site should be considered to avoid valgus with a proximal one-third fracture.

6: Trauma

Bibliography

Baron JA, Karagas M, Barrett J, et al: Basic epidemiology of fractures of the upper and lower limb among Americans over 65 years of age. *Epidemiology* 1996;7:612-618.

Bhattacharyya T, Seng K, Nassif NA, Freedman I: Knee pain after tibial nailing: The role of nail prominence. *Clin Orthop Relat Res* 2006;449:303-307.

Court-Brown CM, Gustilo T, Shaw AD: Knee pain after intramedullary tibial nailing: Its incidence, etiology, and outcome. *J Orthop Trauma* 1997;11:103-105.

Delamarter RB, Hohl M, Hopp E Jr: Ligament injuries associated with tibial plateau fractures. *Clin Orthop Relat Res* 1990;250:226-233.

Dunbar RP, Nork SE, Barei DP, Mills WJ: Provisional plating of Type III open tibia fractures prior to intramedullary nailing. *J Orthop Trauma* 2005;19:412-414.

Egol KA, Weisz R, Hiebert R, Tejwani NC, Koval KJ, Sanders RW: Does fibular plating improve alignment after intramedullary nailing of distal metaphyseal tibia fractures? *J Orthop Trauma* 2006;20:94-103.

Gardner MJ, Yacoubian S, Gellar D, et al: The incidence of soft tissue injury in operative tibial plateau fractures: A magnetic resonance imaging analysis of 103 patients. *J Orthop Trauma* 2005;19:79-84.

Gill TJ, Moezzi DM, Oates KM, Sterett WI: Arthroscopic reduction and internal fixation of tibial plateau fractures in skiing. *Clin Orthop Relat Res* 2001;383:243-249.

Gopal S, Majumder S, Batchelor HG, Knight SL, De Boer P, Smith RM: Fix and flap: The radical orthopaedic and plastic treatment of severe open fractures of the tibia. *J Bone Joint Surg Br* 2000;82:959-966.

Krettek C, Stephan C, Schandelmaier P, Richter M, Pape HC, Miclau T: The use of Poller screws as blocking screws in stabilising tibial fractures treated with small diameter intramedullary nails. *J Bone Joint Surg Br* 1999;81:963-968.

Lansinger O, Bergman B, Korner L, Andersson GB: Tibial condylar fractures: A twenty-year follow-up. *J Bone Joint Surg Am* 1986;68:13-19.

Marsh JL, Smith ST, Do TT: External fixation and limited internal fixation for complex fractures of the tibial plateau. *J Bone Joint Surg Am* 1995;77:661-673.

McQueen MM, Court-Brown CM: Compartment monitoring in tibial fractures: The pressure threshold for decompression. *J Bone Joint Surg Br* 1996;78:99-104.

Muller M: The comprehensive classification of long bones, in Muller ME, Schneider R, Willenegger H (eds): *Manual of Internal Fixation*. Berlin, Germany, Springer-Verlag, 1995, pp 118-158.

Reid JS, Van Slyke MA, Moulton MJ, Mann TA: Safe placement of proximal tibial transfixation wires with respect to intracapsular penetration. *J Orthop Trauma* 2001;15:10-17.

Chapter 59
Foot Trauma

Nelson Fong SooHoo, MD

I. Epidemiology

A. Fractures of the foot are uncommon but often devastating injuries.

B. Calcaneal fractures are the most common tarsal bone fractures; many involve the subtalar joint.

C. Fractures of the talus and fracture-dislocations of the midfoot are uncommon but also have the potential to result in severe functional limitation.

II. Anatomy

A. Bones

1. The foot has 26 bones and numerous joints.

2. The hindfoot includes the talus and calcaneus.

3. The midfoot includes the navicular, cuboid, and cuneiforms and their articulations with the proximal metatarsals.

4. The forefoot includes the phalanges and the distal metatarsals.

B. Joints

1. The key joints to maintain mobility in the foot are the hindfoot joints, including the tibiotalar, subtalar, and talonavicular articulations.

2. The lateral fourth and fifth tarsometatarsal joints are also important for normal foot function.

3. The remaining hindfoot and midfoot joints, including the calcaneocuboid and the first, second, and third tarsometatarsal joints, do not require full range of motion to maintain function.

4. The most important forefoot joints are the metatarsophalangeal (MTP) joints. Interphalangeal joint motion is not critical for normal functioning.

III. Fractures of the Talus

A. Anatomy and blood supply of the talus

1. The talus is divided into a head, neck, and body.

The talus has five articulating surfaces, with 70% covered by cartilage. The only muscle attachment is the extensor digitorum brevis.

2. The talus relies on direct extraosseous blood supply because of the lack of soft-tissue attachments.

3. The limited blood supply to the talus places the talar body at risk for osteonecrosis following talar neck fractures.

a. Most of the blood supply to the body is from the artery of the tarsal canal, a branch of the posterior tibial artery.

b. Most of the blood supply to head and neck is from the artery of the tarsal sinus, a branch of both the anterior tibial artery and peroneal artery.

c. The deltoid artery in the deep portion of the deltoid ligament also supplies blood to the body.

B. Talar neck fractures

1. Mechanisms of injury

a. These fractures occur with dorsiflexion against the tibia, usually the result of a motor vehicle accident or fall.

b. Associated inversion can lead to medial malleolar fracture, whereas eversion may be associated with lateral malleolar fractures.

2. Radiographic evaluation

a. Imaging studies should include three plain radiographic views of the foot.

b. CT is indicated if displacement cannot be ruled out on plain radiographs.

c. MRI can be used postoperatively to detect osteonecrosis.

3. Hawkins fracture classification (**Figure 1**)

a. Guides treatment decisions and is useful in predicting the risk of osteonecrosis

b. Types are based on displacement of the fracture and articulations of the talus.

c. Displaced type II, III, and IV fractures can injure the arteries of the tarsal canal and tarsal

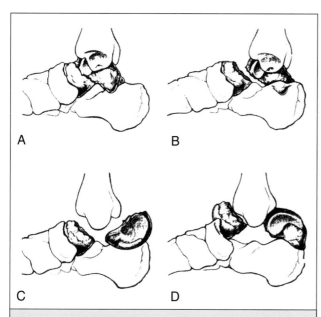

Figure 1 Hawkins classification. **A,** Type I: nondisplaced talar neck fractures. **B,** Type II: displaced talar neck fractures, with subluxation or dislocation of subtalar joint. **C,** Type III: displaced talar neck fractures with associated dislocation of talar body from both subtalar and tibiotalar joints. **D,** Canale and Kelly type IV: displaced talar neck fracture with associated dislocation of talar body from subtalar and tibiotalar joints and dislocation of head/neck fragment from talonavicular joint. *(Reproduced with permission from Sangeorzan BJ: Foot and ankle joint, in Hansen ST Jr, Swiontkowski MF [eds]: Orthopaedic Trauma Protocols. New York, NY, Raven Press, 1993, p 350.)*

Table 1

Complications of Talar Neck Fractures

Fracture Pattern	Osteonecrosis (%)	Posttraumatic Arthritis (%)	Malunion (%)
Type I	0–13	0–30	0–10
Type II	20–50	40–90	0–25
Type III / IV	80–100	70–100	18–27

(Reproduced from Fortin PT, Balazsy JE: Talus fractures: Evaluation and treatment. *J Am Acad Orthop Surg* 2001;9:114-127.)

sinus, placing the talar body at risk of osteonecrosis.

4. Nonsurgical treatment

  a. Closed reduction can be attempted by using plantar flexion with varus or valgus of the heel, depending on the direction of displacement.

  b. Type I fractures can be treated with casting and non–weight bearing. Alternatively, fixation with 6.5-mm posterior-to-anterior lag screws may be used.

5. Surgical treatment

  a. Urgent surgical treatment is required when subluxation or dislocation leads to soft-tissue compromise.

  b. Open reduction and internal fixation (types II, III, IV)

    i. An anteromedial approach is combined with an anterolateral approach (with medial malleolar osteotomy when necessary) for adequate exposure. The anteromedial approach is between the posterior and anterior tibial

tendons. A crossed-screw construct is commonly used with this approach.

    ii. The posterior approach does not allow for open reduction of displaced fractures and is reserved for type I injuries.

    iii. Care is needed to avoid injury to the sural nerve with a posterolateral approach through the interval of the peroneus brevis and flexor hallucis longus (FHL).

  c. The talonavicular joint incongruity seen in type IV injuries should be reduced and pinned.

  d. Medial plating may be useful for comminuted fractures that would collapse with compression screws.

  e. Titanium screws are sometimes advocated to allow MRI evaluation of postoperative osteonecrosis.

6. Complications (**Table 1**)

  a. Osteonecrosis

    i. The limited blood supply at the talar neck places patients at risk for osteonecrosis.

    ii. The risk of osteonecrosis increases by Hawkins fracture type. Restricted weight bearing beyond that needed for fracture healing has not been shown to decrease the risk of osteonecrosis.

    iii. The Hawkins sign, subchondral osteopenia seen at 6 to 8 weeks on plain radiographs, is considered a good prognostic sign because it indicates revascularization of the body. This may occur only medially if the deltoid artery is the only intact blood supply.

    iv. Osteonecrosis may be seen as early as 3 to 6 months postoperatively with sclerosis on plain radiographs. MRI is sensitive for osteonecrosis, with decreased signal on T1-weighted images.

    v. Osteonecrosis usually does not involve the

entire talar body and often does not require further surgery. Tibiotalar fusion is an option when nonsurgical treatment is not successful.

  vi. Extensive osteonecrosis may require excision of the body with tibiotalocalcaneal fusion or Blair fusion. Blair fusion involves resection of the talar body with fusion of the talar head to the tibia and bone grafting of the defect to maintain overall limb length.

 b. Degenerative arthritis is the most common complication and can affect the subtalar and/or tibiotalar joints.

 c. Varus malunion also can occur and limit eversion. This may be treated with osteotomy.

C. Talar body fractures

 1. Fractures involving large portions of the talar body are usually the result of high-energy injuries.

 2. CT provides the best visualization and is used to identify fractures in the transverse, coronal, and sagittal planes.

 3. Open reduction and internal fixation using a dual lateral and medial approach is required when the articular surfaces are displaced more than 2 mm. Medial and/or lateral malleolar osteotomy may be required for adequate visualization.

 4. Complications include osteonecrosis.

D. Osteochondral fractures of the talus

 1. Osteochondral fractures can be seen in association with ankle injuries, including sprains or chronic ankle instability.

 2. Medial osteochondral fractures often are deep and located posterior in the talus.

 3. Lateral osteochondral fractures are more commonly associated with traumatic injuries.

 a. Lateral fractures generally are more shallow and located either in the central or anterior portion of the talus.

 b. Lateral fractures also are more often displaced and symptomatic. Symptoms include pain, swelling, and clicking.

 4. CT or MRI may be useful in imaging these fractures.

 a. MRI is useful as a screening test.

 b. CT is more useful in delineating the extent of lesions already identified by plain radiographs or MRI.

 5. Treatment is guided by symptoms, fragment size, and chronicity of the lesion.

 a. Nonsurgical treatment with non–weight-bearing casting is indicated for nondisplaced fractures.

 b. Open reduction and internal fixation may be indicated for displaced fractures with large fragments (>5 mm).

 c. Arthroscopic débridement and drilling or microfracture is required for acute fractures with large fragments that are not amenable to fixation and for fractures with small fragments. This approach also is indicated for chronic fractures.

 d. Postoperatively, the patient generally is non–weight bearing for up to 6 weeks.

 e. If drilling and microfracture techniques fail, mosaicplasty or autologous chondrocyte transplantation may be options, but the efficacy of these procedures is not well established.

E. Lateral process fractures

 1. These fractures occur with dorsiflexion–external rotation injuries. A common mechanism is a snowboarding injury.

 2. Plain radiographs typically do not show these fractures, but they may be seen on the AP view of the ankle.

 3. CT may be required to adequately visualize these injuries in patients with anterolateral ankle pain and normal plain radiographs following a snowboarding injury.

 4. Nondisplaced fractures can be treated with cast immobilization and non–weight bearing.

 5. Open reduction and internal fixation is indicated for fractures displaced more than 2 mm. Comminuted fractures not amenable to open reduction and internal fixation can be treated with casting. Excision is an option if symptoms persist.

F. Posterior process fractures

 1. The posterior process includes a posteromedial and a posterolateral tubercle. Because plain radiographs may not clearly visualize the area, CT is useful to identify these fractures.

 2. Posteromedial tubercle fractures occur as a result of avulsion of the posterior talotibial ligament or posterior deltoid ligament.

 a. Small fragments are treated with immobilization followed by late excision if symptoms persist.

 b. Large displaced fragments are treated with open reduction and internal fixation.

 3. Posterolateral tubercle fractures occur as a result of avulsion of the posterior talofibular ligament. Pain is aggravated by FHL flexion and extension.

6: Trauma

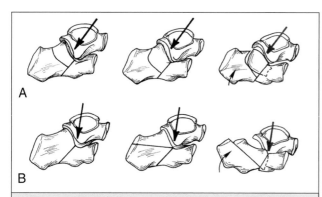

Figure 2 Essex-Lopresti classification of calcaneal fractures and their mechanism of injury. **A,** Joint depression fracture. **B,** Tongue-type fracture. *(Adapted from Burdeaux, BD Jr: Reduction of calcaneal fractures by the McReynolds medial approach technique and its experimental basis.* Clin Orthop Relat Res *1983;177:87-103.)*

    a. Initial nonsurgical management with late excision for symptomatic lesions is indicated with no subtalar involvement.

    b. Open reduction and internal fixation is indicated for fractures with subtalar involvement.

  4. Nonunion is difficult to distinguish from symptomatic os trigonum. Both conditions can be treated with excision.

G. Talar head fractures

  1. Talar head injuries are less common than other areas of the talus.

  2. Nonsurgical treatment consisting of immobilization and non–weight bearing is indicated for nondisplaced fractures.

  3. For displaced fractures, the talonavicular joint should be reduced and the fracture fragments stabilized using screws or pins, depending on fragment size. Small fragments can be excised.

  4. Late talonavicular arthritis can be treated with fusion.

IV. Fractures of the Calcaneus

A. Intra-articular fractures

  1. Mechanisms of injury

    a. The calcaneus is the most frequently fractured of the tarsal bones. Most calcaneus fractures (75%) are intra-articular.

    b. Axial loading is the primary mechanism, with falls from a height and motor vehicle accidents the most common causes.

    c. Oblique shear results in a primary fracture line and two primary fragments: a superomedial fragment and a superolateral fragment.

      i. The superomedial fragment includes the sustentaculum, which is stabilized by strong ligamentous and capsular attachments. This is called the constant fragment because it remains in a stable position, which makes it a useful reference point for anatomic reduction.

      ii. The superolateral fragment has an intra-articular component through the posterior facet.

    d. Secondary fracture lines signal whether there is joint depression or a tongue-type fracture, depending on whether the superolateral fragment and posterior facet are separate from the tuberosity. Fractures in which the superolateral fragment and posterior facet remain attached to the tuberosity posteriorly are tongue-type fractures (**Figure 2**).

  2. Radiographic evaluation

    a. The lateral view can be used to determine the Böhler angle (normal 20° to 40°) to assess loss of height. Double density of the posterior facet indicates subtalar incongruity.

    b. AP and oblique views can visualize the calcaneocuboid joint.

    c. The Broden view is useful intraoperatively to evaluate reduction of the posterior facet.

    d. The axial Harris view visualizes widening, shortening, and varus position of the tuberosity fragment.

    e. An AP view of the ankle also may be useful to assess lateral wall extrusion with impingement against the fibula.

  3. Sanders fracture classification (**Figure 3**)

    a. Used to guide treatment and to predict outcomes of treatment

    b. Based on CT to visualize the subtalar joint at its widest point in the coronal plane. CT also is the most complete and reliable method of visualizing these injuries.

    c. Types are based on the number of articular fragments.

      i. Type I fractures: nondisplaced

      ii. Type II fractures: the posterior facet is in two fragments.

      iii. Type III fractures: the posterior facet is in three fragments.

      iv. Type IV fractures: comminuted, with more than three articular fragments

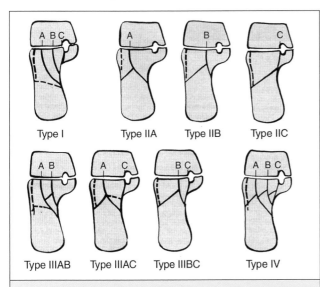

Figure 3 Schematic diagram of Sanders classification. *(Reproduced with permission from Sanders R, Fortin P, Pasquale T, et al: Operative treatment in 120 displaced intra-articular calcaneal fractures: Results using a prognostic computed tomography scan classification.* Clin Orthop Relat Res *1993;290:87-95.)*

d. Other important fracture characteristics include the degree of shortening, widening, and lateral wall impingement, which may result in peroneal tendon pathology.

4. Nonsurgical treatment

   a. Type I fractures are treated nonsurgically.

   b. Patients do not bear weight for 10 to 12 weeks.

   c. Range-of-motion exercises are initiated early, as soon as soft-tissue swelling allows.

5. Surgical treatment

   a. Treatment of type II and III fractures remains controversial. Both open reduction and internal fixation and nonsurgical management have been advocated, with nonsurgical management the same as for type I fractures. Negative prognostic factors for the treatment of these fractures include severity, advanced age, male sex, obesity, bilateral fractures, multiple trauma, and worker's compensation.

   b. Open reduction and internal fixation generally is delayed for 10 to 14 days to allow for resolution of soft-tissue swelling.

      i. An extensile lateral L-shaped incision is the most common approach.

      ii. No-touch retraction techniques are used, a pin is placed in the tuberosity fragment to assist reduction, and a drain is inserted.

iii. Bone grafting has not been shown to have a benefit.

   c. Type IV fractures can be treated using open reduction and internal fixation with possible primary fusion because open reduction and internal fixation alone (as well as nonsurgical treatment) is associated with poor results.

   d. A less invasive sinus tarsi approach combined with an Essex-Lopresti maneuver has become an option recently for intra-articular calcaneal fractures. This approach involves manipulation of the heel to increase the varus deformity, followed by plantar flexion of the forefoot and valgus reduction of the heel to correct the varus deformity. The reduction maneuver can be stabilized with limited percutaneous or open fixation. The depressed posterior facet can also be elevated through the sinus tarsi approach and limited fixation placed.

   e. Outcomes correlate with the accuracy of the reduction and the number of articular fragments. Type II fractures have better outcomes than type III fractures, whereas type IV fractures have the worst outcomes.

6. Complications

   a. A complication rate of up to 40% has been reported. Factors that predict an increased risk of complications include a fall from a height, early surgery, and smoking. Approximately 10% of patients also have associated lumbar spine injuries.

   b. Wound-related complications are the most common. Other potential complications include malunion, subtalar arthritis, and lateral impingement with peroneal tendon pathology.

   c. Compartment syndrome develops in up to 10% of patients and may lead to a hammer toe deformity.

   d. Malunion can also occur, resulting in loss of height, widening, and lateral impingement (**Figure 4**).

      i. The talus may be dorsiflexed, with a decrease in the talar declination angle to less than 20°, which limits ankle dorsiflexion.

      ii. Associated lateral wall impingement may result in peroneal tendon pathology. Subtalar incongruity can also lead to subtalar arthritis. Difficulty with shoe wear also is possible.

   e. Malunion can be classified using CT.

      i. Type I malunion: lateral exostosis with no subtalar arthritis that can be treated with lateral wall resection

      ii. Type II malunion: lateral exostosis with sub-

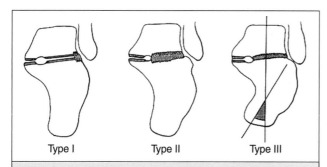

Figure 4 Stephens and Sanders classification of calcaneal malunions. *(Adapted with permission from Stephens HM, Sanders R: Calcaneal malunions: Results of a prognostic computed tomography classification system. Foot Ankle Int 1996;17:395-401.)*

talar arthritis that is treated with lateral wall exostectomy and subtalar fusion

iii. Type III malunion: lateral exostosis with subtalar arthritis and varus malunion that is treated with lateral wall exostectomy and subtalar fusion. The addition of an osteotomy to correct the varus deformity is controversial and has not been proved to improve outcomes.

B. Extra-articular fractures

1. Mechanisms of injury

a. The mechanism of avulsion is the result of strong contraction of the gastrocnemius-soleus complex and avulsion at its insertion.

b. These injuries often occur in patients with osteopenic bone, making secure fixation difficult.

2. Treatment

a. Early reduction is important because displaced fractures can cause pressure necrosis of the overlying skin.

b. Full-thickness skin slough may require flap coverage.

c. Small fragments can be excised, but fractures with larger fragments require open reduction and internal fixation. Note, however, that screw fixation alone may fail in osteopenic bone but can be augmented with tension band fixation.

C. Anterior process fractures

1. Mechanism of injury

a. Anterior process fractures occur with inversion and plantar flexion.

b. They result from avulsion of the bifurcate ligament.

2. Treatment

a. Small extra-articular fragments are treated with immobilization.

b. Larger fragments (>1 cm) can involve the calcaneocuboid joint and require open reduction and internal fixation if joint displacement is present.

c. Late excision is used for chronically painful nonunions.

V. Midfoot Fractures

A. Navicular fractures

1. Anatomy

a. The navicular articulates with the cuneiforms, cuboid, calcaneus, and talus.

b. The talonavicular articulation is critical to maintaining inversion and eversion range of motion.

c. The blood supply is limited in the central portion of the navicular, making this area susceptible to fractures.

2. Radiographic evaluation

a. Plain radiographs including AP, lateral, internal oblique, and external oblique images of the foot are used for initial evaluation.

b. CT is useful for characterizing the fracture pattern. MRI can be used for detection of stress fractures.

3. Avulsion fractures of the navicular

a. Plantar flexion injury is the principal mechanism of injury.

b. Acute treatment consists of immobilization with delayed excision of painful fragments.

c. Open reduction and internal fixation is required for fractures with fragments involving more than 25% of the articular surface.

4. Tuberosity fractures

a. The principal mechanism is eversion and posterior tibial tendon contraction that may result in diastasis of a preexisting accessory navicular.

b. An oblique radiograph at 45° of internal rotation best visualizes the injury.

c. Most tuberosity avulsions can be managed with immobilization.

d. Acute open reduction and internal fixation is indicated with more than 5 mm of diastasis or with large intra-articular fragments.

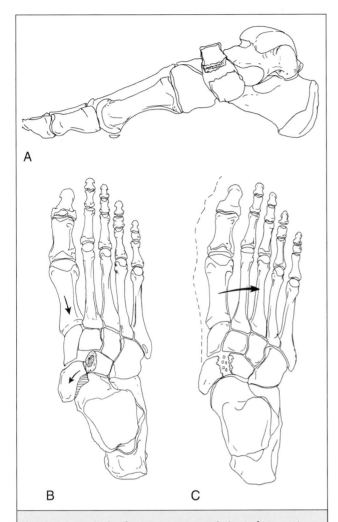

Figure 5 Navicular fractures. **A,** Lateral view of a type I navicular fracture (axial plane fracture line). **B,** AP view of a type II navicular fracture (sagittal plane fracture line). The arrows indicate the direction of applied force. Note also subluxation of the talonavicular joint and proximal migration of the first ray, a common component of type II fractures. **C,** AP view of a type III navicular fracture. Note the comminution, displacement, and incongruity of the talonavicular and naviculocuneiform joints. Arrow indicates the direction of applied force. *(Reproduced from Stroud CC: Fractures of the midtarsals, metatarsals, and phalanges, in Richardson EG [ed]: Orthopaedic Knowledge Update: Foot and Ankle 3. Rosemont, IL, American Academy of Orthopaedic Surgeons, 2003, p 58.)*

e. Symptomatic nonunions are treated with late excision.

5. Body fractures (**Figure 5**)

  a. The mechanism of injury is axial loading.

  b. The Sangeorzan fracture classification is based on the plane of the fracture and degree of comminution (**Table 2**).

Table 2

Sangeorzan Classification of Navicular Fractures

Type	Features
I	Transverse Involves a dorsal fragment <50% of the bone No associated deformity
II	Oblique Most commonly from dorsal-lateral to plantar-medial May be associated with forefoot adduction
III	Central or lateral comminution with abduction May be associated with cuboid or anterior process calcaneal fractures

  c. Minimally displaced type I and II fractures are treated nonsurgically.

  d. Open reduction and internal fixation through a medial incision is used for displaced type I and II fractures or with disruption of the talonavicular joint.

  e. Type III fractures require open reduction and internal fixation with external fixation or primary fusion as needed to maintain lateral column length. Comminution often requires fixation of fragments independently to the cuneiforms if the navicular fragments are too small for open reduction and internal fixation.

6. Stress fractures

  a. These fractures are most common in runners and basketball players.

  b. MRI is a useful screening tool, but CT better visualizes bone when the fracture is visible on plain radiographs.

  c. When acute, these injuries can be treated either nonsurgically or surgically. Nonunions require open reduction and internal fixation. Bone grafting may be used to encourage healing.

B. Tarsometatarsal (Lisfranc) fracture-dislocations

1. Anatomy

  a. The bones of the midfoot include the navicular, cuboid, cuneiforms, and bases of the metatarsals.

  b. The midfoot has osseous stability due to the recessed articulation of the base of the second metatarsal. The trapezoidal shape of the first three metatarsal bases contribute to stability, as do the plantar ligaments. The Lisfranc ligament runs from the base of the second metatarsal to the medial cuneiform.

  c. The lateral tarsometatarsal joints (fourth and

6: Trauma

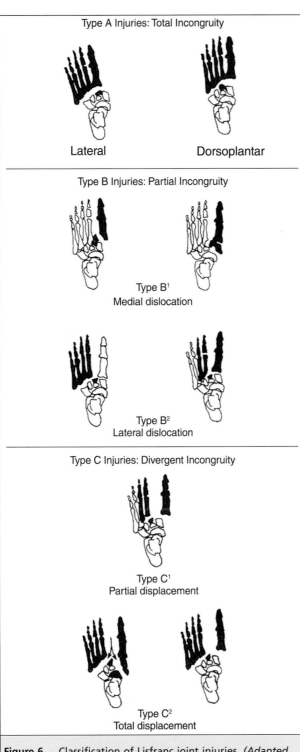

Figure 6 Classification of Lisfranc joint injuries. *(Adapted with permission from Myerson MS, Fisher RT, Burgess AR, Kenzora JE: Fracture dislocations of the tarsometatarsal joints: End results correlated with pathology and treatment.* Foot Ankle *1986;6:228.)*

2. Mechanisms of injury

    a. Direct injuries occur with dorsal force and may result in soft-tissue injuries and compartment syndromes. Both bony and soft-tissue components are common in direct injuries.

    b. Indirect injuries occur with axial loading and twisting on a loaded, plantar flexed foot. Patients commonly report a history of a fixed foot with rotation of the body around the midfoot.

3. Radiographic evaluation

    a. Internal oblique, AP, and lateral views of the foot should be obtained.

    b. Normal anatomic relationships should be maintained.

        i. The medial aspect of the second metatarsal should be aligned with the medial cuneiform.

        ii. The medial aspect of the fourth metatarsal should be aligned with the medial cuboid.

        iii. Diastasis of >2 mm between the base of the first and second metatarsals is pathologic.

        iv. There should be no dorsal subluxation of the metatarsal bases on the lateral view.

    c. The fleck sign is a small avulsed fragment of bone in the interval between the first and second metatarsal bases. This represents avulsion of the Lisfranc ligament from its insertion on the base of the second metatarsal.

    d. Weight-bearing or stress radiographs can be ordered when the results of physical examination and plain radiographs are equivocal.

    e. A 30° internal rotation oblique view best visualizes cuboid compression (nutcracker injury).

4. Fracture classification (**Figure 6**)

    a. Tarsometatarsal injuries are divided into three categories.

        i. Type A injuries: total incongruity of the midfoot joints. The most common direction is lateral, and homolateral injuries may be associated with cuboid compression fractures.

        ii. Type B injuries: partial incongruity of the midfoot joints. Common patterns include medial dislocation of the first metatarsal or lateral dislocation of some or all of the lateral rays.

        iii. Type C injuries: divergent incongruity of the midfoot joints in which the first metatarsal and some or all of the lateral rays displace in opposite directions.

fifth metatarsal-cuboid joints) have 10° to 20° of sagittal plane motion. The medial three tarsometatarsal joints have limited motion.

5. Treatment

a. Open reduction and internal fixation is indicated for displaced midfoot fractures and dislocations.

i. One or two dorsal incisions can be used. The neurovascular bundle is lateral to the first interspace.

ii. Fully threaded cortical screws usually are used because compression across the joint is not necessary.

iii. Percutaneous pins are commonly used in the fourth and fifth tarsometatarsal joints, but screw fixation may be used.

b. Plate fixation or external fixation may be used for cuboid compression (nutcracker injury) to maintain lateral column length.

c. Reduction and screw fixation is indicated to stabilize intercunieform instability.

d. Screws generally are not removed for at least 3 months.

e. Primary fusion has been advocated as an option, particularly in purely ligamentous injuries, which have worse outcomes. However, this option requires further investigation.

f. Late reconstruction of missed injuries (up to 30% of tarsometatarsal injuries) may include fusion of the first three tarsometatarsal joints.

g. Resection arthroplasty with tendon interposition has been advocated in the fourth and fifth tarsometatarsal joints to avoid stiffness and abnormal gait. It is more critical to maintain motion in these joints, and they typically are not symptomatic.

6. Complications

a. Late posttraumatic osteoarthritis is common, occurring in up to 58% of patients. Anatomic reduction, open injury, and comminution predict outcomes.

b. More than 2 mm or 15° of displacement results in a worse prognosis.

c. Purely ligamentous injuries also may have a worse prognosis, leading some to advocate primary fusion as an alternative treatment.

C. Cuboid fractures

1. Compression fractures from a nutcracker mechanism can be part of a Lisfranc fracture-dislocation, whereas isolated cuboid fractures are uncommon.

2. Cuboid fractures with significant compression can result in collapse of the lateral column.

a. External fixation can be used to restore lateral column length and disimpact fragments.

b. Fixation and bone grafting may be required for impacted fractures.

c. Avulsion fractures are treated symptomatically.

D. Cuneiform fractures

1. Isolated cuneiform fractures are uncommon. Avulsion fractures are treated symptomatically.

2. Displaced fractures and intercuneiform instability can occur as part of a Lisfranc fracture-dislocation. These injuries should be reduced and stabilized during fixation of the tarsometatarsal injuries.

VI. Metatarsal and Phalangeal Fractures

A. Metatarsal shaft fractures

1. Mechanisms of injury include a direct blow, avulsion, twisting, or inversion. Repetitive stress also can be a cause.

2. The plantar flexors are the deforming force. A prominent plantar fragment can result in callus formation. A dorsiflexion malunion can result in transfer metatarsalgia.

3. Nonsurgical treatment is appropriate for fractures of the second, third, and fourth metatarsal shafts when there is <3 mm of displacement or <10° of angulation.

4. Indications for surgical treatment

a. Displaced fractures of the first metatarsal. Patients do not tolerate these fractures well because the first ray bears more weight than the lesser metatarsals.

b. Fractures of the second through fourth metatarsals if there is 3 to 4 mm of displacement or >10° of sagittal displacement.

c. Multiple metatarsal fractures

5. Fixation options include Kirschner wires (K-wires), screws, or plates.

B. Metatarsal neck and head fractures

1. Most metatarsal neck fractures can be treated nonsurgically. Metatarsal neck fractures with severe angulation with plantar prominence may require reduction and fixation. Dorsal angulation also may require either closed or open reduction with fixation to prevent transfer metatarsalgia.

2. Metatarsal head fractures are rare and generally can be treated nonsurgically; however, severely displaced fractures may require closed or open reduction and fixation.

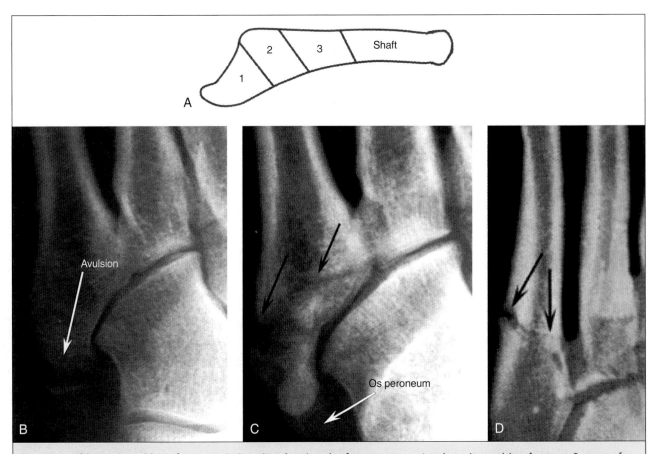

Figure 7   Fifth metatarsal base fractures. **A,** Drawing showing the fracture zones: 1, tuberosity avulsion fracture; 2, zone of metaphyseal-diaphyseal junction; 3, shaft stress fracture zone. **B,** Radiographs showing a displaced tuberosity avulsion fracture: zone 1. **C,** Radiograph showing a displaced metaphyseal-diaphyseal junction fracture: zone 2. **D,** Radiograph showing a diaphyseal shaft stress fracture: zone 3. *(Part A reproduced from Dameron TB: Fractures of the proximal fifth metatarsal: Selecting the best treatment option. J Am Acad Orthop Surg 1995;3:110-114. Parts B through D reproduced with permission from Coughlin MJ, Mann RA [eds]: Surgery of the Foot and Ankle, ed 7. St. Louis, MO, Mosby, 1999, p 1594.)*

C. Fractures of the fifth metatarsal base (**Figure 7**)

1. Type I fractures

   a. Avulsion of the long plantar ligament, the lateral band of the plantar fascia, or contraction of the peroneus brevis may result in these fractures.

   b. Treatment consists of weight bearing as tolerated in a stiff-soled shoe.

   c. Surgery may be necessary, although rarely, for fractures with large displaced intra-articular fragments.

   d. Nonunions also are uncommon but can be treated by excision and repair of the peroneus brevis, as needed.

2. Type II fractures

   a. The metadiaphyseal region is an area of circulatory watershed resulting in limited blood supply. Fractures that occur at the metadiaphyseal junction, approximately 1.5 to 2.5 cm distal to the metatarsal base, are commonly called Jones fractures.

   b. Because of the compromised blood supply in this area, the fracture is at risk of nonunion. Therefore, patients should not bear weight for 6 to 8 weeks.

   c. Acute open reduction and internal fixation using screws is often used in athletes to minimize the possibility of nonunion and prolonged restriction from activity.

   d. Development of postoperative nonunion is associated with a return to activity before evidence of radiographic union and is more common in high-demand athletes.

3. Type III fractures

   a. These are diaphyseal stress fractures. Cavovarus foot deformities increase first tarsometatarsal joint mobility, increasing stress in the lateral column of the foot.

b. Hereditary sensorimotor neuropathy and diabetic neuropathy may result in a patient's inability to sense overload of the bone.

c. Nonsurgical treatment consisting of non–weight-bearing status is used for proximal fractures in the area of the watershed. Pulsed electromagnetic bone stimulators may accelerate healing.

d. Screw fixation is indicated in patients with established sclerosis and nonunion or in athletes.

e. Bone grafting and/or structural correction may be needed to achieve healing and prevent recurrence, particularly in atrophic nonunions.

D. Phalangeal fractures

a. The mechanism of injury is a crush injury or axial loading.

b. Painful subungual hematoma can be evacuated through a hole in the nail.

c. Nonsurgical treatment consisting of closed reduction and buddy taping for 4 weeks generally is indicted for lesser toe injuries. Distal phalanx fractures of the hallux are treated nonsurgically.

d. Surgical treatment is indicated for displaced articular injuries or angulated proximal phalanx fractures of the hallux if closed reduction and percutaneous pinning fail. A failed closed reduction can be converted to open reduction and internal fixation performed through an L-shaped incision dorsally.

E. Sesamoid injuries

a. Injuries can occur by direct impact with compression, through hyperdorsiflexion with a transverse fracture, or with repetitive trauma.

b. Plain radiographs can include a sesamoid view to evaluate the articulation of the sesamoid with the plantar aspect of the metatarsal head. MRI is useful in determining the presence of stress reaction or stress fracture.

c. Acute fractures or stress fractures are treated with padding and immobilization in a hard-soled shoe for 4 to 8 weeks.

d. Excision of the sesamoid is used for chronic symptomatic nonunions. The potential complication of medial sesamoidectomy is hallux valgus, whereas lateral sesamoidectomy may result in hallux varus.

VII. Dislocations of the Foot

A. Subtalar dislocation

1. Mechanism of injury

a. These are high-energy injuries but are closed in 75% of patients.

b. Most dislocations (65% to 80%) are medial, with the talus translated medially. The remaining dislocations generally are lateral; anterior or posterior dislocation is rare.

2. Radiographic evaluation—CT is necessary following reduction to rule out associated fractures, which can occur in up to 44% of patients.

3. Treatment

a. Closed reduction is performed by flexing the knee, recreating the deformity, plantar flexing the foot, and then pushing the talar head; however, up to 32% of dislocations cannot be reduced.

b. Medial dislocations that cannot be reduced are the result of buttonholing of the talus through the extensor digitorum brevis, inferior extensor retinaculum, or talonavicular capsule and/or interposition of the peroneal tendons.

c. Lateral dislocations that cannot be reduced are the result of interposition of the posterior tibial tendon or a bony fragment, with the FHL and flexor digitorum longus less commonly interposed.

d. Open reduction with tendon relocation and stabilization with transarticular pins, as needed, is indicated for dislocations that cannot be reduced.

B. Midtarsal dislocation

1. Midtarsal dislocation involving the talonavicular and calcaneocuboid articulations (Chopart joint) can occur through axial loading (longitudinal), medial stress, lateral stress, plantar stress, or crush injuries.

2. Plain radiographs should be obtained, with CT used if associated fractures are suspected.

3. The prognosis depends largely on the severity of the original injury.

4. Treatment involves prompt reduction to avoid skin necrosis.

a. Nondisplaced and stable injuries can be treated with immobilization and protected weight bearing.

b. Displaced or subluxated joints should be reduced and pinned with K-wires.

C. Isolated tarsal dislocations

1. Isolated dislocations of the talonavicular joint, navicular bone, calcaneocuboid joint, cuboid bone, and cuneiforms are uncommon.

6: Trauma

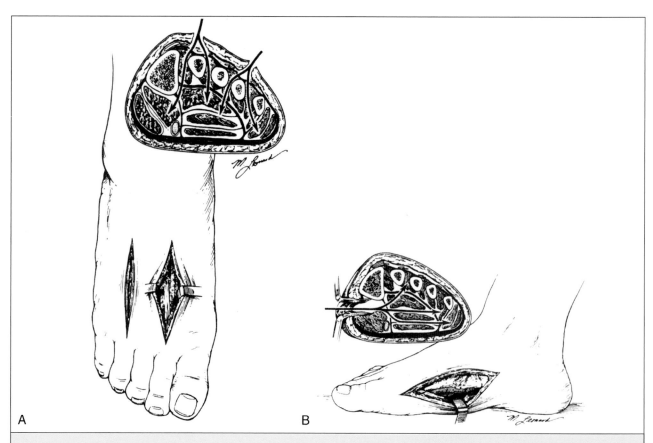

Figure 8   Dorsal (**A**) and medial (**B**) approaches for foot fasciotomies. These approaches can be combined to facilitate decompression. *(Reproduced with permission from Myerson MS: Management of compartment syndromes of the foot.* Clin Orthop Relat Res *1991;271:242-243.)*

2. Treatment involves prompt closed or open reduction to avoid skin necrosis. K-wires may be required to secure anatomic reduction.

D. Forefoot dislocations

1. First MTP joint

a. Dislocations usually are dorsal.

b. Closed reduction usually is attempted first, but may not be possible if the first metatarsal buttonholes through the sesamoid–short flexor complex.

c. A dorsal approach is used for open reduction if necessary.

2. Lesser MTP joints

a. Dislocations usually are dorsal.

b. Closed reduction usually is attempted first but may not be possible if the metatarsal head buttonholes through the plantar plate mechanism.

c. A dorsal incision is used for open reduction if necessary.

3. Interphalangeal joints

a. Dislocations are uncommon and usually dorsal.

b. Closed reduction usually is attempted first but may not be possible if the proximal phalanx buttonholes through the plantar plate.

c. Open reduction is performed through a dorsal approach if necessary.

VIII. Compartment Syndromes

A. Anatomy/pathophysiology

1. The foot has a total of nine compartments divided into four main groups: medial (one compartment), lateral (one compartment), interosseous (four compartments), and central (three compartments, including the deep central, or calcaneal, which communicates with the deep posterior compartment of the leg).

2. Acute trauma to the foot, including calcaneus fractures, Lisfranc injuries, crush injuries, and other high-energy mechanisms can result in compartment syndromes.

B. Clinical evaluation

1. The primary method of diagnosis is clinical.

2. Loss of pulses and capillary refill are unreliable signs.

3. Loss of two-point discrimination and light touch sensation are more reliable than loss of pinprick sensation.

4. Pain with passive dorsiflexion results from stretch of the intrinsic muscles. This decreases compartment volume and increases pressure.

5. Pressure measurements can be helpful in clinically equivocal cases. Pressure thresholds greater than 30 mm Hg or within 30 mm Hg of diastolic blood pressure have been advocated as indications for compartment release.

C. Treatment (**Figure 8**)

1. Fasciotomy is indicated when clinical symptoms are consistent with compartment syndrome.

2. Medial and/or dorsal incisions can be used to release all nine compartments.

a. Two dorsal incisions are commonly used.

   i. The medial incision is used to release the first and second interosseous, medial, and deep central compartments.

   ii. The lateral incision is used to release the two lateral interosseous, superficial and middle central, and lateral compartments.

b. Medial incisions

   i. A single medial incision can be used to release all nine compartments but is technically more difficult.

   ii. A medial incision is sometimes used in conjunction with two dorsal incisions to ensure release of the deep central compartment.

3. Delayed closure should be used because skin closure can increase compartment pressures. A split-thickness skin graft may be required.

Bibliography

Buckley R, Tough S, McCormack R, et al: Operative compared with nonoperative treatment of displaced intraarticular calcaneal fractures: A prospective, randomized, controlled multicenter trial. *J Bone Joint Surg Am* 2002;84:1733-1744.

Canale ST, Kelly FB: Fractures of the neck of the talus: Long-term evaluation of seventy-one cases. *J Bone Joint Surg Am* 1978;60:143-156.

Kelly IP, Glisson RR, Fink C, Easley ME, Nunley JA: Intramedullary screw fixation of Jones fractures. *Foot Ankle Int* 2001;22:585-589.

Kuo RS, Tejwani NC, Digiovanni CW, et al: Outcome after open reduction internal fixation of Lisfranc joint injuries. *J Bone Joint Surg Am* 2000;82:1609-1618.

Larson CM, Almekinders LC, Taft TN, Garret WE: Intramedullary screw fixation of Jones fractures: Analysis of failure. *Am J Sports Med* 2002;30:55-60.

Myerson MS: Experimental decompression of the fascial compartments of the foot: The basis for fasciotomy in acute compartment syndromes. *Foot Ankle* 1988;8:308-314.

Quill GE: Fractures of the proximal fifth metatarsal. *Orthop Clin North Am* 1995;26:353-361.

Sanders R, Fortin P, DiPasquale T, Walling A: Operative treatment in 120 displaced intraarticular calcaneal fractures: Results using a prognostic computed tomography classification. *Clin Orthop Relat Res* 1993;290:87-95.

Schulze W, Richter J, Russe O, Ingelfinger P, Muhr G: Surgical treatment of talus fractures: A retrospective study of 80 cases followed for 1-15 years. *Acta Orthop Scand* 2002;73:344-351.

Shah SN, Knoblich GO, Lindsey DP, Dreshak J, Yerby SA, Chou LB: Intramedullary screw fixation of proximal fifth metatarsal fractures: A biomechanical study. *Foot Ankle Int* 2001;22:581-584.

Teng AL, Pinzur MS, Lomansney L, Mahoney L, Havey R: Funtional outcome following anatomic restoration of tarsal-metatarsal fracture-dislocation. *Foot Ankle Int* 2002;23:922-926.

Thordarson DB, Triffon MJ, Terk MR: Magnetic resonance imaging to detect avascular necrosis after open reduction and internal fixation of talar neck fractures. *Foot Ankle Int* 1996;17:742-747.

Top Testing Facts

Fractures of the Talus

1. The talus is 70% covered by cartilage and the extensor digitorum brevis is the only muscle attachment.

2. The blood supply to the body is mostly from the artery of the tarsal canal, a branch of the posterior tibial artery.

3. The blood supply to the neck is mostly from the artery of the tarsal sinus, a branch formed from the anterior tibial and peroneal arteries.

4. The deltoid artery supplies the medial body.

5. Posttraumatic osteoarthritis is the most common complication of talar neck fracture.

6. Osteonecrosis occurs with increasing frequency as the Hawkins classification for a talar neck fracture increases in severity.

7. Open reduction and internal fixation is required for all displaced talar neck fractures. Open reduction and internal fixation is usually performed through a combined anterolateral and anteromedial approach.

8. The Hawkins sign is subchondral osteopenia seen at 6 to 8 weeks postoperatively after fixation of a talar neck fracture and indicates revascularization and a better prognosis.

9. Varus malunion after a talar neck fracture can lead to loss of eversion.

10. Lateral process fractures of the talus are commonly seen in snowboarders as a result of a dorsiflexion-external rotation mechanism.

Fractures of the Calcaneus

1. Approximately 10% of patients with an intra-articular calcaneal fracture have an associated lumbar spine injury.

2. Approximately 10% of patients with an intra-articular calcaneal fracture have an associated foot compartment syndrome.

3. A superomedial fragment containing the sustentaculum is seen with intra-articular fractures of the calcaneus. This constant fragment is stabilized by ligaments and capsular attachments, making it a useful reference during open reduction and internal fixation.

4. The management of Sanders type II, III, and IV fractures remains controversial.

5. Negative prognostic factors for the surgical treatment of Sanders type II and III fractures include severity, advanced age, male sex, obesity, bilateral fractures, multiple trauma, and worker's compensation.

6. Malunion of calcaneal fractures can result in shortening, widening, and varus position. The symptoms include difficulty with shoe wear and peroneal tendon symptoms.

7. Malunions that result in talar dorsiflexion with loss of talar declination angle to less than 20° can limit ankle dorsiflexion.

8. Malunions of the calcaneus are treated with lateral exostectomy. Fusion is also added for subtalar arthritis.

9. Tension band fixation can be used to avoid failure of screw fixation in avulsion fractures of the calcaneal tuberosity.

10. Anterior process fractures occur with inversion and avulsion of the bifurcate ligament.

Midfoot Fractures

1. The central navicular has limited blood supply and is susceptible to stress fractures.

2. The tarsometatarsal joints are constrained by the recessed articulation of the second metatarsal.

3. The Lisfranc ligament runs from the base of the second metatarsal to the medial cuneiform.

4. The lateral fourth and fifth tarsometatarsal joints have 10° to 20° of sagittal motion, whereas the medial three tarsometatarsal joints have little motion.

5. Lisfranc fracture-dislocations can occur with direct application of force or indirectly through axial loading and twisting on a fixed, plantar flexed foot.

6. Plain radiographs may show a fleck of bone in the proximal first metatarsal interspace. This fleck sign represents the avulsed Lisfranc ligament.

7. Homolateral dislocation of the tarsometatarsal joints may be associated with a compression injury to the cuboid.

8. Intercuneiform instability can be associated with Lisfranc injuries and should be reduced and fixed.

9. Up to 30% of Lisfranc injuries are missed acutely. Weight-bearing or stress radiographs can be used to rule out injury.

10. Fusion of the fourth and fifth tarsometatarsal joints is poorly tolerated, and resection arthroplasty is used in conjunction with fusion of the medial tarsometatarsal joints for missed or late reconstruction of Lisfranc injuries.

Top Testing Facts (cont.)

Metatarsal and Phalangeal Fractures

1. Displacement of first metatarsal fractures is poorly tolerated and is an indication for reduction and fixation.

2. More than 3 mm of displacement, 10° of angulation, or multiple metatarsal fractures are indications for fixation of second, third, or fourth metatarsal fractures.

3. Plantar displacement of metatarsal fractures can lead to callosity.

4. Dorsal displacement of metatarsal fractures can lead to transfer metatarsalgia under adjacent metatarsals.

5. The proximal fifth metatarsal has poor blood supply at the metadiaphyseal junction 1.5 to 2.5 cm distal to the base. Jones fractures occur at this metadiaphyseal junction.

6. High-level athletes may undergo acute fixation of Jones fractures with a screw to avoid delay in the return to activity because of nonunion.

7. Diaphyseal stress fractures of the fifth metatarsal can be caused by cavovarus foot deformities or peripheral neuropathies.

8. Proximal phalanx fractures of the hallux are treated surgically for angulation or displaced intra-articular injuries.

9. Medial sesamoidectomy for nonunion may result in hallux valgus deformity.

10. Lateral sesamoidectomy for nonunion may result in hallux varus deformity.

Dislocations of the Foot

1. Medial subtalar dislocations may be irreducible if the talar head buttonholes through the extensor digitorum brevis, inferior extensor retinaculum, or talonavicular capsule, or with interposition of the peroneal tendons.

2. Lateral subtalar dislocations may be irreducible if the posterior tibial tendon, flexor digitorum longus, or FHL is interposed.

3. Subtalar dislocations are close-reduced by flexing the knee to relax the gastrocnemius-soleus complex, recreating the deformity, plantar flexing the foot, and pushing the talar head.

4. CT is indicated for subtalar dislocations, given the high rate of associated fractures.

5. First MTP joint dislocations may be irreducible because of buttonholing through the sesamoid-short flexor complex.

6. Irreducible first MTP joint dislocations are treated through a dorsal approach.

7. Lesser MTP joint dislocations may be irreducible because of buttonholing through the plantar plate.

8. Irreducible lesser MTP joint dislocations are treated through a dorsal approach.

9. Chopart joints are the talonavicular and calcaneocuboid joints. These joints should be reduced promptly to avoid skin necrosis.

10. Isolated tarsal dislocations are rare but are treated with prompt reduction to avoid skin necrosis.

Compartment Syndromes

1. The foot has a total of nine compartments that comprise four main groups: the medial, lateral, four interosseous, and three central compartments.

2. The central compartment includes the deep central, or calcaneal compartment, which communicates with the deep posterior compartment of the leg.

3. Compartment syndromes result from bleeding and edema that increase the tissue interstitial pressures.

4. Interstitial pressures above the capillary pressure lead to venous occlusion.

5. Irreversible myoneural necrosis and fibrosis occur after 8 hours.

6. Loss of two-point discrimination and light touch are more sensitive signs of compartment syndrome than loss of pinprick sensation. Loss of pulses and capillary refill are unreliable signs.

7. Pain with passive dorsiflexion results from stretch of the intrinsic muscles, resulting in decreased compartment volume and increased pressure.

8. Clinical symptoms are the main indication for compartment release. Pressures greater than 30 mm Hg or within 30 mm Hg of diastolic pressure have been advocated as indications for release in equivocal cases.

9. Two dorsal incisions can be used to release all nine foot compartments.

10. Alternatively, a medial approach can be used to release all nine compartments. The medial approach is more commonly used in conjunction with dorsal incisions to ensure release of the deep central compartment.

I. Fractures of the Ankle

A. Epidemiology

1. Fractures of the ankle are among the most common injuries requiring orthopaedic care.

2. Ankle fractures vary from relatively simple injuries with minimal long-term effects to complex injuries with severe long-term sequelae.

3. Population-based studies have identified an increase in the incidence of ankle fractures. Data from Medicare enrollees suggest the rate of ankle fractures in the United States averages 4.2 fractures per 1,000 Medicare enrollees annually.

4. Rates of surgery vary depending on type of fracture.

   a. For isolated lateral malleolar fractures, the surgical intervention rate is approximately 11%.

   b. For trimalleolar fractures, the surgical intervention rate is 74%.

5. Risk factors for sustaining an ankle fracture include age, increased body mass, and a history of ankle fractures.

6. The highest incidence of ankle fractures occurs in elderly women.

7. Isolated malleolar fractures account for two thirds of ankle fractures.

B. Anatomy of the lower leg

1. Osseous anatomy and ligaments of the ankle joint (**Figure 1**)

   a. The osseous anatomy of the ankle provides stability during weight bearing with mobility in plantar flexion.

   b. The ankle joint behaves like a true mortise in dorsiflexion.

   c. Stability is achieved by articular contact between the medial malleolus, the fibula, the tibial plafond, and the talus.

   d. The talar dome is wider anteriorly than posteriorly, such that as the ankle dorsiflexes, the fibula rotates externally through the tibiofibular syndesmosis to accommodate the talus.

   e. The lateral malleolus is surrounded by multiple strong ligaments.

      i. These include the tibiofibular ligamentous complex of the interosseous membrane and syndesmotic ligaments (anterior inferior tibiofibular ligament, posterior inferior tibiofibular ligament, and the inferior transverse ligament).

      ii. These ligaments are responsible for stability of the ankle in external rotation.

      iii. In addition, the lateral collateral ligaments of the ankle, including the anterior and posterior talofibular ligaments and calcaneofibular ligaments, provide support and resistance to inversion and anterior translation of the talus relative to the fibula.

2. Medial malleolus

   a. The medial malleolar surface of the distal tibia has a larger surface anteriorly than posteriorly.

   b. The posterior border of the medial malleolus includes the groove for the posterior tibial tendon.

   c. The medial malleolus includes the anterior colliculus, which is larger and extends approximately 0.5 cm distal to the smaller posterior colliculus.

   d. The deltoid ligament provides medial ligamentous support of the ankle.

      i. The important deep component of the deltoid ligament arises from the intercollicular groove and posterior colliculus.

      ii. The deep layer of the deltoid ligament is a short, thick ligament inserting on the medial surface of the talus.

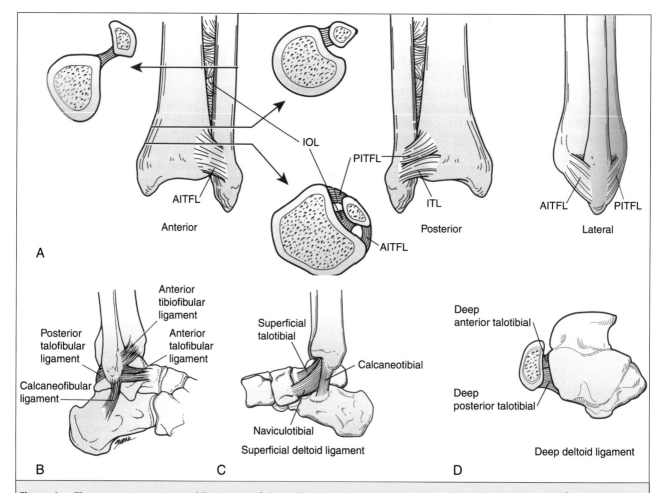

Figure 1   The osseous anatomy and ligaments of the ankle joint. **A,** Anterior, posterior, and lateral views of the tibiofibular syndesmotic ligaments. AITFL = anterior inferior tibiofibular ligament, PITFL = posterior inferior tibiofibular ligament, ITL = inferior transverse ligament, IOL = interosseous ligament. **B,** The lateral collateral ligaments of the ankle and the anterior syndesmotic ligament. Sagittal plane **(C)** and transverse plane **(D)** views of the medial collateral ligaments of the ankle. *(A, C, and D adapted with permission from Browner B, Jupiter J, Levine A [eds]: Skeletal Trauma: Fractures, Dislocations, and Ligamentous Injuries, ed 2. Philadelphia, PA, WB Saunders, 1997. B reprinted with permission from Marsh JL, Saltzman CL, Ankle fractures, in Bucholz RW, Heckman JD, Court-Brown CM [eds]: Rockwood and Green's Fractures in Adults [ed. 6]. Philadelphia, PA, Lippincott Williams & Wilkins, 2006, pp 2147-2247.)*

iii. The superficial deltoid ligament arises from the anterior colliculus of the medial malleolus.

3. Tendinous and neurovascular structures

   a. Posterior group

      i. The posterior group includes the Achilles and plantaris tendons.

      ii. Immediately lateral to the Achilles tendon lies the sural nerve.

   b. Medial group

      i. On the medial side of the ankle, the flexor tendons—including the tibialis posterior, the flexor digitorum longus (FDL), and the flexor hallucis longus—(FHL) course posterior to the medial malleolus.

      ii. The posterior tibial artery and tibial nerve lie between the FDL and FHL tendons.

      iii. The saphenous vein and nerve course superior and anterior to the tip of the medial malleolus and are at risk during surgical repair of malleolar fractures.

   c. Anterior group

      i. On the anterior aspect of the ankle, the extensor retinaculum contains the extensor tendons, including the tibialis anterior, extensor hallucis longus (EHL), extensor digitorum longus (EDL), and peroneus tertius.

      ii. Between the EHL and EDL lie the deep peroneal nerve and the anterior tibial artery.

iii. The superficial peroneal nerve crosses the ankle anterior to the lateral malleolus, superficial to the extensor retinaculum.

iv. Because the superficial peroneal nerve may cross from the lateral compartment to the anterior compartment at varying levels, care must be exercised to avoid injury to this nerve in the treatment of fibular fractures.

d. Lateral group

   i. On the lateral side of the ankle, the peroneal tendons are contained by a stout retinacular structure posterior to the fibula.

   ii. The peroneus longus is more external to the peroneus brevis.

   iii. Lateral approaches to the ankle can injure the superficial nerve more proximally and the sural nerve more distally.

C. Surgical approaches to ankle fractures

1. Direct lateral approach to the fibula

   a. Commonly used to stabilize lateral malleolar fractures

   b. The dissection is anterior to the peroneal tendons at the level of the ankle mortise.

   c. Proximally, the peroneal tendons must be dissected to expose the fibula.

   d. The dissection plane is between the peroneus tertius anteriorly and the peroneus longus and brevis posteriorly.

   e. The superficial peroneal nerve should be considered when more proximal dissection is required for fibular fracture.

   f. The posterior aspect of the lateral malleolus can be approached through this incision; this requires reflection of the peroneal tendons away from the posterior surface of the fibula to facilitate placement of internal fixation on the posterior surface of the fibula.

2. Posterolateral approach to the ankle joint

   a. The posterolateral approach exists between the peroneal tendons and the Achilles tendon.

   b. Direct exposure of the posterior aspect of the tibia is accomplished by elevating the FHL tendon away from the posterior aspect of the tibia in the deep portion of this incision.

   c. This approach is useful for stabilizing a posterior malleolar fracture using direct reduction techniques.

3. Anteromedial approaches to the medial malleolus

   a. The medial malleolus can be approached through a longitudinal incision directly over the malleolus; the saphenous nerve and vein are frequently encountered.

   b. A slightly more anterior incision facilitates direct inspection of the ankle joint and talar dome.

   c. Using a more posteromedial incision, the posterior tibial tendon and neurovascular bundle can be elevated to access the posteromedial portion of the medial malleolus.

4. Percutaneous incisions

   a. In addition to the lateral, posterolateral, and medial approaches, a variety of percutaneous incisions can be used to facilitate hardware placement.

   b. An anterior percutaneus incision often is used to facilitate indirect fixation of a posterior malleolar fracture.

   c. Blunt dissection and placement of retractors and soft-tissue sleeves are required to avoid injury to the neurovascular structures surrounding the ankle.

D. Mechanism of injury

1. Most ankle fractures are low-energy, rotational injuries.

2. Ankle fractures also occur commonly in sports, usually secondary to a rotational mechanism.

3. Fractures with a significant axial loading mechanism are more severe and often result in tibial plafond fractures.

4. Associated injuries

   a. Common with malleolar fractures

   b. Fractures of the talar dome occur in a substantial portion of ankle fractures and are known to compromise long-term outcome.

   c. Associated osseoligamentous injuries such as avulsive injuries of the anterior inferior tibiofibular ligament may occur.

   d. Avulsion fractures in which the anterior inferior tibiofibular ligament avulses from the distal tibia (Chaput tubercle) or fibula (Wagstaffe tubercle) may occur and result in associated external rotation instability.

   e. With adduction-type ankle injuries, impaction injury to the medial distal tibia may occur.

      i. To restore ankle joint congruency, this impaction injury may require treatment in addition to the malleolar fracture.

      ii. This injury pattern should be considered in particular when the medial malleolar fracture has a vertical orientation and is associated with a transverse distal fibular fracture.

6: Trauma

f. The lateral articular surface can be impacted in a pronation-abduction type of mechanism. Reduction and stabilization of the lateral articular impaction can be difficult and may also result in significant long-term outcome problems.

E. Clinical evaluation

1. Clinical evaluation should include a description of the mechanism of injury.

2. An evaluation of medical comorbidities, especially diabetes mellitus, is important. Physical examination should include a thorough inspection for communicating open wounds.

   a. An open ankle fracture is most commonly associated with an open medial wound with a punctate or transverse laceration in communication with the ankle joint.

   b. These fractures should be considered as surgical emergencies.

3. An examination for deformity of the foot relative to the leg and the direction of displacement to the foot should be performed.

4. The complete circulatory and neurologic examination should be documented, including assessment of the superficial peroneal, deep peroneal, sural, and posterior tibial nerves, which can be examined using light touch and sharp/dull discrimination.

5. The condition of the skin must be considered.

6. Soft-tissue swelling should be assessed because it will affect surgical timing.

7. Fracture-dislocations should be reduced to avoid isolated skin and soft-tissue ischemia.

8. In patients without dislocation, the ankle should be palpated for areas of tenderness.

9. Ottawa ankle rules

   a. The Ottawa ankle rules assist physicians in deciding when it is appropriate to obtain radiographs in adults with ankle injuries.

   b. These guidelines are sensitive for ankle fracture, and they reduce the number of radiographs taken, along with associated costs.

   c. According to these rules, ankle radiographs are needed only if there is pain near the malleoli and one or more of the following conditions is present:

      i. Age 55 years or older

      ii. Inability to bear weight

      iii. Bone tenderness at the posterior edge or tip of either malleolus

10. Physical examination and instability

    a. Although physical examination of acute ankle injuries is important, the ability to detect instability by physical examination alone has been questioned.

    b. This is particularly the case for isolated lateral malleolar fractures, in which it is often difficult to determine the degree of instability of the ankle.

    c. In patients with an isolated fibular fracture without talar shift, the ankle should be palpated directly over the deltoid ligament for swelling, ecchymosis, and tenderness as a clue to potential deltoid ligament injury; however, the value of this maneuver to predict ankle instability is comparatively limited.

    d. Stress examination of isolated fibular fractures without talar shift has been advocated recently as a more sensitive examination of ankle instability.

F. Radiographic evaluation

1. Standard radiographs of the ankle include mortise, AP, and lateral views.

   a. The mortise view is obtained by internal rotation of the patient's leg by approximately 15° such that the x-ray beam is perpendicular to the transmalleolar axis.

   b. The AP radiograph is obtained with the x-ray beam in line with the second ray of the foot.

   c. If there is any suggestion of proximal tibial or fibular pain or tenderness or swelling and pain in the foot region, the radiographic evaluation should include full views of the tibia and fibula and foot.

2. Important considerations on standard radiographic views (Figure 2)

   a. The subchondral bone of the tibia and fibula should form a continuous line around the talus on all views.

   b. The talocrural angle (the angle between a line drawn perpendicular to the distal articular surface of the tibia and a line connecting the lateral and medial malleoli) should be 83° ± 4° or within 5° of the contralateral ankle on the mortise view.

   c. The medial clear space (the distance between the medial articular surface of the medial malleolus and the talar dome) should be ≤4 mm and should be equal to the superior clear space between the talus and the distal tibia on the mortise view.

   d. The tibiofibular clear space (the distance between the medial wall of the fibula and the tibial incisural surface) should be ≤6 mm on the mortise view.

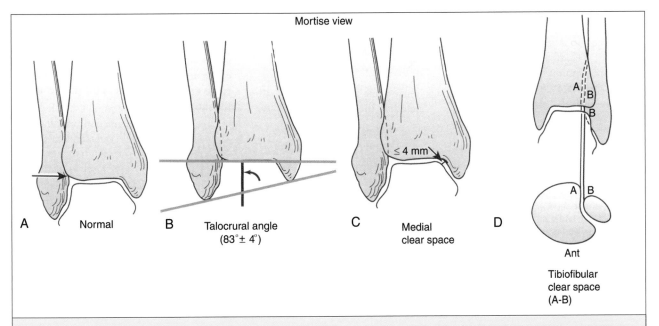

Figure 2   Radiographic appearance of the normal ankle on the mortise view. **A,** The condensed subchondral bone should form a continuous line around the talus. **B,** The talocrural angle should be approximately 83°. **C,** The medial clear space should be equal to the superior clear space between the talus and the distal tibia and ≤4 mm on standard radiographs. **D,** The distance between the medial wall of the fibula and the incisural surface of the tibia, the tibiofibular clear space, should be ≤6 mm. *(A through C adapted with permission from Browner B, Jupiter J, Levine A [eds]: Skeletal Trauma: Fractures, Dislocations, and Ligamentous Injuries, ed 2. Philadelphia, PA, WB Saunders, 1997. D reprinted with permission from Marsh JL, Saltzman CL, Ankle fractures, in Bucholz RW, Heckman JD, Court-Brown CM [eds]: Rockwood and Green's Fractures in Adults [ed. 6]. Philadelphia, PA, Lippincott Williams & Wilkins, 2006, pp 2147-2247.)*

3. In the case of an ankle with an isolated fibular fracture and medial tenderness without evidence of initial talar displacement, a stress view has been recommended.

   a. This may be performed by simple gentle external rotation of the foot with the ankle in dorsiflexion and the leg stabilized, or by supporting the patient's leg with a pillow or cushion and allowing the ankle to rotate with the force of gravity.

   b. In these situations, a widening of the medial clear space of ≥5 mm may occur. This may be indicative of ankle instability secondary to medial ligamentous injury in conjunction with the fibular fracture.

G. Classification—AO/Weber and Lauge-Hansen classifications

   1. AO/Weber classification (**Figure 3**)

      a. Ankle fractures are classified based on the location of the fibular fracture.

      b. The degree of instability depends on the location of the fibular fracture.

      c. Weber A fracture

         i. Occurs when the fibular fracture is located distal to the tibiofibular syndesmosis

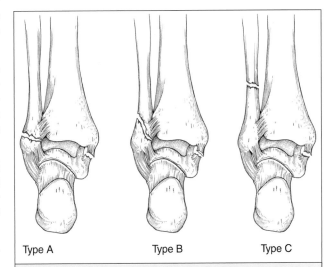

Figure 3   AO/Weber classification of ankle fractures. The staging is determined completely by the level of fibular fracture. Type A occurs below the plafond; type C starts above the plafond. *(Reproduced from Michelson JD: Ankle fractures resulting from rotational injuries. J Am Acad Orthop Surg 2003;11:403-412.)*

      ii. Injury usually occurs according to an inversion mechanism.

Table 1	
Lauge-Hansen Classification of Ankle Fractures	
Fracture Type	**Sequence of Injury**
SAD	Creates an infrasyndesmotic fibular fracture that may be associated with a vertical medial malleolar fracture and medial plafond impaction.
SER	1. Disruption of the anterior inferior tibiofibular ligament 2. Short oblique fracture of the distal fibula analogous to a Weber B-type injury. 3. Injury to the posterior malleolus or posterior tibiofibular ligament 4. Associated fracture of the medial malleolus or a deltoid ligament disruption
PER	1. Medial injury 2. Anterior tibiofibular ligament injury 3. High fibular fracture, analogous to a Weber C–type injury
PAB	1. Medial injury 2. Anterior tibiofibular ligament injury 3. Transverse or laterally comminuted fibular fracture 4. Anterolateral tibial impaction is also possible.

SAD = supination-adduction, SER = supination-external rotation, PER = pronation–external rotation, PAB = pronation-abduction

   iii. Because of the infrasyndesmotic location, Weber A fractures are less likely to result in instability.

   iv. Indications for surgery are therefore dependent on the status of the medial ankle.

  d. Weber B fracture

   i. Most common type of ankle fracture

   ii. Includes a fibular fracture beginning at approximately the level of the ankle syndesmosis (the anterior inferior tibiofibular ligament) and extending proximal and posterior

   iii. May be associated with ankle instability, depending on the status of the medial side of the ankle

  e. Weber C fracture

   i. Associated with a fibular fracture above the level of the ankle syndesmosis

   ii. Usually occurs with an external rotation mechanism

   iii. Weber C ankle fractures are generally unstable because they are usually associated with medial injury.

2. Lauge-Hansen classification (**Figures 4 and 5**)

  a. Roughly corresponds to the Weber classification

  b. In the Lauge-Hansen classification, the ankle fracture is classified according to the mechanism of injury.

   i. Two variables are described, the first being the position of the foot and the second relating to the deforming force applied to the ankle.

   ii. In a cadaveric study, most ankle fracture patterns were reproduced by placing the foot in either supination or pronation and then applying deforming forces in abduction, adduction, or external rotation.

   iii. When the foot is supinated, the medial deltoid ligament is relaxed and the initial injury is lateral.

   iv. When the foot is pronated, the deltoid ligament is tense, and the initial injury occurs medially as either a medial malleolar fracture or deltoid ligament disruption.

  c. The Lauge-Hansen classification describes four major fracture types—supination-adduction (SAD), supination-external rotation (SER), pronation-external rotation (PER), and pronation-abduction (PAB). In each of these, the initial injury is followed in a predictable sequence of further injury to other structures around the ankle (**Table 1**).

  d. As in the Weber classification, the Lauge-Hansen classification requires that particular attention be paid to the specific characteristics of the fibular fracture.

  e. The Lauge-Hansen classification was first designed to assist in determining the forces required to obtain and maintain a closed reduction of an ankle fracture; however, this classification continues to assist with understanding the mechanism of injury of rotational ankle fractures.

H. Nonsurgical treatment

1. Nonsurgical treatment of ankle fractures remains the standard of care in many situations.

2. In stable fibular fractures without associated medial injury, closed treatment leads to excellent function in most cases.

  a. When the fracture is stable, a short leg cast or functional brace can be applied for 4 to 6 weeks.

  b. Weight bearing is permitted when symptoms allow.

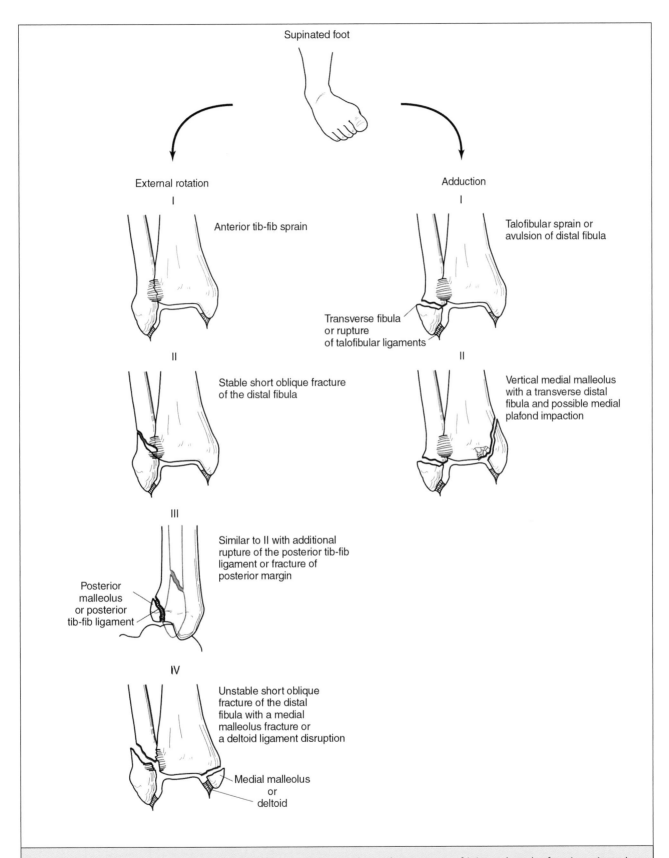

Figure 4   Lauge-Hansen classification of ankle fractures. Drawing shows the sequence of injury when the foot is supinated (SER and SAD injuries). Tib-fib = tibiofibular. *(Reproduced with permission from Marsh JL, Saltzman CL: Ankle fractures, in Bucholz RW, Heckman JD [eds]: Rockwood and Green's Fractures in Adults, ed 5. Philadeplphia, PA, Lippincott Williams & Wilkins, 2001, pp 2001-2090.)*

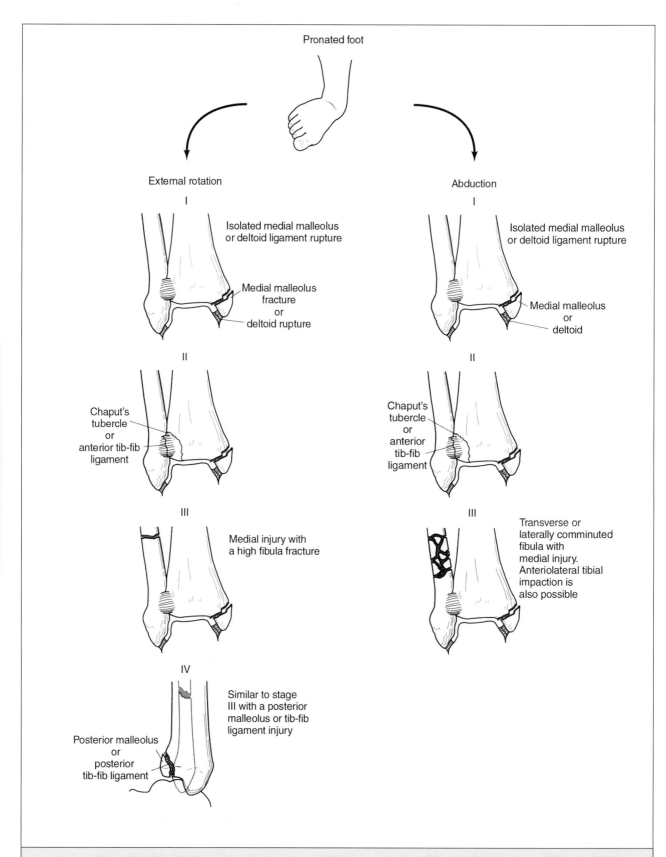

Figure 5   Lauge-Hansen classification of ankle fractures. Drawing shows the sequence of injury when the foot is pronated (PER and PAB injuries). Tib-fib = tibiofibular. *(Reproduced with permission from Marsh JL, Saltzman CL: Ankle fractures, in Bucholz RW, Heckman JD [eds]: Rockwood and Green's Fractures in Adults, ed 5. Philadeplphia, PA, Lippincott Williams & Wilkins, 2001, pp 2001-2090.)*

c. Prolonged immobilization and casting is not necessary.

d. Some studies have reported good results using a simple supportive high–top shoe or elastic bandage.

3. Unstable fractures

a. With an unstable fracture, nonsurgical treatment requires frequent follow-up.

b. Radiographic confirmation that the talus has remained reduced in the mortise is required.

c. Casting and non–weight bearing for a minimum of 4 weeks is required to prevent the ankle from displacing; even so, maintaining the reduction is difficult and has several disadvantages.

i. Prolonged casting presents challenges for elderly or infirm patients.

ii. As swelling diminishes, the reduction may be lost.

iii. Despite the disadvantages, in selected cases such as neuropathic patients or patients too unwell to tolerate surgery, casting is useful.

I. Surgical treatment

1. General issues

a. Surgical treatment is indicated for unstable ankle fractures.

b. Distal tibiofibular diastasis also requires reduction and fixation.

c. The timing of surgery is important.

d. A closed reduction may assist with the resolution of swelling and help to avoid further articular damage.

e. Temporary immobilization and elevation are useful for allowing swelling to resolve.

f. At the time of surgery, perioperative antibiotics are required, and a pneumatic tourniquet to assist with visualization of the surgical field is helpful.

2. Lateral malleolus

a. Fixation of the fibular fracture is usually performed before treatment of the medial or posterior malleolus or syndesmosis. Fixation of the fibula provides stability to the ankle and restores length. Exceptions to the "fibula first" strategy:

i. When the fibular fracture is extensively comminuted, in which case stabilization of the medial side first may assist with positioning the talus within the mortise, therefore helping to achieve an anatomic reduction of the fibula

ii. In many supination–adduction mechanisms, fixation of the fibula provides assistance with stability but is not adequate to reduce the talus within the mortise.

b. Reduction of the fibula may be achieved directly, or indirectly with traction or a push/pull distraction technique.

c. Typically the fibular fracture is stabilized with a one third tubular plate, contoured to the lateral or posterolateral fibula with an additional lag screw to provide fracture compression.

d. Use of a posterior antiglide plate is useful for a very distal fibular fracture, a fracture associated with a posterior dislocation, or osteopenic bone.

e. A posterior plate provides stable fixation in antiglide or buttress mode, even without the use of distal screws.

f. The proximal portion of the plate is fixed with bicortical screws placed from posterior to anterior.

i. Should screws be needed in the distal fragment, they can be placed from posterior to anterior without penetrating the ankle joint.

ii. A lag screw can be placed from posterior to anterior through the plate or, alternatively, from anterior to posterior.

iii. Long oblique fractures of the fibula can be stabilized with lag screws only.

iv. At minimum, two screws placed at least 1 cm apart are required.

v. Additional lag screws or a greater span between the screws provides more stable fixation.

3. Medial malleolus

a. The medial malleolus can be stabilized using a variety of techniques, depending on the fracture pattern.

b. Most fractures are oblique and can be stabilized with two 4.0-mm partially threaded cancellous screws.

i. Exceptions include the anterior colliculus fracture, which can occur with a deep deltoid ligament rupture.

ii. Stabilizing the anterior colliculus may not restore ankle stability.

c. Vertical shear fractures can be associated with articular impaction that may require reduction and bone grafting; as well, antiglide or buttress plate fixation of the vertical shear fracture may be necessary.

4. Posterior malleolus

a. Posterior malleolar fractures involving >25% of the articular surface, or associated with posterior subluxation following fixation of the fibula, require reduction and fixation.

b. The posterior malleolus can be reduced using either direct or indirect techniques.

c. The posterolateral approach described previously is useful for directly visualizing the extra-articular fracture line and facilitates placement of a posterior-to-anterior lag screw or buttress plate.

d. If indirect reduction is used, a reduction tenaculum is placed posteriorly through the fibular incision and anteriorly through a separate small anterior incision.

i. Care should be taken to spread the soft tissues and avoid injuring the vulnerable anterior structures.

ii. A percutaneous anterior-to-posterior screw can then be inserted in lag mode, using fluoroscopic control.

e. Partially threaded screws require care to insert so that the screw threads cross the fracture line for smaller posterior fragments.

5. Tibiofibular syndesmosis

a. Injuries to the tibiofibular syndesmosis are common with rotational ankle injuries.

b. Following fixation of the lateral malleolus, all external rotation and eversion ankle fractures should be evaluated fluoroscopically because syndesmotic instability may be present.

c. Although more common with higher fibular fractures, approximately one third of SER-type ankle fractures are associated with syndesmotic instability after fibular fixation.

d. The syndesmosis is typically stabilized with one or two screws inserted from the fibula into the tibia. The most distal screw should be inserted at the superior margin of the syndesmosis.

e. An accurate anatomic reduction of the syndesmosis is required; overcompression and widening of the syndesmosis as well as anterior translation of the fibula can occur.

f. Achieving an accurate reduction is even more critical when only syndesmosis fixation is used, such as for a proximal fibular fracture associated with interosseous membrane disruption, ankle instability, and fibular shortening. In this instance, an accurate restoration of fibular length and alignment is required before placement of the syndesmosis screw.

g. A variety of implants have been used successfully to stabilize the syndesmosis, including one or two screws, 3.5-mm and 4.5-mm screws, and bioabsorbable implants.

h. Screws can engage either three or four cortices.

i. Screws that engage all four cortices may be more likely to break.

ii. The indications for screw removal remain controversial; however, it seems most important to leave the screws in long enough to ensure ligamentous healing has occurred to prevent redisplacement.

6. Pearls and pitfalls are listed in **Table 2**.

J. Rehabilitation

1. Following fracture fixation, the limb is placed in a bulky cotton dressing incorporating a plaster splint.

2. Progression to weight bearing is based on the fracture pattern, stability of fixation, patient compliance, and philosophy of the surgeon.

K. Complications

1. Nonunion

a. Nonunion is rare and usually involves the medial malleolus when treated closed, associated with residual fracture displacement, interposed soft tissue, or associated lateral instability resulting in shear stresses across the deltoid ligament.

b. If symptomatic, it may be treated with open reduction and internal fixation or electrical stimulation.

c. Excision of the fragment may be necessary if not amenable to internal fixation and the patient is symptomatic.

2. Malunion

a. The lateral malleolus is usually shortened and malrotated.

b. Widened medial clear space and large posterior malleolar fragment are most predictive of poor outcome.

c. The medial malleolus may heal in an elongated position, resulting in residual instability.

3. Wound problems

a. Skin edge necrosis occurs in 3% of patients.

b. Risk is decreased with minimal swelling, no tourniquet, and good soft-tissue technique.

Table 2	
Pearls and Pitfalls of Ankle Fractures	
Site of Fracture	**Pearls**
Lateral malleolus	Restore fibular length. Avoid injury to the superficial peroneal nerve. Fix fibula first unless comminuted PAB mechanism. Check syndesmosis.
Medial malleolus	2 × 4.0-mm partial threaded screws perpendicular to fracture Vertical shear: plate, reduce joint surface Tension band for small fragments
Posterior malleolus	Fix if >25% of articular surface involved
Tibiofibular syndesmosis	Check after fibular fixation. Ensure the fibula is reduced. Leave screws in at least 3 months.

PAB = pronation-abduction

c. In fractures that are operated on in the presence of fracture blisters or abrasions, the complication rate is more than doubled.

4. Infection

a. Occurs in <2% of closed fractures

b. Leave implants in situ if stable, even with deep infection. The implant may be removed after the fracture unites.

c. May require serial débridements with possible arthrodesis as a salvage procedure

5. Posttraumatic arthritis

a. Occurs secondary to damage at the time of injury, altered mechanics, or as a result of inadequate reduction

b. Rare in anatomically reduced fractures, with increasing incidence with articular incongruity

6. Reflex sympathetic dystrophy (rare)—May be minimized by anatomic restoration of the ankle and early return to function.

7. Compartment syndrome of foot (rare)

8. Tibiofibular synostosis—Associated with the use of a syndesmotic screw and is usually asymptomatic.

9. Loss of reduction—Found in 25% of unstable ankle injuries treated nonsurgically.

10. Loss of ankle range of motion

II. Tibial Plafond Fractures

A. Epidemiology

1. A plafond fracture is a distal tibial fracture with intra-articular extension.

2. Tibial plafond fractures account for less than 10% of lower extremity injuries.

3. The average patient age is 35 to 40 years.

4. These injuries are more common in males than in females.

5. The most common mechanisms of injury include motor–vehicle collisions or falls from a height.

6. These fractures appear to be increasing in incidence, similar to other severe lower extremity fractures.

B. Anatomy

1. In the distal part of the calf, the medial border of the tibia lies directly subcutaneously, with a thin layer of skin and subcutaneous tissue covering the bone.

2. Anterior to the tibia lie the tendons of the anterior compartment as well as the anterior tibial vessels and deep peroneal nerve.

3. The fibula sits laterally and relatively posterior to the tibia; in general, only one quarter to one third of the fibula sits anterior to the midline of the tibia.

4. In the posterolateral position lie the peroneal tendons. Directly posterior to the tibia lie the flexor tendons, the Achilles tendon, and the posterior tibial artery and nerve.

5. Fracture anatomy

a. Fractures of the tibial plafond assume a varying course within the cartilage of the distal bone.

b. Fractures may include an impaction of the anterior articular surface, posterior articular surface, or both, as well as central impaction of the articular surface, depending on the exact direction of injury.

c. Careful evaluation of the direction and orientation of the fracture patterns is essential when determining the optimal surgical approach.

C. Surgical approaches

1. Rüedi and Allgöwer described surgical approaches to the distal tibia and fibula: open reduction and internal fixation of the fibula using a lateral approach, and open reduction and internal fixation of the tibia through a medial approach. Over time, this surgical technique has evolved to

6: Trauma

avoid some of the soft-tissue complications potentially associated with open reduction and internal fixation.

2. Some approaches to the distal tibia include skin incisions that do not pass directly over the thin subcutaneous skin of the medial subcutaneous border of the tibia.

3. The anterolateral approach may be useful, particularly when fractures are impacted in valgus and when the fibula is intact or is associated with a very proximal injury.

   a. The anterolateral approach incision is just lateral to the anterior compartment tendons and neurovascular structures and crosses the ankle.

   b. This incision may be long or short as necessary to facilitate reduction.

   c. The superficial peroneal nerve may be at risk with this incision and needs to be carefully avoided.

   d. The skin incision for the anteromedial approach may be placed more anteriorly just adjacent to the anterior tibial tendon to avoid placing this incision directly over the subcutaneous border of the tibia.

   e. The presence of soft-tissue injury and blisters may preclude the use of an anteromedial approach.

   f. When performed, the anteromedial approach should be done with great care to avoid unnecessarily risking further soft-tissue compromise.

4. The lateral incision to the fibula is placed slightly more posteriorly in the case of a tibial plafond fracture. This facilitates a larger skin bridge between the fibular incision and that used for placement of tibial fixation.

   a. Placement of the incision posterior to the peroneal tendons may facilitate visualization, reduction, and fixation of the posterior articular surface of the tibia as well.

   b. This incision courses between the peroneal tendons and the Achilles tendon, care must be taken to protect the sural nerve.

5. External fixation is also described for fractures of the ankle and distal tibia.

   a. The medial subcutaneous border of the tibia is a safe position for wires, and transfibular wires may be safe.

   b. If spanning temporary external fixation is used, the external fixation pins should be placed remote from the fracture site to avoid interference with definitive internal fixation.

D. Mechanism of injury

1. Axial compression—Fall from a height

   a. The force is directed axially through the talus into the tibial plafond, causing impaction of the articular surface; may be associated with significant comminution.

   b. If the fibula remains intact, the ankle is forced into varus with impaction of the medial plafond.

   c. Plantar flexion or dorsiflexion of the ankle at the time of injury results in a primarily posterior or anterior plafond injury, respectively.

2. Shear—Skiing accident

   a. This mechanism is primarily torsion combined with a varus or valgus stress.

   b. It produces two or more large fragments and minimal articular comminution.

   c. There is usually an associated fibular fracture, which is usually transverse or short oblique.

3. Combined compression and shear

   a. These fracture patterns demonstrate components of both compression and shear.

   b. The vector of the two forces determines the fracture pattern.

E. Clinical evaluation

1. Clinical evaluation of fractures of the tibial plafond includes an examination of the neurologic and vascular status of the entire limb.

2. It is useful to examine the stability and alignment of the ankle joint, observing the orientation of the ankle, including its length, alignment, and rotation.

3. The skin may be placed at risk by bone fragments causing pressure on the skin and soft-tissue envelope, and therefore areas of blanching, abrasion, and contusion should be examined.

4. Large blood-filled fracture blisters should be noted, as they frequently preclude immediate open reduction and internal fixation.

F. Radiographic evaluation

1. Plain radiographs

   a. Standard radiographs of the ankle include AP lateral, and mortise view radiographs centered on the joint.

   b. The AP view demonstrates the amount of articular impaction and shortening; the lateral view also demonstrates articular incongruity and is useful for determining the position of the posterior articular segment.

   c. Full-length views of the entire tibia and fibula rule out more proximal injury and assess the extent of metadiaphyseal involvement.

2. Computed tomography

   a. CT is very useful for tibial plafond fractures.

   b. CT aids in identifying fracture fragments not seen on plain radiographs, assists in determining the extent of articular comminution, and is critical for planning surgery and guiding surgical approaches.

   c. CT may assist the surgeon in determining whether a fracture can be reduced percutaneously or whether an open approach is required.

   d. If temporary external fixation is planned, a CT scan done following application of the external fixator and realignment of the limb provides the best information.

G. Classification

   1. There is no universally accepted classification of tibial plafond fractures.

   2. Important characteristics to consider include articular and metaphyseal comminution, shortening of the tibia resulting in proximal displacement of the talus, impaction of individual or multiple joint fragments, and associated soft-tissue injury.

   3. A wide variation in fracture patterns can result, related to the position of the foot and the precise direction and magnitude of the force applied.

   4. The Rüedi-Allgöwer classification considers three variations of tibial plafond fractures (**Figure 6**).

      a. Type I fractures—Nondisplaced

      b. Type II fractures—Displaced but minimally comminuted

      c. Type III fractures—Highly comminuted and displaced. The comminution and displacement of this classification refers to the articular surface.

   5. The OTA classification system is more precise (**Figure 7**).

      a. Distal tibial fractures are divided into type A fractures, which are extra-articular; type B, or partial articular fractures; and type C, or total articular fractures.

      b. Each category is further subdivided into three groups based upon the amount and degree of comminution.

      c. Other characteristics of the fracture, such as the location and direction of fracture lines or the presence of metaphyseal impaction, are also included in further subdivisions.

      d. Types B, C1, C2, and C3 are the fractures commonly considered to be tibial plafond fractures.

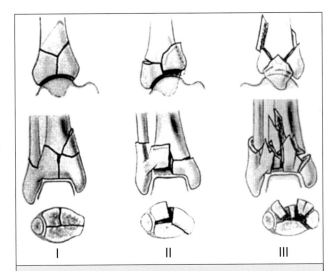

Figure 6 Rüedi-Allgöwer classification of tibial plafond fractures. *(Reproduced with permission from Rüedi TP, Allgöwer M: Fractures of the lower end of the tibia into the ankle joint: Results 9 years after open reduction.* Injury *1973;5:130.)*

6. The soft-tissue injury is also important. The most vulnerable skin for tibial plafond fractures is the anteromedial side of the tibia.

   a. Grade 0—Closed fractures without appreciable soft-tissue injury.

   b. Grade 1—Abrasions or contusions of skin and subcutaneous tissue.

   c. Grade 2—A deep abrasion with some muscle involvement

   d. Grade 3—Extensive soft-tissue damage and severe muscle injury. Compartment syndrome and arterial rupture are also considered grade 3 injuries.

H. Nonsurgical treatment

   1. Nonsurgical care is less common for tibial plafond fractures than for ankle fractures.

   2. Indications

      a. Stable fracture patterns without displacement of the articular surface are treated nonsurgically because nonsurgical treatment of fractures with articular displacement has generally yielded poor results.

      b. Nonambulatory patients or patients with significant neuropathy may be treated nonsurgically as well.

   3. Nonsurgical treatment consists of a long leg cast for 6 weeks followed by a fracture brace and range-of-motion exercises versus early range-of-motion exercises.

      a. Manipulation of displaced fractures is unlikely

6: Trauma

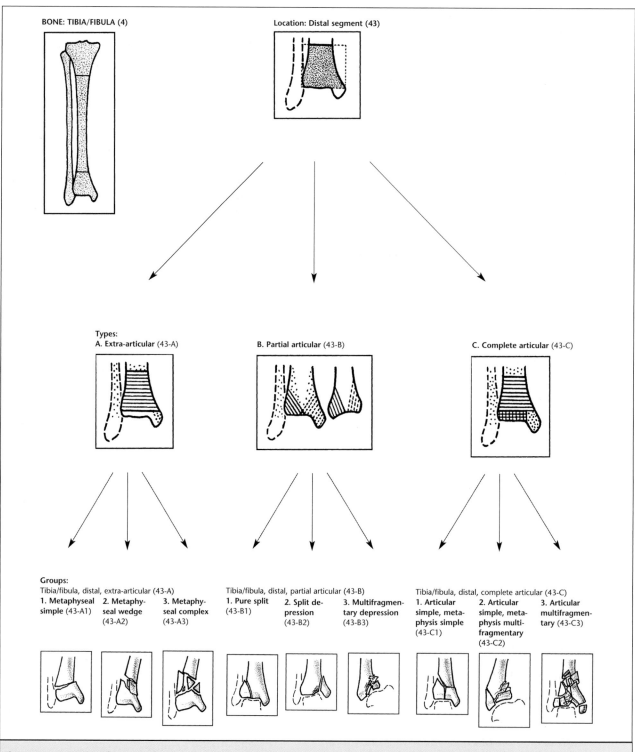

Figure 7 OTA classification of distal tibial fractures. Type A fractures are extra-articular, type B are partial articular, and type C are total articular. Types B3, C1, C2, and C3 are the fractures commonly considered tibial plafond fractures.

to result in reduction of intra-articular fragments.

b. Loss of reduction is common.

c. Inability to monitor soft-tissue status and swelling is a major disadvantage.

I. Surgical treatment

1. Most treatment strategies for tibial plafond fractures currently are related to safe management of the soft tissues.

2. Either external or internal fixation is used.

3. External fixation—As definitive treatment, uses limited approaches to reduce the articular surface with minimal internal fixation of the joint surface.

   a. General

      i. May bridge the ankle or may be localized to the distal tibia

      ii. External fixation that spans the ankle may involve less disruption of the zone of injury but has the disadvantage of rigidly immobilizing the ankle.

      iii. External fixation applied to a single side of the ankle joint allows greater motion at the ankle. However, it cannot be used for all fractures, and in this case, the placement of pins and wires will commonly disrupt the zone of injury.

      iv. An additional alternative includes articulated fixation, which allows some motion at the ankle but may be difficult to apply because the axis of the hinge of the fixator must correspond to the axis of the ankle joint.

   b. Techniques for application of definitive external fixation

      i. When using an ankle bridging technique, pins are placed initially in the calcaneus and talar neck while proximal pins are placed in the medial subcutaneous border of the tibia.

      ii. A fixator is then placed and the articular surface is provisionally reduced with ligamentotaxis.

      iii. Fracture reduction forceps or clamps can then be placed percutaneously directly over the fracture lines to reduce displaced fragments.

      iv. Articular fragments are stabilized using lag screws.

      v. The external fixator is used to maintain length, alignment, and rotation of the extremity and to protect the joint as fracture healing occurs.

      vi. This technique preserves soft tissues and can be performed on a staged basis if necessary when the zone of injury is felt to be unsafe to tolerate the limited approaches required for reduction.

4. Internal fixation

   a. General

      i. Internal fixation using definitive plate fixation of high-energy tibial plafond fractures continues to evolve.

      ii. Initial successes using this technique described by Rüedi and Allgöwer were followed by many reports of failure with the incidence of wound complications approaching 40% in large series of patients sustaining high-energy tibial plafond fractures.

   b. Techniques

      i. Various techniques have been recommended for minimizing the complications of plating, including delaying definitive surgical treatment using spanning external fixation until the soft tissues have settled; use of lower profile implants; avoiding anteromedial incisions; indirect reduction techniques that minimize soft-tissue stripping; patient selection based upon the injury pattern as necessary.

      ii. With consideration of these principles, the rate of wound complications reported in more recent series ranges from 0% to 6%.

      iii. The use of locked plates and percutaneously applied plates may also be of use to further improve results.

   c. Definitive internal fixation—Performed in stages.

      i. Stage 1—Includes fibular plating to regain lateral column length and application of a simple spanning external fixator.

        (a) Two proximal half-pins placed on the anterior tibia are used.

        (b) Care should be taken to keep these pins well proximal to the fracture line to avoid compromising definitive fixation.

        (c) A 5- or 6-mm centrally threaded pin can be placed across the calcaneus and attached to the proximal half-pins using a combination of struts. This technique is simple to apply and maintains stability and alignment. Extra care is necessary to avoid pressure from bony fragments on soft tissues, prevent shortening, and maintain forefoot positioning.

      ii. Typically a delay of approximately 2 weeks then ensues, to allow the soft tissues to settle.

      iii. Stage 2—Includes formal articular reduction and internal fixation.

        (a) Once open reduction and internal fixation is performed, incisions are only as large as required to anatomically reduce the articular surface. Periosteal stripping is performed only at the edges of the fracture to achieve visualization of the reduction while preserving blood supply.

Table 3

Pearls and Pitfalls of Tibial Plafond Fractures

Treatment Step	Pearls
Soft-tissue management	Avoid surgery when swollen Use spanning fixator to control alignment and soft tissues
Spanning fixator	Simple construct Tibial pins should avoid future surgical site Reestablish length and alignment
Definitive open reduction and internal fixation	Approach guided by CT Limited incisions, avoid periosteal stripping Restore alignment and anatomically reduce joint. Use distractor intraoperatively to facilitate reduction. Low-profile implants

(b) Precontoured plates may be useful; both anteromedial and anterolateral plates facilitate percutaneous placement. Locking plates may be of benefit, particularly when articular surface comminution is present.

(c) Bone grafting with bone graft substitutes or chips of allograft to fill metaphyseal voids was once described as a standard step in fixation of a tibial plafond fracture; however, with less extensive dissection in the metaphyseal region, the indications for grafting have become less routine.

5. Pearls and pitfalls are described in **Table 3**.

J. Rehabilitation

1. Rehabilitation of tibial plafond fractures is prolonged, and patients should be counseled that weight bearing may be contraindicated for 3 months or more.

2. In patients treated by external fixation, the healing time has generally been 12 to 16 weeks.

3. Tibial plafond fractures have a significant deleterious long-term effect on patients' ankle function and quality of life. Worse outcomes are seen if complications occur.

4. Where possible, motion of the ankle joint should be permitted and facilitated.

5. The use of a removable boot or brace may be of benefit as the patient transitions from immobilization and non–weight bearing to mobilization and protected weight-bearing status.

K. Complications

1. Malunion

   a. Malalignment of the tibia is relatively common.

   b. Articular malunion is probably even more common than recognized.

   c. Series using definitive external fixation have reported an increased incidence of fair or poor articular reduction compared with formal open reduction and internal fixation.

   d. Angular malalignment may also occur. Loss of alignment following treatment occurs in particular if union is delayed and implant failure occurs.

2. Nonunion and delayed union

   a. The rate of delayed union and nonunion for tibial plafond fractures is difficult to determine because surgical implants obscure radiographic visualization of the fracture.

   b. Some series report nonunion rates of approximately 5%.

   c. It is likely that more comminuted fractures, and those with greater devascularization of the fracture fragments, are more likely to lead to nonunion, and for this reason soft-tissue dissection should be minimized.

3. Infection and wound breakdown

   a. Infection and wound breakdown is a devastating complication.

   b. Wound breakdown is almost always severe and frequently leads to unfavorable outcomes.

   c. The cost of treating this complication is extremely high because multiple surgical procedures are required and amputation may be the result.

   d. Although the use of modern techniques of soft-tissue preservation whenever possible appears to have substantially decreased the rate of infection and wound breakdown, some risk of infection and wound breakdown remains, and patients should be counseled regarding this risk before undertaking surgical treatment of the tibial plafond fracture.

4. Ankle arthritis

   a. Significant arthrosis of the ankle joint is common after tibial plafond fractures.

      i. In one study, arthrosis was found in 74% of patients from 5 to 11 years postinjury.

      ii. Arthrosis most commonly begins within 1 or 2 years postinjury.

   b. The presence of radiographic arthritis does not

always correlate well with subjective clinical results, and despite the devastating impact to the articular surface and problems associated

with fracture of the tibial plafond, arthrodesis is not commonly required until many years after the injury.

Top Testing Facts

1. The talar dome is wider anteriorly than posteriorly.

2. The superficial deltoid arises from the anterior colliculus and the deep deltoid from the posterior colliculus of the medial malleolus.

3. According to the Ottawa ankle rules, ankle radiographs are indicated if the patient has an ankle injury and is older than 55 years, unable to bear weight, or has tenderness at the posterior edge or tip of either malleolus.

4. Fractures of the fibula are usually fixed prior to the medial malleolus, lateral malleolus, or syndesmosis in order to obtain length

5. Exceptions to the "fibula first" rule include (1) extensively comminuted fibular fractures in which stabilization at the medial side first may facilitate positioning of the talus within the mortise an d(2) supination-adduction injuries.

6. An SER type IV injury is associated with an unstable short oblique fracture at the distal fibula and a medial malleolus fracture or deltoid ligament disruption.

7. Posterior malleolar fractures involving >25% of the articular surface should be reduced and stabilized.

8. Tibial plafond (pilon) fractures result from either axial compression or shear.

9. Internal fixation of high-energy tibial plafond fractures usually should be achieved approximately 2 weeks after the injury, preceded by a period of temporary external fixation.

10. The superficial peroneal nerve may be injured when using an anterolateral approach to treat a tibial plafond fracture.

Bibliography

Brage ME, Bennett CR, Whitehurst JB, Getty PJ, Toledano A: Observer reliability in ankle radiographic measurements. *Foot Ankle Int* 1997;18:324-329.

Court-Brown CM, Walker C, Garg A, et al: Half-ring external fixation in the management of tibial plafond fractures. *J Orthop Trauma* 1999;13:200-206.

Egol KA, Amirtharajah M, Tejwani NC, Capla EL, Koval KJ: Ankle stress test for predicting the need for surgical fixation of isolated fibular fractures. *J Bone Joint Surg Am* 2004;86: 2393-2398.

Honkanen R, Tuppurainen M, Kroger H, et al: Relationships between risk factors in fractures differ by type of fracture: A population based study of 12,192 perimenopausal women. *Osteoporos Int* 1998;8:25-31.

Jenkinson RJ, Sanders DW, Macleod MD, Domonkos A, Lydestadt J: Intraoperative diagnosis of syndesmosis injuries in external rotation ankle fractures. *J Orthop Trauma* 2005;19: 604-609.

Kannus P, Palvanenm P, Niemi S, et al: Increasing number and incidence of low trauma ankle fractures in elderly people: Finnish statistics during 1970 to 2000 and projections for the future. *Bone* 2002;31:430-433.

Koval KJ, Lurie J, Zhou W, et al: Ankle fractures in the elderly: What you get depends on where you live and who you see. *J Orthop Trauma* 2005;19:635-639.

Lauge-Hansen N: Fractures of the ankle: Combined experimental-surgical and experimental roentgenologic investigations. *Arch Surg* 1950;60:957-985.

Makwana NK, Bhowal B, Harper WM, Hui AW: Conservative versus operative treatment for displaced ankle fractures in patients over 55 years of age: A prospective, randomized study. *J Bone Joint Surg Br* 2001;83:525-529.

McConnell T, Creevy W, Tornetta P III: Stress examination of supination external rotation-type fibular fractures. *J Bone Joint Surg Am* 2004;86:2171-2178.

Michelson JD, Varner KE, Checcone M: Diagnosing deltoid injury in ankle fractures: The gravity stress view. *Clin Orthop Relat Res* 2001;387:178-182.

Patterson MJ, Cole JD: Two-stage delayed open reduction and internal fixation of severe pilon fractures. *J Orthop Trauma* 1999;13:85-91.

Pollak AN, McCarthy ML, Bess RS, et al: Outcomes after treatment of high-energy tibial plafond fractures. *J Bone Joint Surg Am* 2003;85:1893-1900.

Sirkin M, Sanders R, DiPasquale T, et al: A staged protocol for soft tissue management in the treatment of complex pilon fractures. *J Orthop Trauma* 1999;13:78-84.

Stiell IG, McKnight RD, Greenburg GH, et al: Implementation of the Ottawa rules. *JAMA* 1994;271:827-832.

Steill I, Wells G, Laupacis A, et al: Multi-centred trial to introduce the Ottawa rules for use for radiography in acute ankle injuries: Multi-centred ankle study group. *BMJ* 1995;311: 594-597.

Tornetta P III: Competence of the deltoid ligament in bimalleolar ankle fractures after medial malleolar fixation. *J Bone Joint Surg Am* 2000;82:843-848.

Tornetta P III, Creevy W: Lag screw only fixation of the lateral malleolus. *J Orthop Trauma* 2001;15:119-121.

Tornetta P III, Weiner L, Bergman M, et al: Pilon fractures: Treatment with combined internal and external fixation. *J Orthop Trauma* 1993;7:489-496.

6: Trauma

Chapter 61

Nonunions, Osteomyelitis, and Limb Deformity Analysis

*David W. Lowenberg, MD

I. Nonunions

A. Definitions

1. Nonunions—A nonunion represents an arrest of the bone healing process. Classically, nonunion of a long bone is defined by the US Food and Drug Administration as a fracture that has failed to show progressive evidence of healing over a 4- to 6-month period. In reality, once a fracture has lost the potential to progress with healing, it is a nonunion.

2. Delayed unions—Delayed union has been defined as a fracture that has failed to achieve full bony union by 6 months after the injury. This definition generally applies to long bones, however, and is therefore incomplete. To include fractures that would generally heal much more quickly (eg, distal radial fractures), the definition of a delayed union is now a fracture taking longer to show progression toward healing than would normally be expected.

3. Fractures with large segmental defects—These fractures clearly are functionally nonunions from the time of the injury and should be treated as such.

B. Etiology

1. Common factors—Often the cause of nonunions is multifactorial; however, there are usually a host of common denominators that contribute to the development of a nonunion (**Table 1**). Of all potential causes, inadequate fracture stabilization and lack of adequate blood supply are the most common.

2. Infection—Infection in and of itself does not preclude a fracture from healing; however, it can certainly be a contributing factor to a fracture failing to progress to union. Clearly, even if the fracture does heal, the osteomyelitis must be treated. Hence, eradicating infection should be a concomitant goal along with achieving bony union.

3. Fracture location—Location of the fracture can be an important contributing factor, as certain areas of the skeleton (eg, carpal navicular, distal tibal diaphyseal-metaphyseal junction, proximal diaphysis of the fifth metatarsal) are more prone to the development of nonunion.

4. Fracture pattern—Fracture pattern can influence the development of nonunion, especially when the fracture occurs in the diaphysis of a long bone. Segmental fractures and fractures with large butterfly fragments are more prone to nonunion, probably because of devascularization of the intermediary segment.

C. Evaluation

1. History

Table 1

Causes of Nonunion

I. Excess motion: Due to inadequate immobilization
II. Gap between fragments
  A. Soft tissue interposition
  B. Distraction by traction or hardware
  C. Malposition, overriding, or displacement of fragments
  D. Loss of bone substance
III. Loss of blood supply
  A. Damage to nutrient vessels
  B. Excessive stripping or injury to periosteum and muscle
  C. Free fragments, severe comminution
  D. Avascularity due to hardware
IV. Infection (?)
  A. Bone death (sequestrum)
  B. Osteolysis (gap)
  C. Loosening of implants (motion)
V. General—Age, nutrition, steroids, anticoagulants, radiation, burns, etc, predispose but do not cause nonunion

(Reproduced with permission from Rosen H: Treatment of nonunions: General principles, in Chapman MW [ed]: Operative Orthopaedics, Philadelphia, PA, JB Lippincott, 1988, p 491.)

David W. Lowenberg, MD, is a consultant for or an employee of Stryker and Biotech.

6: Trauma

Table 2

Forces Involved in Four Common Mechanisms of Injury*

Fall off curb	100 ft-lb
Skiing (20 mph)	300-500 ft-lb
Gunshot wound	2,000 ft-lb
Bumper injury (20 mph)	100,000 ft-lb

*Based on the equation $E = 1/2mv^2$
(Adapted with permission from Chapman M, Yaremchuk MJ, et al: Acute and definitive management of traumatic and osteocutaneous defects of the lower extremity. Plast Reconstr Surg 1987;80:1.)

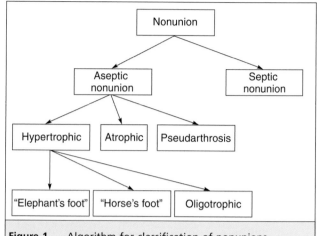

Figure 1   Algorithm for classification of nonunions.

a. The mechanism of injury (**Table 2**), prior surgical as well as nonsurgical interventions, host quality (ie, underlying metabolic, nutritional, or immunologic disease), and use of nonsteroidal anti-inflammatory drugs (NSAIDs) or tobacco are vital factors in determining proper treatment of the patient.

b. Additional important factors are pain at the fracture site with axial loading of the involved extremity, as well as motion at the fracture site perceived by the patient.

2. Physical examination

a. The examination should include a detailed evaluation of distal pulses and patency of vessels as well as motor and sensory function in the limb.

b. Actual mobility of the nonunion, or lack thereof, is another important factor in deciding on treatment.

c. The limb should be evaluated for deformity, including rotational deformity and any resultant limb-length discrepancy, as this might affect treatment decisions.

3. Imaging studies

a. High-quality radiographs are the gold standard in evaluating fracture healing. To assess for a nonunion, four views of the limb segment in question are the first essential study.

b. If these radiographs fail to clearly determine union, then a CT scan with reformations reconstruction can be quite helpful. The value of CT can be diminished, however, if there is significant hardware at the fracture site.

c. If limb-length discrepancy or deformity is a potential issue in the lower limb, a 51-in, full-length, weight-bearing view of both lower extremities is required.

d. Bone scanning can be a helpful adjuvant; however, it is rarely used as a sole determinant of whether a nonunion exists.

4. Laboratory studies—If deep infection or chronic osteomyelitis is suspected, then screening laboratory studies (complete blood cell count [CBC], erythrocyte sedimentation rate [ESR], and C-reactive protein [CRP]) are warranted.

D. Classification—An algorithm for basic classification of nonunions is provided in **Figure 1**.

E. General treatment issues—Nontreatment is a viable option in a small percentage of patients because some nonunions can be asymptomatic (eg, hypertrophic clavicular shaft nonunions). Also, in some instances, the treatment can cause greater morbidity than the consequences of leaving the nonunion untreated.

F. Nonsurgical treatment

1. Fracture brace immobilization with axial loading of the limb is a viable treatment option for certain rigid/stable nonunions.

2. Bone growth stimulators (inductive or capacitive coupling devices) are an option in some patients. Published controlled clinical studies remain scarce, however, and the use of these devices is essentially limited to the United States. Clear contraindications to electrical stimulation include synovial pseudarthroses, mobile nonunions, and a fracture gap >1 cm.

G. Surgical treatment—The basic goal of surgery for nonunions is to create a favorable environment for fracture healing. This includes stable fixation with preservation of blood supply to the bone and soft-tissue envelope, the minimization of shear forces, especially in nonunions with a high degree of fracture obliquity, and good bony apposition.

1. Hypertrophic nonunions

a. The defining factor in hypertrophic nonunions is that they have viable bone ends; these are usually stiff in nature.

b. Generally, these fractures "want to heal" and have the proper biology to heal, but they lack stable fixation.

c. Treatment is therefore generally aimed at providing appropriate stabilization and is most easily achieved with internal fixation (plates and screws, locked intramedullary rods, etc).

d. The nonunion itself does not generally need to be taken down, unless required for proper fracture reduction.

2. Oligotrophic nonunions

a. Oligotrophic nonunions are generally lacking in callus. They often resemble atrophic nonunions radiographically but in fact have viable bone ends.

b. Oligotrophic nonunions occasionally require further biologic stimulus and can behave like atrophic nonunions.

3. Atrophic nonunions

a. The defining factor in atrophic nonunions is often the presence of avascular or hypovascular bone ends. These are usually mobile, and so atrophic nonunions are often called mobile nonunions.

b. Occasionally, oligotrophic fractures that go on to nonunion because of muscle interposition can look and behave like atrophic nonunions despite having viable bone ends.

c. Treatment objectives for atrophic nonunions

i. The apposition of well-vascularized bone ends

ii. Stable fixation with the use of hardware, be it internal or multiplanar external fixation if the need exists

iii. Grafting to fill bony defects and provide osteoinductive agents to the local environment. Autogenous iliac crest bone grafting is the gold standard for osteoinductive agents. The recombinant bone morphogenetic proteins (BMPs) are promising alternatives. Other graft materials (eg, crushed cancellous allograft, demineralized allogenic bone matrix) are, for all practical purposes, osteoconductive only.

iv. Preservation or creation of a healthy, well-vascularized local soft-tissue envelope

4. Pseudarthrosis

a. A pseudarthrosis, which is in effect a "false joint," is often present if infection exists, and the bone ends are always atrophic with impaired vasculature.

b. When a pseudarthrosis is exposed surgically,

an actual joint capsule with enclosed synovial fluid is found.

c. To heal a pseudarthrosis requires complete surgical takedown with excision of the atrophic bone ends, followed by proper surgical stabilization with preservation of the remaining bone and soft-tissue vascularity.

5. Infected nonunions

a. Although infection does not prevent a fracture from healing, if a fracture goes on to a nonunion and becomes infected, the chance of healing is low if the infection is not eradicated.

b. Infected nonunions are often pseudarthroses and should be treated as such.

c. Treatment goals

i. Remove all infected and devitalized bone and soft tissue.

ii. Sterilize the local wound environment with the use of local wound management techniques (antibiotic bead pouch, vacuum-assisted closure [VAC] sponge, etc).

iii. Create healthy, bleeding bone ends with a well-vascularized soft-tissue envelope.

iv. Provide fracture stability.

d. Achieving the treatment goals most often requires a staged approach, with multiple surgeries.

e. Because the treatment often results in a significant amount of bone loss, bone transport or later limb lengthening using the Ilizarov method is often beneficial.

f. Placement of a free muscle flap can be crucial in the management of the local soft-tissue environment if the soft-tissue envelope becomes deficient after treatment or the soft-tissue envelope is overly scarred and dysvascular.

g. The surgeon must be well versed in the use of free tissue transfers to successfully treat difficult nonunions.

H. Pearls and pitfalls

1. It is best to achieve as stable a fixation as possible to allow for joint mobilization above and below the nonunion. Because these limbs have already been through much trauma, the periarticular regions are prone to stiffness.

2. A healthy, well-vascularized soft-tissue envelope is necessary for healing of tenuously vascularized diaphyseal bone ends. The generous use of free or rotational muscle transfers enhances the healing environment by providing more vascular access.

6: Trauma

3. If union fails despite optimal treatment, metabolic or other endogenous problems that can inhibit fracture healing should be sought.

   a. NSAIDs—One of the most common culprits is a patient's use of NSAIDs. These medications can inhibit fracture healing by preventing calcification of the osteoid matrix.

   b. Tobacco use—Smoking has been shown to play a role in the inhibition of bone healing, with an increased risk of nonunion in those who smoke or use tobacco-based products. Nicotine causes arteriolar vasoconstriction, thereby further inhibiting blood flow to bone and the already compromised area about an injury. This, in effect, acts as a secondary insult to the already compromised site of bone and soft-tissue injury.

II. Osteomyelitis

A. Etiology

   1. Classically, osteomyelitis occurs via hematogenous seeding or direct inoculation, most typically secondary to trauma.

   2. Hematogenous osteomyelitis (see chapter 28, Osteoarticular Infection) is most commonly seen in the pediatric population. It occurs with seeding of the bacteria at metaphyseal end arterioles.

   3. Possible pathogens include not only bacteria but also fungi and yeasts, but *Staphylococcus*, *Streptococcus*, *Enterococcus*, and *Pseudomonas* represent the preponderance of cases.

B. Types of osteomyelitis—Osteomyelitis is further subcategorized as acute or chronic.

   1. Acute osteomyelitis

      a. Acute osteomyelitis generally represents the first episode of infection of the bone.

      b. It is characterized by a rapid presentation and a rapidly evident purulent infection.

      c. Acute osteomyelitis can become chronic over time.

   2. Chronic osteomyelitis

      a. Chronic osteomyelitis can be present for decades.

      b. It can convert from a dormant to an active state without a known antecedent event or as a result of a local or systemic change in the host.

C. Biofilm-bacteria complex

   1. The biofilm-bacteria complex that develops in orthopaedic infections, whether osteomyelitis or hardware infections, makes these infections difficult to treat.

   2. The biofilm-bacteria complex is the entity comprising the bacteria in an extracellular matrix with a glycocalyx.

   3. This matrix is avascular, making it difficult for bacteria to penetrate.

D. Evaluation

   1. Clinical

      a. A draining sinus tract with abscess formation is the classic presentation of osteomyelitis. Often, the sinus tracts are multifocal in nature.

      b. In acute osteomyelitis secondary to trauma, the clinical manifestation of the disease is exposed bone or a nonhealing, soupy, soft-tissue envelope over the bone.

      c. Indolent infections might present with only chronic swelling and induration; occasionally, recurrent bouts of cellulitis accompany this.

   2. Imaging

      a. Radiographic evaluation with four views of the affected extremity is necessary to initially evaluate for osteomyelitis.

      b. Osteomyelitis can present acutely as areas of osteolysis, then chronically with areas of dense sclerotic bone because of the avascular, necrotic nature of osteomyelitic bone.

      c. When a necrotic segment of free, devascularized, infected bone is left in a limb over time, it becomes radiodense on radiographs and is called a sequestrum (**Figure 2**). Occasionally, this will be engulfed and surrounded or walled off by healthy bone; it is then called an involucrum.

   3. Laboratory studies

      a. Hematologic profiles can be useful in the workup for osteomyelitis. In chronic osteomyelitis, however, it is not uncommon for all laboratory indices to be normal.

      b. The common blood tests that should be ordered include a CBC with differential, an ESR, and a CRP.

      c. In acute osteomyelitis, an elevated white blood cell count (WBC) along with elevated platelet count, ESR, and CRP level may be present; a "left shift" of the differential is often present as well.

      d. In chronic osteomyelitis, the WBC and platelet count are usually normal. Often the ESR is normal as well, and occasionally the CRP level is also normal.

e. Surgery or trauma can also elevate the platelet count, ESR, and CRP level. In this setting, the platelet count generally returns to normal once the hemoglobin level has stabilized to a more normal range; however, the CRP value normalizes within 3 weeks, and the ESR returns to normal within 3 to 4 months.

4. Tissue culture

a. The diagnosis of osteomyelitis is dependent on obtaining appropriate culture specimens.

b. The gold standard for proper diagnosis is obtaining good tissue samples for culture. If an abscess cavity exists, this can sometimes be performed adequately with needle aspiration.

c. Appropriate bacterial and fungal plating of the specimen is of paramount importance.

E. Classification

1. The most widely accepted clinical staging system for osteomyelitis is the Cierny-Mader system (Table 3).

2. This system first considers the anatomy of the bone involvement (see Figure 3), then subclassifies the disease according to the physiologic status of the host (Table 4).

3. This staging method helps define the lesion being treated as well as the host's ability to deal with the process.

4. Prognosis has been well correlated with the physiologic host subclassification.

F. General treatment principles

1. Once the osteomyelitis has been staged and the host's condition has been defined and optimized, a treatment plan individualized to the patient's condition and goals can be determined.

2. Ideally, the goal of treatment is complete eradication of the osteomyelitis with a preserved soft-tissue envelope, a healed bone segment, and preserved limb length and function.

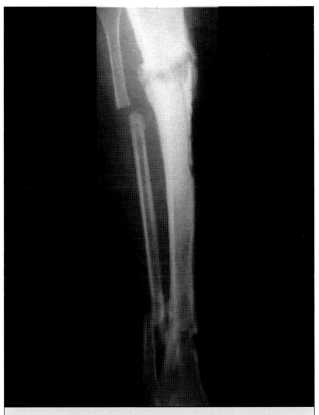

Figure 2 Radiograph of a 24-year-old male 2 years after an open tibia fracture. The dense, necrotic cortical bone at the medial border of his tibia represents a sequestrum.

6: Trauma

Table 3

Cierny-Mader Staging System for Osteomyelitis

Stage	Anatomic Type	Typical Etiology	Treatment
1	Medullary	Infected intramedullary nail	Removal of the infected implant and isolated intramedullary débridement
2	Superficial; no full-thickness involvement of cortex	Chronic wound, leading to colonization and focal involvement of a superficial area of bone under the wound	Remove layers of infected bone until viable bone is identified
3	Full-thickness involvement of a cortical segment of bone; endosteum is involved, implying intramedullary spread	Direct trauma with resultant devascularization and seeding of the bone	Noninvolved bone is present at same axial level, so the osteomyelitic portion can be excised without compromising skeletal stability.
4	Infection is permeative, involving a segmental portion of the bone.	Major devascularization with colonization of the bone	Resection leads to a segmental or near-segmental defect, resulting in loss of limb stability.

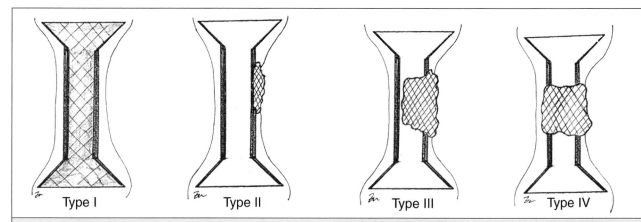

Figure 3 Schematic illustration of the Cierny-Mader anatomic classification of osteomyelitis. Type I is intramedullary osteomyelitis; type II is superficial osteomyelitis with no intramedullary involvement; type III is invasive localized osteomyelitis with intramedullary extension, but with a maintained, stable, uninvolved segment of bone at the same axial level; and type IV is invasive diffuse osteomyelitis, with involvement of an entire axial segment of bone, such that excision of the involved segment leaves a segmental defect of the limb. *(Reproduced from Ziran BH, Rao N: Infections, in Baumgaertener MR, Tornetta P III [eds]: Orthopaedic Knowledge Update: Trauma 3. American Academy of Orthopaedic Surgeons, Rosemont, IL, 2005, p 132.)*

Table 4

Physiologic Host Classification Used with the Cierny-Mader Osteomyelitis Classification System

Type	Infection Status	Factors Perpetuating Osteomyelitis	Treatment
A	Normal physiologic responses to infection	Little or no systemic or local compromise; minor trauma or surgery to affected part	No contraindications to surgical treatment
B (local)	Locally active impairment of normal physiologic responses to infection	Cellulitis, prior trauma (such as open fracture, compartment syndrome, and free flap), or surgery to area; chronic sinus; free flap	Consider healing potential of soft tissues and bone, and anticipate the need for free-tissue transfer and hyperbaric oxygen.
B (systemic)	Systemically active impairment of normal physiologic responses to infection	Diabetes, immunosuppression, vascular disease, protein deficiency, or metabolic disease	Consider healing potential of soft tissues and treat correctable metabolic or nutritional abnormalities.
C	Severe infection	Severe systemic compromise and stressors	Because treatment of condition is worse than the condition itself, suppressive treatment or amputation is recommended.

(Reproduced from Ziran BH, Rao N: Infections, in Baumgaertener MR, Tornetta P III [eds]: Orthopaedic Knowledge Update: Trauma 3. Rosemont, IL, American Academy of Orthopaedic Surgeons, 2005, p 133.)

G. Surgical treatment

1. Surgical débridement

   a. Surgical débridement is the cornerstone of osteomyelitis treatment.

   b. Aggressive débridement is often required to remove all infected and devitalized bone and tissue.

   c. The single most common mistake in treatment is inadequate débridement with residual devitalized tissue remaining in the wound bed.

   d. Débridement of any dense fibrotic scar is also necessary because this is often quite avascular and represents a poor soft-tissue bed for healing.

   e. Atrophic skin that has become adherent to the bone (eg, the medial border of the tibia) also requires débridement because of its impaired blood supply and compliance.

2. Skeletal stabilization

   a. Skeletal stabilization of the affected limb is necessary for all type 4 lesions as well as some type 3 lesions where a large amount of bone has been removed.

b. Stabilization is most often accomplished with external fixation or a short course of external fixation followed by internal fixation. It also can be accomplished with antibiotic bone cement–impregnated nails.

c. If a segmental defect is created with the débridement, then proper planning in skeletal stabilization must occur from the start, with a clear and comprehensive plan established to gain bony stability of the limb.

d. For small defects (<2 cm), acute shortening remains a reasonable option for treatment; defects can also be stabilized with rods or plates once infection is eradicated, then the defect eliminated with bone grafting or osteomyocutaneous free tissue transfer.

e. For some large osseous defects, the best option remains bone transport.

3. Dead space management

a. Débridement creates a dead space; this space requires appropriate management while the infection is being eradicated.

b. The dead space can be filled by means of local muscle mobilization, a rotational muscle flap, or a free muscle flap.

c. The VAC sponge is a useful short-term adjunct to assist in dead-space management until definitive soft-tissue coverage is achieved; however, its long-term use is questionable, and if placed directly over cortical bone for an extended period, it can lead to desiccation and resultant death of the cortical bone in contact with it.

d. Antibiotic-impregnated polymethylmethacrylate (PMMA) beads are a time-honored method of dead-space management; they also provide an effective means of local, high-dose antibiotic delivery. Most surgeons make their own beads by mixing PMMA with tobramycin and vancomycin powder. Other antibiotics used include gentamycin, erythromycin, tetracycline, and colistin. Resorbable materials including calcium sulfate, calcium phosphate, and hydroxyapatite ceramic beads with antibiotic impregnation have recently been introduced, but their clinical efficacy has not yet been well established.

i. Antibiotic-impregnated PMMA beads can be used effectively with or without a closed soft-tissue envelope.

ii. With an open soft-tissue envelope, the beads can be placed, then the limb and wound can be wrapped with an adhesive-coated plastic film laminate. This provides a biologic barrier with high-dose local antibiotic delivery and classically does well for 4 to 6 days before requiring changing because of leakage.

iii. With a closed soft-tissue envelope, the beads can be left in for an extended period to further ensure that infection has been controlled.

4. Soft-tissue coverage

a. A close working relationship with a microsurgeon experienced in soft-tissue mobilization and free-tissue transfer is imperative in managing these complex problems.

b. Microvascular free muscle transfer is the gold standard for restoration of a well-vascularized soft-tissue envelope after infection, trauma, or osteomyelitis.

c. Rotational muscle flaps are a good adjuvant for certain soft-tissue defects or when access to a microsurgeon is not possible. Rotational muscle flaps are particularly useful about the pelvis, thigh, and shoulder girdle.

d. Flap coverage combined with bone transport to fill large bone and soft-tissue defects can be performed safely and effectively with good long-term results.

5. Antibiotic coverage

a. An infectious disease consult and parenteral antibiotics are mainstays of the treatment of osteomyelitis.

b. Classic treatment protocols involve a 6-week course of an intravenous antibiotic regimen; however, no empiric data have shown that this is necessary. Recent data suggest that with proper and meticulous débridement, dead-space management, and soft-tissue management, a shorter duration of intravenous antibiotic delivery is as efficacious as a longer course of treatment.

c. With the sharp increase in organisms developing resistance to standard antibiotic protocols, such as methicillin-resistant *Staphylococcus aureus* and vancomycin-resistant *Enterococcus*, care must be taken in choosing an appropriate antibiotic regimen. Newer antibiotics such as daptomycin have been incorporated into the antibiotic armamentarium for the treatment of such pathogens.

d. In certain instances (C hosts), long-term antibiotic suppression can be the treatment of choice. The choice between a single and a multidrug regimen should be made carefully, with consultation with an infectious disease specialist, to minimize the chances of further development of pathogen resistance.

III. Limb Deformity Analysis

A. General principles

1. To understand whether a deformity exists, the parameters of a normal limb must be known.

2. Generally, the contralateral limb can be used as a control; however, with certain conditions (eg, metabolic bone disorders), the contralateral limb is usually abnormal.

3. Many nonunions develop a resultant deformity, and malunions, by definition, have a deformity.

4. Limb deformity is more of an issue in the lower extremity than the upper extremity.

5. Normal lower extremity alignment values have been established and are provided in **Figure 4**. The mechanical axis of the lower extremity passes from the center of the hip to the center of the talar dome. Ideal limb alignment is defined as when this mechanical axis line passes through the center of the knee.

B. Mechanical parameters (**Figure 4**, *A*)—Essential mechanical parameters that must be compared between limbs are the absolute limb segment lengths as well as comparative limb segment and total limb rotation. Limb lengths and deformity parameters are independent of each other, as are rotational deformities, and all must be measured separately. The nonrotational deformity parameters that must be measured and compared with the contralateral limb on appropriate radiographic views include the following:

1. Lateral proximal femoral angle (LPFA)

2. Mechanical lateral distal femoral angle (mLDFA)

3. Joint line convergence angle (JLCA)

4. Medial proximal tibial angle (MPTA)

5. Lateral distal tibial angle (LDTA)

C. Anatomic parameters (**Figure 4**, *B*)—Anatomic limb measurement parameters define the alignment of the bones themselves and do not have to mirror the mechanical axis. In the normal limb, however, the mechanical and anatomic parameters should yield the same measurements at a level from the knee distally. The unique anatomic parameters of the lower extremity are the following:

1. Medial neck-shaft angle (MNSA)

2. Medial proximal femoral angle (MPFA)

3. Anatomic lateral distal femoral angle (aLDFA)

D. Evaluating lower limb alignment

1. The gold standard for evaluating lower limb alignment is a weight-bearing radiograph of both lower extremities from the hips to the ankles on a

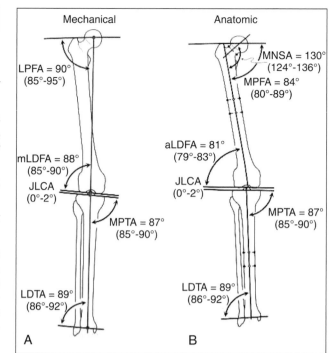

Figure 4   Standard mean values (with ranges) for normal lower extremity limb alignment. **A**, Mechanical alignment values. **B**, Anatomic alignment values. MNSA = medial neck-shaft angle; MPFA = medial proximal femoral angle; aLDFA = anatomic lateral distal femoral angle; JLCA = joint line convergence angle; LDTA = lateral distal tibial angle; MPTA = medial proximal tibial angle; LPFA = lateral proximal femoral angle; mLDFA = mechanical lateral distal femoral angle. (*Reproduced with permission from Paley D:* Principles of Deformity Correction. *Berlin, Germany, Springer-Verlag, 2002, pp 1-17.*)

51-inch cassette, as well as true AP and lateral views of the affected limb segment(s) (**Figure 5**).

a. The mechanical and anatomic axis angles described above are measured on the radiographs. This allows determination of the segment level of deformity (whether it is at the level of the femur, tibia, or joint line due to soft-tissue laxity), degree of deformity, and type of deformity.

b. To locate the exact site of the deformity, the mechanical and often the anatomic axis of each limb segment must be plotted.

2. Mechanical axis deviation (MAD)

a. The MAD is defined as a distance that the mechanical axis has deviated from the normal position through the center of the knee (**Figure 6**, *A*).

b. This measurement is particularly helpful when treating the common ailments of genu varum and genu valgus.

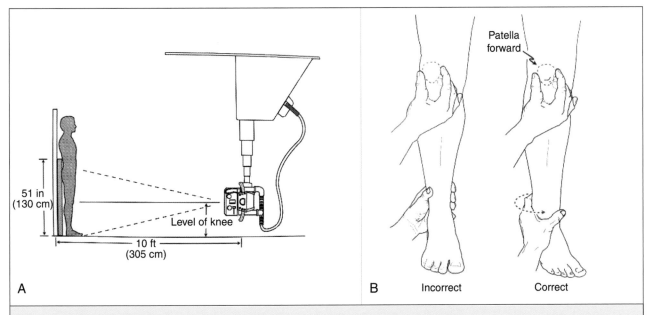

Figure 5   **A,** Illustration showing method for correctly obtaining weight-bearing AP radiograph of both lower extremities. **B,** Correct technique for obtaining consistent, true orthogonal views of the leg. (*Reproduced with permission from Paley D: Principles of Deformity Correction. Berlin, Germany, Springer-Verlag, 2002, pp 1-17.*)

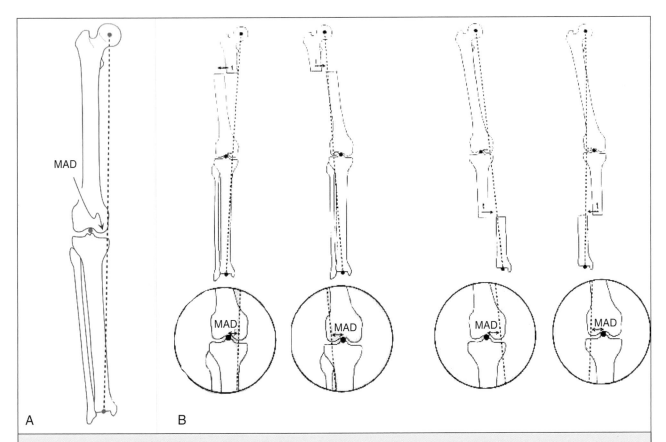

Figure 6   **A,** Mechanical axis deviation (MAD) is measured at the level of the knee joint and represents the distance that the mechanical axis is displaced from the normal for that limb. The "normal for the limb" is defined as the point that the mechanical axis passes in the contralateral, unaffected limb or a point in a range of 0 to 6 mm medial to the center of the knee, depending on what information is available. **B,** Illustrative examples of the effect of femoral and tibial translation on the mechanical axis of the limb. (*Reproduced with permission from Paley D: Principles of Deformity Correction. Berlin, Germany, Springer-Verlag, 2002, pp 31-60.*)

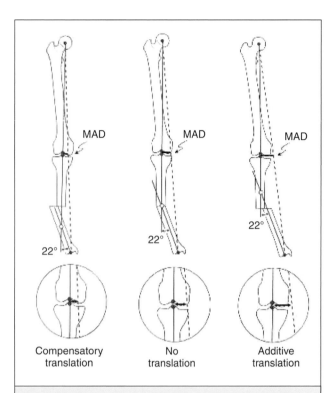

Figure 7 Translation of a limb segment can have a compensatory or an additive effect on an angulatory deformity depending on the directional plane of the translation. (*Reproduced with permission from Paley D:* Principles of Deformity Correction. *Berlin, Germany, Springer-Verlag, 2002, pp 31-60.*)

MAD

22°

Compensatory translation

MAD

22°

No translation

MAD

22°

Additive translation

c. The measurement of the MAD combined with the measurement of the accompanying joint orientation angles is particularly useful in the treatment of any juxta-articular deformity about the knee.

3. Diaphyseal deformities

a. These deformities, especially those that are posttraumatic, are often not simply just an angulatory problem. More often than not, there is an accompanying translational or rotatory deformity.

b. Translational deformities can contribute at least as much to mechanical axis deformity as do angulatory deformities (**Figure 6**, *B*).

c. Translational deformities with accompanying angulatory deformities can either be compensatory, whereby the translation is away from the concavity of the deformity, or additive, whereby the translated distal segment is toward the side of concavity. Hence, a limb with an angulatory deformity with an accompanying compensatory translational component can in effect have no or negligible mechanical axis deviation of the overall limb (**Figure 7**).

4. Center of rotation and angulation (CORA)

a. To determine the true site of deformity, and not just the limb segment involved, the CORA must be plotted.

b. The CORA represents the point in space where the axis of mechanical deformity exists and the virtual point in space where the virtual apex of correction should occur.

c. The CORA is plotted out by drawing the mechanical axes for the limb segments (**Figure 8**).

d. When the affected limb has no translational deformity and no other accompanying juxta-articular deformity or additional site of deformity, then the CORA is at the site of apparent deformity.

e. If a deformity exists secondary to angulation and translation (eg, malunion), then the CORA will be at a site other than that of the apparent angulatory deformity. This is the result of the contributory effect (regardless of whether it is a compensatory or additive translational compononent) of the translated limb segment.

5. Evaluation in the sagittal plane—All the measurements and plotting of limb axes done in the coronal (AP) plane can also be done in the sagittal (lateral) plane, although sagittal plane deformities are better tolerated in the lower extremity.

6. Upper extremity deformities—These same methods of deformity analysis also can be applied to the upper extremity. Common sites of posttraumatic deformity are at the elbow, secondary to malreduction of supracondylar fractures, and at the wrist, due to shortening and deformity secondary to malreduction of distal radial fractures.

E. Treatment

1. General principles

a. Order of correction—Alignment deformities should be corrected in the following order: angulation, translation, length, then rotation. In correcting the rotation, especially if an external fixator is used, a resultant residual translation can be encountered. If this is the case, then this residual translation must now be corrected. Utilizing this progression of correction of deformity parameters leads to the most predictable proper restoration of limb alignment.

b. Rotational malalignment is the most common posttraumatic deformity encountered; however, it is the least precise of the variables that can be measured. It is most often assessed clinically by comparing the affected limb with the contralateral limb.

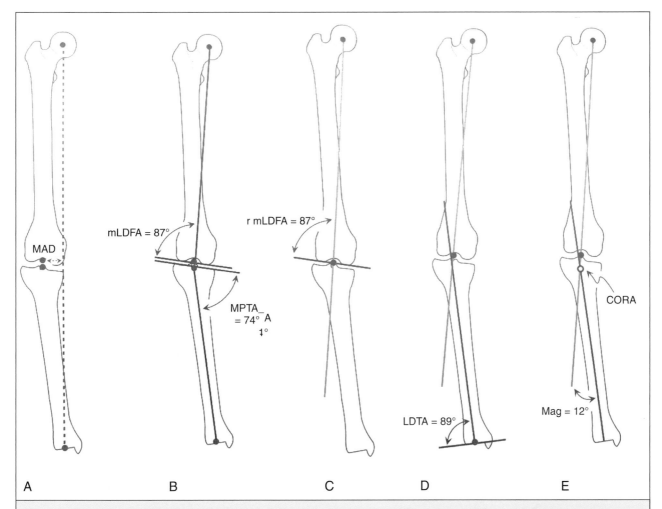

Figure 8 Determination of the center of rotation of angulation (CORA). **A,** The mechanical axis of the limb is drawn, and the MAD determined. **B,** The mLDFA, JLCA, and MPTA for the limb are determined. Because the mLDFA is in the range of normal, and the JLCA is parallel, then the deformity exists in the tibia, as the MPTA is abnormal at 74°. **C,** Because the mechanical axis of the femur is normal, the mechanical axis line of the femur can then be extended down the limb to represent the mechanical axis of the tibia. **D,** The distal mechanical axis is defined as a line from the center of the ankle and parallel to the shaft of the tibia. The LDTA is found to be normal. **E,** The CORA is now defined as the intersection of the proximal mechanical axis line with the distal mechanical axis line. Imagine translating the distal segment at this level and see how the point of the CORA changes. Mag = magnitude of deformity. (*Reproduced with permission from Paley D:* Principles of Deformity Correction. *Berlin, Germany, Springer-Verlag, 2002, pp 195-234.*)

c. Various values of acceptable lower extremity malalignment have been published, but there is no definitive value as to the maximum acceptable rotatory deformity tolerated in the lower limb. Most experts do concede, however, that any rotatory deformity of the leg >10° is poorly tolerated in most individuals.

2. Surgical technique

a. Order of correction—Alignment deformites should be corrected in the following order: angulation, translation, length, and then rotation.

b. Newer versions of external fixation allow simultaneous correction of all deformity parameters without the need for the residual translation correction. However, the need to follow the classic order of correction remains.

c. Simple deformities without clinically significant limb-length inequality can usually successfully be corrected with the use of locked rodding or plate and screw osteosynthesis.

d. Regardless of the method of fixation used, the need for proper preoperative planning and templating remains.

6: Trauma

Top Testing Facts

Nonunions

1. Stable fixation is of extreme importance in treating all nonunions. Particular attention should be paid to the elimination of shear in nonunions with a large degree of fracture obliquity.

2. It is best to achieve as stable a fixation as possible to allow for joint mobilization above and below a nonunion. These limbs have already been through much trauma, and hence the periarticular regions are prone to stiffness.

3. A healthy, well-vascularized soft-tissue envelope is necessary for healing of tenuously vascularized diaphyseal bone ends. The generous use of free or rotational muscle transfers enhances the healing environment by bringing in more vascular access.

4. If union fails despite optimal treatment, one should look for metabolic or other endogenous problems that are inhibiting fracture healing.

Osteomyelitis

1. For a successful cure, all necrotic bone and soft tissue must be meticulously débrided.

2. Proper dead-space management and soft-tissue coverage are equally important to achieve a satisfactory outcome.

3. Properly stage the host and the bone involvement at the beginning of treatment so that an appropriate treatment plan can be established.

Limb Deformity Analysis

1. The types of deformity that can exist in a limb are angulation, translation, length, and rotation. Rotation is generally measured clinically, whereas the other parameters are measured on appropriate radiographs.

2. Translation deformities can be as deleterious to limb alignment as angulatory deformities. Translation deformities can be either compensatory or additive to an angulatory deformity, and it is important to recognize this.

3. Because angulation is a phenomenon independent of translation, an apparent site of deformity might not actually be the true CORA. Therefore, this site must be precisely determined by making the measurements on long radiographs.

Bibliography

Bhandari M, Tornetta P III, Sprague S, et al: Predictors of reoperation following operative management of fractures of the tibial shaft. *J Orthop Trauma* 2003;17:353-361.

Bosse MJ, McCarthy ML, Jones AL, et al; The Lower Extremity Assessment Project (LEAP) Study Group: The insensate foot following severe lower extremity trauma: An indication for amputation? *J Bone Joint Surg Am* 2005;87:2601-2608.

Cierny G, Zorn KL: Segmental tibial defects, comparing conventional and Ilizarov methodologies. *Clin Orthop Relat Res* 1994;301:118-133.

Hak DJ, Lee SS, Goulet JA: Success of exchange reamed intramedullary nailing for femoral shaft nonunions or delayed union. *J Orthop Trauma* 2000;14:178-182.

Lowenberg DW, Feibel RJ, Louie KW, Eshima I: Combined muscle flap and Ilizarov reconstruction for bone and soft tissue defects. *Clin Orthop Relat Res* 1996;332:37-51.

MacKenzie EJ, Bosse MJ, Kellam JF, et al: Early predictors of long-term work disability after major limb trauma. *J Trauma* 2006;61:688-694.

Mahaluxmivala J, Nadarajah R, Allen PW, Hill RA: Ilizarov external fixator: Acute shortening and lengthening versus bone transport in the management of tibial non-unions. *Injury* 2005;36:662-668.

Marsh JL, Prokuski L, Biermann JS: Chronic infected tibial nonunions with bone loss: Conventional techniques versus bone transport. *Clin Orthop Relat Res* 1994;301:139-146.

McKee MD, DiPasquale DJ, Wild LM, Stephen DJ, Kreder HJ, Schemitsch EH: The effect of smoking on clinical outcome and complication rates following Ilizarov reconstruction. *J Orthop Trauma* 2003;17:663-667.

Milner SA, Davis TR, Muir KR, Greenwood DC, Doherty M: Long term outcome after tibial shaft fracture: Is malunion important? *J Bone Joint Surg Am* 2002;84:971-980.

Paley D: *Principles of Deformity Correction.* Berlin, Germany, Springer-Verlag, 2002.

Rao N, Santa E: Anti-infective therapy in orthopedics. *Op Tech Orthop* 2002;12:247-252.

Rubel IF, Kloen P, Campbell D, et al: Open reduction and internal fixation of humeral nonunions: A biomechanical and clinical study. *J Bone Joint Surg Am* 2002;84:1315-1322.

Watson JT: Distraction osteogenesis. *J Am Acad Orthop Surg* 2006;14(10 Suppl):S168-S174.

Watson JT, Anders M, Moed BR: Management strategies for bone loss in tibial shaft fractures. *Clin Orthop Relat Res* 1995;315:138-152.

Weresh MJ , Hakanson R , Stover MD , Sims SH , Kellam JF, Bosse MJ: Failure of exchange reamed intramedullary nails for ununited femoral shaft fractures. *J Orthop Trauma* 2000; 14:335-358.

Ziran B, Rao N: Treatment of orthopedic infections. *Op Tech Orthop* 2003;12:225-314.

Index

Page numbers followed by *f* indicate figures.
Page numbers followed by *t* indicate tables.

A

A-bands, 84*f*, 85, 85*f*
A-type fibers, 80
abandonment, definition, 135
Abbreviated Injury Scale (AIS), 541
abdominal compression test, 817
abdominal injuries, sports-related, 517–518
abductor digiti minimi (ADM), 1149
abductor hallucis (AbH), 1149
abductor pollicis longus (APL) muscle, 909*t*, 910
abrasion arthroplasty, 1011–1012
abscesses, 732, 733*f*, 1213–1214. *see also* infections
absolute risk reduction (ARR), 199, 208
acceleration, definition of, 16
accessory navicular, 355–356, 356*f*
accessory ossicles, foot, 289*f*
Accreditation Council for Continuing Medical Education (ACCME), 126
accuracy, definition, 204
acetabular components
    cemented, 1025
    cementless, 1027–1028
    options, 1037–1038
    revision, 1033, 1035
acetabular dysplasia, 1006*t*
acetabular index, 322–323, 323*f*
acetabular labral tears, 1005
acetabular osteotomy, 1006
acetabular version, 1009*f*
acetabulum
    anatomy of, 583, 583*f*
    defects, 1035-1038
    fractures, 583–588
        classification, 585, 586*f*
        clinical evaluation, 584
        complications, 587–588
        epidemiology, 583
        mechanisms of injury, 584
        periprosthetic, 1075–1077, 1076*t*
        radiography, 584–585, 585*f*
        rehabilitation, 586–587
        treatment, 585–586, 586*t*
    metastatic bone disease, 485, 485*f*
    roof arc measurement, 585*f*
    surgical approaches, 584, 587*t*
acetylcholine (ACh), 72, 85–86
acetylcholinesterase inhibitors, 86
Achilles tendon
    acute ruptures, 1194–1195, 1195*f*
    anatomy, 1193
    ankle anatomy and, 660
    chronic ruptures, 1195
    disorders, 1193, 1193*f*
    lengthening of, 1198
    reflexes, 703
    tendinosis, 1194*f*
achondrogenesis, 54
achondroplasia, 359, 361–362

characteristics, 6*t*
description, 32–33
features, 360*t*
genetic abnormalities, 32*t*, 37*t*, 360*t*
radiograph, 361*f*
Achterman and Kalamchi classification, 348
acidic fibroblast growth factor (aFGF), 48
acne mechanica, 519
acral metastasis, 929
acromioclavicular (AC) joint
    anatomy of, 794
    arthrosis, 824–825
    biomechanics of repair, 854
    modified Weaver-Dunn transfer, 853–854
    separations, 852–856
acromion
    anatomy of, 793
    fractures, 855*t*
    ossification center, 793
actin, sarcomere composition and, 84
Actinomyces isrealii, 731
action potentials, 72
acute hematogenous osteomyelitis (AHO), 97, 267, 268–269
acute lateral ankle instability, 1179-1180
acute normovolemic hemodilution, 159
Acute Physiology and Chronic Health Evaluation (APACHE), 541
adalimumab, 12
adamantinoma, 388, 434—435, 434*f*
adaptive immunity, 10
adductor brevis muscle, 611
adductor longus muscle, 193, 611
adductor magnus muscle, 611
adductor muscles, release of, 192
adenosine diphosphate (ADP), 88–89
adenosine monophosphate (AMP), 89
adenosine triphosphate (ATP), 88–89
adhesions, tendon, 949–950
adolescent patients. *see also* pediatric patients
    Blount disease in, 341*t*, 343
    developmental dysplasia of the hip in, 321
adrenal corticoids, 34–35
adult respiratory distress syndrome (ARDS), 544, 616
adult spinal deformity (ASD), 721-725
advance directives, 127
advanced cardiac life support (ACLS), 516
Advanced Trauma Life Support (ATLS)
    components
        primary survey, 542
        secondary survey, 542
    in femoral shaft fractures, 611
    field assessments, 540
    in on-field injuries, 516
aerobic metabolism, 89, 195–196
aerobic training, 90, 715
Aeromonas hydrophilia, 960
afferent dorsal roots, 73
afferent nerves, 71, 73, 75, 75*t*
age/aging. *see also* elderly persons
    articular cartilage changes in, 59, 60*t*
    bone mass during, 24
    cervical myelopathy and, 755

health care appropriate in, 128
intervertebral disks and, 94
tendon biomechanics and, 66
Agency for Healthcare Research and Quality (AHRQ), 119
aggrecan, 54, 54*f*, 55*f*, 58*f*, 65
ALARA (as low as reasonably achievable) dosing, 142
Albers-Schönberg disease. *see* osteopetrosis
alcohol intake, preoperative assessments, 145
alendronate, 493
Alexander disease, 151*t*
alkaline phosphatase, 493
Allen-Ferguson classification of subaxial cervical fractures, 743, 744*f*
Allis test, 321
allograft prosthetic composites (APCs), 1038, 1040*f*
allografts
    bone, 112–114
allopurinol, 498
alloys, definition of, 25
alumina, 27, 1021
alveolar rhabdomyosarcoma, 385*t*
American Academy of Orthopaedic Surgeons (AAOS)
    Committee on the Hip, 1035–1036, 1036*f*
    femoral deficiency classification, 1035–1036
    Sign Your Site program, 120
American Joint Commission for Cancer classifications, 382, 383*t*, 384*t*
American Spinal Injury Association (ASIA), 189*t*, 190, 735, 736*f*, 739
amino acids, use by athletes, 521
aminoglycosides, 105*t*, 107*t*, 962
amniotic band syndrome, 316–317, 317*f*
amniotic disruption sequence. *see* amniotic band syndrome
amphotericin, 108, 732
AMPLE history, in the field, 540
amputation
    after bone tumor treatment, 388
    after total knee arthroplasties, 1065
    ankle, 179
    complications, 178–179
    hallux, 179
    hindfoot, 179
    indications for, 184, 389
    levels of, metabolic costs, 183*t*
    limb salvage *versus*, 537
    lower limb, 177–179
    for malignant tumors, 389
    painful residual limb, 183, 187
    in patients with diabetes, 1220–1221
    for pediatric limb deficiencies, 346
    in periprosthetic infections, 1071
    replantation, 183–184, 975–978
    for soft-tissue sarcomas, 459
    of toes, 179
    transfemoral, 179
    traumatic, 183–184, 541
        care of body parts, 541
    upper limb, 183–185, 184–185